Avin Mauran

January 21, 199

British Columbia

Cancer Agency

LUNG TUMORS

LUNG BIOLOGY IN HEALTH AND DISEASE

Executive Editor

Claude Lenfant
Director, National Heart, Lung and Blood Institute
National Institutes of Health
Bethesda, Maryland

The opinions expressed in these volumes do not necessarily represent the views of the National Institutes of Health.

LUNG TUMORS

FUNDAMENTAL BIOLOGY AND CLINICAL MANAGEMENT

Edited by

Christian Brambilla
Elisabeth Brambilla

Institut Albert Bonniot
Centre Hospitalier Universitaire de Grenoble
Grenoble, France

MARCEL DEKKER, INC.   NEW YORK · BASEL · HONG KONG

Library of Congress Cataloging-in-PublicationData

Lung tumors: fundamental biology and clinical management / edited by Christian Brambilla,
  Elisabeth Brambilla.
      p.   cm. — (Lung biology in health and disease; v. 124)
  Includes bibliographical references and indexes.
  ISBN: 0-8247-0160-7 (alk. paper)
    1. Lungs—Tumors—Treatment. 2. Lungs—Tumors—Molecular aspects. [DNLM: 1.
  Lung Neoplasms—genetics. 2. Lung Neoplasms—diagnosis. 3. Lung Neoplasms—
  therapy. 4. Molecular Biology.   W1 LU62 v. 124 1999/ WF 658 L9643 1999]
  RC280.L8L866   1999
  616.99'424—dc21
  DNLM/DLC
  For Library of Congress

This book is printed on acid-free paper.

Headquarters
Marcel Dekker, Inc.
270 Madison Avenue, New York, NY 10016
tel: 212-696-9000; fax: 212-685-4540

Eastern Hemisphere Distribution
Marcel Dekker AG
Hutgasse 4, Postfach 812, CH-4001 Basel, Switzerland
tel: 44-61-261-8482; fax: 44-61-261-8896

World Wide Web
http://www.dekker.com

The publisher offers discounts on this book when ordered in bulk quantities. For
more information, write to Special Sales/Professional Marketing at the
headquarters address above.

Current printing (last digit)
10 9 8 7 6 5 4 3 2 1

PRINTED IN THE UNITED STATES OF AMERICA

INTRODUCTION

There is evidence that as early as the year 2000 BC Egyptian healers knew about the presence and development of tumors; there is also evidence that they knew of no treatment and that they thought tumors should be left alone.

The nineteenth century marked the beginning of a growing interest in the biology and pathology of tumors. Julius Cohnheim, in his famous lectures at the University of Leipzig, talked extensively about tumors. In one of his lectures on morbid embryology, he introduced a rather fascinating term: *monstra per excessum*. This, of course, had nothing to do with cancer but nonetheless the expression is quite representative!

Cohnheim knew about neoplasms. He once posed the question, "What is the ultimate destiny of a tumor?" The answer he gave was "a neoplasm never spontaneously recedes and disappears." He further commented about "malignant tumors":

> These tumors, as I already pointed out, ruthlessly invade the neighboring tissues; nay more, secondary growth in remote localities, which present physiological differences, may arise under their influence.

Although at that time lung tumors were not even part of the vocabulary, these comments describe their natural history.

Today, looking back on the acquisition and evaluation of new knowledge in the field of cancer, one can only marvel at how much has been accomplished. Granted, if these accomplishments are judged by the mortality rate, enthusiasm may not be so great, but this would be a very limited view of reality. The disciplines of cell biology, microbiology, virology, and, more recently, molecular biology and genetics have greatly expanded our knowledge of the field of cancer.

Indeed, these disciplines have contributed to research on lung tumors. Thus, no reader familiar with the Lung Biology in Health and Disease series should be surprised to see this new volume on lung cancer, because it is so different from previous books on the same subject. In this book, Drs. Elisabeth and Christian Brambilla, who served as editors as well as contributors, combine the perspectives of a distinguished team of investigators. They assembled a roster of international contributors whose work has been central to the advances made in this field. John Minna, himself a pioneer in lung cancer research, has provided a Foreword that describes this volume most comprehensively.

It is with gratitude to all the contributors and to the editors that I present this volume, *Lung Tumors: Fundamental Biology and Clinical Management,* to the readership of this series.

Claude Lenfant, M.D.
Bethesda, Maryland

FOREWORD

Lung cancer represents a major cancer challenge in both the Western world and Asia. As we all know, it is preventable by interdicting cigarette smoking. Therefore, the first line of attack should be preventing the initiation of smoking and developing new aids for smoking cessation. This is particularly important because addiction to nicotine and cigarette smoking usually occurs before age 20, and smoking cessation is difficult once addiction occurs. In the United States, potential landmark financial settlements between tobacco companies and various state governments or the federal government are occurring. However, these settlements, despite the large financial figures being discussed, only make sense if they have an impact on reducing smoking in children and preventing the export of American tobacco products abroad. It will be interesting to see if similar settlements with tobacco companies occur in western Europe.

However, even if smoking levels decline, we would still be forced to deal with a large number of lung cancer cases developing because of prior cigarette smoking over the next 50 years. In fact, in the United States, about 50% of new lung cancer cases occur in former smokers. Currently, the optimal application of the best staging tools and integration of surgery, radiotherapy, and chemotherapy gives an overall 5-year survival rate of approximately 15% of all newly diagnosed lung cancer patients. We need to do much better than this and a status report on these efforts is given in detail in several chapters in this volume. In part this will require modification of our histological classification (Chap. 1), identification of new (Chap. 2), rare (Chap. 6), metastatic (Chap. 7) tumors, and development of tumor markers for aid in diagnosis and following therapy (Chap. 27). Nevertheless, the sophistication of initial staging with CT scans (Chap. 30), of determining resectability of non-small-cell lung cancer (NSCLC) and prognostic factors in unresectable NSCLC (Chap. 36), of thoracic surgery and pre- and postoperative care, and chest radiotherapy, including new approaches (Chap. 37), have all improved dramatically over the past 20 years. New forms of radiotherapy are being developed (Chaps. 31 and 33), while photodynamic therapy is being tested as a new tool (Chap. 32). The role of surgery is being defined for lung metastases and second lung cancers (Chap. 42). There have also been successes with chemotherapy (Chap. 35). This was first dramatically seen in small-cell lung cancer (SCLC), where it can be curative (Chap. 38), and, more recently, in NSCLC, where randomized trials have shown its benefits with surgery in both adjuvant and neoadjuvant settings (Chap. 34). In addition, the integration of chemotherapy and chest radiotherapy has been demonstrated to be of clinical survival benefit in both SCLC (Chap. 39) and NSCLC (Chap. 34). However, all experts in the field agree that significantly improved chemotherapy agents are needed, and several new agents have been and will be introduced into clinical care (Chap. 41). Finally, the successes have led to studies of long-term survivors where we must learn of the late effects of treatment and be aware of the very high frequency of developing a second lung cancer (Chap. 40).

There have been important advances in basic research concerning the molecular pathogenesis of lung cancer and these are covered in detail in this volume. Lung cancer occurs because of mutations in dominant and recessive oncogenes, development of genetic instability (Chap. 15), activation of a cellular immortalization program involving the RNA-enzyme complex telomerase (Chap. 16), activation of paracrine and autocrine growth factor loops (Chap. 22), activation of tumor angiogenesis (Chaps. 23 and 24), disruption of host immunity against the tumor, and development of molecular expression programs allowing metastases (Chaps. 25 and 26). Some of the best-characterized recessive oncogenes are those of p53 (Chaps. 28 and 10), RB (Chap. 11), p16 (Chap. 12), the newly discovered FHIT gene and other changes on chromosome 3 (Chap. 9), as well as deregulation of cell cycle control (Chap. 12) and regulation of gene expression by methylation (Chap. 13). The most frequently abnormal dominant oncogenes include *ras* (Chap. 8) and *myc*. There is also considerable evidence that smoking induces mutations in these specific genes (Chap. 8). These aspects are all discussed in detail in several chapters in this volume.

Is there a way to translate these basic research observations from the laboratory to the clinic? As many of the chapters review in detail, there are multiple paths for this translation. We now know that 10 to 20 mutations are required to develop a clinically evident lung cancer. These represent absolute differences between the lung cancer and normal tissues. We also know that correcting even one of these mutations appears to either reverse the malignant phenotype or cause the lung cancer to undergo programmed cell death (apoptosis). Thus, one general strategy is to develop new treatments based on these differences. The specific mutated or expressed genes representing these genetic alterations are rapidly being identified and there should be a multitude of such translational targets. These would include drugs or antibodies directed against oncogene products or pathways, angiogenesis, or autocrine/ paracrine growth factors; gene replacement therapy, such as for p53, already successfully accomplished in lung cancer by local injection (Chap. 45); and tumor-specific vaccine therapy and/or correcting the host cellular immune deficits caused by tumor products (Chap. 44).

A second general approach is to use this information for early cancer detection and for designing and monitoring chemoprevention efforts (Chaps. 14 and 21). If there are 10 to 20 lesions, can we detect one or two of these before a full-fledged cancer develops? The answer appears to be "yes." An amazing finding to come out recently has been the discovery of multiple clones of cells in preneoplastic lesions (hyperplasia, dysplasia, carcinoma in situ) or histologically normal respiratory epithelium of current and former smokers containing loss of alleles at recessive oncogene (tumor suppressor gene) loci (Chaps. 17 and 18). In contrast, such clones are rarely, if ever, found in lifetime nonsmokers. In retrospect, this could be predicted from the field cancerization theory. The development of technology for the precise microdissection of these preneoplastic lesions, including new laser capture technology as well as a variety for PCR-based markers for genetic analysis, has hastened progress in this area. There have also been advances in histologically identifying preneoplastic lesions, including the identification of atypical adenomatous hyperplasia (AHH) (Chap. 4). Other advances have occurred in the area of developing very sensitive assays for detecting rare mutant cells in a field of normal cells (Chaps. 8 and 15). There have also been new advances in fiberoptic bronchoscopy, such as fluorescent bronchoscopy, which allows identification of these lesions (Chap. 29). Twenty years ago there were large, randomized trials testing chest x-rays and sputum cytologies as screening tools for early lung cancer detection. While these methods detected early-stage lung cancer, the screening failed to alter the survival of this screened population. This was because lung cancer metastasized at a relatively early stage from the primary lesion. These molecular markers offer the hope of early molecular detection before a lesion can be seen on a chest x-ray. In addition, they provide rational biomarkers for monitoring the effectiveness of chemoprevention. Currently, there is much interest and several randomized clinical trials of various retinoid compounds and antioxidants as chemopreventative agents (Chaps. 19 and 20). These have been shown to prevent the development of second aerodigestive tract malignancies in head and neck and lung cancer patients. It will be very important to document the reversal of all the genetic changes in the respiratory epithelium of patients without active lung cancer. Several randomized trials are currently addressing these issues.

This volume thus covers a broad range of topics and up-to-the-minute information pertinent to lung cancer etiology, diagnosis, staging, treatment, prognosis, early detection, prevention, and the development of new treatments.

John D. Minna
University of Texas
Southwestern Medical Center
Dallas, Texas

PREFACE

In the field of lung tumors new biological concepts have recently emerged leading to new diagnostic, prognostic, and therapeutic approaches. Clinical management of lung cancer has also progressed with both clinically established and more controversial ways of taking care of patients. For these reasons it seems a good time to review the situation. This book address new approaches to the diagnosis and treatment of lung tumors with contributions from fundamental biologists, surgical pathologists, and clinicians.

The latest concepts on classification of lung tumors and particularly preinvasive lesions and new entities are described using sophisticated tools now available to pathologists for the diagnosis. The reader will get a deep insight into the process of cycle control and molecular pathology following a comprehensive pathway to describe the key factors of lung tumor carcinogenesis. New tumor suppressor genes, new concepts in the clonal relationship between distant preinvasive lesions in field cancerization, and the complex connections between host and tumors are the discoveries of today for the clinical applications of tomorrow. Clinical management closely follows biological advances, and using new diagnostic imaging and therapeutic approaches provides molecular biologists with new opportunities to work on human samples. Multimodality treatments using powerful and aggressive chemotherapy and fractionated radiotherapy protocols need to be evaluated because even a small increase in the percentage of lung cancer cure leads to a large number of patients benefiting without ignoring the induced iatrogenicity.

For all of these reasons, *Lung Tumors* will be a valuable reference for all those interested in finding a cure.

Christian Brambilla
Elisabeth Brambilla

CONTRIBUTORS

Rodrigo Arriagada   Institut Gustave-Roussy, Villejuif, France

David Beer   Department of Surgery, University of Michigan Medical School, Ann Arbor, Michigan.

Isabelle Bolon   Scientific Researcher, CJF INSERM 97-01, Institut Albert Bonniot, Centre Hospitalier Universitaire de Grenoble, Grenoble, France

Christian Brambilla, M.D.   Professor, CJF INSERM 97-01, Institut Albert Bonniot, Centre Hospitalier Universitaire de Grenoble, Grenoble, France

Elisabeth Brambilla, M.D.   Professor, CJF INSERM 97-01, Institut Albert Bonniot, Centre Hospitalier Universitaire de Grenoble, Grenoble, France

Gianfranco Buccheri, M.D.   Thoracic Oncologist, Department of Pulmonary Medicine, Azienda Ospedaliera "S. Croce e Carle," Cuneo, Italy

Philip T. Cagle, M.D.   Department of Pathology, Baylor College of Medicine, Houston, Texas

B. Chauvet   Clinique Sainte Catherine, Avignon, France

Grace Chung, Ph.D.   MRC Laboratory of Molecular Biology, Cambridge, England

Thomas V. Colby, M.D.   Department of Pathology, Mayo Clinic Scottsdale, Scottsdale, Arizona

Jean-Luc Coll   Scientific Researcher, CJF INSERM 97-01, Institut Albert Bonniot, Centre Hospitalier Universitaire de Grenoble, Grenoble, France

Denis A. Cortese, M.D.   Mayo Medical School and May Clinic, Jacksonville, Florida

Max Coulomb, Ph.D.   Professor, Service de Radiologie, Institut Albert Bonniot, Centre Hospitalier Universitaire de Grenoble, Grenoble, France

Frank Cuttitta, Ph.D.   Intervention Section, Department of Cell and Cancer Biology, Medicine Branch, National Cancer Institute, National Institutes of Health, Bethesda, Maryland

Pascal Demoly, M.D., Ph.D.   Maladies Respiratoires, Centre Hospitalier Universitaire, Montpellier, France

Alain Depierre, M.D.   Professor, Chest Disease Department, University Hospital, Besançon, France

Eric S. Edell, M.D.   Associate Professor of Medicine, Mayo Medical School; Consultant, Pulmonary and Critical Care Medicine, Mayo Clinic, Rochester, Minnesota

Fabrizio M. Facchini   Research Fellow, Department of Respiratory Medicine, Middlesex Hospital, London, England

Marie Favrot   Professor, CJF INSERM 97-01, Institut Albert Bonniot, Centre Hospitalier Universitaire de Grenoble, Grenoble, France

Gilbert R. Ferretti, M.D.   Service de Radiologie et Imagerie Médicale, Institut Albert Bonniot, Centre Hospitalier Universitaire de Grenoble, Grenoble, France

J.K. Field, M.D., Ph.D., B.D.S., M.R.C. Path.   Director, Roy Castle International Centre for Lung Cancer Research and The University of Liverpool, Liverpool, England

R. Garcia   Clinique Sainte Catherine, Avignon, France

Kevin C. Gatter   Oxford University, Oxford, England

Adi F. Gazdar, M.D.   Hamon Center for Therapeutic Oncology Research, University of Texas Southwestern Medical Center, Dallas, Texas

Sylvie Gazzeri, Ph.D.   Scientific Researcher, CJF INSERM 97-01, Institut Albert Bonniot, Centre Hospitalier Universitaire de Grenoble, Grenoble, France

Valérie Gouyer   Scientific Researcher, CJF INSERM 97-01, Institut Albert Bonniot, Centre Hospitalier Universitaire de Grenoble, Grenoble, France

Samir M. Hanash   Department of Pediatrics, University of Michigan Medical School, Ann Arbor, Michigan

Fred R. Hirsch, M.D.   Chief Physician, Department of Oncology, Finsen Center, Rigshospitalet, Copenhagen, Denmark

Walter N. Hittelman, M.D.   Professor, University of Texas M.D. Anderson Cancer Center, Houston, Texas

Daniel R. Jacobson, M.D.   Department of Medicine, New York University School of Medicine and Department of Veterans Affairs Medical Center, New York, New York

Pascale Jacoulet, M.D.   Pneumologist, Chest Diseases Department, Centre Hospitalier Universitaire, Besançon, France

Yashima Kazuo   University of Texas Southwestern Medical Center, Dallas, Texas

Stephen C. Lam, M.D., F.R.C.P.C., F.C.C.P.   Professor, Department of Medicine, University of British Columbia and the British Columbia Cancer Agency, Vancouver, British Columbia, Canada

Thierry Le Chevalier, M.D.   Head, Lung Unit, Department of Medicine, Institut Gustave-Roussy, Villejuif, France

Cécile Le Péchoux   Institut Gustave-Roussy, Villejuif, France

Calum MacAulay   University of British Columbia and British Columbia Cancer Agency, Vancouver, British Columbia, Canada

Nadine Martinet, Ph.D. Université Henri-Poincaré, Vandoeuvre-les-Nancy, France

Yves Martinet, M.D., Ph.D. Professor, Pneumologie A, Université Henri-Poincaré, Vandoeuvre-les-Nancy, France

R. J. A. M. Michalides, Ph.D. Department of Tumor Biology, The Netherlands Cancer Institute, Amsterdam, The Netherlands

Cesar A. Moran Department of Pulmonary and Mediastinal Pathology, Armed Forces Institute of Pathology, Washington, D.C.

François Mornex Professor, Department of Radiation Oncology, Centre Hospitalier Lyon Sud, Pierre-Bénite, France

Denis Moro, M.D. Department of Respiratory Medicine, Institut Albert Bonniot, Centre Hospitalier Universitaire de Grenoble, Grenoble, France

Jean-Jacques Moulin INRS, Vandoeuvre-les-Nancy, France

James L. Mulshine, M.D. Head, Intervention Section, Department of Cell and Cancer Biology, Medicine Branch, National Cancer Institute, National Institutes of Health, Bethesda, Maryland

Nevin Murray, M.D., F.R.C.P. Clinical Professor, Department of Medical Oncology, British Columbia Cancer Agency, Vancouver, British Columbia, Canada

Adrien Negoescu, M.D., Ph.D. CJF INSERM 97-01, Institut Albert Bonniot, Centre Hospitalier Universitaire de Grenoble, Grenoble, France

Andrew G. Nicholson, M.R.C.Path., D.M. Consultant Histopathologist/Honorary Senior Lecturer, Department of Histopathology, Royal Brompton Hospital, London, England

Silvia Novello Department of Clinical and Biological Sciences, University of Turin, Turin, Italy

Naoyoshi Onuki University of Texas Southwestern Medical Center, Dallas, Texas

Kell Østerlind, M.D. Consultant, Medical Department F, Hillerød Sygehus, Hillerød, Denmark

Ugo Pastorino, M.D. European Institute of Oncology, Milan, Italy

Francesco Pezzella, M.D., M.R.C.Path.   Senior Lecturer, Department of Histopathology, University College London, London, England

Jean-Louis Pujol, M.D.   Professor, Chest Department, Centre Hospitalier Universitaire, Montpellier, France

E. Quoix, M.D.   Professor, Pavillon Laennec, Hôpitaux Universitaires, Strasbourg, France

Pamela Rabbitts, B.Sc., Ph.D.   Department of Oncology, University of Cambridge, Cambridge, England

Asha Rathi   University of Texas Southwestern Medical Center, Dallas, Texas

François L. Reboul, M.D.   Medical Director, Department of Thoracic Oncology, Clinique Sainte Catherine, Avignon, France

Bruce Richardson   Department of Internal Medicine, University of Michigan Medical School, Ann Arbor, Michigan

Catherine Robert   CJF INSERM 97-01, Institut Albert Bonniot, Centre Hospitalier Universitaire de Grenoble, Grenoble, France

Giorgio V. Scagliotti, M.D.   Department of Clinical and Biological Sciences, University of Turin, Turin, Italy

Philippe Scheid, M.D.   Pneumologie A, Université Henri-Poincaré, Vandoeuvre-les-Nancy, France

Fabrice Soncin   CNRS EP 560, Institut de Biologie de Lille, Lille, France

Jean-Charles Soria   Institut Gustave-Roussy, Villejuif, France

Thierry Soussi   Directeur de Recherche, INSERM U301, Institut Curie, Paris, France

Gabriella Sozzi, Ph.D.   Department of Experimental Oncology A, Istituto Nazionale Tumori, Milan, Italy

Stephen G. Spiro, B.Sc., M.D., F.R.C.P.   Department of Respiratory Medicine, Middlesex Hospital, London, England

Saul Suster, M.D. Director of Anatomic Pathology, Baptist Hospital of Miami and Clinical Professor of Pathology, University of Miami School of Medicine, Miami, Florida

M. Taulelle, M.D. Clinique Sainte Catherine, Avignon, France

Melvyn S. Tockman, M.D., Ph.D. Professor of Medicine, University of South Florida, Tampa, Florida

William D. Travis, M.D. Co-Chair, Department of Pulmonary and Mediastinal Pathology, Armed Forces Institute of Pathology, Washington, D.C.

Anthony M. Treston, Ph.D. Intervention Section, Department of Cell and Cancer Biology Medicine Branch, National Cancer Institute, National Institutes of Health, Bethesda, Maryland

Bernard Vandenbunder, Ph.D. Directeur de Recherches, Developpement et Cancérisation, CNRS EP 560, Institut de Biologie de Lille, Lille, France

Paul Van Houtte, M.D. Professor, Department of Radiotherapy, Jules Bordet Institute, Brussels, Belgium

L. van't Veer Department of Molecular Pathology, Netherlands Cancer Institute, Amsterdam, The Netherlands

Nico van Zandwijk, M.D., Ph.D., F.C.C.P. Head, Department of Thoracic Oncology, Netherlands Cancer Institute, Amsterdam, The Netherlands

Jean-Michel Vignaud, M.D. Professor, Laboratoire d'Anatomie Pathologique, and INSERM U14 Faculté de Médecine, Université Henri-Poincaré, Vandoeuvre-les-Nancy, France

P. Vincent Clinique Sainte Catherine, Avignon, France

Arvind Virmani University of Texas Southwestern Medical Center, Dallas, Texas

Jean-Philippe Vuillez, M.D., Ph.D. Research on Radiopharmaceuticals Laboratory, Faculty of Medicine, Institut Albert Bonniot, Centre Hospitalier Universitaire de Grenoble, Grenoble, France

Patrick Weynants, M.D. Professor, Department of Pneumology, Université Catholique de Louvain, Yvoir, Belgium

CONTENTS

1

The Need for a New Classification for Lung and Pleural Tumors

WILLIAM D. TRAVIS

Armed Forces Institute of Pathology
Washington, D.C.

THOMAS V. COLBY

Mayo Clinic Scottsdale
Scottsdale, Arizona

Tumor classification systems need to be updated periodically as progress is made in understanding of the clinical, epidemiological, histogenetic, and molecular aspects of various tumors. It has been 30 years since the first classification of lung tumors was proposed by the World Health Organization (WHO) (1) and 17 years since the WHO classification was updated in 1981 (2). During the subsequent period, substantial progress has been made in our understanding of lung tumors. In 1988, a major change in 1981 WHO proposal for subclassification of small-cell lung carcinoma (SCLC) was suggested by the pathology panel of the International Association for the Study of Lung Cancer (IASLC) (3). In 1994, WHO adopted the IASLC pathology panel to comprise the core membership of the WHO committee to develop a new revised classification of lung and pleural tumors. In addition to the IASLC pathology panel members, an extended panel of reviewers were asked to serve on the WHO committee to help develop this new classification (Table 1). This chapter is a brief preliminary overview of the new classification proposed by the WHO pathology panel (Table 2) (4). The formal blue book *Histological Classification of Lung and Pleural Tumors* with more detailed discussion and illustrations should be published in 1998 (4). This classification is also adopted by the IASLC. Because of the work by the IASLC pathology panel and the support contributed by the IASLC to this project, we

1

Table 1 WHO Pathology Panel Members

Chair
  William D. Travis, M.D.*
    Washington, D.C.
Coordinators
  Thomas V. Colby, M.D.*
    Scottsdale, AZ
  Bryan Corrin MD, MRCPath*
    London, England
  Yukio Shimosato, M.D.*
    Tokyo, Japan
Core Panel Members
  Emilio Alvarez Fernandez, M.D.*
    Madrid, Spain
  Professor E. Brambilla, M.D.*
    Grenoble, France
  Samuel P. Hammar, M.D.*
    Bremerton, WA
  Dr. Philip S. Hasleton*
    Manchester, England
  Fred R. Hirsch, M.D., Ph.D.*
    Copenhagen, Denmark
  Bruce Mackay, M.D., Ph.D.*
    Houston, TX
  Helmut Popper, M.D.*
    Graz, Austria
  Richard H. Steele, M.B., Ch.B., Ph.D., F.R.C.P.A., F.A.F.O.M.*
    Woolloongabba, Australia
Contribution on preinvasive lesions by Wilbur Franklin, M.D. *
    Denver, CO (Chair, International Association for the Study of Lung Cancer/National Cancer
    Institute SPORE Pathology Working Group for Classification of Preinvasive Epithelial
    Abnormalities of Lung)
Extended Panel of Reviewers
  Seena Aisner, M.D.*
    Newark, NJ
  Andrew Churg, M.D.
    Vancouver, British Columbia, Canada
  Louis P. Dehner, M.D.
    St. Louis, MO
  Adi F. Gazdar, M.D.*
    Dallas, TX
  Douglas W. Henderson, MBBS, MRCPath, FRCPA
    Bedford Park, South Australia
  N. A. Jambhekar, M.D.
    Parel Bombay, India
  Michael N. Koss, M.D.
    Los Angeles, CA
  Prof. Dr. Klaus-Michael Müller
    Bochum, Germany
  Prof. Nicolai Petrovitchev
    Moscow, Russia
  Dr. Paulo Saldiva
    Sao Paulo, Brazil
  Mary Sheppard, BSc, MD, MRCPath*
    London, England
  Dr. Sjoerd Sc. Wagenaar
    Amsterdam, The Netherlands
  Dr. Li Wei-hua
    Beijing, P.R. China

*IASLC Pathology Panel Members.

Table 2 1998 WHO/IASLC Histological Classification of Lung and Pleural Tumors

1. Epithelial Tumors
   1.1   Benign
      1.1.1   Papillomas
         1.1.1.1   Squamous cell papilloma
            1.1.1.1.1   Exophytic
            1.1.1.1.2   Inverted
         1.1.1.2   Glandular papilloma
         1.1.1.3.   Mixed squamous cell and glandular papilloma
      1.1.2   Adenomas
         1.1.2.1   Alveolar adenoma
         1.1.2.2   Papillary adenoma
         1.1.2.3.   Adenomas of salivary gland type
            1.1.2.3.1   Mucous gland adenoma
            1.1.2.3.2   Pleomorphic adenoma
            1.1.2.3.3   Other
         1.1.2.4   Mucinous cystadenoma
         1.1.2.5   Others
   1.2   Preinvasive lesions
      1.2.1   Squamous dysplasia/carcinoma in situ
      1.2.2   Atypical adenomatous hyperplasia
      1.2.3   Diffuse idiopathic pulmonary neuroendocrine cell hyperplasia
   1.3   Invasive malignant
      1.3.1   Squamous cell carcinoma
         Variants
         1.3.1.1   Papillary
         1.3.1.2   Clear cell
         1.3.1.3   Small-cell
         1.3.1.4   Basaloid
      1.3.2   Small-cell carcinoma
         Variant
         1.3.2.1   Combined small-cell carcinoma
      1.3.3   Adenocarcinoma
         1.3.3.1   Acinar
         1.3.3.2   Papillary
         1.3.3.3   Bronchioloalveolar carcinoma
            1.3.3.3.1   Nonmucinous (Clara cell/type II pneumocyte type)
            1.3.3.3.2   Mucinous (Goblet cell type)
            1.3.3.3.3   Mixed mucinous and nonmucinous (Clara cell/type II pneumocyte and goblet cell type) or indeterminate
         1.3.3.4   Solid adenocarcinoma with mucin formation
         1.3.3.5   Mixed
         1.3.3.6   Variants:
            1.3.3.6.1   Well-differentiated fetal adenocarcinoma
            1.3.3.6.2   Mucinous ("colloid")
            1.3.3.6.3   Mucinous cystadenocarcinoma
            1.3.3.6.4   Signet ring
            1.3.3.6.5   Clear cell

Table 2 Continued

        1.3.4.   Large cell carcinoma
                Variants
                1.3.4.1   Large-cell neuroendocrine carcinoma
                        1.3.4.1.1   Combined large-cell neuroendocrine carcinoma
                1.3.4.2   Basaloid carcinoma
                1.3.4.3   Lymphoepithelioma-like carcinoma
                1.3.4.4   Clear cell carcinoma
                1.3.4.5   Large-cell carcinoma with rhabdoid phenotype
        1.3.5.   Adenosquamous carcinoma
        1.3.6   Carcinomas with pleomorphic, sarcomatoid, or sarcomatous elements
                1.3.6.1   Carcinomas with spindle and/or giant cells
                        1.3.6.1.1   Pleomorphic carcinoma
                        1.3.6.1.2   Spindle cell carcinoma
                        1.3.6.1.3   Giant cell carcinoma
                1.3.6.2   Carcinosarcoma
                1.3.6.3   Blastoma (Pulmonary blastoma)
        1.3.7   Carcinoid tumor
                1.3.7.1   Typical carcinoid
                1.3.7.2   Atypical carcinoid
        1.3.8   Carcinomas of salivary gland type
                1.3.8.1   Mucoepidermoid carcinoma
                1.3.8.2   Adenoid cystic carcinoma
                1.3.8.3   Others
        1.3.9   Unclassified carcinoma
2.   Soft Tissue Tumors
    2.1   Localized fibrous tumor
    2.2   Epithelioid hemangioendothelioma
    2.3   Pleuropulmonary blastoma
    2.4   Chondroma
    2.5   Calcifying fibrous pseudotumor of the pleura
    2.6   Congenital peribronchial myofibroblastic tumor
    2.7   Diffuse pulmonary lymphangiomatosis
    2.8   Desmoplastic small round cell tumor
    2.9   Other
3.   Mesothelial Tumors
    3.1   Benign
        3.1.1   Adenomatoid tumor
    3.2   Malignant
        3.2.1   Epithelioid mesothelioma
        3.2.2   Sarcomatoid mesothelioma
                3.2.2.1   Desmoplastic mesothelioma
        3.2.3   Biphasic mesothelioma
        3.2.4   Other

Table 2 Continued

4. Miscellaneous Tumors
    4.1 Hamartoma
    4.2 Sclerosing hemangioma
    4.3 Clear cell tumor
    4.4 Germ cell neoplasms
        4.4.1 Teratoma, mature or immature
        4.4.2 Malignant germ cell tumor
    4.5 Thymoma
    4.6 Melanoma
    4.7 Others
5. Lymphoproliferative Diseases
    5.1 Lymphoid interstitial pneumonia
    5.2 Nodular lymphoid hyperplasia
    5.3 Low-grade marginal zone B-cell lymphoma of the mucosa-associated lymphoid tissue
    5.4 Lymphomatoid granulomatosis
6. Secondary Tumors
7. Unclassified Tumors
8. Tumor-like Lesions
    8.1 Tumorlet
    8.2 Multiple meningothelioid nodules
    8.3 Langerhans cell histiocytosis
    8.4 Inflammatory pseudotumor (Inflammatory myofibroblastic tumor)
    8.5 Organizing pneumonia
    8.6 Amyloid tumor
    8.7 Hyalinizing granuloma
    8.8 Lymphangioleiomyomatosis
    8.9 Multifocal micronodular pneumocyte hyperplasia
    8.10 Endometriosis
    8.11 Bronchial inflammatory polyp
    8.12 Others

refer to it as the WHO/IASLC Histological Classification of Lung and Pleural Tumors (Table 2).

    Tumor classification systems provide the foundation for tumor diagnosis and patient therapy (5). Therefore, they provide a critical basis for epidemiologic and clinical studies. In developing this classification, we tried to adhere to the principles of reproducibility, clinical significance, and simplicity. We also tried to minimize the number of unclassifiable lesions (2). Whenever possible, changes in classification were based on newly available published data. However, in some cases, such data were not available and decisions had to be made based on the collective experience and wisdom of the panel members. In general, certain time-honored terms were retained unless new concepts had emerged, necessitating a change.

I. Preinvasive Lesions

In addition to the categories of squamous dysplasia and carcinoma in situ, two additional lesions were added to the category of preinvasive lesions: atypical adenomatous hyperplasia (AAH) and diffuse idiopathic pulmonary neuroendocrine cell hyperplasia.

Many publications on the subject of atypical adenomatous hyperplasia suggest that it is a precursor to adenocarcinoma (6–10). Multiple terms have been used for this lesion, including alveolar cell hyperplasia, atypical alveolar hyperplasia, bronchioloalveolar cell adenoma, alveolar atypical hyperplasia, and atypical alveolar cuboidal cell hyperplasia. However, most studies have examined these lesions as incidental findings in lung specimens resected for lung cancer. Therefore, the opportunity to investigate the biology of this lesion as a precursor to carcinoma has been limited. The concept that AAH is a precursor to invasive carcinoma is largely an assumption based on the concurrent finding of these lesions in the lung parenchyma adjacent to lung carcinomas, primarily adenocarcinomas. In addition, some have attempted to identify AAH within the same mass of carcinoma as it merges with an adenocarcinoma. Only rare cases have been documented where AAH was identified and there was subsequent progression to invasive carcinoma. Extensive multicentric AAH appears to be a potential setting for progression to occur (9), although a recent study suggests that the prognosis of lung carcinoma is not affected by the presence of coexisting AAH (6).

Diffuse idiopathic neuroendocrine cell hyperplasia is a very rare lesion that can be associated with multiple carcinoid tumors (11). Neuroendocrine cell hyperplasia occurs most commonly as a reactive hyperplasia in the setting of airway fibrosis and/or inflammation (12,13). Up to two thirds of patients with peripheral carcinoid tumors may have neuroendocrine cell hyperplasia in the adjacent bronchiolar epithelium (14). A subset of these patients will have airway fibrosis, and a smaller number may have obstructive pulmonary function. In 1992, Aguayo et al. identified a small group of patients who presented with interstitial lung disease characterized by obstructive pulmonary function and histologic evidence of bronchiolar fibrosis associated with neuroendocrine cell hyperplasia (11). Some of these patients also had multiple tumorlets, and some had carcinoid tumors (11). Since neuroendocrine cells produce bombesin and other mediators that can act as fibroblast growth factors, it was proposed that the neuroendocrine cells are the cause of the fibrosis rather than a secondary reaction to the airway fibrosis. These observations suggest that diffuse idiopathic neuroendocrine cell hyperplasia is a condition in which neuroendocrine cell hyperplasia may progress to carcinoid tumors.

II. Adenocarcinomas

Since adenocarcinoma is now the predominant histologic subtype in many countries (15,16), issues relating to subclassification of adenocarcinoma are very important.

Adenocarcinoma subclassification was one of the most difficult problems faced in revising the classification of lung carcinomas. One of the biggest problems with lung adenocarcinomas is the frequent histologic heterogeneity (17). In fact, mixtures of adenocarcinoma histologic subtypes are more common than tumors consisting purely of a single pattern of acinar, papillary, bronchioloalveolar, and solid adenocarcinoma with mucin formation.

Another problem has been the imprecise application of criteria for diagnosis of bronchioloalveolar carcinoma. Since it has been shown that patients with solitary, noninvasive bronchioloalveolar carcinomas measuring less than 2.0 cm can be cured (18), we have restricted the definition of this tumor to only noninvasive tumors. If stromal, vascular, or pleural invasion are identified in an adenocarcinoma that has an extensive bronchioloalveolar carcinoma component, it would be classified as an *adenocarcinoma, mixed subtype* with predominant bronchioloalveolar pattern and either a focal acinar, solid, or papillary pattern depending on which pattern is seen in the invasive component. Criteria for diagnosis of bronchioloalveolar carcinoma have varied widely in the past, and the tumor described above would have been labeled as bronchioloalveolar carcinoma in many series. This definition is much more restrictive than any previously used by many pathologists.

Several variants of adenocarcinoma are recognized in the new classification including well-differentiated fetal adenocarcinoma (19–21), mucinous ("colloid") adenocarcinoma (22), mucinous cystadenocarcinoma (23), signet ring adenocarcinoma (24), and clear cell adenocarcinoma (25).

III. Neuroendocrine Tumors

Since 1981 there has been substantial evolution of concepts of neuroendocrine lung tumor classification. These issues are discussed in more detail in Chapter 3. Large-cell neuroendocrine carcinoma (LCNEC) is now recognized as a histologically high-grade non–small-cell carcinoma (26). It has a very poor prognosis, similar to that of SCLC. Atypical carcinoid is recognized as an intermediate-grade neuroendocrine tumor with a prognosis that falls between typical carcinoid and the high-grade SCLC and LCNEC (27). In addition, it has become well recognized that neuroendocrine differentiation can be demonstrated by immunohistochemistry or electron microscopy in 10–20% of common non–small-cell lung carcinomas (NSCLC) that do not have any neuroendocrine morphology (28–31). These tumors are not formally recognized within the WHO/IASLC classification scheme since the clinical and therapeutic significance of neuroendocrine differentiation in NSCLC is not firmly established. These tumors are referred to collectively as NSCLC with neuroendocrine differentiation.

IV. Large-Cell Carcinoma

In addition to the general category of large-cell carcinoma, several uncommon variants are recognized including LCNEC (26), basaloid carcinoma (32,33), lymphoepithelioma-like carcinoma (34,35), clear cell carcinoma (25), and large-cell carcinoma with rhabdoid phenotype (36). Basaloid carcinoma is also recognized as a variant of squamous cell carcinoma, and rarely adenocarcinomas may have a basaloid pattern. However, in tumors without either of these features, they are regarded as a variant of large-cell carcinoma (32,33).

V. Carcinomas with Pleomorphic, Sarcomatoid, or Sarcomatous Elements

Although immunohistochemical, ultrastructural, and molecular studies can all be helpful in analyzing these tumors, we have proposed a classification scheme based solely on light microscopy.

This is a very difficult group of tumors to classify for several reasons. First, they are rare tumors and few pathologists have the opportunity to study very many cases. Spindle and giant cell carcinomas and carcinosarcomas comprise only 0.4% and 0.1% of all lung malignancies, respectively (15). In addition, this group of tumors reflects a continuum in histologic heterogeneity as well as epithelial and mesenchymal differentiation (37,38). Biphasic pulmonary blastoma is regarded as part of the spectrum of carcinomas with pleomorphic, sarcomatoid, or sarcomatous elements based on clinical and molecular data (21,39,40).

It is rare to encounter a pure spindle or giant cell carcinoma (37). More commonly, these patterns are mixed with other histologic subtypes of lung carcinoma and frequently the spindle cell and giant cell pattern are seen together. Carcinosarcoma is arbitrarily defined as a biphasic tumor with carcinomatous and sarcomatous components only if the latter demonstrate heterologous elements such as malignant bone, cartilage, or skeletal muscle. Pleomorphic carcinoma is diagnosed in a biphasic tumor showing carcinomatous as well as spindle and/or giant cell components even if epithelial differentiation cannot be demonstrated in the spindle cell component by immunohistochemistry or electron microscopy.

VI. Immunohistochemistry and Electron Microscopy

While immunohistochemistry and electron microscopy are invaluable techniques for diagnosis and subclassification of lung tumors, we have attempted to establish a classification that is simple, practical, and able to be used even in surgical pathology laboratories where these techniques may not be available.

Nevertheless, immunohistochemistry and/or electron microscopy are required for definitive diagnosis of large-cell neuroendocrine carcinoma and malignant mesothelioma. The intent of our emphasis on light microscopy is not meant to discourage the use of these techniques. The distinctive immunostaining characteristics of certain tumors can be very useful, such as HMB-45 positivity in clear cell tumors and lymphangioleiomyomatosis and EMA staining in sclerosing hemangiomas.

VII. Molecular Studies

The advent of molecular biology has also allowed a new depth of insight into the understanding of many lung tumors. It has allowed molecular demonstration of the neoplastic nature of certain lesions such as alveolar adenoma (41), chondroid hamartoma (42,43), and inflammatory pseudotumors (inflammatory myofibroblastic tumor) (44). It has also provided insights into genetic abnormalities that have contributed to histologic classification of lung tumors and preinvasive lesions (40,45–48).

Similar to our comments on immunohistochemistry and electron microscopy, our emphasis on light microscopic criteria for diagnosis of lung tumors is not intended to discourage the use of molecular techniques as diagnostic aids and research tools.

VIII. Conclusion

Most lung tumors can be classified by light microscopic criteria. Although special techniques are necessary to classify a few tumors, the advantage of the emphasis on light microscopic criteria for most tumors in this classification system is the potential for widespread and worldwide application.

Future studies should clarify some of the difficult problems in lung tumor classification, especially for preinvasive lesions, adenocarcinoma subtyping, large-cell neuroendocrine carcinoma, and carcinomas with pleomorphic, sarcomatoid, or sarcomatous elements.

References

1. World Health Organization. Histological Typing of Lung Tumours. 1st ed. Geneva: World Health Organization, 1967.
2. World Health Organization. Histological Typing of Lung Tumors. 2d ed. Geneva: World Health Organization, 1981.
3. Hirsch FR, Matthews MJ, Aisner S, Campobasso O, Elema JD, Gazdar AF, Mackay B, Nasiell M, Shimosato Y, Steele RH. Histopathologic classification of small cell lung cancer. Changing concepts and terminology. Cancer 1988; 62:973–977.
4. World Health Organization. Histological Typing of Lung and Pleural Tumors, 3rd ed. International Histological Classification of Tumours. No. 1. In press.
5. Colby TV, Koss MN, Travis WD. Tumors of the Lower Respiratory Tract; Armed Forces Institute of Pathology Fascicle, Third Series. Washington, DC: Armed Forces Institute of Pathology, 1995.
6. Suzuki K, Nagai K, Yoshida J, Yokose T, Kodama T, Takahashi K, Nishimura M, Kawasaki H, Yokozaki M, Nishiwaki Y. The prognosis of resected lung carcinoma associated with atypical adenomatous hyperplasia: a comparison of the prognosis of well-differentiated ad-

enocarcinoma associated with atypical adenomatous hyperplasia and intrapulmonary metastasis. Cancer 1997; 79:1521–1526.

7. Kitamura H, Kameda Y, Nakamura N, Inayama Y, Nakatani Y, Shibagaki T, Ito T, Hayashi H, Kimura H, Kanisawa M. Atypical adenomatous hyperplasia and bronchoalveolar lung carcinoma. Analysis by morphometry and the expressions of p53 and carcinoembryonic antigen. Am J Surg Pathol 1996; 20:553–562.

8. Mori M, Tezuka F, Chiba R, Funae Y, Watanabe M, Nukwa T, Takahashi T. Atypical adenomatous hyperplasia and adenocarcinoma of the human lung. Their heterology in form and analogy in immunohistochemical characteristics. Cancer 1996; 77:665–674.

9. Miller RR. Bronchioloalveolar cell adenomas. Am J Surg Pathol 1990; 14:904–912.

10. Kodama T, Biyajima S, Watanabe S, Shimosato Y. Morphometric study of adenocarcinomas and hyperplastic epithelial lesions in the peripheral lung. Am J Clin Pathol 1986; 85:146–151.

11. Aguayo SM, Miller YE, Waldron JA, Jr, Bogin RM, Sunday ME, Staton GW, Jr, Beam WR, King TE, Jr. Brief report: idiopathic diffuse hyperplasia of pulmonary neuroendocrine cells and airways disease. N Engl J Med 1992; 327:1285–1288.

12. Aguayo SM, King TE, Jr, Waldron JA, Jr, Sherritt KM, Kane MA, Miller YE. Increased pulmonary neuroendocrine cells with bombesin-like immunoreactivity in adult patients with eosinophilic granuloma. J Clin Invest 1990; 86:838–844.

13. Gosney JR, Sissons MC, Allibone RO, Blakey AF. Pulmonary endocrine cells in chronic bronchitis and emphysema. J Pathol 1989; 157:127–133.

14. Miller RR, Muller NL. Neuroendocrine cell hyperplasia and obliterative bronchiolitis in patients with peripheral carcinoid tumors. Am J Surg Pathol 1995; 19:653–658.

15. Travis WD, Travis LB, Devesa SS. Lung cancer [published erratum appears in Cancer 1995; 75(12):2979]. Cancer 1995; 75:191–202.

16. Takeshima Y, Nishisaka T, Kawano R, Kishizuchi K, Fujii S, Kitaguchi S, Inai K. p16/CDKN2 gene and p53 gene alterations in Japanese non-smoking female lung adenocarcinoma. Jpn J Cancer Res 1996; 87:134–140.

17. Roggli VL, Vollmer RT, Greenberg SD, McGavran MH, Spjut HJ, Yesner R. Lung cancer heterogeneity: a blinded and randomized study of 100 consecutive cases. Hum Pathol 1985; 16:569–579.

18. Noguchi M, Morikawa A, Kawasaki M, Matsuno Y, Yamada T, Hirohashi S, Kondo H, Shimosato Y. Small adenocarcinoma of the lung. Histologic characteristics and prognosis. Cancer 1995; 75:2844–2852.

19. Nakatani Y, Kitamura H, Inayama Y, Ogawa N. Pulmonary endodermal tumor resembling fetal lung. The optically clear nucleus is rich in biotin. Am J Surg Pathol 1994; 18:637–642.

20. Kodama T, Shimosato Y, Watanabe S, Koide T, Naruke T, Shimase J. Six cases of well-differentiated adenocarcinoma simulating fetal lung tubules in pseudoglandular stage. Comparison with pulmonary blastoma. Am J Surg Pathol 1984; 8:735–744.

21. Koss MN, Hochholzer L, O'Leary T. Pulmonary blastomas. Cancer 1991; 67:2368–2381.

22. Moran CA, Hochholzer L, Fishback N, Travis WD, Koss MN. Mucinous (so-called colloid) carcinomas of lung. Mod Pathol 1992; 5:634–638.

23. Dixon AY, Moran JF, Wesselius LJ, McGregor DH. Pulmonary mucinous cystic tumor. Case report with review of the literature. Am J Surg Pathol 1993; 17:722–728.

24. Kish JK, Ro JY, Ayala AG, McMurtrey MJ. Primary mucinous adenocarcinoma of the lung with signet-ring cells: a histochemical comparison with signet-ring cell carcinomas of other sites. Hum Pathol 1989; 20:1097–1102.

25. Katzenstein AL, Prioleau PG, Askin FB. The histologic spectrum and significance of clear-cell change in lung carcinoma. Cancer 1980; 45:943–947.

26. Travis WD, Linnoila RI, Tsokos MG, Hitchcock CL, Cutler GB, Jr, Nieman L, Chrousos G, Pass H, Doppman J. Neuroendocrine tumors of the lung with proposed criteria for large-cell neuroendocrine carcinoma. An ultrastructural, immunohistochemical, and flow cytometric study of 35 cases. Am J Surg Pathol 1991; 15:529–553.

27. Arrigoni MG, Woolner LB, Bernatz PE. Atypical carcinoid tumors of the lung. J Thorac Cardiovasc Surg 1972; 64:413–421.

28. Schleusener JT, Tazelaar HD, Jung SH, Cha SS, Cera PJ, Myers JL, Creagan ET, Goldberg

RM, Marschke RF, Jr. Neuroendocrine differentiation is an independent prognostic factor in chemotherapy-treated non small cell lung carcinoma. Cancer 1996; 77:1284–1291.

29. Linnoila RI, Piantadosi S, Ruckdeschel JC. Impact of neuroendocrine differentiation in non-small cell lung cancer. The LCSG experience. Chest 1994; 106:367S–371S.

30. Carles J, Rosell R, Ariza A, Pellicer I, Sanchez JJ, Fernandez-Vasalo G, Abad A, Barnadas A. Neuroendocrine differentiation as a prognostic factor in non-small cell lung cancer. Lung Cancer 1993; 10:209–219.

31. Neal MH, Kosinski R, Cohen P, Orenstein JM. Atypical endocrine tumors of the lung: a histologic, ultrastructural, and clinical study of 19 cases. Hum Pathol 1986; 17:1264–1277.

32. Brambilla E, Moro D, Veale D, Brichon PY, Stoebner P, Paramelle B, Brambilla C. Basal cell (basaloid) carcinoma of the lung: a new morphologic and phenotypic entity with separate prognostic significance. Hum Pathol 1992; 23:993–1003.

33. Moro D, Brichon PY, Brambilla E, Veale D, Labat F, Brambilla C. Basaloid bronchial carcinoma. A histologic group with a poor prognosis. Cancer 1994; 73:2734–2739.

34. Butler AE, Colby TV, Weiss L, Lombard CM. Lymphoepithelioma-like carcinoma of the lung. Am J Surg Pathol 1989; 13:632–639.

35. Chan JK, Hui PK, Tsang WY, Law CK, Ma CC, Yip TT, Poon YF. Primary lymphoepithelioma-like carcinoma of the lung. A clinicopathologic study of 11 cases. Cancer 1995; 76:413–422.

36. Cavazza A, Colby TV, Tsokos M, Rush W, Travis WD. Lung tumors with a rhabdoid phenotype. Am J Clin Pathol 1996; 105:182–188.

37. Fishback NF, Travis WD, Moran CA, Guinee DG, Jr, McCarthy WF, Koss MN. Pleomorphic (spindle/giant cell) carcinoma of the lung. A clinicopathologic correlation of 78 cases. Cancer 1994; 73:2936–2945.

38. Nappi O, Glasner SD, Swanson PE, Wick MR. Biphasic and monophasic sarcomatoid carcinomas of the lung. A reappraisal of 'carcinosarcomas' and 'spindle-cell carcinomas.' Am J Clin Pathol 1994; 102:331–340.

39. Bodner SM, Koss MN. Mutations in the p53 gene in pulmonary blastomas: immunohistochemical and molecular studies. Hum Pathol 1996; 27:1117–1123.

40. Holst VA, Finkelstein S, Colby TV, Myers JL, Yousem SA. p53 and K-ras mutational genotyping in pulmonary carcinosarcoma, spindle cell carcinoma, and pulmonary blastoma: implications for histogenesis. Am J Surg Pathol 1997; 21:801–811.

41. Roque L, Oliveira P, Martins C, Carvalho C, Serpa A, Soares J. A nonbalanced translocation (10;16) demonstrated by FISH analysis in a case of alveolar adenoma of the lung. Cancer Genet Cytogenet 1996; 89:34–37.

42. Xiao S, Lux ML, Reeves R, Hudson TJ, Fletcher JA. HMGI(Y) activation by chromosome 6p21 rearrangements in multilineage mesenchymal cells from pulmonary hamartoma [comment]. Am J Pathol 1997; 150:901–910.

43. Kazmierczak B, Wanschura S, Rosigkeit J, Meyer-Bolte K, Uschinsky K, Haupt R, Schoenmakers EF, Bartnitzke S, Van de Ven WJ, Bullerdiek J. Molecular characterization of 12q14–15 rearrangements in three pulmonary chondroid hamartomas. Cancer Res 1995; 55:2497–2499.

44. Snyder CS, 'Aquila MD, Haghighi P, Baergen RN, Suh YK, Yi ES. Clonal changes in inflammatory pseudotumor of the lung. A case report. Cancer 1995; 76:1545–1549.

45. Miller YE, Franklin WA. Molecular events in lung carcinogenesis. Hematol Oncol Clin North Am 1997; 11:215–234.

46. Harris CC. p53 tumor suppressor gene: at the crossroads of molecular carcinogenesis, molecular epidemiology, and cancer risk assessment. Environ Health Perspect 1996; 104(suppl 3):435–439.

47. Brambilla E, Negoescu A, Gazzeri S, Lantuejoul S, Moro D, Brambilla C, Coll JL. Apoptosis-related factors p53, Bcl2, and Bax in neuroendocrine lung tumors. Am J Pathol 1996; 149:1941–1952.

48. Fong KM, Biesterveld EJ, Virmani A, Wistuba I, Sekido Y, Bader SA, Ahmadian M, Ong ST, Rassool FV, Zimmerman PV, Giaccone G, Gazdar AF, Minna JD. FHIT and FRA3B 3p14.2 allele loss are common in lung cancer and preneoplastic bronchial lesions and are associated with cancer-related FHIT cDNA splicing aberrations. Cancer Res 1997; 57:2256–2267.

2

Basaloid Carcinoma of the Lung

ELISABETH BRAMBILLA and DENIS MORO

Institut Albert Bonniot
Centre Hospitalier Universitaire de Grenoble
Grenoble, France

I. Definition

Basaloid carcinoma is one of the rarest forms of non–small-cell non-neuroendocrine carcinoma of the lung, since it accounts for about 5% of surgically treated cases. Although its incidence is higher than that of uncommon tumors described in the World Health Organization's most recent histological classification of lung tumors (1), such as carcinoid tumors, it was described in this classification among "other malignant epithelial neoplasms" as presenting as "tumors resembling the basal cell carcinoma of the skin." Spencer (2) in 1985 described two cases he had observed where removal of the endobronchial tumor was followed by long survival. He consequently expected that these tumors would have a good prognosis. With the exception of these brief comments, basaloid carcinoma, which shares several morphological characteristics with basal cell carcinoma of skin, was not fully described as a distinct morphological entity in the lung until recently (3).

Similar basal cell tumors had been recognized previously in the upper aerodigestive tract (4–6) as a variant of squamous cell carcinoma (basaloid squamous carcinoma) and in the anal canal, where they are described as a rare poorly differentiated form of cloacogenic carcinoma (7–9). Basaloid carcinoma has also been reported in the esophagus (10) and in the uterine cervix (11,12), where it is considered as a solid form of adenoid cystic carcinoma and is regarded to have a worse prognosis than classical adenoid cystic carcinoma of the same locations.

Basaloid carcinoma of the lung was precisely identified and fully described in 1992 (3) following review of a large series of cases that had been surgically treated and previously classified as poorly differentiated squamous cell carcinoma or indifferentiated large cell carcinoma. The first description was based on 38 cases among 700 surgically treated tumors, and the present description is based on 50 cases identified during review of 1011 lung tumors in our institution over an 11-year period. After its initial description, basaloid carcinoma has been described in several books on lung tumor pathology (13–15) as a variant of squamous cell carcinoma. Thus, basaloid carcinoma is now well recognized as a specific histopathological entity with prognostic significance.

II. Clinical Features

All 50 patients presenting basaloid carcinoma were men aged 36–84 years (median 60 years). The clinical presentation included weight loss, respiratory symptoms of obstructive pneumonia, hemoptysis, cough, and chest pain. In the vast majority of the cases (85%) the tumor was located in lobar or segmental bronchi; it was more distally situated in the other 15% of cases. They were all single tumors. The TNM (16) stages after surgery were as follows: 40% were stage I, 30% stage II, and 30% stage III. Therapy was by surgery alone in half of the cases and surgery followed by radiation therapy in the other half. There was no statistical difference between basaloid and squamous carcinoma in regard to male prevalence, smoking habits, clinico-pathologic presentation (17), location, or postoperative staging.

III. Macroscopic Appearance

Exophytic endobronchial growth in proximal lobar to segmental bronchi is observed in 85% of cases (3,17) and is always associated with bronchial wall invasion. Endobronchial tumors frequently grow along the bronchial lumen and infiltrate the glandular ducts in a finger-like fashion. In other cases the tumor infiltrates the bronchial wall without causing obstruction. The frequent proximal situation of basaloid carcinoma is responsible for invasion of mediastinal pleural or adipose tissue in 30% of cases with subsequent classification into stage III of the TNM classification. Tumors range in size from 1 to 7 cm in diameter, but half of the cases are <3 cm in diameter and are thus stage T1 at the time of surgery.

IV. Histopathology

Basaloid carcinoma may present as a monomorphic variety, implying that 80% of the tumor cells have the histopathologic features defining the basaloid component.

This basaloid component may be mixed with other tumors of another histological pattern in the mixed basaloid variety.

The cardinal histopathologic features defining the basaloid component include a solid lobular or anastomotic trabecular pattern, growing invasively in a finger-like fashion from the bronchial and/or glandular duct lining (Fig. 1); small rather monomorphic cuboidal to fusiform cells of 12–15 μm mean diameter, with moderately hyperchromatic nuclei showing a finely granular chromatin, no prominent nucleoli, and scanty to moderate amounts of cytoplasm; peripheral palisading with radially arranged cells at the periphery of lobules (Fig. 2, 3); and a high rate of mitosis ranging from 25 to 60 per 10 high power fields (Fig. 3).

The following features, although less common, are highly characteristic of basaloid carcinoma. Sixty percent of tumors show centrilobular coagulative comedo-type necrosis. One third of the cases display small cystic spaces, sometimes containing mucinous-like material occasionally stained with diastase digested PAS and/or alcian blue (Fig. 3). Rosettes are present in one third of the cases, which, in combination with palisading, can create differential diagnosis difficulties with neuroendocrine lung tumors, as we will discuss later (Fig. 4). Papillary structures are seen in 20% of the cases when there is endobronchial growth. Despite the absence of individual cell keratinization within the basal cell component and intercellular bridging, abrupt keratin pearl formation, mimicking hair follicles (keratin pearls), is encountered in 25% of the cases. These figures of pilous differentiation do not deserve classification of a given case under the mixed form in itself.

Modification of the stroma is observed in half of the cases, under the form of

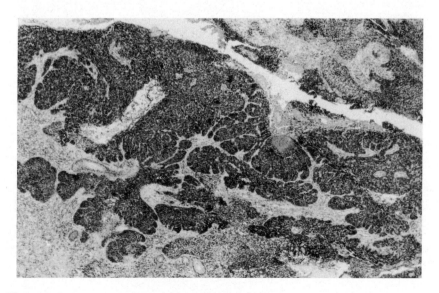

Figure 1   Invasive growth from bronchial and glandular duct lining in a finger-like fashion. (HES ×40)

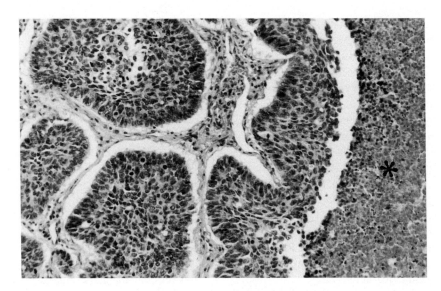

Figure 2 Lobular pattern with peripheral palisading (arrow) and comedo-type necrosis (asterisk). (HES ×250)

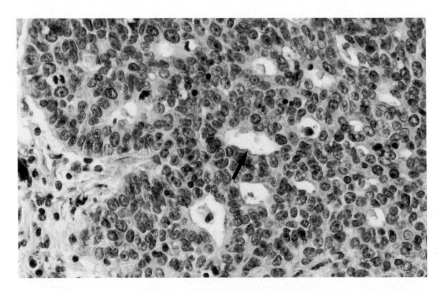

Figure 3 Small monomorphic basaloid cells with hyperchromatic nuclei, finely granular chromatin, and scanty cytoplasm. Note the high rate of mitosis and small cystic spaces (arrow). (HES ×400)

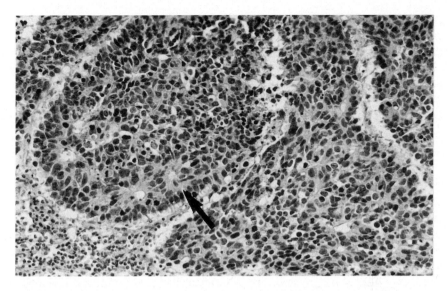

Figure 4   Peripheral palisading and numerous rosettes (arrow) in a case resembling large-cell neuroendocrine carcinoma. Neuroendocrine stains were negative. (HES ×250)

hyalinosis sometimes dissociating tumor lobules in irregular cell rows (one third of the cases) or myxoid basophilic stroma in 20% of the cases. Rare cases (<10%) show osseous or chondroid metamorphism of the stroma.

In the pure type of basaloid carcinoma (half of the cases), more than 80% of cells show basaloid appearance. In the other half of cases, the basaloid component accounts for at least 60% of the tumor bulk and is juxtaposed or admixed in more intimate fashion with another tumor type of larger cell size. In the mixed forms, the second component is a well- or moderately well-differentiated squamous carcinoma showing classical intercellular bridging and true individual cell keratinization in 80% of the cases, a large-cell carcinoma showing neither intercellulaire bridging nor keratin production and resembling transitional cell carcinoma of urinary bladder in 10%, a mucus-secreting adenocarcinoma of acinar or tubular architecture in 5%, and both adeno and squamous differentiation in the last 5%.

Overlying and adjacent carcinoma in situ extending far from the primary tumor site is extremely frequent (50%), often seen in lobar, segmental, or subsegmental bronchi in continuity or not with the invasive tumor. These long extended carcinoma in situ are of special concern with respect to curative surgery and management of preinvasive bronchial lesions.

The distinctive and characteristic histolopathologic features of basaloid carcinoma in its pure form are thus similar to those of basal cell carcinoma of the skin and the basaloid form of cloacogenic anal carcinoma (7,8). When associated with squamous cell carcinoma in a mixed basaloid carcinoma, they resemble tumors described in the upper aerodigestive tract (4–6,18) as basaloid-squamous carcinoma.

Pure basaloid carcinoma is far more frequent in the lung than in the upper aero-digestive tract. Alternatively, when the basaloid component is associated with glandular differentiation, it bears some resemblance to the solid forms of adenoid cystic carcinoma and when the basaloid carcinoma is admixed with an undifferentiated large-cell component, the tumor resembles the transitional type of cloacogenic carcinoma (19).

V.   Immunohistochemical Phenotype

A.   Cytokeratins

Basaloid carcinoma cells consistently express low molecular weight acidic keratins CK18, 19, and the basic cytokeratin 7 and 8 of the Moll catalog (17), although the staining may sometimes be weak and heterogeneous. In half of the cases they also express cytokeratins 13 and 16. The cytokeratin distribution thus mimics that of the normal basal cells of pseudostratified and squamous normal epithelia and of non-keratinizing squamous carcinoma (20,21). In at least some tumor cells, cytokeratins 5, 6, and 14 are also expressed. These last cytokeratins are restricted to the basal cells of stratified epithelia and are not seen in glandular epithelia, neuroendocrine carcinoma, or adenoid cystic carcinoma. Remnants of normal structures entrapped within the basaloid component, such as normal gland ducts, are always more intensely stained for cytokeratins than the basaloid tumor component itself, which often displays light and focal staining. In contrast, high molecular weight cytokeratins 4, 10, and 11, which are characteristic of well-differentiated squamous carcinoma showing keratinization, are never expressed in the basaloid component unless in keratin pearls.

B.   Neuroendocrine Markers

Particular attention has been paid to neuroendocrine markers in basaloid carcinoma since they can show palisading and rosette formation, which is also a common feature of large-cell neuroendocrine carcinoma, a recently identified class of high-grade neuroendocrine lung tumor (22). In contrast, neuroendocrine markers such as chromogranine A, Leu 7 (CD57), synaptophysin, and neural cell adhesion molecule (NCAM) and NCAM PSA (a polysyalilated form of NCAM) are all negative in most cases (95%). In the last 5% of basaloid carcinoma, a minority of tumor cells (5–20%) expresses one of these markers. This limited focal expression of neuroendocrine markers was observed with the same frequency in the associated component in the mixed basaloid tumors more often in the adenocarcinomatous component than in the squamous cell component. Any basaloid tumor, pure or mixed, expressing multiple neuroendocrine markers in more than 20% of the basaloid component should be excluded from this class as representing, depending on the presence or absence of distinctive neuroendocrine features, whether large-cell neuroendocrine carcinoma or non–small-cell carcinoma with neuroendocrine differentiation, despite their basaloid-like pattern. When frozen tumor tissue is available, several neuroendocrine markers should be sought, the most distinctive being the NCAM molecules (23,24) (one of which—123C3—is also reactive on paraffin sections) (25). Synaptophysin and neurofilament reactivities are always negative in basaloid carcinoma. Finally, only tumors with no more than one neuroendocrine marker on less than 20% of the tumor cells should be called basaloid carcinoma. This of course emphasizes the requirement for neuroendocrine marker negativity, especially in pure basaloid cases where rosettes and palisading are obvious. Since basaloid carcinoma are composed of poorly differentiated cells with the phenotype of totipotent stem cells, their ability to adopt neuroendocrine differentiation is not surprising. Accordingly, 5–20% of non–small-cell lung carcinomas, depending on the studies and the markers chosen, were shown to express neuroendocrine markers (26,27) despite lacking obvious neuroendocrine features such as palisading and rosettes. These are now classified as non–small-cell carcinomas with neuroendocrine differentiation according to the new proposal of Travis et al. (22). Whether or not these carcinomas differ in their behavior from their non-neuroendocrine counterparts has yet to be definitively assessed. Most previous studies have assumed the prognostic influence of neuroendocrine markers in non–small-cell carcinoma with no consideration for the new classification of neuroendocrine lung tumors. Some of the cases included in this category because of large-cell morphology were true large-cell neuroendocrine carcinoma, which are high-grade tumors of dismal prognosis. This could have overcome the real prognostic value of the expression of neuroendocrine markers in non–small-cell lung carcinoma. Consequently, there is no good reason at the present time to separate basaloid carcinoma showing partial neuroendocrine expression from carcinoma that lacks such differentiation unless the prognostic significance of this partial neuroendocrine expression is recognized after reappraisal of the cases according to the new WHO classification.

C. Proliferation Markers

In keeping with their mitotic rate, basaloid tumors show a high proliferation index as indicated by a mean of 30% labeled cells with Ki67 antibody (28) or MIB1 effective on paraffin sections. This proliferation index is in the range of that observed in large-cell neuroendocrine carcinoma and in some small-cell lung carcinoma. It is far above the mean percentage of Ki67-labeled cells observed in non–small-cell lung carcinoma of adeno or squamous type (10–15%).

D. Other Markers

On frozen material, positive immunostaining for epidermal growth factor receptor (29) is observed in 90% of the cases as is immunoreactivity for histocompatibility antigens HLA type I and II (unpublished data). This is of interest because neuroendocrine tumors are always negative for these markers (30). No other marker is of real value in the identification of basaloid carcinoma. Epithelial membrane antigen is expressed in two thirds of the cases, but there is no expression of S100 protein, smooth muscle actin, and α-smooth muscle actin, in contrast to adenoid cystic carcinoma. Phenotypic markers referring to abnormal expression of oncogenes or tumor-suppressor genes are of no help in the positive or differential diagnosis of basaloid carcinoma.

VI. Ultrastructural Features

Most basaloid carcinoma appears as poorly differentiated proliferations at the ultra-structural level. Tumor cells within the basaloid component are polygonal or elon-gated, their nuclear chromatin is finally dispersed, and the nuclear envelope is free of indentation. The cytoplasm generally contains a large number of free ribosomes, polyribosomes, and mitochondria. Strands of rough endoplasmic reticulum are fre-quently seen and can be numerous. The cell borders are smooth or lightly interdigi-tated. In all cases the cells are connected by small, well-defined desmosomes con-nected in short tonofilament bundles. Scanty tonofilament bundles are infrequently seen in the cytoplasm (Fig. 5). In a few cases, acini formation or microvilli are ob-served, whereas true acinar formation with protruding microvilli and tripartite junc-

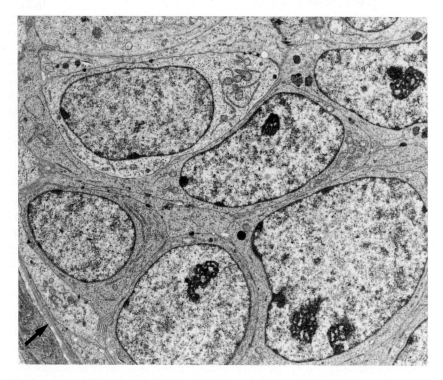

Figure 5 Ultrastructure of basaloid carcinoma showing small elongated cells joined by small desmosomes containing strands of rough endoplasmic reticulum. Amorphous basal ma-terial is deposited at the periphery of cell nests (arrow). (E.M. ×6750)

tional complexes are rare. No dense core neurosecretory granules are seen, nor are typical mucus granules, although small mucus granules are sometimes noted. Dense lysosomes, somewhat evocative of Clara cell granules, are also encountered. Perilobular basal lamina is observed in all cases, which is sometimes discontinuous or abnormally thick or mixed with microfibrils or amorphous material. Reduplicated and multilayered basal lamina, a prominent feature of adenoid cystic carcinoma, are not observed in basaloid carcinoma.

The overall ultrastructural features of basaloid carcinoma are those previously described in this type of tumor at other sites (5,9,10,31,32) and are comparable with normal intermediate bronchial cells immediately located suprabasally to the anchoring basal cells of the large bronchi. According to previous descriptions (33,34), normal basal bronchial epithelial cells contain more dense and numerous tonofilaments than intermediate suprabasal cells and basaloid tumor cells, which exhibit long profiles of rough endoplasmic reticulum, tenuous tonofilaments, and a few microvilli (34). The presence of small mucus granules in both intermediate cells of normal and regenerative bronchial epithelia (33) and basaloid tumor cells is consonant with this common lineage. Basal and intermediate (small mucus granule) cells are pluripotent reserve cells with regenerative and proliferative function, which make them good candidates for malignant transformation. This is consistent with basaloid carcinoma being regarded as a stem cell proliferation.

VII. Differential Diagnosis

Differential diagnosis of basaloid carcinoma has to be assessed in regard to adenoid cystic carcinoma, poorly differentiated carcinoma, and large-cell neuroendocrine carcinoma.

Similarities between basaloid carcinoma and adenoid cystic carcinoma in its solid form reside in the presence of small cystic spaces where mucin stains can be focally positive. Their distinction is even more difficult when the basaloid component is associated, in the mixed forms, with a glandular-like component. The absence of cylindromatous pattern and the presence of necrosis as well as a high mitotic index (>25 mitoses per 10 high-power fields) distinguish basaloid carcinoma from adenoid cystic carcinoma.

The main differential diagnosis is from poorly differentiated squamous cell carcinoma, since basaloid carcinoma has been proposed to be part or a variety of the former. Since basaloid carcinoma has a significantly worse prognosis than poorly differentiated squamous carcinoma, we believe that they should be distinguished as separate histological classes. Centrilobular keratin pearls are sometimes observed within pure basaloid carcinoma, and squamous cell carcinoma is a frequent component associated with the basaloid component in the mixed form. However, the absence of intercellular bridging and of progressive or individual cell cornification in the basaloid component, the smaller cell size, a higher nuclear-to-cytoplasmic ratio, and low pleiomorphism are characteristic features of basaloid carcinoma that help to distinguish it from squamous cell carcinoma. The most difficult differential diagnosis is distinguishing the pure form of basaloid carcinoma, forming palisades and rosettes, from large-cell neuroendocrine carcinoma. However, most large-cell neuroendocrine carcinoma has larger cell size, more cellular pleiomorphism, a mosaic pattern, a coarsely granular or vesicular chromatin, and more prominent nucleoli than basaloid carcinoma. However, neuroendocrine markers are required to separate both entities when a neuroendocrine-like pattern is present. Expression of several neuroendocrine markers (at least three) is the hallmark of large-cell neuroendocrine carcinoma in association with obvious endocrinoid pattern, which allows its separation from basaloid carcinoma. Moreover, neurosecretory granules, which are observed in large-cell neuroendocrine when searched for, are never detected in basaloid carcinoma by electron microscopy.

Much easier is the differential diagnosis between basaloid carcinoma and intermediate-type small-cell lung carcinoma. Basaloid carcinoma shares with this type of carcinoma a small nuclear size and a finely packed granular chromatin pattern. However, basophilia and compaction of the chromatin are always much higher in small-cell lung carcinoma, and nuclear molding is almost specific for this last entity. More importantly, the diffuse pattern of small-cell lung carcinoma and its paucity of stroma are in great contrast to the well-defined lobular and trabecular pattern of basaloid carcinoma, where basal lamina is easily identified at the periphery of lobules and trabeculae and heavily stained for collagen IV and laminin. Furthermore, necrosis is focal and punctate or comedo-type in basaloid carcinoma rather than widespread, poorly limited, and infarct-like in small-cell lung carcinoma. The Azzopardi effect (on basophilia of vascular walls) is a typical feature of small-cell lung carcinoma and is never seen in basaloid carcinoma.

VIII. Histogenesis and Oncogenesis

Basaloid carcinoma as shown by morphological, immunophenotypic, and ultrastructural features is reminiscent of totipotent reserve or basal cells, which have the expected propensity for further multidirectional differentiation along squamous, glandular, or even neuroendocrine pathways. Carcinoma in situ and extension into the gland ducts suggest an origin of basaloid carcinoma from transformed basal cells of the surface epithelium or gland ducts (37,38). Interestingly, occasional cases of small-cell carcinoma that lack neurosecretory granules but show features of squamous differentiation have been described (35–39) under various names, such as small-cell squamous carcinoma, undifferentiated carcinoma of small-cell type, or reserve cell carcinoma, illustrating the fact that some carcinomas of small-cell appearance lack the characteristic neurosecretory granules, which is the hallmark of neuroendocrine differentiation. A large proportion of such tumors, negative for neuroendocrine markers or lacking neurosecretory granules, should probably be regarded as basaloid carcinomas.

Basal or suprabasal intermediate cells (small mucus granule cells) appear to be the best candidate for malignant transformation in bronchi based on their undifferentiated phenotype and their capacity for cell renewal and division: 1% of them are cycling cells as demonstrated by the Ki67 or PCNA labeling of normal bronchi. Their malignant transformation under the effect of environmental and tobacco smoke or asbestosis carcinogenic factors likely depends on the type of mutation acquired on key genes controlling proliferation, differentiation, and apoptosis. These genetic events create genomic instability and diversification resulting in different tumor types (40). The high frequency and wide extent of dysplasia and carcinoma in situ observed in the vicinity of basaloid carcinoma (50%), which is far higher than the frequency observed in association with squamous cell carcinoma (20%), strongly suggest progressive malignant transformation from preinvasive states. The sequence of the molecular and genetic events and their temporal association with the morphological steps of the transformation pathway is far from clear. However, p53 mutation (41–44), chromosome 3 deletion (45), and aneuploidy (46) have been documented in early preinvasive bronchial lesions of patients with synchronous lung cancer. We studied p53 expression and the expression of target genes of its downstream transcription pathway in several preinvasive lesions associated with seven cases of surgically treated basaloid carcinoma. p53 stabilization was found in one third of the areas of dysplasia and two thirds of the areas of carcinoma in situ, and exclusively when accompanying basaloid carcinoma also displayed p53 stabilization. This suggested that the p53 disorder is an early genetic event and precedes invasion in basaloid carcinoma. We demonstrated an early imbalance of bax and bcl2 protein expression. Equilibrium of bax with bcl2 in cell cytoplasm is believed to regulate susceptibility to cell death. Interestingly, bax and bcl2 genes are target genes of p53 transcription. However, the bcl2/bax imbalance, which was present in one third of the preinvasive lesions and was mainly maintained in the invasive basaloid carcinoma, was not related to p53 status. This suggests an early resistance to apoptosis conferred by a high bcl2 : bax ratio in one third of the preinvasive lesions associated or preceding basaloid carcinoma. More interestingly, 80% of basaloid carcinoma express bcl2 more intensely than bax, in contrast with other non–small-cell lung carcinoma, where bax highly predominates on bcl2. This tendency toward high bcl2 and low bax expression in basaloid tumors and one third of their precursor lesions is likely to allow escape from programmed cell death, which, in addition to increased proliferation, may explain the rapid rate of progression of this particular tumor type.

Retinoblastoma gene expression was maintained in 90% of basaloid carcinoma cases and was constantly retained in precursor bronchial lesions. In contrast, 20% of moderate and severe dysplasia and in situ carcinoma showed loss of expression of cyclin-dependent kinase (CdK) inhibitor p16[INK4], the protein products of which prevent Rb from phosphorylating in normal cells to allow G1 arrest. Since 75% of basaloid carcinomas have lost p53 function, 60% have lost Rb function through inappropriate phosphorylation, and the majority have a high bcl2 : bax ratio in favor of bcl2, basaloid carcinoma clones seem to have selected strong means for growth control evasion at the G1 restriction point and apoptosis inhibition as com-

pared with other non–small-cell lung carcinomas. High proliferation rate and reduced apoptosis could be responsible for their more aggressive behavior.

IX. Prognosis

Basaloid carcinoma of the lung has a poor prognosis (14). The 5-year actuarial survival rate of 10% in stage I and II as compared with 47% in the same stages of
poorly differentiated squamous cell carcinoma definitely differentiate basaloid carcinoma from squamous cell carcinoma. The median survival of stage I–II patients
is 600 days for basaloid carcinoma against 1200 days in poorly differentiated squamous cell carcinoma. Capewell et al. (47) showed a 35% 5-year survival rate for
stage I and stage II resected lung tumors: 55% and 31% for adenocarcinoma and
squamous carcinoma, respectively. The worse prognosis for basaloid carcinoma is
probably attributable to its poor differentiation. However, the prognostic influence
of the degree of differentiation in other non–small-cell carcinomas remains controversial. Some authors found a poor prognosis or higher recurrence rate in poorly
differentiated resected lung carcinoma as compared with well-differentiated forms
(48–50), but this difference was not confirmed in other larger series (51–53). Kaplan
Meier analysis (Fig. 6) shows a significant difference ($p = 0.004$) in the rate of cumulative survival, corrected for the cause of death, between basaloid carcinoma and

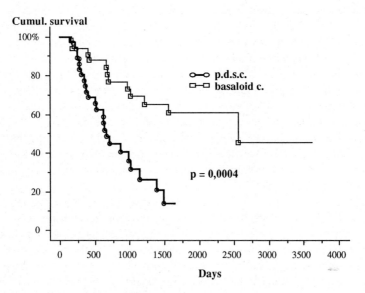

Figure 6   Survival rate (Kaplan Meier) analysis in basaloid carcinoma as compared with
poorly differentiated squamous carcinoma (p.d.s.c).

poorly differentiated squamous cell carcinoma, showing that poor differentiation alone does not account for the poor prognosis of basaloid carcinoma. In contrast, there is no difference in survival rates between pure and mixed basaloid carcinoma. That the basaloid carcinoma has unique prognostic significance among non–small-cell non-neuroendocrine carcinomas justifies its recognition as a distinct entity. The more aggressive pattern of the basaloid carcinoma has been shown in other tumor locations, such as the upper aerodigestive tract. Wain et al. (4) pointed out a high frequency of metastatic spread. Basaloid carcinoma shows an especially high number of brain metastases. Thus, basal cell carcinoma has prognosis somewhere between small-cell carcinoma and resectable non–small-cell lung carcinoma. The presence of a high mitotic index and a high rate of proliferation markers (mean Ki67 = 30%) probably contribute to this poor prognosis. The proximity to the stem cell of the point of differentiation arrest, evident for both small-cell carcinoma and basaloid carcinoma, could allow active proliferation and rapid tumor progression. Because a diagnosis of basaloid carcinoma is of prognostic significance, it could be helpful to identify them on small biopsies. However, the diagnostic criteria include mitotic rate, architecture, and evaluation of the size of the basaloid component, which could be difficult to assess on bronchial biopsy, which may only sample small, superficial parts of the tumors. In addition, the high frequency of overlying carcinoma in situ may confound the diagnosis. If a basal cell pattern is present on a bronchial biopsy, differentiation from an intermediate small-cell carcinoma or other neuroendocrine tumor could be difficult and would require examination for neuroendocrine markers. However, it is reasonable to reach this diagnosis on lymph node biopsy or other metastatic site if all methods of characterization are available.

We are very aware that the requirement of at least 60% basal cells in order to classify a tumor as basaloid carcinoma is arbitrary and that basal cells occur in a small proportion of all squamous cell carcinomas and in carcinoma in situ. Since we found no clear-cut difference in survival time between pure and mixed basal cell carcinoma, further investigation is needed to clarify what proportion of basal cells in carcinoma influences the prognosis.

There are no conclusive data about the pattern of relapse of basal cell carcinoma, but the more aggressive behavior of these tumors may justify a more thorough workup, including brain computed tomography and bone scanning, before surgical treatment. The best therapeutic procedure for basal cell carcinoma as well as non–small-cell lung carcinoma remains to be defined. Surgery alone is obviously not sufficient to cure most basaloid carcinoma stage I–II patients. Therapeutic response rates to different modalities and studies of survival of other larger series of basaloid carcinoma could clarify their clinical relevance. In conclusion, basaloid carcinoma is a malignant proliferation of primitive cells that displays unique and specific histopathological features and molecular abnormalities. Because these tumors bear a poorer prognosis than other operable lung cancers, they merit recognition as a separate entity.

References

1. World Health Organization. Histological typing of lung tumors. 2d ed. Am J Clin Pathol 1982; 123–136.
2. Spencer H. Carcinoma of the lung. In: Spencer H, ed. Pathology of the Lung. 4th ed. Oxford: Pergamon, 1985:907.
3. Brambilla E, Moro D, Veale P, Brichon PY, Paramelle B, Brambilla C. Basal cell (basaloid) carcinoma of the lung: a new morphologic and phenotypic entity with separate prognostic significance. Hum Pathol 1992; 23:993–1003.
4. Wain SL, Kier R, Vollmer RT, Bossen EH. Basaloid squamous carcinoma of the tongue, hypopharynx and larynx: report of 10 cases. Hum Pathol 1996; 17:1158–1166.
5. McKay MJ, Bilous AM. Basaloid squamous carcinoma of the hypopharynx. Cancer 1989; 63:2528–2531.
6. Banks ER, Frierson HF, Mills SE, George E, Zarbo RJ, Swanson PE. Basaloid squamous cell carcinoma of the head and neck. Am J Surg Pathol 1992; 16:939–946.
7. Klotz RG, Pamukoghout T, Souilliard DH. Transitional cloacogenic carcinoma of the anal canal. Clinicopathologic study of three hundred seventy three cases. Cancer 1967; 20:1727–1745.
8. Kheir S, Hickley RC, Martin RG; McKay B, Gallager HS. Cloagenic carcinoma of the anal canal. Arch Surg 1972; 104:407–415.
9. Gillepsie JJ, McKay B. Histogenesis of cloagenic carcinoma: fine structure of anal transitional epithalium and cloagnic carcinoma. Hum Pathol 1978; 9:579–587.
10. Benisch B, Toker C. Esophageal carcinomas with adenoid cystic differentiation. Arch Otolaryngol 1972; 96:260–263.
11. Gallager HS, Simpson CB, Alberto GA. Adenoid cystic carcinoma of the uterine cervix: report of 4 cases. Cancer 1971; 27:1398–1402.
12. Mos LD, Collins DN. Squamous and adenoid cystic basal cell carcinoma of the cervix uteri. Am J Obstet Gynecol 1964; 88:86–90.
13. Saldana M. Pathology of Pulmonary Disease. Philadelphia: Lippincott, 1993.
14. Hasleton P. Spencer's Pathology of the Lung. New York: 1996.
15. Colby TV, MN Koss, WD Travis. Atlas of Tumor Pathology. Tumors of the Lower Respiratory Tract. Washington, DC: AFIP, 1995.
16. Mountain CF. A new international staging system for lung cancer. Chest 1986; 89:225–233.
17. Moro D, Brichon PY, Brambilla E, Veale D, Labat F, Brambilla C. Basaloid bronchial carcinoma. A histologic group with a poor prognosis. Cancer 1994; 73:2734–2739.
18. Luna MA, Naggar AE, Parichatikanon P, Weber RS, Batsakis JG. Basaloid squamous carcinoma of the upper aerodigestive tract: clinicopathologic and DNA flow cytometric analysis. Cancer 1990; 66:537–542.
19. Levin SE. Cooperman. H, Freilich M, Lomas M, Kaplan L. Transitional cloagenic carcinoma of the anus. Dis Col 1977; 20:17–23.
20. Moll R, Franke NW, Schiller DL, Geiger B, Krepler R. The catalog of human cytokeratins: patterns of expression in normal epithelia, tumors and cultured cells. Cell 1982; 31:11–24.
21. Blobel GA, Moll R, Franke NW, Vogt-Moykopf I. Cytokeratins in normal lung and lung carcinomas. Virch Arch B Cell Pathol 1984; 45:407–427.
22. Travis WD, Linnoila RI, Tsokos MG, et al. Neuroendocrine tumors of the lung with proposed criteria for large cell neuroendocrine carcinoma. An ultrastructural immunohistochemical and flow cytometric study of 35 cases. Am J Surg Pathol 1991; 15:529–553.
23. Patel K, Moore SE, Dickson G, et al. Neural cell adhesion molecule (NCAM) is the antigen recognized by monoclonal antibodies of similar specificity in small cell lung carcinoma and neuroblastoma. Int J Cancer 1989; 44:573–578.
24. Brambilla E, Veale D, Moro D, Morel F, Dubois F, Brambilla C. Neuroendocrine phenotype in lung cancers. Comparison of immunohistochemistry with biochemical determination of enolase isoenzymes. Am J Clin Pathol 1992; 98:88–97.
25. Michalides R, Springall D, Zandwijk N, Koopman J, Hilkens J, Mooi W. NCAM and lung cancer. Int J Cancer 1994; 8:34–37.

26. Linnoila RI, Mushine JL, Steinberg, et al. Neuroendocrine differentiation in endocrine and nonendocrine lung carcinoma. Am J Pathol 1988; 90:641–652.
27. Berendsen H, De Leij L, Poppema S, et al. Clinical characterization of non small cell lung cancer tumors showing neuroendocrine differentiation features. J Clin Oncol 1989; 7:1614–1620.
28. Gerdes J, Schwab V, Lemke H, Stein H. Production of a mouse monoclonal antibody reactive with a human nuclear antigen associated with cell proliferation. Int J Cancer 1983; 32:13–20.
29. Cerny T, Barnes DH, Hasleton C, et al. Expression of epidermal growth factro receptor (EGFr) in human lung tumours. Br J Cancer 1986; 54:259–265.
30. Doyle A, Martin NJ, Funa R, et al. Markedly decreased expression of class I histocompatibility antigens, protein and mRNA in human small cell lung cancer. J Exp Med 1985; 161:1135–1151.
31. Ho KJ, Herrera GA, Jones JM, Alexander CB. Small cell carcinoma of the esophagus: evidence for a unified histogenesis. Hum Pathol 1984; 15:460–468.
32. Hewan-Lowe D, Dardick I. Ultrastructural distinction of basaloid squamous carcinoma and adenoid cystic carcinoma. Ultrastructural Pathol 1995; 19:371–381.
33. McDowell EH, Barrett LA, Glavin F, Harris CC, Trump BF. The respiratory epithelium in human bronchus. J Natl Respir Inst 1978; 61:587–606.
34. Breeze RG, Wheeldon EB. The cells of the pulmonary airway. Am Rev Respir Dis 1977; 116:705–777.
35. Churg A, Johnston WH, Stulbarg M. Small cell squamous and mixed small cell squamous small cell anaplastic carcinomas of the lung. Am J Pathol 1980; 4:255–263.
36. Li W, Hammar SP, Jolly PC, Hill LD, Anderson RP. Unpredictible course of small cell undifferentiated carcinoma. J Thorac Cardiovasc Surg 1981; 81:34–43.
37. Gould VE, Memoli VA, Dardi LE. Multidirectional differentiation in human epithelial cancers. J Submicrosc Cytol 1981; 13:97–115.
38. Bolen JW, Thorning D. Histogenic classification of lung carcinomas. Small cell carcinomas studied by light and electron microscopy. J Submicrosc Cytol 1982; 14:499–514.
39. Nomori H, Shimosato Y, Kodama T, Morinaga S, Nakajima T, Watanabe S. Subtypes of small cell carcinoma of the lung: morphometric, ultrastructural and immunohistochemical analyses. Hum Pathol 1986; 17:604–613.
40. Minna JD. The molecular biology of lung cancer pathogenesis. Chest 1993; 103:449–456.
41. Sozzi G, Mliozzo H, Donghi R, et al. Deletion of 17p and p53 mutations in preneoplastic lesions of the lung. Cancer Res 1992; 52:6079–6082.
42. Nuorva K, Soini Y, Kamel D, et al. Concurrent p53 expression in bronchial dysplasias and squamous cell lung carcinomas. Am J Pathol 1993; 142:725–732.
43. Bennett WP, Colby TV, Travis WD, et al. P53 protein accumulates frequently in early bronchial neoplasia. Cancer Res 1993; 53:4817–4822.
44. Fontanini G, Vignati S, Bigini D, et al. Human non small cell lung cancer: p53 protein accumulation is an early event and persists during metastatic progression. J Pathol 1994; 174:23–31.
45. Sundaresan V, Ganly P, Hasleton P, et al. P53 and chromosome 3 abnormalities, characteristic of malignant lung tumours, are detectable in preinvasive lesions of the bronchus. Oncogene 1992; 7:1989–1997.
46. Gazdar AF, Hung J, Walker L, et al. Extensive areas of dysplasia and aneuploidy of the entire bronchial mucosal tract accompanies non small cell lung cancers and provides evidence for the field cancerization theory. Proc Am Soc Clin Oncol 1993; 12:334–340.
47. Capewell S, Sudlow MF. Performance and prognosis in patients with lung cancer. Thorax 1990; 45:951–956.
48. Sellman M, Henze A, Peterffy A. Extended intrathoracic resection for lung cancer. Scand J Thorac Cardiovasc Surg 1987; 21:69–72.
49. The Ludwig Cancer Study Group. Patterns of failure in patients with resected stage I and II non–small-cell carcinoma of the lung. Ann Surg 1987; 205:67–71.
50. Read RC, Schaefer R, North N, Walls R. Diameter, cell type, and survival in stage I primary non-small-cell lung cancer. Arch Surg 1988; 123:446–449.

51. Smyth JF. The surgical management of bronchial carcinoma-prognostic indices. In: Smyth-Edward Arnold JF, eds. The Management of Lung Cancer. London: Edward Arnold, 1984:81–90.
52. Feld R, Rubinstein LV, Weisenberger TH. Sites of recurrences in resected stage I non-small-cell lung cancer: a guide for future studies. J Clin Oncol 1984; 2:1352–1358.
53. Little AG, Demeester TR, Ferguson MK. Modified stage I (T1NOM0, T2NOM0) non small-cell lung cancer: treatment results, recurrence patterns, and adjuvant immunotherapy. Surgery 1986; 100:621–628.

3

Neuroendocrine Tumors of the Lung

WILLIAM D. TRAVIS

Armed Forces Institute of Pathology
Washington, D.C.

Neuroendocrine (NE) tumors of the lung represent one of the most difficult problems in lung tumor diagnosis for the surgical pathologist. One of the reasons this group of tumors is so important is that small-cell carcinoma (SCLC) comprises the vast majority of NE lung tumors and has the most distinctive clinical features and therapeutic implications. Although the other NE tumors such as typical carcinoid (TC) and atypical carcinoid (AC) as well as large-cell neuroendocrine carcinoma (LCNEC) are much rarer, they frequently enter into the differential diagnosis of SCLC. For this reason, NE tumors are often discussed as a spectrum. In this chapter we will present the concept that TC and AC represent low- and intermediate-grade NE tumors that are closely related. In addition, diffuse idiopathic pulmonary neuroendocrine cell hyperplasia (DIPNECH) has recently been recognized as a preoplastic lesion for both TC and AC. In contrast, high-grade LCNEC and SCLC are closely related to each other, but their relationship to NE cell hyperplasia and the carcinoids is more distant.

This chapter will begin by discussing the pulmonary NE cells, NE cell hyperplasia, and tumorlets. Then each major type of pulmonary NE tumors will be addressed specifically.

I. Neuroendocrine Cells

Fröhlich described neuroendocrine cells in the human bronchus as clear cells *(helle Zelle)* due to their frequently clear cytoplasm (Fig. 1) (1). Solitary neuroendocrine cells are usually situated at the base of the respiratory mucosa near the basement membrane, and they often do not reach the bronchial lumen. The normal function of these cells is not understood, although they are known to produce numerous hormonal substances including bombesin-like peptides (BLPs) (2). Recent studies have shown that one BLP, gastrin-releasing peptide (GRP), plays an important role in lung development (3–5) and migration of epithelial cells (6), an essential process in repair following airway injury (7,8).

   Neuroendocrine cells exist in the normal bronchial and bronchiolar mucosa mostly as solitary cells and rarely as small clusters of four to eight cells called NE bodies (Fig. 1) (9–13). Solitary NE cells and NE bodies are prominent in fetal lungs, reaching a peak in the second trimester of gestation and gradually decreasing in number as the lungs mature (14–16). These NE cells are markedly increased in lungs

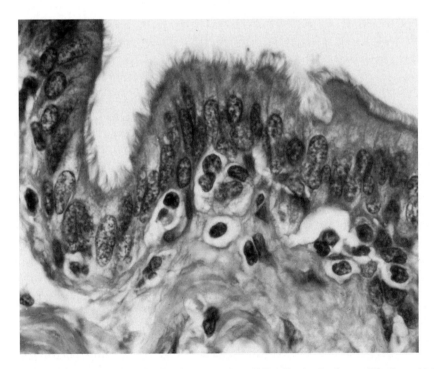

Figure 1   Neuroendocrine (NE) body and solitary NE cells. At the base of the bronchial epithelium are several solitary NE cells with clear cytoplasm and finely granular nuclear chromatin. In the center is a cluster of 4–5 NE cells forming a NE body. (×1000)

of premature infants with advanced chronic lung disease associated with broncho-pulmonary dysplasia (BPD) (16). The finding of prominent NE cells in fetal lung and in bronchopulmonary dysplasia is consistent with the concept that NE cells are important in lung development and repair.

II. Neuroendocrine Cell Hyperplasia and Tumorlets

One can regard NE cell proliferations in the lung as a spectrum of NE cell hyperpla-sia and tumorlets (Table 1) (17,18). The cytologic appearance of the NE cells in these lesions is basically the same: a round to oval-shaped cell with a moderate amount of eosinophilic cytoplasm and finely granular nuclear chromatin. NE cell hyperplasia and tumorlets are incidental microscopic findings usually lacking clini-cal significance. Carcinoid tumors represent one extreme end of the spectrum of NE cell proliferations since there is a continuum between tumorlets and carcinoid tu-mors and also a frequent association between carcinoid tumors and both NE cell hy-perplasia and tumorlets. However, the high-grade NE tumors of SCLC and LCNEC are part of a different spectrum of NE differentiation that occurs in carcinomas of the lung (Table 1). The relationship of these high-grade tumors to NE cell hyperplasia/ tumorlets and both the typical and atypical carcinoids (TC and AC) is more distant.

Table 1   Spectrum of Neuroendocrine Proliferations and Neoplasms

---

   I. NE cell hyperplasia and tumorlets
      A. NE cell hyperplasia
         1. NE cell hyperplasia associated with fibrosis and/or inflammation
         2. NE cell hyperplasia adjacent to carcinoid tumors
         3. Diffuse idiopathic pulmonary NE cell hyperplasia with or without
            airway fibrosis/obstruction
      B. Tumorlets (<0.5 cm)
  II. Tumors with NE morphology
      A. Typical carcinoid (0.5 cm or >)
      B. Atypical carcinoid
      C. Large cell neuroendocrine carcinoma
      D. Small cell carcinoma
 III. Non–small-cell carcinoma with NE differentiation
      Lung carcinomas lacking NE morphology that have NE markers by
      immunohistochemistry or NE granules by electron microscopy
 IV. Other tumors with NE properties
      A. Pulmonary blastoma
      B. Primitive neuroectodermal tumor
      C. Desmoplastic round cell tumor
      D. Carcinomas with rhabdoid phenotype
      E. Paraganglioma

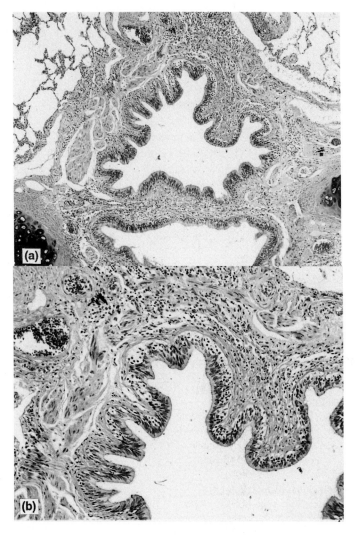

Figure 2   (a) Linear and nodular hyperplasia of NE cells. There is a continuous linear and nodular proliferation of NE cells within the bronchial epithelium. This bronchus was situated adjacent to a carcinoid tumor. (×75) (b) The NE cells are situated at the base of the bronchial mucosa along the basement membrane. The NE cells have prominent clear cytoplasm and they are numerous, forming a continuous arrangement of nodules and single cells. (×150)

There are three patterns of NE cell hyperplasia: (1) increased numbers of solitary NE cells, (2) linear arrangements of NE cells along the bronchiolar epithelium, and (3) nodular hyperplasia consisting of numerous NE bodies (Fig. 2) (19). Any combination of the above patterns may also occur (Fig. 2B). NE cell hyperplasia occurs in conditions associated with chronic inflammation of airways such as bronchiectasis (20), bronchopulmonary dysplasia (16,21,22), Wilson-Mikity syndrome (21), Langerhans cell histiocytosis (23), respiratory bronchiolitis (24,25), and bronchopulmonary dysplasia (16). It also occurs in association with carcinoid tumors (26). Interestingly, in lungs with honeycomb fibrosis, Wilson et al. could not find any NE cells (27).

Tumorlets are millimeter-sized nodular proliferations of NE cells that extend beyond the subepithelial basement membrane and often through the bronchiolar wall into surrounding lung parenchyma (Fig. 3) (19,28–31). Frequently the proliferating NE cells are embedded in a dense fibrous stroma (Fig. 3). The architecture of the bronchioles is commonly distorted and may be obliterated. At the larger end of the spectrum they may become visible on gross exam. There is a continuum in size between tumorlets and carcinoid tumors. Arbitrarily a NE proliferation measuring 0.5 cm or larger is regarded as a carcinoid tumor and any smaller NE lesion is regarded as a tumorlet (28). Occasionally the distinction between a tumorlet and a

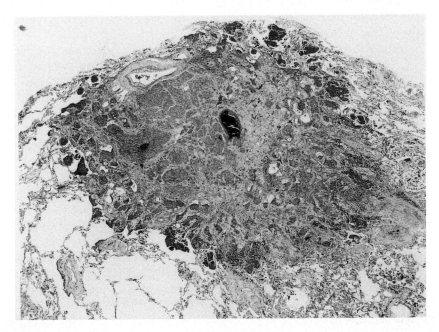

Figure 3 Diffuse idiopathic pulmonary NE cell hyperplasia. A dense fibrous scar obliterates the bronchiolar lumen. The residual airway lumen is replaced by a linear and circumferential arrangement of NE cells. (×30)

carcinoid tumor may be difficult when the tumorlet spreads along airways rather than forming a discrete mass.

Tumorlets have been reported to occur in the setting of bronchiectasis or interstitial fibrosis (31,32). However, Churg and Warnock found that only one third of tumorlets were in diseased lungs (30). For decades the traditional concept has maintained that NE cell hyperplasia and tumorlets are reactions secondary to underlying airway inflammation or fibrosis.

This concept was reversed in 1992 when Aguayo et al. reported six patients with obstructive airways disease who had unexplained diffuse pulmonary NE cell hyperplasia and airway fibrosis in their lung biopsies (33). Since NE cells produce a number of substances including bombesin that can act as a fibroblast growth factor (34), Aguayo et al. proposed that in this clinical setting NE cell proliferation could be a primary lesion that is the underlying cause for airway fibrosis rather than a secondary reaction (33). This entity was called diffuse idiopathic pulmonary NE cell hyperplasia (DIPNECH) with obstructive airways disease.

Patients with DIPNECH present with cough and exertional dyspnea, reticulonodular infiltrates on chest radiographs, and obstructive pulmonary function (33). Histologically, the bronchial and bronchiolar epithelium shows diffuse NE cell hyperplasia with numerous NE bodies. Scattered bronchioles show an obliterative type of fibrosis (Fig. 4). Occasionally the fibrosis consists of a focal scar situated immediately beneath a focus of NE cell hyperplasia. The rarity of DIPNECH is reflected by the paucity of subsequent reports (35,36).

Four of the six patients reported by Aguayo et al. had one or more carcinoid tumors (33). The occurrence of carcinoid tumors in this setting suggests that DIPNECH may be a preneoplastic lesion. Since the vast majority of NE cell hyperplasias appear occur as reactive lesions, only the very rare cases of DIPNECH should be regarded as preneoplastic. This is recognized as a new category of preinvasive lesions in the new World Health Organization and International Association for the Study of Lung Cancer proposal for histologic classification of lung and pleural tumors.

Miller and Müller studied a series of peripheral carcinoids and demonstrated NE hyperplasia and obliterative bronchiolar fibrosis in the airways surrounding 76% and 32% of peripheral carcinoids, respectively (26). A subset of these patients had obstructive pulmonary function, some with and others without a history of smoking (26). While this suggests that NE cell hyperplasia is frequently found in association with peripheral carcinoids, it is not clear whether these cases represented DIPNECH or just a localized NE cell hyperplasia adjacent to the carcinoid tumors. It is possible that the obstructive pulmonary function in some of the patients correlated with the presence of DIPNECH. It would be difficult to consider NE cell hyperplasia to be idiopathic in airways distal to endobronchial carcinoids, since it could occur as a secondary reaction associated with postobstructive pneumonia or bronchiectasis.

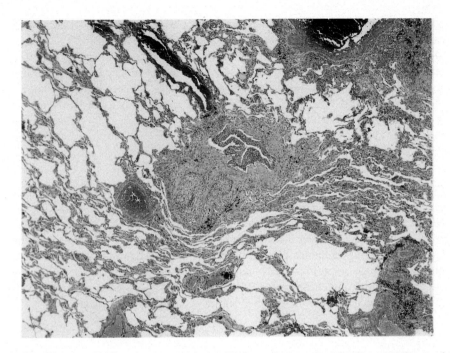

Figure 4 Tumorlet. This millimeter-sized subpleural nodule consists of organoid nests of NE cells proliferating within a dense fibrous stroma. (×100)

III. Tumors with Neuroendocrine Morphology

Lung tumors with neuroendocrine morphology by light microscopy include the low-grade TC, intermediate-grade AC, and high-grade LCNEC and SCLC (37). All of these tumors express similar neuroendocrine morphologic features by light micros-copy such as organoid nesting, palisading, a trabecular pattern, or rosette-like struc-tures.

A. Typical and Atypical Carcinoid

Clinical Features

Carcinoid tumors are low- and/or intermediate-grade malignant neoplasms of neu-roendocrine cells, which comprise 1–2% of all lung malignancies (38,39). They are divided into TC and AC, with the latter possessing more malignant histologic and clinical features (18,40,41).

The indolent nature of carcinoid tumors is reflected by the finding that 51% of patients are asymptomatic at presentation (42). The most common pulmonary mani-festations include hemoptysis in 18%, postobstructive pneumonitis in 17%, and dyspnea in 2% of patients (42). A variety of paraneoplastic syndromes can occur with carcinoid tumors, including the carcinoid syndrome (42,43), Cushing's syndrome (44,45), multiple endocrine neoplasia type 1 (46), and acromegaly (47). The male-to-female ratio varies in different studies of bronchial carcinoids, with some studies showing more males and others more females, while some show no sex predominance (41,42,48–52). Carcinoids can occur at any age, but the mean age is 55 years (42). Bronchial carcinoids are the most common lung malignancy in childhood (53).

Pathologic Features

Carcinoid tumors are frequently divided into central and peripheral tumors. The percentage of peripheral tumors has been reported to be from 16 to 40% (42,54,55). However, if one examines the location of carcinoid tumors by CT scan, they are equally distributed between the periphery, mid-portion, and central aspects of the lung (18). Central carcinoids frequently invade the bronchial lumen as a polypoid mass and may cause postobstructive pneumonia and bronchiectasis. Carcinoids are circumscribed but not encapsulated. TC are typically solid, smooth and tan or yellow, while the cut surface of AC often shows necrosis or hemorrhage.

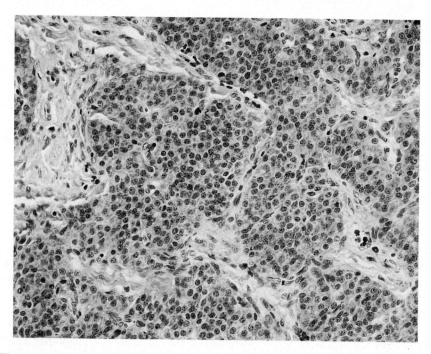

Figure 5   Typical carcinoid. The tumor consists of organoid nests of uniform cells with a delicate fibrovascular stroma. Necrosis is absent. (×150)

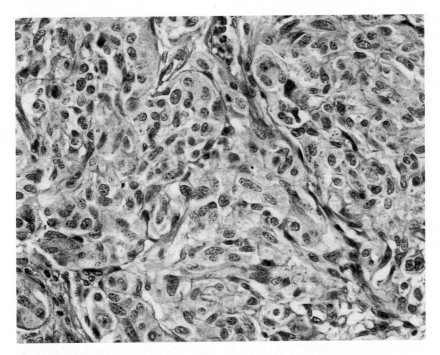

Figure 6 Typical carcinoid. The organoid nesting arrangement of these tumors cells is prominent. The cells show a moderate amount of eosinophilic cytoplasm and finely granular nuclear chromatin. (×400)

Table 2 Histologic Criteria for Lung Carcinoid Tumors

Typical carcinoid: A tumor with carcinoid morphology and less than two mitoses per 2 mm² (10 HPF) and lacking necrosis.

Atypical carcinoid: A tumor with carcinoid morphology and mitoses of two or more and less than 10 per 2 mm² (10 HPF) *or* necrosis (often punctate).

Central carcinoids tend to be larger than peripheral tumors, with a mean diameter of 3.1 cm versus 2.4 cm, respectively (42). AC are larger than TC, with a mean diameter of 3.6 cm compared to 2.3 cm for TC (42).

Both TC and AC are characterized histologically by neuroendocrine morphologic patterns such as organoid nesting (Figs. 5 and 6), trabecular, palisading and rosette-like structures. Cytologically the tumor cells are uniform with a moderate amount of finely granular eosinophilic cytoplasm and finely granular nuclear chromatin (Table 2; Fig. 6). Nucleoli can be seen in both TC and AC, but they tend to be more conspicuous in AC. Both TC and AC can show a variety of histologic patterns including spindle cell (56,57), papillary (58), glandular, paraganglioma-like

(59), and follicular patterns (18). The tumor cells of pulmonary carcinoid tumors may have oncocytic (60–65), acinic cell–like, signet-ring, clear cell, mucin-producing, or melanocytic features (28,59,66). Stromal changes such as amyloid (67–69), ossification (61,70), and sclerosis may also be seen. The latter may be detected radiographically. Dense fibrous stroma is common. Rarely it may be mistaken for amyloid.

AC, as defined by Arrigoni et al., is distinguished from TC by the following criteria: (1) increased mitotic activity with 1 mitotic figure per 1–2 high-power fields (or 5–10 mitoses/10 HPF), (2) nuclear pleomorphism, hyperchromatism, and an abnormal nuclear:cytoplasmic ratio, (3) areas of increased cellularity with disorganization of the architecture, and (4) tumor necrosis (40).

However, Arrigoni et al. did not specify whether one or all of these criteria were necessary to make a diagnosis of AC, and the criteria were not based on any statistical analysis. For this reason we recently used statistical survival analysis to show that the number of mitoses is the most important histologic predictor of prognosis (41). Based on this study, it was proposed that the criteria for diagnosis of AC be modified to the following: a tumor with neuroendocrine morphology with either mitotic counts of 2 or more and 10 or less per 2 mm^2 area (or per 10 HPF with 1 HPF = 0.2 mm^2 area) *or* with coagulative necrosis.

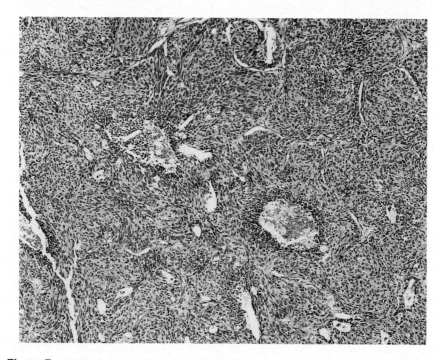

Figure 7   Atypical carcinoid. Within the organoid nests of cells are punctate foci of necrosis. (×75)

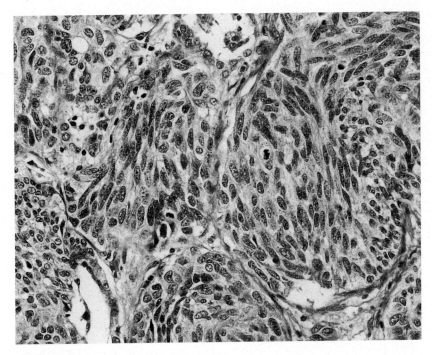

Figure 8 Atypical carcinoid. The tumor cells are round, oval, and spindle-shaped. Two mitoses are present in this field (arrowheads). There is moderate eosinophilic cytoplasm, and the chromatin is finely granular. (×300)

The necrosis in AC usually consists of small foci centrally located within organoid nests of tumor cells (Fig. 7); uncommonly the necrosis may form larger confluent zones. In contrast, TC may have focal cytologic pleomorphism, but necrosis is absent and mitotic figures are rare (less than 2 per 2 mm^2) (Fig. 8) (41). Criteria for separation of TC from AC are summarized in Table 3. The method used for counting mitoses is discussed below.

Prognosis

A study of 200 AFIP NE lung tumors revealed 5- and 10-year survival of 56 and 35% for AC, respectively. This is significantly worse than the 87% 5- and 10-year survival for TC ($p < 0.001$) (Fig. 9) (41). Survival analysis of histologic features for both TC and AC together demonstrated worse prognosis for patients with tumors having increased numbers of mitoses per 2 mm^2 (10 HPF) as well as the presence of necrosis, vascular invasion, pleomorphism, and nucleoli (41).

Other studies have correlated prognosis in carcinoid tumors with a variety of clinical and pathologic features including advanced stage, lymph node metastases, large tumor size (>3 cm), vascular invasion, AC versus TC, intraluminal versus ex-

Table 3 Typical and Atypical Carcinoid: Distinguishing Features

Histologic or clinical feature	Typical carcinoid	Atypical carcinoid
Histologic patterns: organoid, trabecular, palisading, and spindle cell	Characteristic	Characteristic
Mitoses	<2 per 2 mm^2	≥ 2 and ≤ 10 per 2 mm^2
Necrosis	Absent	Characteristic, usually focal or punctate
Nuclear pleomorphism, hyperchromatism	Usually absent, not sufficient by itself for diagnosis of AC	Often present
Regional lymph node metastases at presentation	5–15%	40–48%
Distant metastases at presentation	Rare	20%
Disease-free survival at 5 years	100%	69%
Disease-free survival at 10 years	87%	52%

trabronchial spread, aneuploidy, S-phase, and integrated optical density measurement of nuclear DNA content (41,42,71–73).

The optimal therapy for AC is not known. Surgery is the primary therapeutic approach for TC and probably also for AC (74,75). Sleeve resections may be possible in some carcinoids (74,75). However, due to the rarity of AC and the problems with diagnostic criteria, it is not known if chemotherapy or radiation are effective approaches to management of AC. Chemotherapy and radiation therapy are often considered in patients with advanced-stage AC or unresectable metastases (76–79). One must critically assess the histologic criteria used in studies attempting to address the issue of adjunctive therapy for AC. Inclusion of LCNEC or paucity of histologic detail regarding the tumors are serious problems. Patients with TC have an excellent prognosis and rarely die of tumor (42,80). However, regional lymph node metastases can occur in 5–20% of TC. Therefore the presence of metastases should not be used as a criterion for distinguishing TC from AC (42). Lung carcinoids, even TC can recur, metastasize, and kill patients many years after presentation (80,81).

Ultrastructure, Immunohistochemistry, and Flow Cytometry

By electron microscopy (EM), TC have numerous dense core granules with heterogeneity in shape and size. In addition to dense core granules, numerous cytoplasmic mitochondria are present in oncocytic carcinoids (64). AC have fewer dense core granules than TC. The NE granules tend to be smaller with less variation in size (18).

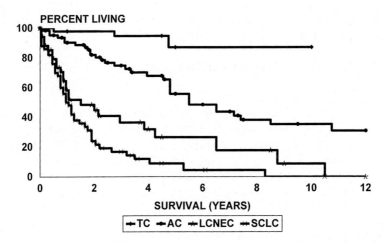

Figure 9 Survival of NE lung tumors. Survival for AC is significantly worse than that for TC ($p < 0.001$). Survival for SCLC and LCNEC is significantly worse than that for AC ($p < 0.001$). The survival for SCLC and LCNEC is not significantly different. Kaplan-Meier survival curves based on 200 NE tumors, most of which were surgically resected.

TC tend to express stronger immunohistochemical staining for neuroendocrine and hormonal markers than other NE tumors. The most useful immunohistochemical marker of neuroendocrine differentiation is chromogranin followed by synaptophysin and Leu 7 (18).

Aneuploidy can occur in both TC and AC. Aneuploidy is significantly more frequent in AC than TC (48,82). It has been found in 5–32% of TC and 16–79% of AC (18,48,72,82–84). In addition, aneuploidy correlates with poor prognosis (82–84). However, aneuploidy does not always correlate with poor prognosis, since Jones et al. found that 58% of patients with aneuploid carcinoid tumors survived 5 years (82).

Differential Diagnosis

Separation of TC from AC (and occasionally SCLC) can be difficult, especially in small, crushed biopsy specimens. Unless mitosis or necrosis is present in a transbronchial biopsy it may be impossible to separate TC from AC until the resected specimen is examined. Due to the many histologic patterns of carcinoids, there is a broad differential diagnosis. Spindle cell carcinoids can be confused with other non-neuroendocrine tumors composed of spindle-shaped cells such as smooth muscle tumors (leiomyoma, leiomyosarcoma), chemodectoma, or spindle cell carcinoma. Oncocytic carcinoids can raise the consideration of oncocytoma, acinic cell carcinoma, or mucoepidermoid carcinoma. Glandular patterns can be confused with adenocarcinomas. In most cases recognition of the carcinoid tumor can be achieved by detecting an organoid pattern, finely granular nuclear chromatin, and positive immunohistochemical staining for neuroendocrine markers or dense core granules by EM.

B. Large Cell Neuroendocrine Carcinoma

Clinical Features

A recent study revealed the median age for patients with LCNEC to be 60 years (range 33–80 yr), 80% of whom are men (85). In this study staging information was available in 67 patients with stage I, II, III, and IV disease in 49, 12, 25, and 13% of patients, respectively. All 23 patients with available smoking histories were smokers, 84% with >40 pack-years (85). Ectopic hormone production is uncommon in cases of LCNEC (18). One patient is reported to have had Eaton-Lambert syndrome (86).

Pathologic Features

The median tumor size is 3.3 cm (range 1–9 cm). Most LCNEC are peripheral, but they may also be central lung tumors. The average size is 3.0 cm with a range of 1.3–8 cm. They are usually circumscribed, nodular masses with a necrotic, tan, red cut surface.

LCNEC are defined by the following histologic criteria (Table 4): (1) light microscopic features commonly associated with neuroendocrine tumors such as organoid, palisading, trabecular, or rosette-like growth patterns (Figs. 10 and 11);

Table 4   Histologic Criteria for Large-Cell Neuroendocrine Carcinoma and Small-Cell Carcinoma

---

Large Cell Neuroendocrine Carcinoma
1. A tumor with a neuroendocrine morphology (organoid nesting, palisading, rosettes, trabeculae)
2. High mitotic rate: ≥11 per 2 mm^2 (10 HPF), median of 70 per 2 mm^2 (10 HPF)
3. Necrosis (often large zones)
4. Cytologic features of a large-cell carcinoma: large cell size, low nuclear to cytoplasmic ratio, vesicular or fine chromatin, and/or frequent nucleoli—some tumors have fine nuclear chromatin and lack nucleoli, but qualify as non–small-cell carcinoma based on other criteria such as large cell size and abundant cytoplasm
5. NE granules by electron microscopy or positive immunohistochemical staining for one or more NE immunohistochemical markers (other than NSE)

Small-Cell Carcinoma[a]
1. Small size (generally less than the diameter of three small resting lymphocytes)
2. Scant cytoplasm
3. Nuclei: finely granular nuclear chromatin; absent or faint nucleoli
4. High mitotic rate: ≥10 per 2 mm^2 (10 HPF), median of 80 per 2 mm^2 (10 HPF)
5. Frequent necrosis, often in large zones

---

[a] From Refs. 95, 96.

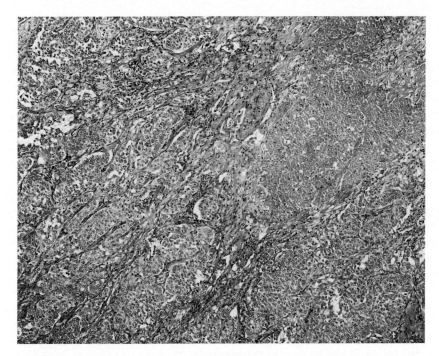

Figure 10 Large cell neuroendocrine carcinoma. A large infarct-like zone of necrosis is present and the tumor cells are arranged in organoid nests with peripheral palisading. (×30)

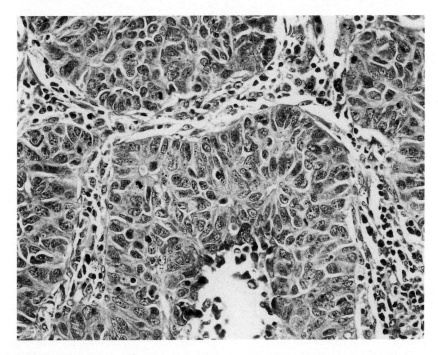

Figure 11 Large cell neuroendocrine carcinoma. In addition to peripheral palisading, several rosette-like structures are present (arrows). (×300)

(2) cytologic features of a NSCLC: large cell size, polygonal shape, low N/C ratio, coarse or vesicular (occasionally finely granular) nuclear chromatin, and frequent nucleoli (Fig. 12); (3) a high mitotic rate ($\geq 11/2$ mm^2), (4) necrosis, frequently extensive; and (5) neuroendocrine features by immunohistochemistry or electron microscopy (Fig. 13) (18,41). The mitotic rate averages 75/2 mm^2, and the necrosis tends to consist of large infarct-like zones. A small percentage of tumors lack nucleoli or have finely granular chromatin but qualify as NSCLC based on other cytologic features such as large cell size.

The original criteria for LCNEC proposed in 1991 defined the mitotic range based on counts per 10 HPF (18). The recent revision of criteria for mitotic counts bases the mitotic range on counts per 2 mm^2 area (41). This emphasizes the importance of counting mitoses in high-power fields filled with viable tumor as well as the variation in area seen in the high-power fields of microscopes made by different manufacturers (see Sec. V).

There is a spectrum of NE morphology within LCNEC, with some tumors having very prominent trabecular, palisading, or rosette-like patterns. In such cases the NE pattern is readily appreciated. In other cases the NE features are more subtle, and the NE morphology may be easily overlooked. Palisading is not specific for NE differentiation. It can be seen in the basaloid variant of squamous cell carcinoma

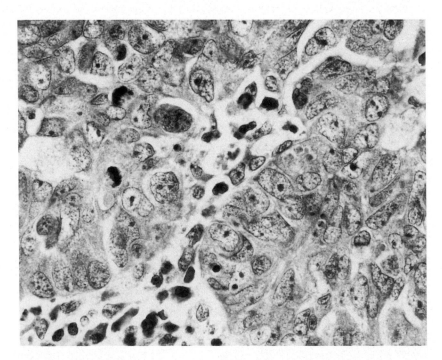

Figure 12 Large cell neuroendocrine carcinoma. At higher magnification the tumor cells are relatively large and many have distinct nucleoli. Several mitoses are present. ($\times 720$)

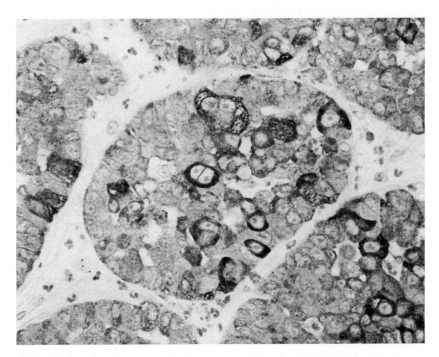

Figure 13 Large cell neuroendocrine carcinoma. Synaptophysin strongly stains many of the tumor cells. (Immunohistochemistry for synaptophysin ×300)

(87) and basaloid carcinomas (88,89). Nevertheless, palisading in a poorly differentiated carcinoma is often a clue to NE differentiation and should prompt the consideration to perform immunohistochemical stains for NE markers.

It is very difficult to establish the diagnosis of LCNEC based on transbronchial biopsy, needle biopsy, or cytology specimens. Recognition of the NE morphology is an essential criterion, and it can be very difficult to appreciate on small tissue samples. For this reason the diagnosis of LCNEC is less likely to be made in patients with unresectable disease where only small biopsy samples are obtained. This differs substantially from SCLC where the diagnosis is readily established on cytology and small biopsy samples.

The term "large cell carcinoma with NE morphology" can be used for tumors resembling LCNEC by light microscopy if tissue samples are not available for special studies to confirm the diagnosis. More studies are needed to see if there are clinical differences between LCNEC and large-cell carcinomas with NE morphology.

LCNEC may also be associated with mixtures of other histologic types of lung carcinoma including adenocarcinoma, squamous cell carcinoma, spindle cell carcinoma, giant cell carcinoma, and small-cell carcinoma. Adenocarcinoma is the most common other histologic type associated with LCNEC. Since LCNEC appears closely related to SCLC, we have proposed that LCNEC mixed with other NSCLC components be called combined LCNEC, similar to combined SCLC.

Ultrastructure, Immunohistochemistry, and Flow Cytometry

By electron microscopy dense core granules in LCNEC tend to be few in number as well as focal or patchy (18). Features of glandular and/or squamous differentiation may also be identified (18).

LCNEC stain immunohistochemically with chromogranin A in 54/73 (74%), synaptophysin in 48/62 (77%), and leu-7 in 28/54 (52%) (85). The immunohistochemical staining is often focal. In 75% of LCNEC, aneuploidy may be demonstrated (18).

Treatment and Prognosis

Patients with LCNEC have a very poor prognosis. The 5- and 10-year survival is 27 and 9%, respectively, with no survivors at 12 years (Fig. 9) (85). This is a significantly worse prognosis than that for AC ($p < 0.001$), but it is not significantly different from patients with SCLC, even after stratification by stage (41,85).

How LCNEC patients should be treated remains to be determined. The tumors should be surgically resected if possible. This not only provides an important therapeutic step in management of the patients, it also allows for a definitive diagnosis. To date anecdotal experience indicates that some patients with advanced-stage LCNEC show a response to chemotherapy. It is possible that adjunctive chemotherapy may be of benefit following surgery.

Recently Dresler et al. reported a study attempting to determine the survival and response to therapy for LCNEC (90). Although the title of Dresler's article implies a study of LCNEC, if one examines carefully the histologic details of the tumors, it appears that cases of AC and combined SCLC with large cell carcinoma were also included. Rather than providing much-needed information, the study further confuses the issue. A prospective multi-institutional study based on carefully classified NE tumors is needed to determine the optimal therapy for these tumors. Without studies based on careful pathologic diagnosis, the confusion about the clinical management of these tumors will persist.

Differential Diagnosis

The differential diagnosis of LCNEC includes AC, SCLC, large cell carcinoma and large-cell carcinoma with NE differentiation (LCC-ND), and large cell carcinoma with NE morphology. AC and LCNEC are best distinguished based on mitotic counts (18). Large cell carcinoma with NE morphology may overlap with those tumors called basaloid carcinoma by Brambilla et al., since a subset of the tumors they reported have a rosette-like pattern (88,89). However, immunohistochemistry or electron microscopy does not detect NE differentiation. This is an important area for future study. The lack of a NE morphologic pattern distinguishes large cell carcinoma with NE differentiation from LCNEC.

The most difficult NE tumor to separate from LCNEC is SCLC (91). A constellation of criteria should be used to separate LCNEC from SCLC rather than a single criterion such as the issue of nucleoli (Table 5).

C. Small-Cell Carcinoma

Clinical

SCLC accounts for 20–25% of all lung cancers, and approximately 30,000 new cases occur in the United States each year (39,92). Due to its distinctive clinical characteristics and its responsiveness to chemotherapy, SCLC is separated from all other NSCLC (93). The median age for patients with SCLC is 60 years (range 32–79 years). There is a strong male predominance.

SCLC frequently has extensive metastases. Paraneoplastic syndromes are relatively common compared to other histologic types of lung cancer.

Table 5 Light Microscopic Criteria for Distinguishing Small Cell Carcinoma and Large Cell Neuroendocrine Carcinoma

Histologic feature	Small cell carcinoma	Large cell neuroendocrine carcinoma[a]
Cell size	Smaller (less than diameter of three lymphocytes)	Larger
Nuclear/Cytoplasmic ratio	Higher	Lower
Nuclear chromatin	Finely granular, uniform	Coarsely granular or vesicular; less uniform
Nucleoli	Absent or faint	Often (not always) present; may be prominent or faint
Nuclear molding	Characteristic	Uncharacteristic
Fusiform shape	Common	Uncommon
Polygonal shape with ample pink cytoplasm	Uncharacteristic	Characteristic
Nuclear smear	Frequent	Uncommon
Mitotic counts	High (average 70/2 mm^2)	High (average 70/2 mm^2)
Basophilic staining of vessels and stroma	Occasional	Rare

[a]Modified from Ref. 111.

Pathologic Features

A perihilar mass is seen at presentation in about two thirds of patients. Mediastinal lymph node involvement is often extensive. SCLC rarely present as a peripheral coin lesion (94).

The 1981 WHO proposal subclassified SCLC into three subtypes: (1) oat cell carcinoma, (2) intermediate cell type, and (3) combined oat cell carcinoma (95). This was modified by the pathology panel of the International Association for the Study of Lung Cancer in 1988, who proposed that the terms "oat cell carcinoma" and "intermediate cell type" be dropped and that SCLC be divided into three categories: SCLC, mixed small cell/large cell carcinoma, and combined SCLC, which also has components of squamous cell and/or adenocarcinoma (96).

Since there is conflicting data regarding the prognosis of mixed SCLC/large-cell carcinoma compared to pure SCLC (96–98), the new WHO/IALSC Histologic Classification of Lung and Pleural Tumors has eliminated this category and reduces the subclassification of SCLC to only two major categories: SCLC for all tumors consisting purely of SCLC and combined SCLC for tumors showing a mixture of

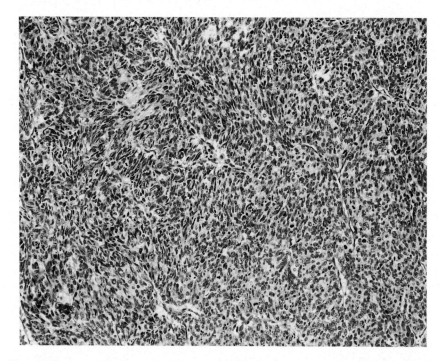

Figure 14 Small cell carcinoma. The tumor consists of a sheet of small, round to spindle-shaped cells with scant cytoplasm. Numerous mitoses are visible even at this low magnification. (×150)

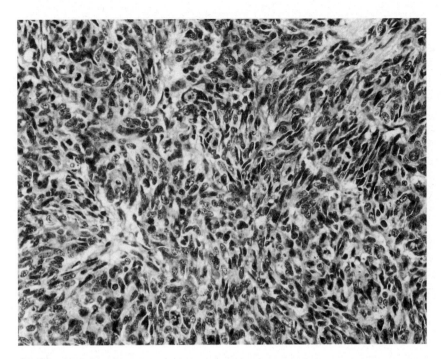

Figure 15 Small cell carcinoma. This tumor is very cellular due to the small size and scant cytoplasm of the tumor cells. (×300)

SCLC and any other NSCLC component such as adenocarcinoma, squamous cell carcinoma, large cell carcinoma, spindle cell carcinoma (89), or giant cell carcinoma.

SCLC is defined by light microscopy as a tumor with small cells (usually less than the diameter of three small resting lymphocytes), scant cytoplasm, a round to fusiform shape, finely granular nuclear chromatin, and absent or inconspicuous nucleoli (Figs. 14–16; Table 4) (96). Nuclear molding is often present. Necrosis is common and often extensive. Mitotic rates are high, averaging 80 mitoses per 2 mm². Vascular encrustation of vascular walls with basophilic staining, known as the Azzopardi effect, is often present in areas of necrosis (100).

Combined SCLC with large cell carcinoma is seen in 4–5% of SCLC (98). Combined SCLC with adenocarcinoma or squamous cell carcinoma occur in approximately 1–3% of SCLC (96–98). SCLC can also occur with spindle cell carcinoma (99) and giant cell carcinoma. It also can occur as a component of carcinosarcoma in association with malignant heterologous elements such as malignant bone, cartilage, or skeletal muscle.

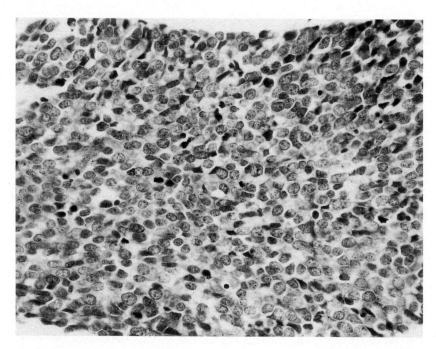

Figure 16   Small cell carcinoma. The tumor cells are small with scant cytoplasm and finely granular nuclear chromatin. Nucleoli are absent and nuclear molding is focally present. Mitoses are prominent. (×450)

Ultrastructure, Immunohistochemistry, and Flow Cytometry

SCLC express many neuroendocrine, hormonal, and other markers that can be detected by immunohistochemistry (18). Chromogranin A and synaptophysin are the most useful NE markers (18). Immunostaining for neuron specific enolase (NSE) is not a very useful neuroendocrine marker, since it stains up to 60% of NSCLCs (18,101). Some neural cell adhesion molecule (NCAM) antibodies may be useful (102–104). A recent study indicated that negative immunohistochemical staining for cathepsin B, cathepsin D, carcinoembryonic antigen, and neu oncoprotein was associated with prolonged survival in small cell carcinoma of the lung (105). MIB1 staining is higher in SCLC than in AC or TC and correlates with poor survival (106).

Dense core NE granules can be found in 67–90% of SCLC (107,108). They are usually few in number, small in size (100–130 nm), and occasionally situated in small dendritic cytoplasmic processes (108).

Aneuploidy is found in up to 85% of SCLC (18,72,109). However, it does not appear to correlate well with prognosis (72,109). High nucleolar organizer region values in lung neuroendocrine tumors also correlate with poor prognosis (110).

Therapy and Prognosis

Patients with SCLC who have limited-stage and extensive-stage disease have a median survival of 3 and 1.5 months, respectively, if they do not receive therapy (93). The median survival for SCLC patients treated with combination chemotherapy and chest radiotherapy is improved to 10–16 months for those with limited-stage disease and 6–11 months for those with extensive-stage disease (93).

Study of 200 NE tumors from AFIP revealed a 5- and 10-year survival of 9 and 5% for SCLC, respectively (with no survivors at 10.5 years) (Fig. 9) (41). Many of the SCLCs in this series were low stage, since they were obtained by surgical resection.

Differential Diagnosis

The most common and important differential diagnosis for SCLC is NSCLC, especially large-cell carcinoma and LCNEC. Separation of these tumor types depends on a set of criteria rather than a single feature. This should not rest on a single criterion such as cell size or nucleoli, but multiple additional features including nuclear to cytoplasmic ratio, nuclear chromatin, nucleoli, nuclear molding, cell shape (fusiform vs. polygonal), and hematoxylin vascular staining (Table 5) (18,111). In 5–7% of cases there is disagreement among expert lung cancer pathologists over the diagnosis of SCLC (112,113).

One should be careful in attempting to make the diagnosis of SCLC based on biopsies with marked crush artifact unless areas of preserved tumor cells are seen. The diagnosis of SCLC can be very difficult if histologic sections are too thick or darkly stained. In such cases it can be very difficult to see the nuclear detail and assess for the presence or absence of nucleoli. This problem is often resolved by obtaining additional good-quality 5-μm sections that are well stained.

Other lesions that can be confused with SCLC include carcinoid tumors and lymphoid infiltrates, whether due to small lymphocytic lymphoma or chronic inflammation. SCLC differ from lymphoid lesions by the cohesiveness of the tumor cells, often reflected by nuclear molding. Immunohistochemistry for keratin and lymphoid markers such as common leukocyte antigen can be very useful in the distinction of lymphoid lesions from SCLC.

Occasionally the differential of SCLC and metastatic Merkel cell carcinoma is encountered. Merkel cell carcinomas are more likely to stain with neurofilament protein (100,114) and cytokeratin 20 (115). Rarely primitive neuroectodermal tumors (PNET) may also present as a primary tumor in the lung. They differ from SCLC in that the tumor cells are discohesive and they usually stain negative or only focally for keratin but strongly positive with antibodies to CD99 (MIC2) (116).

D. NSCLC with Neuroendocrine Differentiation

It has been recognized for several decades that neuroendocrine differentiation can be shown by immunohistochemistry in 10–20% of ordinary squamous cell carcinomas, adenocarcinomas, or large-cell carcinomas (117–123). NE differentiation is found more often in adenocarcinomas than in large-cell or squamous cell carcinomas. In the new WHO/IASLC classification, these tumors are referred to as NSCLC with neuroendocrine differentiation (NSCLC-ND) (Table 1), however, they have not been given a formal place in the classification scheme for the following reasons. While NSCLC-NE have drawn much interest, there is controversy whether these tumors have worse or better survival (117–119). In addition, it is not clear whether they are more or less responsive to chemotherapy than NSCLC lacking neuroendocrine differentiation (124–126). More definitive data, hopefully obtained in prospective clinical trials, is needed to address this issue.

IV. Overall Survival Analysis for All NE Tumors

We recently showed that for the four major histologic types of NE lung tumors, stage, mitoses, necrosis, vascular invasion, and the presence of nucleoli were significant predictors of survival, but pleomorphism was not (41). After stratification for stage, using a Cox-multivariate survival analysis including certain histologic features—average number of mitoses per 2 mm^2 (10 HPF) (as a continuous variable), necrosis, vascular invasion, and nucleoli—we found prognostic significance for mitoses, necrosis, and vascular invasion (41).

Multivariate analysis was then performed using average number of mitoses per 2 mm^2 (10 HPF) (collapsed into three categories: <2, 2–10, ≥ 11). By this analysis, mitotic counts were the only independent predictor of prognosis, and the other variables including necrosis, vascular invasion, and nucleoli were not significant (41).

V. Mitosis Counting

Mitosis counting is the most important criteria for distinguishing AC from TC and from the high-grade NE tumors LCNEC and SCLC. If done carefully with attention to morphologic criteria and methodology, mitotic counts have been shown to be reproducible and prognostically useful in a variety of tumors (127–130). The quality of the specimen is important. Mitoses can be very difficult to assess if sections are too thick, suboptimally stained, or if there is extensive necrosis, fibrous or inflammatory stroma, and crush artifact. In some cases it may be necessary to prepare additional well-stained 5-μm sections. One should count the areas of highest mitotic activity and exclude areas of necrosis and prominent stroma (127).

The criteria listed above were established using an Olympus BH2 microscope at a HPF magnification of 40× with a standard eyepiece (field of view number 20), which resulted in an area of 0.2 mm^2/10 HPF. Since there is considerable variation in the area viewed by different microscopes, the surgical pathologist should either calculate the number of HPF necessary to view 2 mm^2 or use a calibrated eyepiece grid in order to apply our criteria.

VI. Summary

NE tumors of the lung are best classified within a three-grade, four-category scheme for classification of NE tumors, with TC representing a low-grade tumor, AC an intermediate-grade tumor, and LCNEC and SCLC high-grade tumors. We recently showed that this classification scheme has substantial reproducibility with an overall kappa value of 0.70 (91). This reproducibility study was based on the original Arrigoni criteria of a mitotic range between 5 and 10 mitoses per 10 HPF (2 mm^2) for AC and revealed that the areas of greatest disagreement between observers were LCNEC versus SCLC and TC versus AC (91). We recently modified the criteria for separating TC from AC in an attempt to sharpen this distinction (41). It also showed that there was a high degree of reproducibility in distinguishing between the categories of AC and the high-grade tumors of LCNEC and SCLC (91). Due to the complexity of this group of tumors, occasional cases may be difficult to fit precisely into this scheme. However, it does not seem practical to expand the scheme due to problems in reproducibility. Hopefully these criteria will be tested in prospective clinical trials, especially to study the rare AC and LCNEC.

Acknowledgment

The author would like to thank Robin-Anne Ferris for assistance in photography.

References

1. Frölich F. Die "Helle Zelle" der Bronchialschleimhaut und ihre Beziehungen zum Problem der Chemoreceptoren. Frankfurter Z Pathol 1949; 60:517.
2. Gosney JR. Pulmonary Endocrine Pathology. Boston: Butterworth-Heinemann, 1992.
3. Wang D, Yeger H, Cutz E. Expression of gastrin-releasing peptide receptor gene in developing lung. Am J Respir Cell Mol Biol 1996; 14:409–416.
4. Sunday ME, Hua J, Reyes B, Masui H, Torday JS. Anti-bombesin monoclonal antibodies modulate fetal mouse lung growth and maturation in utero and in organ cultures. Anat Rec 1993; 236:25–34.
5. Sunday ME, Hua J, Dai HB, Nusrat A, Torday JS. Bombesin increases fetal lung growth and maturation in utero and in organ culture. Am J Respir Cell Mol Biol 1990; 3:199–205.
6. Kim JS, McKinnis VS, White SR. Migration of guinea pig airway epithelial cells in response to bombesin analogues. Am J Respir Cell Mol Biol 1997; 16:259–266.
7. Spurzem JR, Rennard SI, Romberger DJ. Bombesin-like peptides and airway repair: a recapitulation of lung development? Am J Respir Cell Mol Biol 1997; 16:209–211.
8. Spindel ER. Roles of bombesin-like peptides in lung development and lung injury. Am J Respir Cell Mol Biol 1996; 14:407–408.
9. Gosney JR, Sissons MC, O'Malley JA. Quantitative study of endocrine cells immunoreactive for calcitonin in the normal adult human lung. Thorax 1985; 40:866–869.
10. Gosney JR, Sissons MC, Allibone RO. Neuroendocrine cell populations in normal human lungs: a quantitative study. Thorax 1988; 43:878–882.
11. Lauweryns JM, Goddeeris P. Neuroepithelial bodies in the human child and adult lung. Am Rev Respir Dis 1975; 111:469–476.

12. Lauweryns JM, Cokelaere M, Theunynck P. Neuro-epithelial bodies in the respiratory mucosa of various mammals. A light optical, histochemical and ultrastructural investigation. Z Zellforsch Mikrosk Anat 1972; 135:569–592.

13. Boers JE, den BJ, Koudstaal J, Arends JW, Thunnissen FB. Number and proliferation of neuroendocrine cells in normal human airway epithelium. Am J Respir Crit Care Med 1996; 154:758–763.

14. Lauweryns JM, Peuskens JC. Neuro-epithelial bodies (neuroreceptor or secretory organs?) in human infant bronchial and bronchiolar epithelium. Anat Rec 1972; 172:471–481.

15. Stahlman MT, Jones M, Gray ME, Kasselberg AG, Vaughn WK. Ontogeny of neuroendocrine cells in human fetal lung. III. An electron microscopic immunohistochemical study. Lab Invest 1987; 56:629–641.

16. Johnson MD, Gray ME, Stahlman MT. Calcitonin gene-related peptide in human fetal lung and in neonatal lung disease. J Histochem Cytochem 1988; 36:199–204.

17. Gould VE, Linnoila RI, Memoli VA, Warren WH. Neuroendocrine components of the bronchopulmonary tract: hyperplasias, dysplasias, and neoplasms. Lab Invest 1983; 49:519–537.

18. Travis WD, Linnoila RI, Tsokos MG, Hitchcock CL, Cutler GB, Jr, Nieman L, Chrousos G, Pass H, Doppman J. Neuroendocrine tumors of the lung with proposed criteria for large-cell neuroendocrine carcinoma. An ultrastructural, immunohistochemical, and flow cytometric study of 35 cases. Am J Surg Pathol 1991; 15:529–553.

19. Sheppard MN, Luna R, Horiba K, Galateau-Salle F, Gal A, Franklin WA, Miller YE, Fleming MV, Liotta LA, Stetler-Stevenson WG, Ferrans VJ, Travis WD. Extracellular matrix (ECM) remodelling in neuroendocrine (NEC) proliferations of the lung: idiopathic diffuse hyperplasia of pulmonary neuroendocrine cells (IDHPNEC), tumorlets (TL), and carcinoid tumors (CT). Mod Pathol 1998; 11:179 (abstr).

20. Pilmane M, Luts A, Sundler F. Changes in neuroendocrine elements in bronchial mucosa in chronic lung disease in adults. Thorax 1995; 50:551–554.

21. Gillan JE, Cutz E. Abnormal pulmonary bombesin immunoreactive cells in Wilson-Mikity syndrome (pulmonary dysmaturity) and bronchopulmonary dysplasia. Pediatr Pathol 1993; 13:165–180.

22. Johnson DE, Kulik TJ, Lock JE, Elde RP, Thompson TR. Bombesin-, calcitonin-, and serotonin-immunoreactive pulmonary neuroendocrine cells in acute and chronic neonatal lung disease. Pediatr Pulmonol 1985; 1:S13–S20.

23. Aguayo SM, King TE, Jr, Waldron JA, Jr, Sherritt KM, Kane MA, Miller YE. Increased pulmonary neuroendocrine cells with bombesin-like immunoreactivity in adult patients with eosinophilic granuloma. J Clin Invest 1990; 86:838–844.

24. Aguayo SM. Pulmonary neuroendocrine cells in tobacco-related lung disorders. Anat Rec 1993; 236:122–128.

25. Aguayo SM. Determinants of susceptibility to cigarette smoke. Potential roles for neuroendocrine cells and neuropeptides in airway inflammation, airway wall remodeling, and chronic airflow obstruction. Am J Respir Crit Care Med 1994; 149:1692–1698.

26. Miller RR, Müller NL. Neuroendocrine cell hyperplasia and obliterative bronchiolitis in patients with peripheral carcinoid tumors. Am J Surg Pathol 1995; 19:653–658.

27. Wilson NJ, Gosney JR, Mayall F. Endocrine cells in diffuse pulmonary fibrosis. Thorax 1993; 48:1252–1256.

28. Colby TV, Koss MN, Travis WD. Tumors of the Lower Respiratory Tract; Armed Forces Institute of Pathology Fascicle, Third Series. Washington, DC: Armed Forces Institute of Pathology, 1995.

29. Whitwell F. Tumourlets of the lung. J Pathol Bacteriol 1955; 70:529–541.

30. Churg A, Warnock ML. Pulmonary tumorlet. A form of peripheral carcinoid. Cancer 1976; 37:1469–1477.

31. Ranchod M. The histogenesis and development of pulmonary tumorlets. Cancer 1977; 39:1135–1145.

32. Bonikos DS, Archibald R, Bensch KG. On the origin of the so-called tumorlets of the lung. Hum Pathol 1976; 7:461–469.

33. Aguayo SM, Miller YE, Waldron JA, Jr, Bogin RM, Sunday ME, Staton GW, Jr, Beam WR,

King TE, Jr. Brief report: idiopathic diffuse hyperplasia of pulmonary neuroendocrine cells and airways disease. N Engl J Med 1992; 327:1285–1288.

34. Rozengurt E, Sinnett-Smith J. Bombesin stimulation of DNA synthesis and cell division in cultures of Swiss 3T3 cells. Proc Natl Acad Sci USA 1983; 80:2936–2940.

35. Sheerin N, Harrison NK, Sheppard MN, Hansell DM, Yacoub M, Clark TJ. Obliterative bronchiolitis caused by multiple tumourlets and microcarcinoids successfully treated by single lung transplantation. Thorax 1995; 50:207–209.

36. Brown MJ, English J, Muller NL. Bronchiolitis obliterans due to neuroendocrine hyperplasia: high-resolution CT—pathologic correlation. AJR Am J Roentgenol 1997; 168:1561–1562.

37. Travis WD, Linder J, Mackay B. Classification, histology, cytology, and electron microscopy. In: Pass HI, Mitchell JB, Johnson DH, Turrisi AT, eds. Lung Cancer, Principles and Practice. Philadelphia: Lippincott-Raven, 1996:361–395.

38. Carter D, Eggleston JC. Tumors of the Lower Respiratory Tract. Atlas of Tumor Pathology, Second Series, Fascicle 17. Washington, DC: Armed Forces Institute of Pathology, 1980.

39. Travis WD, Travis LB, Devesa SS. Lung cancer [published erratum appears in Cancer 1995; 75(12):2979]. Cancer 1995; 75:191–202.

40. Arrigoni MG, Woolner LB, Bernatz PE. Atypical carcinoid tumors of the lung. J Thorac Cardiovasc Surg 1972; 64:413–421.

41. Travis WD, Rush W, Flieder D, Fleming MV, Gal A, Falk R, et al. Survival analysis of 200 pulmonary neuroendocrine tumors: with clarification of criteria for atypical carcinoid and its separation from typical carcinoid large cell neuroendocrine carcinoma and small cell carcinoma. Am J Surg Pathol (in press).

42. McCaughan BC, Martini N, Bains MS. Bronchial carcinoids. Review of 124 cases. J Thorac Cardiovasc Surg 1985; 89:8–17.

43. Ricci C, Patrassi N, Massa R, Mineo C, Benedetti-Valentini F. Carcinoid syndrome in bronchial adenoma. Am J Surg 1973; 126:671–677.

44. Pass HI, Doppman JL, Nieman L, Stovroff M, Vetto J, Norton JA, Travis WD, Chrousos GP, Oldfield EH, Cutler GB, Jr. Management of the ectopic ACTH syndrome due to thoracic carcinoids. Ann Thorac Surg 1990; 50:52–57.

45. Oliaro A, Filosso PL, Casadio C, Ruffini E, Mazza E, Molinatti M, Cianci R, Porrello C, Rastelli M, Oliveri F. Bronchial carcinoid associated with Cushing's syndrome. J Cardiovasc Surg (Torino) 1995; 36:511–514.

46. Nakhoul F, Kerner H, Levin M, Best LA, Better OS. Carcinoid tumor of the lung and type-1 multiple endocrine neoplasia associated with persistent hypercalcemia: a case report. Miner Electrolyte Metab 1994; 20:107–111.

47. Scheithauer BW, Carpenter PC, Bloch B, Brazeau P. Ectopic secretion of a growth hormone-releasing factor. Report of a case of acromegaly with bronchial carcinoid tumor. Am J Med 1984; 76:605–616.

48. el-Naggar AK, Ballance W, Karim FW, Ordóñez NG, McLemore D, Giacco GG, Batsakis JG. Typical and atypical bronchopulmonary carcinoids. A clinicopathologic and flow cytometric study. Am J Clin Pathol 1991; 95:828–834.

49. Rush W, Zeren H, Griffin JL, Hitchcock C, Becker RL, Przygodzki RM, Gal A, Koss M, Travis WD. Histologic subtypes of pulmonary neuroendocrine carcinomas: prognostic correlations. Mod Pathol 1995; 8:153A.

50. Rea F, Binda R, Spreafico G, Calabró F, Bonavina L, Cipriani A, Di Vittorio G, Fassina A, Sartori F. Bronchial carcinoids: a review of 60 patients. Ann Thorac Surg 1989; 47:412–414.

51. Brandt B, Heintz SE, Rose EF, Ehrenhaft JL. Bronchial carcinoid tumors. Ann Thorac Surg 1984; 38:63–65.

52. Akiba T, Naruke T, Kondo H, Goya T, Tsuchiya R, Suemasu K, Noguchi M, Sakurai K. Carcinoid tumor of the lung: clinicopathological study of 32 cases. Jpn J Clin Oncol 1992; 22:92–95.

53. Lack EE, Harris GB, Eraklis AJ, Vawter GF. Primary bronchial tumors in childhood. A clinicopathologic study of six cases. Cancer 1983; 51:492–497.

54. Stamatis G, Freitag L, Greschuchna D. Limited and radical resection for tracheal and bron-

chopulmonary carcinoid tumour. Report on 227 cases. Eur J Cardiothorac Surg 1990; 4:527–532.

55. Abdi EA, Goel R, Bishop S, Bain GO. Peripheral carcinoid tumours of the lung: a clinico-pathological study. J Surg Oncol 1988; 39:190–196.

56. Geller SA, Gordon RE. Peripheral spindle-cell carcinoid tumor of the lung with type II pneumocyte features. An ultrastructural study with comments on possible histogenesis. Am J Surg Pathol 1984; 8:145–150.

57. Gillespie JJ, Luger AM, Callaway LA. Peripheral spindled carcinoid tumor: a review of its ultrastructure, differential diagnosis, and biologic behavior. Hum Pathol 1979; 10:601–606.

58. Mark EJ, Quay SC, Dickersin GR. Papillary carcinoid tumor of the lung. Cancer 1981; 48:316–324.

59. Carlson JA, Dickersin GR. Melanotic paraganglioid carcinoid tumor: a case report and review of the literature. Ultrastruct Pathol 1993; 17:353–372.

60. Matsumoto S, Muranaka T, Hanada K, Takeo S. Oncocytic carcinoid of the lung. Radiat Med 1993; 11:63–65.

61. McLendon RE, Roggli VL, Foster WL, Jr, Becsey D. Carcinoma of the lung with osseous stromal metaplasia. Arch Pathol Lab Med 1985; 109:1051–1053.

62. Kuwahara T, Maruyama K, Mochizuki S, Seki Y, Sawada K. Oncocytic carcinoid of the lung. An ultrastructural observation. Acta Pathol Jpn 1984; 34:355–359.

63. Sajjad SM, Mackay B, Lukeman JM. Oncocytic carcinoid tumor of the lung. Ultrastruct Pathol 1980; 1:171–176.

64. Sklar JL, Churg A, Bensch KG. Oncocytic carcinoid tumor of the lung. Am J Surg Pathol 1980; 4:287–292.

65. Scharifker D, Marchevsky A. Oncocytic carcinoid of lung: an ultrastructural analysis. Cancer 1981; 47:530–532.

66. Gal AA, Koss MN, Hochholzer L, DeRose PB, Cohen C. Pigmented pulmonary carcinoid tumor. An immunohistochemical and ultrastructural study. Arch Pathol Lab Med 1993; 117:832–836.

67. Abe Y, Utsunomiya H, Tsutsumi Y. Atypical carcinoid tumor of the lung with amyloid stroma. Acta Pathol Jpn 1992; 42:286–292.

68. Al-Kaisi N, Abdul-Karim FW, Mendelsohn G, Jacobs G. Bronchial carcinoid tumor with amyloid stroma. Arch Pathol Lab Med 1988; 112:211–214.

69. el-Gatit A, Al-Kaisi N, Moftah S, Olling S, al-Khaja N, Belboul A, Roberts D. Atypical bronchial carcinoid tumour with amyloid deposition. Eur J Surg Oncol 1994; 20: 586–587.

70. Thomas CP, Morgan AD. Ossifying bronchial adenoma. Thorax 1958; 13:286–293.

71. Paladugu RR, Benfield JR, Pak HY, Ross RK, Teplitz RL. Bronchopulmonary Kulchitzky cell carcinomas. A new classification scheme for typical and atypical carcinoids. Cancer 1985; 55:1303–1311.

72. Jackson-York GL, Davis BH, Warren WH, Gould VE, Memoli VA. Flow cytometric DNA content analysis in neuroendocrine carcinoma of the lung. Correlation with survival and histologic subtype. Cancer 1991; 68:374–379.

73. Smolle-Jüttner FM, Popper H, Klemen H, Pinter H, Pongratz-Roeger M, Smolle J, Friehs G. Clinical features and therapy of "typical" and "atypical" bronchial carcinoid tumors (grade 1 and grade 2 neuroendocrine carcinoma). Eur J Cardiothorac Surg 1993; 7:121–124.

74. Bueno R, Wain JC, Wright CD, Moncure AC, Grillo HC, Mathisen DJ. Bronchoplasty in the management of low-grade airway neoplasms and benign bronchial stenoses. Ann Thorac Surg 1996; 62:824–828.

75. Cerfolio RJ, Deschamps C, Allen MS, Trastek VF, Pairolero PC. Mainstem bronchial sleeve resection with pulmonary preservation. Ann Thorac Surg 1996; 61:1458–1462.

76. Costes V, Marty-Ane C, Picot MC, Serre I, Pujol JL, Mary H, Baldet P. Typical and atypical bronchopulmonary carcinoid tumors: a clinicopathologic and KI-67-labeling study. Hum Pathol 1995; 26:740–745.

77. Grote TH, Macon WR, Davis B, Greco FA, Johnson DH. Atypical carcinoid of the lung. A distinct clinicopathologic entity. Chest 1988; 93:370–375.

78. Wilkins EW, Jr, Grillo HC, Moncure AC, Scannell JG. Changing times in surgical management of bronchopulmonary carcinoid tumor. Ann Thorac Surg 1984; 38:339–344.
79. Tsutsumi Y, Yazaki K, Yoshioka K. Atypical carcinoid tumor of the lung, associated with giant-cell transformation in bone metastasis. Acta Pathol Jpn 1990; 40:609–615.
80. Warren WH, Gould VE. Long-term follow-up of classical bronchial carcinoid tumors. Clinicopathologic observations. Scand J Thorac Cardiovasc Surg 1990; 24:125–130.
81. Schreurs AJ, Westermann CJ, van den Bosch JM, Vanderschueren RG, Brutel de la Rivière A, Knaepen PJ. A twenty-five-year follow-up of ninety-three resected typical carcinoid tumors of the lung. J Thorac Cardiovasc Surg 1992; 104:1470–1475.
82. Jones DJ, Hasleton PS, Moore M. DNA ploidy in bronchopulmonary carcinoid tumours. Thorax 1988; 43:195–199.
83. Caulet S, Capron F, Ghorra C, Brechot JM, Lebeau B, Diebold J. Flow cytometric DNA analysis of 20 bronchopulmonary neuroendocrine tumours. Eur Respir J 1993; 6:83–89.
84. Padberg BC, Woenckhaus J, Hilger G, Beccu L, Jochum W, Range U, Kastendieck H, Schroder S. DNA cytophotometry and prognosis in typical and atypical bronchopulmonary carcinoids. A clinicomorphologic study of 100 neuroendocrine lung tumors. Am J Surg Pathol 1996; 20:815–822.
85. Okby N, Flieder D, Rush W, Brambilla E, Hasleton P, Steele R, Gal AA, Koss MN, Fleming MV, Hammar S, Colby TV, Sheppard M, Falk R, Travis WD, Travis J. Large cell neuroendocrine carcinoma (LCNEC): a clinicopathologic study of 76 cases. Mod Pathol 1998; 11:178 Abstract.
86. Demirer T, Ravits J, Aboulafia D. Myasthenic (Eaton-Lambert) syndrome associated with pulmonary large-cell neuroendocrine carcinoma. South Med J 1994; 87:1186–1189.
87. Lin O, Harkin TJ, Jagirdar J. Basaloid-squamous cell carcinoma of the bronchus. Report of a case with review of the literature. Arch Pathol Lab Med 1995; 119:1167–1170.
88. Moro D, Brichon PY, Brambilla E, Veale D, Labat F, Brambilla C. Basaloid bronchial carcinoma. A histologic group with a poor prognosis. Cancer 1994; 73:2734–2739.
89. Brambilla E, Moro D, Veale D, Brichon PY, Stoebner P, Paramelle B, Brambilla C. Basal cell (basaloid) carcinoma of the lung: a new morphologic and phenotypic entity with separate prognostic significance. Hum Pathol 1992; 23:993–1003.
90. Dresler CM, Ritter JH, Patterson GA, Ross E, Bailey MS, Wick MR. Clinical-pathologic analysis of 40 patients with large cell neuroendocrine carcinoma of the lung. Ann Thorac Surg 1997; 63:180–185.
91. Travis WD, Colby TV, Gal AA, Klimstra DS, Falk R, Koss MN. Reproducibility of neuroendocrine lung tumor classification. Hum Pathol 1998; 29:272–279.
92. Parker SL, Tong T, Bolden S, Wingo PA. Cancer statistics, 1997 [published erratum appears in Cancer J Clin 1997; 47(2):68]. Cancer J Clin 1997; 47:5–27.
93. Minna JD, Pass HI, Glatstein E, Ihde DC. Cancer of the lung. In: DeVita VT, Hellman S, Rosenberg SA, eds. Cancer. Principles and Practice of Oncology. 3rd ed. Philadelphia: J.B. Lippincott Co., 1989:591–705.
94. Gephardt GN, Grady KJ, Ahmad M, Tubbs RR, Mehta AC, Shepard KV. Peripheral small cell undifferentiated carcinoma of the lung. Clinicopathologic features of 17 cases. Cancer 1988; 61:1002–1008.
95. World Health Organization. Histological Typing of Lung Tumors. 2d ed. Geneva: World Health Organization, 1981.
96. Hirsch FR, Matthews MJ, Aisner S, Campobasso O, Elema JD, Gazdar AF, Mackay B, Nasiell M, Shimosato Y, Steele RH. Histopathologic classification of small cell lung cancer. Changing concepts and terminology. Cancer 1988; 62:973–977.
97. Radice PA, Matthews MJ, Ihde DC, Gazdar AF, Carney DN, Bunn PA, Cohen MH, Fossieck BE, Makuch RW, Minna JD. The clinical behavior of mixed: small cell/large cell bronchogenic carcinoma compared to pure: small cell subtypes. Cancer 1982; 50:2894–2902.
98. Fraire AE, Johnson EH, Yesner R, Zhang XB, Spjut HJ, Greenberg SD. Prognostic significance of histopathologic subtype and stage in small cell lung cancer. Hum Pathol 1992; 23:520–528.
99. Tsubota YT, Kawaguchi T, Hoso T, Nishino E, Travis WD. A combined small cell and

spindle cell carcinoma of the lung. Report of a unique case with immunohistochemical and ultrastructural studies. Am J Surg Pathol 1992; 16:1108–1115.

100. Azzopardi JG. Oat-cell carcinoma of the bronchus. J Pathol Bacteriol 1959; 78:513–519.

101. Said JW, Vimadalal S, Nash G, Shintaku IP, Heusser RC, Sassoon AF, Lloyd RV. Immunoreactive neuron-specific enolase, bombesin, and chromogranin as markers for neuroendocrine lung tumors. Hum Pathol 1985; 16:236–240.

102. Broers JL, Mijnheere EP, Rot MK, Schaart G, Sijlmans A, Boerman OC, Ramaekers FC. Novel antigens characteristic of neuroendocrine malignancies. Cancer 1991; 67:619–633.

103. Souhami RL, Beverley PC, Bobrow LG. Antigens of small-cell lung cancer. First International Workshop. Lancet 1987; 2:325–326.

104. Tome Y, Hirohashi S, Noguchi M, Shimosato Y. Preservation of cluster 1 small cell lung cancer antigen in zinc-formalin fixative and its application to immunohistological diagnosis. Histopathology 1990; 16:469–474.

105. Sloman A, D'Amico F, Yousem SA. Immunohistochemical markers of prolonged survival in small cell carcinoma of the lung. An immunohistochemical study. Arch Pathol Lab Med 1996; 120:465–472.

106. Bohm J, Koch S, Gais P, Jutting U, Prauer HW, Hofler H. Prognostic value of MIB-1 in neuroendocrine tumours of the lung. J Pathol 1996; 178:402–409.

107. Hammar SP, Bockus D, Remington F, Friedman S. Small cell undifferentiated carcinomas of the lung with nonneuroendocrine features. Ultrastruct Pathol 1985; 9:319–330.

108. Mackay B, Ordóñez NG, Bennington JL, Dugan CC. Ultrastructural and morphometric features of poorly differentiated and undifferentiated lung tumors. Ultrastruct Pathol 1989; 13:561–571.

109. Oud PS, Pahlplatz MM, Beck JL, Wiersma-Van Tilburg A, Wagenaar SJ, Vooijs GP. Image and flow DNA cytometry of small cell carcinoma of the lung. Cancer 1989; 64:1304–1309.

110. Böhm J, Kacic V, Gais P, Präuer HW, Höfler H. Prognostic value of nucleolar organizer regions in neuroendocrine tumours of the lung. Histochemistry 1993; 99:85–90.

111. Vollmer RT. The effect of cell size on the pathologic diagnosis of small and large cell carcinomas of the lung. Cancer 1982; 50:1380–1383.

112. Roggli VL, Vollmer RT, Greenberg SD, McGavran MH, Spjut HJ, Yesner R. Lung cancer heterogeneity: a blinded and randomized study of 100 consecutive cases. Hum Pathol 1985; 16:569–579.

113. Vollmer RT, Birch R, Ogden L, Crissman JD. Subclassification of small cell cancer of the lung: the Southeastern Cancer Study Group experience. Hum Pathol 1985; 16:247–252.

114. Shah IA, Netto D, Schlageter MO, Muth C, Fox I, Manne RK. Neurofilament immunoreactivity in Merkel-cell tumors: a differentiating feature from small-cell carcinoma. Mod Pathol 1993; 6:3–9.

115. Chan JK, Suster S, Wenig BM, Tsang WY, Chan JB, Lau AL. Cytokeratin 20 immunoreactivity distinguishes Merkel cell (primary cutaneous neuroendocrine) carcinomas and salivary gland small cell carcinomas from small cell carcinomas of various sites. Am J Surg Pathol 1997; 21:226–234.

116. Lumadue JA, Askin FB, Perlman EJ. MIC2 analysis of small cell carcinoma. Am J Clin Pathol 1994; 102:692–694.

117. Berendsen HH, de Leij L, Poppema S, Postmus PE, Boes A, Sluiter HJ, The H. Clinical characterization of non-small-cell lung cancer tumors showing neuroendocrine differentiation features. J Clin Oncol 1989; 7:1614–1620.

118. Kibbelaar RE, Moolenaar KE, Michalides RJ, Van Bodegom PC, Vanderschueren RG, Wagenaar SS, Dingemans KP, Bitter-Suermann D, Dalesio O, Van Zandwijk N. Neural cell adhesion molecule expression, neuroendocrine differentiation and prognosis in lung carcinoma. Eur J Cancer 1991; 27:431–435.

119. Turnbull AD, Huvos AG, Goodner JT, Foote FW, Jr. Mucoepidermoid tumors of bronchial glands. Cancer 1971; 28:539–544.

120. Schleusener JT, Tazelaar HD, Jung SH, Cha SS, Cera PJ, Myers JL, Creagan ET, Goldberg RM, Marschke RF, Jr. Neuroendocrine differentiation is an independent prognostic factor in chemotherapy-treated nonsmall cell lung carcinoma. Cancer 1996; 77:1284–1291.

121. Kiriakogiani-Psaropoulou P, Malamou-Mitsi V, Martinopoulou U, Legaki S, Tamvakis N, Vrettou E, Fountzilas G, Skarlos D, Kosmidis P, Pavlidis N. The value of neuroendocrine markers in non-small cell lung cancer: a comparative immunohistopathologic study. Lung Cancer 1994; 11:353–364.
122. Linnoila RI, Piantadosi S, Ruckdeschel JC. Impact of neuroendocrine differentiation in non-small cell lung cancer. The LCSG experience. Chest 1994; 106:367S–371S.
123. Carles J, Rosell R, Ariza A, Pellicer I, Sanchez JJ, Fernandez-Vasalo G, Abad A, Barnadas A. Neuroendocrine differentiation as a prognostic factor in non-small cell lung cancer. Lung Cancer 1993; 10:209–219.
124. Linnoila RI, Jensen SM, Steinberg SM, Minna JD, Gazdar AF, Mulshine JL. Neuroendocrine (NE) differentiation in non-small cell lung cancer (NSCLC) correlates with favorable response to chemotherapy. Proc Am Soc Clin Oncol 1989; 8:248 Abstract.
125. Graziano SL, Mazid R, Newman N, Tatum A, Oler A, Mortimer JA, Gullo JJ, DiFino SM, Scalzo AJ. The use of neuroendocrine immunoperoxidase markers to predict chemotherapy response in patients with non-small-cell lung cancer. J Clin Oncol 1989; 7:1398–1406.
126. Gazdar AF, Kadoyama C, Venzon D, Park JG, Tsai CM, Linnoila RI, Mulshine JL, Ihde DC, Giaccone G. Association between histological type and neuroendocrine differentiation on drug sensitivity of lung cancer cell lines. Monogr Natl Cancer Inst 1992; 191–196.
127. van DP, Baak JP, Matze-Cok P, Wisse-Brekelmans EC, van GC, Kurver PH, Bellot SM, Fijnheer J, van GL, Kwee WS. Reproducibility of mitosis counting in 2,469 breast cancer specimens: results from the Multicenter Morphometric Mammary Carcinoma Project. Hum Pathol 1992; 23:603–607.
128. Norris HJ. Editorial: Mitosis counting—III. Hum Pathol 1976; 7:483–484.
129. Kempson RL. Editorial: Mitosis counting—II. Hum Pathol 1976; 7:482–483.
130. Scully RE. Editorial: Mitosis counting—I. Hum Pathol 1976; 7:481–482.

4

Precursor Lesions to Pulmonary Neoplasia

THOMAS V. COLBY

Mayo Clinic Scottsdale
Scottsdale, Arizona

I. Introduction

There are a number of putative precursor lesions to lung tumors; terms such as pre-neoplastic, premalignant, preinvasive, and others have been applied. No one term is universally agreed upon, and conceptual problems arise with some of them. For example, is squamous carcinoma in situ premalignant or simply preinvasive? Does the term preinvasive imply that a lesion will necessarily become invasive if followed over time? Is dysplasia neoplastic or preneoplastic? The World Health Organization (WHO) uses the term "preinvasive" for "epithelial abnormalities that are cytologically neoplastic but do not penetrate the basement membrane" (1). However, conceptual problems aside, histologists and cytologists have for decades recognized mucosal lesions in the large airways that precede lung carcinomas or are more common in patients with lung carcinoma, and for the purpose of this review, the less committal designation of "precursor lesions to pulmonary neoplasia" will be applied.

Mucosal changes in the large airways that may precede or accompany invasive squamous carcinoma have included hyperplasia, metaplasia, dysplasia, and squamous carcinoma in situ (2). Recently, a putative precursor to some adenocarcinomas of the lung has been recognized; atypical adenomatous hyperplasia is the term most commonly used, but there are a number of other synonyms (see below) (2). Less well recognized but also within the spectrum of precursors to pulmonary neoplasia is bronchiolar neuroendocrine cell hyperplasia associated with peripheral carcinoid tumors (3).

II. Changes in the Large Bronchi That May Accompany or Precede Squamous Carcinoma

Many histologic and cytologic studies have confirmed an association between mucosal proliferations in the large airways and the development of squamous carcinoma of the lung. Hyperplastic lesions (basal cell hyperplasia/reserve cell hyperplasia), metaplastic lesions (primarily squamous metaplasia), squamous dysplasia, and squamous carcinoma in situ have all been implicated as precursors to squamous carcinoma (2). Most of the seminal studies in this area occurred two to three decades ago, but there has been a revival in interest in dysplastic lesions in the large airways with the advent of fluorescence bronchoscopy and technical advances in the study of molecular and genetic aspects of lung carcinogenesis.

Hyperplasia of the bronchiolar epithelium (basal/reserve cell hyperplasia) and squamous metaplasia have generally been considered reversible, and not premalignant in the sense of squamous dysplasia or carcinoma in situ (2–4). Squamous metaplasia is an extremely common finding, especially as a response to cigarette smoking. Peters et al. studied bronchoscopic biopsies from six sites in 106 heavy cigarette smokers: squamous metaplasia was noted at one or more biopsy sites in approximately two thirds, and one quarter showed squamous metaplasia in three or more biopsy sites (5). The incidence of squamous metaplasia increased with smoking history and was highest in individuals who had smoked more than two packs of cigarettes per day. Auerbach et al. noted similar findings in autopsy tissues: basal cell hyperplasia and squamous metaplasia are increased in smokers in proportion to smoking history (4,6).

Two studies have suggested that squamous metaplasia may harbor some genetic abnormalities similar to those found in lung carcinoma (7,8); however, it appears from the illustrations that dysplastic lesions (squamous metaplasia with dysplasia) were being studied.

Dysplasia and carcinoma in situ are the changes most frequently associated with squamous carcinomas of the lung. In a large longitudinal study of sputum cytology specimens, Saccomanno et al. studied more than 50,000 samples from approximately 6000 men, many of whom had worked in the uranium mining industry (9). Four groups were recognized: smoking uranium miners, nonsmoking uranium miners, smoking nonminers, and nonsmoking nonminers. Both smoking and uranium mining were found to be associated with an increased incidence of dysplasia, carcinoma in situ, and invasive carcinoma. Interestingly, dysplastic squamous cells in the sputum were seen in cases that on follow-up ultimately developed another form of carcinoma of the lung, such as small-cell carcinoma. The studies of Saccomanno et al. documented that increasing degrees of cytologic dysplasia may be recognized an average of 4–5 years prior to the development of frank carcinoma of the lung.

Meticulous histologic studies of the bronchi, primarily in cases of lung carcinoma, have also confirmed an association of dysplastic changes in the bronchial mucosa with carcinoma. In some instances, a direct continuity can be shown between the invasive carcinoma and increasing degrees of dysplasia and carcinoma in situ in the adjacent mucosa. Auerbach et al. studied serial bronchial sections from large numbers of patients including those who died of lung cancer, those who had a smoking history but did not die of lung cancer, and those who had never smoked regularly (6). Cases were evaluated for basal cell hyperplasia, squamous metaplasia, and carcinoma in situ. These changes were found least frequently in individuals who had never smoked regularly and showed a progressive increase in moderate to heavy smokers. The changes were most extensive in individuals who died of carcinoma of the lung.

In another study, Auerbach et al. showed that dysplastic changes and carcinoma in situ tended to be distributed irregularly throughout *all* segments of the tracheobronchial tree in individuals who died of lung cancer; the lesions were found just as frequently in the lung free of cancer as in the one involved by cancer (10). Early invasive carcinoma was found in regions of carcinoma in situ suggesting origin from the carcinoma in situ.

In a follow-up study, Auerbach et al. compared the occurrence of dysplastic and in situ carcinomatous lesions in the large airways in individuals who died between 1955 and 1960 and those who died between 1970 and 1977 (4). In both periods, dysplasia and carcinoma in situ were seen less frequently in nonsmokers compared to cigarette smokers and both increased in frequency according to the amount of smoking (adjusted for age). The cases from 1970 to 1977 showed significantly less basal cell hyperplasia, less loss of ciliated cells, and fewer dysplastic changes for all groups according to the number of cigarettes smoked. Dysplastic changes were more frequent in those dying between 1955 and 1960: 0% for nonsmokers, 2.6% of those who smoked 1–19 cigarettes, 13.2% for those who smoked 20–39 cigarettes, and 22.5% for those who smoked 40+ cigarettes per day. Corresponding figures from patients dying between 1970 and 1977 were 0, 0.1, 0.8, and 2.2%, respectively. The changes were thought to reflect changes in smoking habits and types of cigarettes smoked.

The presumed sequence of events in the development of squamous carcinoma in the large airways is that a carcinogen (e.g., cigarette smoke) leads to a series of morphologic changes, which ultimately lead to carcinoma (2,4,6,10). These changes initially include goblet cell hyperplasia, squamous metaplasia, and reserve cell/basal cell hyperplasia. Metaplasia and hyperplasia are thought to be reversible. These are followed by varying degrees of squamous dysplasia and ultimately squamous carcinoma in situ, from which an invasive carcinoma may develop. Dysplastic cells are thought to be indicative of a significant abnormality with morphologic features (and molecular features—see below) akin to carcinoma. The full sequence of events is

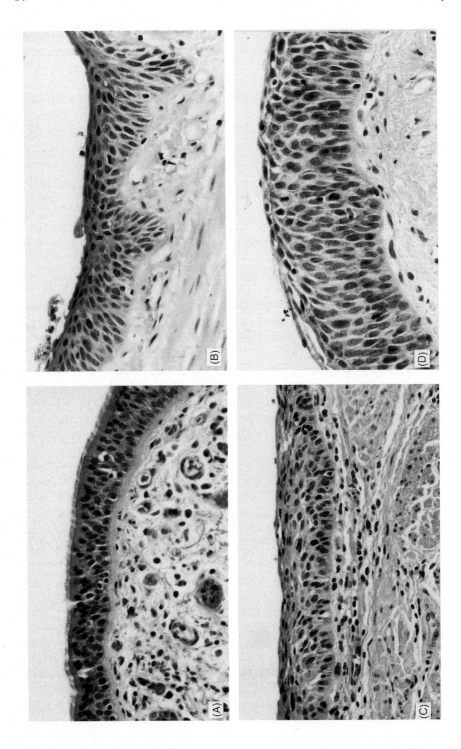

rarely seen, and carcinomas may even arise in the setting of normal adjacent bronchial mucosa or in association with mucosa that does not show fully developed features of carcinoma in situ. These abnormalities are illustrated in Figures 1 through 5, and criteria for their recognition are shown in Table 1.

Some of the distinctions between grades of dysplasia are arbitrary and, as such, subjectively determined. In addition to the histologic and cytologic changes in the mucosal epithelial cells themselves, there are basement membrane changes, increase in submucosal lymphocytes and vascularity, as well as some architectural abnormalities (irregular thickening—see Fig. 3) that may be identified in dysplasia and carcinoma in situ. Fisseler-Eckhoff et al. showed in studies of collagen types I and III and the glycoproteins laminin and fibronectin that there was increasing basement membrane matrix derangement associated with increasing degrees of dysplasia (11). This was associated with neoangiogenesis in severe dysplasia and carcinoma in situ in which disintegration of some of the extracellular matrix components was noted. The authors interpreted the results as reflecting a loss of function of the abnormal basal cells.

Nagamoto et al. (12) have shown the proximity of minute squamous carcinomas to foci showing what they termed "basal cells with marked atypia." The authors identified atypical cells in the basal layer and distinguished this change from basal cell hyperplasia. The authors believed that basal cells with marked atypia "could develop into dysplasia." From their figures, atypical basal cells are shown beneath ciliated columnar epithelium, and such a change is not recognized in Table 1, but I believe that this change should be included as a form of dysplasia.

Carcinoma in situ and microinvasive carcinoma in the large airways have usually fallen into the category of occult carcinomas, i.e., carcinomas that are not radiographically identifiable (13–17). Most are early squamous carcinomas of the large airways that are recognized on the basis of an abnormal sputum cytology. The definition of occult carcinoma is predicated on the radiologic methods available and lesions that are not visible on routine chest radiographs may be apparent with more sensitive radiologic techniques. Be that as it may, the data of Woolner et al. (15) are representative of occult squamous carcinomas of the lung (Table 2). It is apparent that only a minority of occult squamous cancers are in situ.

Figure 1 Bronchial dysplasia. (A) Normal (baseline) ciliated columnar epithelium as seen in surgical resection specimen. There is surface maturation, intercellular edema, and disorganization of the basal layer. (B) Squamous metaplasia with mild dysplasia with nuclear variation and hyperchromasia, disorganization of the basal layer, and superficial maturation. (C) Squamous metaplasia with moderate dysplasia. There is marked variation in nuclei, relatively little maturation, and disorganization of the basal layer. (D) Severe dysplasia with loss of the normal basal layer, nuclear variation, and minimal maturation; some might consider Fig. 1D as showing carcinoma in situ. Note that the thickness of these lesions varies and that significant dysplasia may be relatively thin. (Figures 1B and 1D from Ref. 76.)

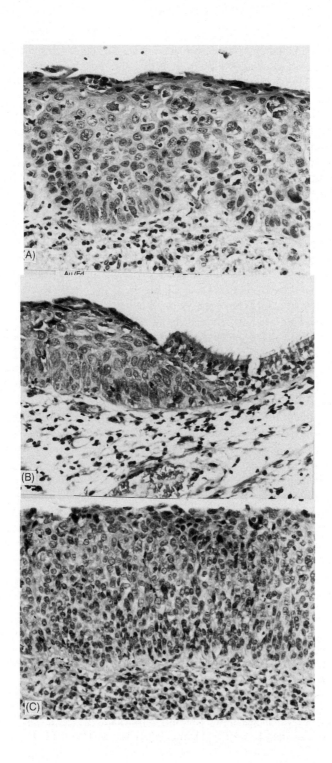

Many studies have provided insights into early squamous carcinoma of the lung (13–18). Extensive sampling of resected lesions is necessary for full appreciation of the lesions. In resected specimens it is recommended that the bronchial tree be blocked in a serial fashion so that the lesions can be fully studied and early foci of invasion identified. In situ carcinoma may be multifocal and found to arise at any site in the bronchial tree, but it shows a predilection to occur at carinae in the upper lobes at the segmental or subsegmental levels. Dysplastic and in situ carcinomatous lesions are commonly invisible to the naked eye; once microinvasive carcinoma has developed, some degree of abnormality such as mucosal thickening or roughening is usually apparent with careful naked eye examination. Individual lesions of carcinoma in situ may be extremely small, 13 of the 19 cases studied by Nagamoto et al. were ≤4 mm in size (18).

Dysplasia and carcinoma in situ frequently extend down the ducts of submucosal glands (Fig. 3). Among individual cases of carcinoma in situ, there is often apparent histologic variation in the differentiation: some foci may show better squamous differentiation than others, the latter being poorly differentiated or even anaplastic in appearance. The mucosa at the margins of carcinoma in situ may be normal, or there may be a gradual transformation to normal epithelium through decreasing grades of dysplasia and squamous metaplasia. In an individual case, the mucosa directly adjacent to squamous carcinoma in situ may be normal, hyperplastic, metaplastic, or show any grade of dysplasia.

The recognition of invasive carcinoma arising in carcinoma in situ may be extremely difficult, analogous to the similar situation in the cervix, particularly in regards to separating extension down submucosal gland ducts versus stromal invasion. The distinction is complicated by the fact that invasion may actually arise from the foci of extension of squamous carcinoma in situ down submucosal gland ducts. Stromal fibroplasia, irregular cell nests, and keratin pearl formation are clues to invasion.

The rate of progression of dysplasia and carcinoma in situ in the large airways varies; longitudinal studies show that the period of time from a positive sputum (from an occult squamous carcinoma) to a recognizable lesion on a chest x-ray may take many months or even years (9,13–16).

Nagamoto et al. have suggested that there may be subtypes among occult squamous carcinomas of the bronchus (17). The majority, corresponding to those studied by Woolner et al. (15), Carter (14), and Melamed et al. (13), may be relatively indolent carcinomas and are referred to as the "creeping type." These tumors tend to show a tendency for lateral spread in the mucosa in contrast to the less com-

---

Figure 2 Bronchial squamous carcinoma in situ. (A) Full thickness change with cells showing cytologic features of squamous carcinoma. (B) Abrupt transition between squamous carcinoma in situ normal mucosa (right). (C) Carcinoma in situ composed predominantly of small cells without obvious squamous differentiation. (From Ref. 76.)

(3A)

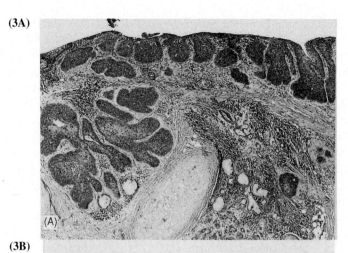

(3B)

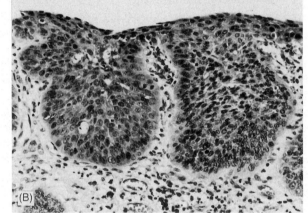

(4)

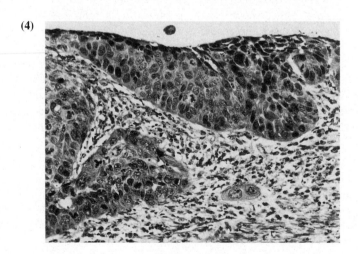

mon but more aggressive "penetrating type," which tends to show early downward invasive growth. Not surprisingly, the latter type would tend to produce a mass and/or obstruction much sooner than the more indolent type and, as such, at the time of recognition be a frank carcinoma of the lung.

Occult squamous carcinomas represent an unusual subtype of lung cancer, and in the routine practice of surgical pathology involvement of the bronchial margin of resection in lung cancer specimens is relatively uncommon. The data of Rilke et al. are representative (19). In a consecutive series of 215 cases, there were 68 in which the bronchial margin was specifically evaluated. The bronchial margin was negative in 53 of the 68 (78%), and among the remaining 22% the bronchial margin showed dysplasia in 7.3% and carcinoma in situ in 4.4%. Direct infiltration of the margin by carcinoma occurred in 10.3%. Of the 8 cases (11.7%) that showed dysplasia or carcinoma in situ at the margin, seven were squamous carcinomas.

Recently, the use of the fluorescence bronchoscope has increased the recognition of, and interest in, dysplastic lesions of the large airways. Since dysplastic lesions tend to show less autofluorescence than normal mucosa, they may be visible with fluorescence bronchoscopy when invisible with conventional white light. In a study by Lam et al., sensitivity was improved by 50% over white light bronchoscopy (20). Three hundred and twenty-eight biopsies from 53 patients and 41 volunteers were studied; in 15% of patients with lung cancer, a synchronous separate carcinoma in situ was found; 40% of the smokers were found to have dysplasia that was severe in 12%; 25% of the exsmokers had moderate dysplasia, 6% severe dysplasia, and 13% carcinoma in situ (20). These relatively high frequencies reflect the increased sensitivity of the fluorescence bronchoscope for detecting these lesions.

Studies using fluorescence bronchoscopy have commenced in high-risk patients (i.e., smokers) for the purposes of recognition and serial study of dysplastic lesions as well as assessing the effects of cancer chemoprevention agents. In one report, serial study of a site of bronchial carcinoma in situ that was treated with 13 *cis*-retinoic acid showed persistence of deletions of 3p and 9p despite apparent regression of the lesion to a lower histologic grade following the therapy (21).

Molecular and genetic advances in the study of carcinogenesis have engendered a renewed interest in precursor lesions in the large airways. In keeping with a multistage model of carcinogenesis, the number and degree of genetic abnormalities identified correlate with the histologic grade of dysplasia; high-grade dysplasia

---

Figure 3 Bronchial squamous carcinoma in situ with involvement of submucosal glands. (A) Irregular thickening of the mucosa with bulbous cell nests protruding beneath the surface. Involvement of submucosal glands is apparent at the left. (B) Full thickness cytologic abnormality with minimal squamous maturation at the surface. (From Ref. 76.)

Figure 4 Squamous carcinoma in situ with early stromal invasion. There is full thickness cytologic atypia with cells showing features of squamous carcinoma. The submucosa shows early invasion by a single cell nest (right lower center). (From Ref. 76.)

Table 1 Mucosal Lesions of the Large Airways

I. Hyperplasias and Metaplasias

Goblet cell hyperplasia	Increase in the number of goblet cells in the bronchial mucosa so that goblet cells are frequently adjacent to one another.
Basal cell (reserve cell) hyperplasia	Expansion of basilar zone of bronchial mucosa. Nuclei are stratified in lower levels of the mucosa, but cilia and goblet cells are maintained at luminal surface.
Immature squamous metaplasia	Similar to basal cell hyperplasia except that epithelium occupies nearly full thickness of epithelium. Cells in this condition have less cytoplasm that in mature squamous metaplasia and are nonkeratinized. Ciliated cell may be retained on the epithelial surface, but goblet cells are depleted.
Squamous metaplasia	Transformation of columnar epithelial surface to squamous. There is progressive maturation of epithelial cells from the basal zone through a well-defined intermediate (prickle) cell zone to a desquamating superficial zone in which keratinized epithelial cells are oriented parallel to the basement membrane. There is minimal cellular pleomorphism or cytological atypia.

II. Dysplasia and Carcinoma In Situ

Abnormality	Thickness	Cell size	Maturation/orientation	Nuclei
Mild dysplasia	Mildly increased	Mild increase Mild anisocytosis, pleomorphism	Continuous progression maturation from base to luminal surface Basilar zone expanded with cellular crowding in lower third Distinct intermediate (prickle cell) zone present Superficial flattening of epithelial cells	Mild variation of N/C ratio Finely granular chromatin Minimal angulation Nucleoli inconspicuous or absent Nuclei vertically oriented in lower third Mitoses absent or very rare
Moderate dysplasia	Moderately increased	Mild increase in cell size; cells often small	Partial progression of maturation from base to luminal surface	Moderate variation of N/C ratio Finely granular chromatin

		Markedly increased	May have moderate anisocytosis, pleomorphism	Basilar zone expanded with cellular crowding in lower two thirds of epithelium Intermediate zone confined to upper third of epithelium Superficial flattening of epithelial cells	Nuclear angulations, grooves, lobulations Nucleoli inconspicuous or absent Nuclei vertically oriented in lower two thirds Mitotic figures present in lower third
Severe dysplasia	Markedly increased	Markedly increased	May have marked anisocytosis, pleomorphism	Little progression of maturation from base to luminal surface Basilar zone expanded with cellular crowding well into upper third Intermediate zone greatly attenuated Superficial flattening of epithelial cells	N/C ratio often high and variable Chromatin coarse and uneven Nuclear angulations and folding prominent Nucleoli frequently present and conspicuous Nuclei vertically oriented in lower two thirds Mitotic figure present in lower two thirds
Carcinoma in situ	May or may not be increased	May be markedly increased	May have marked anisocytosis, pleomorphism	No progression of maturation from base to luminal surface; epithelium could be inverted with little change in appearance Basilar zone expanded with cellular crowding throughout epithelium Intermediate zone absent Surface flattening only of most superficial cells	N/C ratio often high and variable Chromatin coarse and uneven Nuclear angulations and folding prominent Nuclei frequently present and conspicuous No consistent orientation of nuclei in relation to epithelial surface Mitotic figures present through full thickness

N/C = nuclear to cytoplasmic.
Source: Adapted from Ref. 1.

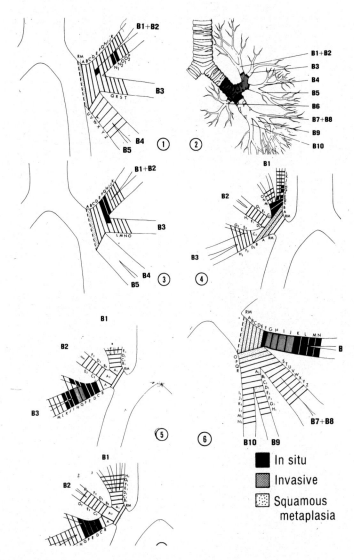

Figure 5 Mapping bronchial mucosal dysplasia and carcinoma in situ. The extent of squamous carcinoma in situ, invasive carcinoma, and squamous metaplasia (including dysplasia) are illustrated from seven cases of early squamous carcinoma. (From Ref. 13.)

Table 2 Occult Squamous Carcinomas

Category	Depth of invasion (cm)	Number	%
In situ carcinoma	0	23	34
Intramucosal invasion	<0.10	12	18
Invasion to bronchial cartilages	0.11–0.30	11	16
Deep invasion to full thickness of bronchial wall	0.31–0.50	10	14
Extrabronchial invasion	>0.50	12	18
Total		68	100

Source: Adapted from Ref. 15.

and carcinoma in situ show most or all of the genetic abnormalities that can be identified in invasive carcinomas (22–24).

Several studies have shown increasing p53 immunoreactivity (usually reflective of p53 mutations) in increasing grades of dysplasia in the bronchial tree (7,8,25–29). The data of Bennett are representative and are shown in Table 3. Other genetic abnormalities identified in dysplasia and carcinoma in situ include c-myc oncogene expression (30), abnormal Bcl.2 overexpression (32), deletions in the short arm of chromosome 3 (3p deletions) (26,28,29,32,33), chromosome 17p (25), and chromosomes 5 and 9 (29,33,34). Loss of heterozygosity at 9p loci is thought to be an early event in lung carcinogenesis (34). Genetic damage may exist in the absence of morphologic abnormalities (35).

Cellular proliferation and ploidy analysis have been studied in dysplasia and carcinoma in situ of the bronchi. In moderate and severe dysplasia, Pendleton et al. showed that there was an increase in number of PCNA positive cells indicating abnormal growth control (36). PCNA score correlated with mitotic counts. Smith et al. showed the presence of extensive regions of aneuploidy in the respiratory epithelium of patients with lung cancer; aneuploidy in dysplasia and carcinoma in situ were present only in the cases in which the accompanying carcinoma was aneuploid and not found in association with the four diploid tumors studied (37). Aneuploid mucosal lesions were more frequent in the peripheral parts of the lung, and both the degree and incidence of aneuploidy increased with the severity of the dysplasia. The authors concluded that their findings supported the concept of field cancerization (37). Abe et al. studied nucleolar organizer regions using the silver staining technique (Ag-NOR) and found that there were significantly fewer Ag-NOR counts in dysplasia (called "atypical squamous metaplasia" by the authors) and those in carcinoma in situ (38).

Viral infection has generally not been implicated in squamous metaplasia and dysplasia in the large airways. Bejui-Thivolet et al. studied 10 cases of squamous metaplasia and 33 cases of squamous carcinoma of the lung with in situ hybridiza-

Table 3 p53 Protein Accumulation at Multiple
Stages of Bronchial Carcinogenesis

Mucosal pattern	% Positive
Normal (u = 22)	0
Metaplasia (u = 15)	7
Mild dysplasia (u = 11)	30
Moderate dysplasia (u = 17)	27
Severe dysplasia (u = 18)	60
Carcinoma in situ (u = 25)	58
Microinvasive carcinoma (u = 10)	68

Source: Ref. 27.

tion for human papilloma virus types 6, 11, 16, and 18 (39). The authors confirmed that human papilloma virus could be identified in squamous metaplastic lesions of the bronchial mucosa as well as in squamous carcinomas: 1 of 10 cases of squamous metaplasia showed positivity for HPV type 6, and 6 of 33 squamous carcinomas showed positivity for HPV types 6 (1), 11 (1), 16 (1), and 18 (3). The significance of these findings remains to be clarified.

The expression of the various cytokeratins was studied by Pendleton et al. in normal bronchial epithelium and bronchial dysplasia (40). The pattern of keratin expression varied between normal and dysplasia and the phenotypic heterogeneity of the dysplastic lesions for cytokeratins was similar to that seen in lung carcinomas. Dysplasia tended to show a loss of cytokeratin 6 expression with concomitant increase in expression in cytokeratin 14 and involucrin.

The histologic differential diagnosis of dysplasia and carcinoma in situ includes:

1. Inflammatory and regenerative bronchial mucosal atypia—the presence of neutrophils, ulceration, fibrin, and history of known inflammatory process (such as "bronchitis") are all important clues to reactive atypia.
2. The effects of radiation and/or chemotherapy—knowledge of the history is extremely helpful; the nuclei tend to be large and bizarre and the cytoplasm abundant.

In these instances the situation should be very carefully evaluated, and a conservative approach is appropriate. In some cases, follow-up cytologic studies (after the inflammatory process has cleared) is the only way to be sure that a given lesion is inflammatory rather than dysplastic.

III. Atypical Adenomatous Hyperplasia

Atypical adenomatous hyperplasia (AAH) has been proposed as a precursor of adenocarcinoma of the lung, analogous to the concept of adenomas as precursors of adenocarcinoma of the colon (1,2,41–43). Definitions for the proliferative lesions in bronchioles and alveoli are less clear-cut than in the large airways, and there are some differences in the definitions used in the various series described below. Nevertheless, two types of lesions can be recognized. The first is a proliferation of type 2 alveolar lining cells that has been called pneumocyte hyperplasia, alveolar cell hyperplasia, and alveolar epithelial hyperplasia, and most investigators recognize this lesion as a benign proliferative reaction with reparative epithelium occurring as a response to injury; it is extremely common and unlikely to have any malignant or premalignant potential. The second type, which many investigators believe to be a precursor to adenocarcinoma, has gone under the names atypical adenomatous hyperplasia (the most commonly used term) (41,44–53), bronchioloalveolar tumor of uncertain malignant potential (42), bronchioloalveolar cell adenoma (43), atypical alveolar epithelial hyperplasia (54), atypical bronchioloalveolar cell hyperplasia (55), alveolar atypical hyperplasia (56), atypical pneumocyte hyperplasia (57), atypical alveolar hyperplasia (58,59), and atypical alveolar cell hyperplasia (60). Some studies have compared these two types of alveolar cell proliferation, but most research interest has centered on atypical adenomatous hyperplasia and its relationship to adenocarcinoma, particularly nonmucinous bronchioloalveolar cell carcinoma.

For many years, lung scarring was thought to be a precursor to an appreciable percentage of peripheral adenocarcinomas of the lung, particularly cases showing central sclerosis with overlying pleural puckering. A number of recent studies have confirmed that the fibrosis in most cases is a secondary event (i.e., they are sclerosing carcinomas) rather than a precursor to the adenocarcinoma (45,46,61–65). Nevertheless, there remain occasional well-documented cases of "scar carcinoma" in which an adenocarcinoma develops around a site of well-documented scarring, such as an old infectious granuloma (66).

The concept of scar carcinoma remains valid for carcinomas that develop in the setting of diffuse pulmonary fibrosis such as idiopathic pulmonary fibrosis, progressive systemic sclerosis, pulmonary histiocytosis X, and asbestosis (67). In the case of carcinoma of the lung associated with pulmonary histiocytosis X, concomitant cigarette smoking may also be a contributing factor (68).

Atypical adenomatous hyperplasia was implicated as a precursor to adenocarcinoma by Miller et al. in studies that eventually labeled this lesion "bronchioloalveolar cell adenoma" (42,43). Among 62 consecutive resections for adenocarcinoma of the lung, there were 12 cases (19%) in which more than one adenocarcinoma was found; in 4 of the 50 cases with single adenocarcinomas and one of the cases with more than one adenocarcinoma, multiple 0.1–0.2 cm nodules were interpreted as "bronchioloalveolar tumors of uncertain malignant potential" (42). The authors drew an analogy between their findings and the multiplicity and premalignant potential of adenomas in the large intestine. Miller subsequently labeled these lesions bronchioloalveolar cell adenomas (43). The occurrence and malignant potential of bronchioloalveolar cell adenomas was thought to explain the relatively common occurrence of multiple adenocarcinomas of the lung. In another study of 240 consecu-

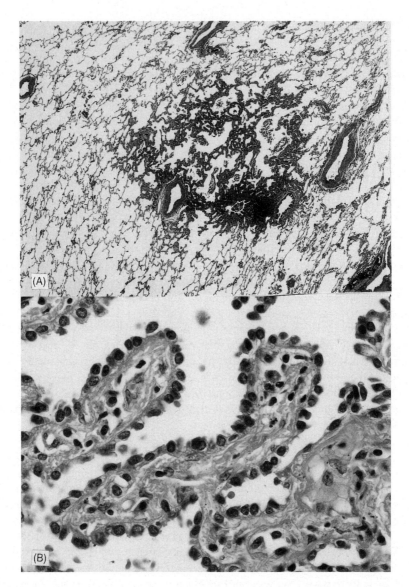

Figure 6 Atypical adenomatous hyperplasia. (A) A discrete nodule 3 mm in diameter. (B) The uniform proliferation of cells with slightly hyperchromatic nuclei along alveolar walls that themselves show slight thickening and fibrosis. (Case courtesy of M. Noguchi, M.D., Tokyo, Japan)

tive resections for carcinoma, Miller identified 23 cases (9.3%) that had a total of 41 grossly identified bronchioloalveolar cell adenomas 1–7 mm in diameter (43). In Miller's studies, the lungs were inflated with Bouin's fixative and sectioned at 1- to 1.5-cm intervals. Bouin's fixation highlighted the small nodules so they were easily grossly identified (42,43). The frequency with which Miller identified these nodules (see below) was in part a reflection of these methods.

Most other investigators have chosen to use the term atypical adenomatous hyperplasia (41,44–52), but many other synonyms have been used. The incidence of AAH in resection specimens is a function of the methods of tissue examination and varies with the extent of sampling of lung tissue and fixation. The Bouin's fixation used by Miller allowed for relatively easy gross identification of AAH (42,43). In addition, the study population will show some variation in the incidence of AAH, since AAH is more frequently associated with adenocarcinoma (55) than other types of lung carcinoma. In six series reviewed, the incidence varied from 5.7 to 16% of cases (42,43,53–56). A figure of 10% in resection specimens is reasonable (53). It is not surprising that the incidence of AAH in unselected autopsy material is less. Sterner et al. reviewed 100 consecutive autopsies and found 2 cases of AAH, for an incidence of 2% (69).

AAH is a focal lesion in the lung parenchyma that tends to be less than 5 mm in diameter, although some may be as large as a centimeter in diameter (Figs. 6, 7). These lesions are recognizable at scanning power microscopy. AAH may center on respiratory bronchioles having associated pigmented (smoker's) macrophages and as such may be part of the spectrum of respiratory bronchiolitis. The lining cells of AAH are cuboidal with moderate cytoplasm. They lack nuclear crowding and columnar shape. The nuclei are mildly hyperchromatic without prominent nucleoli. Intranuclear cytoplasmic inclusions, typical of type 2 pneumocytes in general, may be seen (42,43). The degree of nuclear atypia increases centrally as the lesions enlarge; this is in keeping with the notion that these lesions are precursors to carcinoma and that, as they enlarge, the development of carcinoma becomes more likely.

The concept of the adenoma/carcinoma sequence as it applies to AAH and adenocarcinoma of the lung suggests that there is a continuum from AAH to bronchioloalveolar carcinoma and that along this continuum there is a spectrum of progressively abnormal cytologic changes, histologic changes, immunohistochemical changes, morphometric changes, and genetic changes toward the bronchioloalveolar carcinoma end of the spectrum (41–59) (Fig. 8). This concept explains the frequent occurrence of AAH and a bronchioloalveolar adenocarcinomatous pattern at the edge of less differentiated adenocarcinomas of the lung and the relatively common "satellite lesions" in cases of bronchioloalveolar carcinoma. The concept of AAH also explains the occurrence of multiple adenocarcinomas which can be histologically similar, and this has both theoretical (i.e., multicentricity of carcinoma as a reflection of field cancerization) and practical implications in management (i.e., local resection of multiple primary tumors). The presence of more than one such tumor need not necessarily be taken as evidence of metastasis and therefore preclude resection(s) for cure (70).

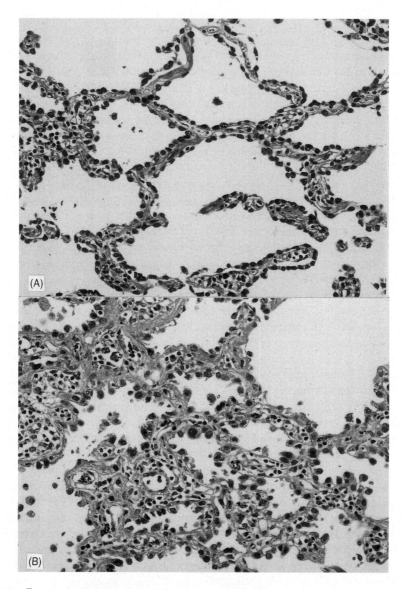

Figure 7 Atypical adenomatous hyperplasia with possible early carcinoma. Most of this lesion showed features of AAH as seen in Fig. 7A with a uniform proliferation of cells along slightly thickened alveolar septa. Focally, however, the cells showed increased and nuclear size and atypia, which may represent the earliest changes of carcinoma. Figures 7A and 7B taken at same magnification. (Case courtesy of M. Noguchi, M.D., Tokyo, Japan.)

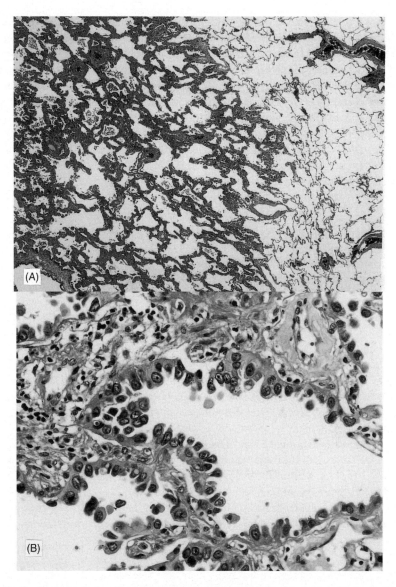

Figure 8 Bronchioloalveolar carcinoma resembling atypical adenomatous hyperplasia. The nodule (A) measured 2 cm in diameter. At low power there is a distinct resemblance to atypical adenomatous hyperplasia. Cytologically, however (B), there is significant nuclear atypia with prominent nucleoli and marked crowding of cells. (Case courtesy of M. Noguchi, M.D., Tokyo, Japan.)

A number of other observations support an association of AAH with adeno-carcinoma beyond the mere observation that these lesions are frequently associated with one another. AAH has been shown to have immunohistochemical staining features more akin to carcinoma (than to typical alveolar cell hyperplasia) (45,46,50,51,60,71), aneuploidy (45,46,52), morphometric features that overlap with adenocarcinoma (48,52), abnormalities in p53 and c-erb-B-2 expression similar to those shown in adenocarcinoma, growth fraction (by Ki67 labeling) intermediate between (typical) alveolar cell hyperplasia and carcinoma (58) and evidence of *K-ras* mutations (28,72,73). Loss of heterozygosity at 9p loci has been found in pre-invasive foci associated with adenocarcinoma (34). The association is nicely summarized by Noguchi and Shimosato (46):

> Stepwise progression in malignancy can be disclosed not only by cytologic and histologic examination but also by proliferative activity of the tumor, such as mitotic activity, the percentage of DNA-synthesizing cells and the frequency of proliferating cell nuclear antigen positive cells, the mean nuclear DNA content of tumor cells and occurrence of aneuploid cell lines, and abnormalities of oncogenes (c-*Ki-ras*, myc- family and c-erbB-2), such as point mutation, rearrangement, amplification, and tumor suppressor genes (point mutation and deletion) such as p53.

In one interesting study, Mao et al. showed with a polymerase chain reaction–based assay that archival sputum samples could be examined for the presence of oncogene mutations (72). Of a total of 15 adenocarcinomas studied, 10 had either a *ras* or p53 gene mutation. In 8 of these 10, an identical mutation could be detected in at least one sputum sample obtained a year or more prior to the clinical diagnosis. The authors suggested that this technique might allow early detection of lung cancer.

The immunohistochemical differences demonstrable between typical alveolar cell hyperplasia, atypical adenomatous hyperplasia, and adenocarcinoma are of potential diagnostic importance, and the data of Rao and Fraire (60) are shown in Table 4. According to Rao and Fraire, negative immunostaining for Leu-M1, CEA, and B72.3 may be helpful in distinguishing atypical adenomatous hyperplasia (or alveolar cell hyperplasia) from adenocarcinoma (60).

Recent studies of adenocarcinoma of the lung and its precursor lesions confirm a number of common morphologic observations in adenocarcinomas of the

Table 4 Immunohistochemical Staining Patterns for Alveolar Cell Hyperplasia, Atypical Adenomatous Hyperplasia, and Adenocarcinoma

Lesion	CAM5.2	AE1/AE3	Leu-M1	CEA	B72.3
Alveolar cell hyperplasia	17/23	17/23	0/23	4/22	1/23
Atypical adenomatous hyperplasia	6/6	6/6	0/6	1/6	0/6
Adenocarcinoma	23/23	22/23	17/23	22/23	18/23

Source: Ref. 60.

lung. Many adenocarcinomas, particularly bronchioloalveolar carcinoma, have cells lining peripheral alveoli that appear less atypical than the cells near the center of the lesion; these could be cells of (precursor) AAH. The center of the lesion is where invasive carcinoma typically develops, and the cytologic features are more atypical. When invasion occurs, there is significantly more cellular anaplasia and a fibroblastic stromal reaction.

The concept of AAH and its relationship to adenocarcinoma raises an issue that has not been addressed in adenocarcinoma of the lung, namely the concept of carcinoma in situ. This is a well-recognized concept in the large airways (discussed above) with a dysplasia–carcinoma in situ–microinvasive carcinoma–frank invasive carcinoma sequence sometimes recognizable in squamous carcinomas involving the bronchi. The atypical adenomatous hyperplasia–BAC sequence is analogous and raises the question whether AAH and/or bronchioloalveolar carcinoma should be considered dysplastic or "in situ" processes. This issue is unresolved at this point, and by convention bronchioloalveolar carcinomas are classified among carcinomas, whereas squamous carcinoma in situ is classified as a preinvasive lesion (1).

The differential diagnosis of AAH includes a number of lesions:

1. Type 2 cell proliferations associated with organizing inflammatory processes: This is extremely common in acute and chronic forms of lung injury; co-existing evidence of acute lung injury (fibrin, hyaline membranes, organization) or chronic injury (fibrosis and honeycombing) are usually present; prior chemotherapy may be associated bizarre cytologic features of the type 2 cells.
2. Respiratory (smoker's) bronchiolitis: Some cases overlap with AAH; RB is centered on respiratory bronchioles and is associated with slight interstitial inflammation, proliferation of cytologically benign type 2 cells, and prominent increase in pigmented airspace macrophages in and around respiratory bronchioles.
3. Peribronchiolar metaplasia: This may also be called bronchiolarization of alveoli; epithelium showing features of bronchiolar epithelium (including ciliated cells) is seen as a metaplastic reaction involving alveoli around a bronchiole that usually shows co-existing evidence of peribronchiolar scarring.
4. Rare benign tumors such as alveolar adenoma and papillary adenoma of type 2 cells: These are *solitary* lesions that tend to be radiographically identified, whereas *AAH is a multifocal process* only identified histologically.
5. Nonmucinous bronchioloalveolar carcinoma (discussed below).

The practical issue regarding the separation between AAH and nonmucinous BAC has obvious management implications. Nodules of AAH tend to be 5 mm or smaller in diameter and to have mild atypia, cuboidal cells, and relatively little cell crowding and nuclear molding. Bronchioloalveolar carcinomas tend to be >1 cm in diameter (and, as such, radiographically visible) and to have cuboidal to columnar cells that show crowding and moderate or greater nuclear atypia. Bronchioloalveolar carcinomas tend to have the greatest degree of histologic and cytologic abnormality near the center, and it is these regions that should be studied for differential diagnosis as opposed to the periphery, where cytologic features identical to AAH may be present. The presence of a stromal invasion is indicative of frank adenocarcinoma. Stromal invasion typically manifests with marked cytologic atypia and irregular cell nests in a fibroblastic stroma (and not elastotic sclerosis of preexisting alveolae, which may be seen in sclerosing BAC).

The distinction between AAH and BAC is not always straightforward, and some cases must be individualized. The above guidelines leave some gray zones (e.g., occasional lesions of AAH are larger than 0.5 cm and some BAC are smaller than 1.0 cm in diameter). In general, a conservative approach is recommended, particularly for small lesions that are entirely included within a wedge biopsy (with negative margins). In a recent study of resected lung cancers, the presence of AAH (in addition to the carcinomas) did not adversely affect prognosis (53).

IV.   Bronchiolar Neuroendocrine Cell Proliferation as a Precursor to Peripheral Carcinoid Tumors

The frequent association of bronchiolar neuroendocrine cell hyperplasia (carcinoid tumorlets) with peripheral carcinoid tumors (3) suggests that it may be a precursor to these tumors.

Bronchiolar neuroendocrine cell hyperplasia represents a proliferation of neuroendocrine cell in and around small airways (3,74–76). It is first recognized as an intramucosal microproliferation just above the basement membrane; lesions expand to produce nodules up to 0.5 cm in diameter (Fig. 9). Nodules larger than 0.5 cm are arbitrarily considered carcinoid tumors (76).

In a study of peripheral carcinoid tumors, Miller and Müller showed that there was a frequent association of bronchiolar neuroendocrine cell hyperplasia (carcinoid tumorlets) in the surrounding lung tissue, suggesting that these proliferations were a precursor to the carcinoid tumor (3). Other reports have confirmed this association (77,78), and it is reasonable to assume that bronchiolar neuroendocrine cell hyperplasia does indeed represent a precursor to carcinoid tumors in the sense that once they have attained the size of ≥0.5 cm, they are arbitrarily classified as carcinoid tumors.

Carcinoid tumorlets have long been thought to be an incidental finding associated with scarred airways and, as such, were recognized with some frequency in lobectomies for bronchiectasis (76). Recently it has been suggested that bronchiolar neuroendocrine cell hyperplasia itself may lead to airway scarring, and a number of instances of airflow obstruction due to scarring in the small airways have been reported (77–79).

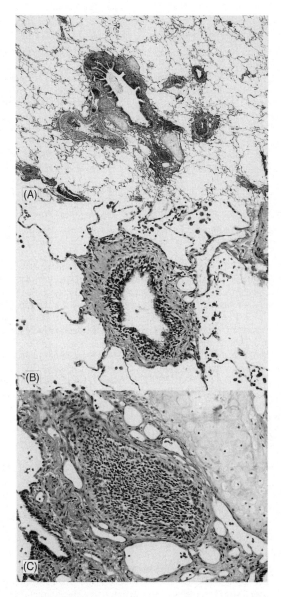

Figure 9 Bronchiolar neuroendocrine cell hyperplasia. There is a spindle cell proliferation involving a small bronchus (A, center) and two adjacent bronchioles (center right). Mural thickening of a bronchiole with associated proliferation of small spindled hyperchromatic cells in the basal layer is apparent (B). The neuroendocrine features of the proliferating cells are apparent in a cell nest adjacent to cartilage (C). There is peripheral palisading and basaloid features. (Case courtesy of Dr. Joanne Wright of Vancouver, British Columbia.)

References

1. Histologic Classification of Lung and Pleural Tumors. 3rd ed. Geneva: World Health Organization. In preparation.
2. Franklin WA, Travis WD. Preinvasive epithelial abnormalities of the lung. IASLC/NCI SPORE Pathology Working Group Meeting, February 1, 1996.
3. Miller R, Müller NL. Neuroendocrine cell hyperplasia and obliterative bronchiolitis in patients with peripheral carcinoid tumors. Am J Surg Pathol 1995; 19:653–658.
4. Auerbach O, Hammond C, Garfinkel L. Changes in bronchial epithelium in relation to cigarette smoking, 1955–1960 vs. 1970–1977. NEJM 1979; 300:381–386.
5. Peters EJ, Morice R, Benner SE, Lippman S, Lukeman J, Lee JS, Ro JL, Hong WK. Squamous metaplasia of the bronchial mucosa and its relationship to smoking. Chest 1993; 103:1429–1432.
6. Auerbach O, Gere B, Forman JB, Petrick TG, Smolin HJ, Muchsam GE, Kassouny DY, Stout AP. Changes in the bronchial epithelium in relation to smoking and cancer of the lung. NEJM 1957; 256:97–104.
7. Klein N, Vignaud JM, Sadmi M, Plenat F, Borelly J, Duprez A, Martinet Y, Martinet N. Squamous metaplasia expression of proto-oncogenes and p53 in lung cancer patients. Lab Invest 1993; 68:26–32.
8. Boers JE, Ten Velde G, Thunnissen FBJM. p53 in squamous metaplasia: a marker for risk of respiratory tract carcinoma. Am J Respir Crit Care Med 1996; 153:411–416.
9. Saccomanno G, Archer VE, Auerbach O, Saunders RP, Brennan LM. Development of carcinoma of the lung as reflected in exfoliated cells. Cancer 1974; 32:256–270.
10. Auerbach O, Gere B, Pawlowski JM, Muehsam GE, Smolin HJ, Purday Stout A. Carcinoma-in-situ and early invasive carcinoma occurring in the tracheobronchial trees in cases of bronchial carcinoma. J Thorac Surg 1957; 34:298–309.
11. Fisseler-Eckhoff A, Prebeg M, Voss B, Müller K-M. Extracellular matrix in preneoplastic lesions and early cancer of the lung. Path Res Pract 1990; 186:95–101.
12. Nagamoto N, Saito Y, Sato M, Sagawa M, Kanma K, Takahashi S, Usuda K, Endo C, Fujimura S, Nakada T. Lesions preceding squamous cell carcinoma of the bronchus and multicentricity of canceration: serial slicing of minute lung cancers smaller than 1 mm. Tohoku J Exp Med 1993; 170:11–23.
13. Melamed MR, Zaman MB, Flehinger BJ, Martini N. Radiologically occult in situ and incipient invasive epidermoid lung cancer. Detection by sputum cytology in a survey of asymptomatic cigarette smokers. Am J Surg Pathol 1977; 1:5–16.
14. Carter D. Pathology of early squamous cell carcinoma of the lung. Pathol Annu 1978; 13:131–147.
15. Woolner LB, Fontana RS, Cortese DA, Sanderson DR, Bernatz PE, Payne WS, Pairolero PC, Piehler JM, Taylor WF. Roentgenographically occult lung cancer; pathologic findings and frequency of multicentricity during a ten-year period. Mayo Clin Proc 1984; 59:453–466.
16. Woolner LB. The lung. In: Henson DE, Albores-Saavedra J, eds. The Pathology of Incipient Neoplasia. Philadelphia: WB Saunders, 1986:57–85.
17. Nagamoto N, Saito Y, Suda H, Imai T, Sato M, Ohta S, Kanma K, Sagawa M, Takahashi S, Usuda K, Nakada T, Sato H, Hashimoto K. Relationship between length of longitudinal extension and maximal depth of transmural invasion in roentgenographically occult squamous cell carcinoma of the bronchus (nonpolypoid type). Am J Surg Pathol 1989; 13:11–20.
18. Nagamoto N, Saito Y, Sato M, Sagawa M, Kanma K, Takahashi S, Usuda K, Endo C, Fujimura S, Nakada T. Clinicopathological analysis of 19 cases of isolated carcinoma in situ of the bronchus. Am J Surg Pathol 1993; 17:1234–1243.
19. Rilke F, Carbone A, Clemente C, Pilotti S. Surgical pathology of resectable lung cancer. In: Muggia F, Rozencweig M, eds. Lung Cancer: Progress in Therapeutic Research. New York: Raven Press, 1979:129–142.
20. Lam S, MacAulay C, Hung J, LeRiche J, Profio AE, Palcic B. Detection of dysplasia and car-

cinoma in situ with a lung imaging fluorescence endoscope device. J Thorac Cardiovasc Surg 1993; 105:1035–1040.

21. Thiberville L, Payne P, Metayer J, Vielkinds J, LeRiche J, Palcic B, Lam S. Molecular follow-up of a preinvasive bronchial lesion treated by 13-cis-retinoic acid. Hum Pathol 1997; 28:108–110.

22. Gazdar AF, Bader S, Hung J, Kishimoto Y, Sekido Y, Sugio K, Virmani A, Fleming J, Carbone DP, Minna JD. Molecular genetic changes found in human lung cancer and its precursor lesions. Cold Spring Harbor Symp Quant Biol 1994; 109:565–572.

23. Gazdar AF. Molecular changes preceding the onset of invasive lung cancer. Lung Cancer 1994; 11(suppl 2):16–17.

24. Franklin WA. The biology of bronchial premalignancy. Sem Respir Crit Car Med 1996; 17:309–321.

25. Sozzi G, Miozzo M, Donghi R, Pilotti S, Cariani CT, Pastorino U, Della Porta G, Pierotti MA. Deletions of 17p and p53 mutations in preneoplastic lesions of the lung. Cancer Res 1992; 52:6079–6082.

26. Sundaresan V, Ganly P, Hasleton P, Rudd R, Sinha G, Bleehen NM, Rabbitts P. p53 and chromosome 3 abnormalities, characteristic of malignant lung tumours, are detectable in preinvasive lesions of the bronchus. Oncogene 1992; 7:1989–1997.

27. Bennett WP, Colby TV, Travis WD, Borkowski A, Jones RT, Lane DP, Metcalf RA, Samet JM, Takeshima Y, Gu JR, Vähäkangas KH, Soini Y, Pääkkö P, Welsh JA, Trump BF, Harris CC. p53 protein accumulates frequently in early bronchial neoplasia. Cancer Res 1993; 53:4817–4822.

28. Sozzi G, Miozzo M, Pastorino U, Pilotti S, Donghi R, Giarola M, De Gregorio L, Manenti G, Radice P, Minoletti F, Della Porta G, Pierotti MA. Genetic evidence for an independent origin of multiple preneoplastic and neoplastic lung lesions. Cancer Res 1995; 55:135–140.

29. Sundaresan V, Heppell-Parton A, Coleman N, Miozzo M, Sozzi G, Ball R, Cary N, Hasleton P, Fowler W, Rabbits P. Somatic genetic changes in lung cancer and precancerous lesions. Ann Oncol 1995; 6(suppl 1):S27–S32.

30. Lee JD, Lee DH, Park SS, Shin DH, Chung HC, Lee JH. Oncogene expressions detected by in situ hybridization of squamous metaplasia, dysplasia and primary lung cancer in human. J Korean Med Sci 1989; 4:121–127.

31. Walker C, Robertson L, Myskow M, Dixon G. Expression of the BCL-2 protein in normal and dysplastic bronchial epithelium and in lung carcinomas. Br J Cancer 1995; 72:164–169.

32. Hung J, Kishimoto Y, Sugio K, Virmani A, McIntire DD, Minna JD, Gazdar AF. Allele-specific chromosome 3p deletions occur at an early stage in the pathogenesis of lung carcinoma. JAMA 1995; 273:558–563.

33. Thiberville L, Payne P, Vielkinds J, LeRiche J, Horsman D, Nouvet G, Palcic B, Lam S. Evidence of cumulative gene losses with progression of premalignant epithelial lesions to carcinoma of the bronchus. Cancer Res 1995; 55:5133–5139.

34. Kishimoto Y, Sugio K, Hung JY, Virmani AK, McIntire DD, Minna JD, Gazdar AF. Allele-specific loss in chromosome 9p loci in preneoplastic lesions accompanying non-small-cell lung cancer. JNCI 1995; 87:1224–1229.

35. Brambilla E. Early detection. In: Hirsch F, ed. Clinical and Biologic Basis of Lung Cancer Prevention. Copenhagen: Birkhauser, In press.

36. Pendleton N, Dixon GR, Green JA, Myskow MW. Expression of markers of differentiation in normal bronchial epithelium and bronchial dysplasia. J Pathol 1996; 178:146–150.

37. Smith AL, Hung J, Walker L, Rogers TE, Vuitch F, Lee E, Gazdar AF. Extensive areas of aneuploidy are present in the respiratory epithelium of lung cancer patients. Br J Cancer 1996; 73:203–209.

38. Abe S, Ogura S, Kunikane H, Suko N, Watanabe N, Nakajima I, Kawakami Y, Inoue K. Nucleolar organizer regions in precancerous and cancerous lesions of the bronchus. Cancer 1991; 67:472–475.

39. Bejui-Thivolet F, Liagre N, Chignol MC, Chardonnet Y, Patricot LM. Detection of human papillomavirus DNA in squamous bronchial metaplasia and squamous cell carcinomas of the

lung by in situ hybridization using biotinylated probes in paraffin-embedded specimens. Hum Pathol 1990; 21:111–116.

40. Pendleton N, Dixon GR, Burnett HE, Occleston NL, Myskow MW, Green JA. Expression of proliferating cell nuclear antigen (PCNA) in dysplasia of the bronchial epithelium. J Pathol 1993; 170:169–172.

41. Kodama T, Biyajima S, Watanabe S, Shimosato Y. Morphometric study of adenocarcinomas and hyperplastic epithelial lesions in the peripheral lung. Am J Clin Pathol 1986; 85:146–151.

42. Miller RR, Nelems B, Evans KG, Müller NL, Ostrow DN. Glandular neoplasia of the lung. A proposed analogy to colonic tumors. Cancer 1988; 61:1009–1014.

43. Miller RR. Bronchioloalveolar cell adenomas. Am J Surg Pathol 1990; 14:904–912.

44. Nakayama H, Noguchi M, Tsuchiya R, Kodama T, Shimosato Y. Clonal growth of atypical adenomatous hyperplasia of the lung: Cytofluorometric analysis of nuclear DNA content. Mod Pathol 1990; 3:314–320.

45. Shimosato Y, Noguchi M, Matsuno Y. Adenocarcinoma of the lung: its development and malignant progression. Lung Cancer 1993; 9:99–108.

46. Noguchi M, Shimosato Y. The development and progression of adenocarcinoma of the lung. In: Hansen HH, ed. Lung Cancer. Dordrecht: Kluwer Academic Publishers, 1994:131–142.

47. Weng S, Tsuchiya E, Satoh Y, Kitagawa T, Nakagawa K, Sugano H. Multiple atypical adenomatous hyperplasia of type II pneumonocytes and bronchiolo-alveolar carcinoma. Histopathology 1990; 16:101–103.

48. Mori M, Chiba R, Takahashi T. Atypical adenomatous hyperplasia of the lung and its differentiation from adenocarcinoma. Cancer 1993; 72:2331–2340.

49. Kitamura H, Kameda Y, Nakamura N, Nakatani Y, Inayama Y, Iida M, Noda K, Ogawa N, Shibagaki T, Kanisawa M. Proliferative potential and p53 overexpression in precursor and early stage lesions of bronchioloalveolar lung carcinoma. Am J Pathol 1995; 146:876–887.

50. Kitamura H, Kameda Y, Nakamura N, Inayama Y, Nakatani Y, Shibagaki T, Ito T, Hayashi H, Kimura H, Kanisawa M. Atypical adenomatous hyperplasia and bronchoalveolar lung carcinoma. Analysis by morphometry and the expressions of p53 and carcinoembryonic antigen. Am J Surg Pathol 1996; 20:553–562.

51. Mori M, Tezuka F, Chiba R, Funae Y, Watanabe M, Nukiwa T, Takahashi T. Atypical adenomatous hyperplasia and adenocarcinoma of the human lung. Their heterology in form and analogy in immunohistochemical characteristics. Cancer 1996; 77:665–674.

52. Yokozaki M, Kodama T, Yokose T, Matsumoto T, Mukai K. Differentiation of atypical adenomatous hyperplasia and adenocarcinoma of the lung by use of DNA ploidy and morphometric analysis. Mod Pathol 1996; 9:1156–1164.

53. Suzuki K, Nagai K, Yoshida J, Yokose T, Kodama T, Takahashi K, Nishimura M, Kawasaki H, Yokozaki M, Nishiwaki Y. The prognosis of resected lung carcinoma associated with atypical adenomatous hyperplasia. Cancer 1997; 79:1521–1526.

54. Nakanishi K. Alveolar epithelial hyperplasia and adenocarcinoma of the lung. Arch Pathol Lab Med 1990; 114:363–368.

55. Weng S-Y, Tsuchiya E, Kasuga T, Sugano H. Incidence of atypical bronchioloalveolar cell hyperplasia of the lung: relation to histological subtypes of lung cancer. Virch Arch A Pathol Anat 1992; 420:463–471.

56. Carey FA, Wallace WAH, Fergusson RJ, Kerr KM, Lamb D. Alveolar atypical hyperplasia in association with primary pulmonary adenocarcinoma: a clinicopathological study of 10 cases. Thorax 1992; 47:1041–1043.

57. Gollowitsch F, Pailer S, Popper HH. Atypical pneumocyte hyperplasia a probable precursor lesion of bronchioloalveolar adenocarcinoma of the lung. Eur Respir J 1991; 7:1355.

58. Kerr KM, Carey FA, King G, Lamb D. Atypical alveolar hyperplasia: relationship with pulmonary adenocarcinoma, p53, and c-erbB-2 expression. J Pathol 1994; 174:249–256.

59. Westra WH, Baas IO, Hruban RH, Askin FB, Wilson K, Offerhaus GJA, Siebos RJC. K-ras oncogene activation in atypical alveolar hyperplasia of the human lung. Cancer Res 1996; 56:2224–2228.

60. Rao SK, Fraire A. Alveolar cell hyperplasia in association with adenocarcinoma of lung. Mod Pathol 1995; 8:165–169.

61. Shimosato Y, Hashimoto T, Kodama T, Kameya T, Suzuki A, Nishiwaki Y. Prognostic implications of fibrotic focus (scar) in small peripheral lung cancers. Am J Surg Pathol 1980; 4:365–373.
62. Madri JA, Carter D. Scar cancers of the lung: origin and significance. Hum Pathol 1984; 15:625–631.
63. Cagle PT, Cohle SD, Greenberg SD. Natural history of pulmonary scar cancers. Clinical and pathologic implications. Cancer 1985; 56:2031–2035.
64. Kung ITM, Lui IOL, Loke SL, Khin A, Mok CK, Kam WK, So SY. Pulmonary scar cancer. The pathologic reappraisal. Am J Surg Pathol 1985; 9:391–400.
65. Kolin A, Koutoulakis T. Role of arterial occlusion in pulmonary scar cancers. Hum Pathol 1988; 19:1161–1167.
66. Yoneda K. Scar carcinomas of the lung in a histoplasmosis endemic area. Cancer 1990; 65:164–168.
67. Schwarz MI, King TE Jr, eds. Interstitial Lung Disease. St. Louis: Mosby Year Book, 1993:345.
68. Lombard CM, Medeiros LJ, Colby TV. Pulmonary histiocytosis X and carcinoma. Arch Pathol Lab Med 1987; 111:339–341.
69. Sterner DJ, Masuko M, Roggli VL, Fraire AE. Prevalence of pulmonary atypical alveolar cell hyperplasia in an autopsy population: a study of 100 cases. Mod Pathol 1997; 10(5):469–473.
70. Barsky SH, Grossman DA, Ho J, Holmes EC. The multifocality of bronchioloalveolar lung carcinoma: evidence and implications of a multiclonal origin. Mod Pathol 1994; 7:633–640.
71. Barekman CL, Adair CF. Immunohistochemistry of pneumocytes in hyperplasia and neoplasia. Appl Immunohistochem 1996; 4:61–65.
72. Mao L, Hruban RH, Boyle JO, Tockman M, Sidransky D. Detection of oncogene mutations in sputum precedes diagnosis of lung cancer. Cancer Res 1994; 54:1634–1637.
73. Sugio K, Kishimoto Y, Virmani AK, Hung JY, Gazdar AF. K-*ras* mutations are a relatively late event in the pathogenesis of lung carcinomas. Cancer Res 1994; 54:5811–5815.
74. Churg A, Warnock ML. Pulmonary tumorlet. A form of peripheral carcinoid. Cancer 1976; 37:1469–1477.
75. Ranchod M. The histogenesis and development of pulmonary tumorlets. Cancer 1977; 39:1135–1145.
76. Colby TV, Koss MN, Travis WD. Tumors of the lower respiratory tract. In: AFIP Atlas of Tumor Pathology. Washington, DC: Armed Forces Institute of Pathology, 1995.
77. Miller MA, Mark GJ, Kanarek D. Multiple peripheral pulmonary carcinoids and tumorlets of carcinoid type, with restive and obstructive lung disease. Am J Med 1978; 65:373–380.
78. Sheerin N, Harrison NK, Sheppard MN, Hansell DM, Yacoub M, Clark TJH. Obliterative bronchiolitis caused by multiple tumorlets and microcarcinoids successfully treated by single lung transplantation. Thorax 1995; 50:207–209.
79. Aguayo SM, Miller YE, Waldron JA, Bogin RM, Sunday ME, Staton GW, Beam WR, King TE. Idiopathic diffuse hyperplasia of pulmonary neuroendocrine cells and airway disease. NEJM 1992; 327:1285–1288.

5

Pulmonary Lymphoproliferative Disorders

ANDREW G. NICHOLSON

Royal Brompton Hospital
London, England

I. Introduction

Disorders that fall under the heading of pulmonary lymphoproliferative disease have provoked considerable debate over the past three and a half decades, principally as to which should be considered reactive and which neoplastic. However, with the recognition of extranodal lymphomas as a distinct type of non-Hodgkin's lymphoma, coupled with both widespread availability of immunohistochemistry and access to molecular biology, considerable advances have been made in clarifying the nature of these disorders. This chapter documents current views on these disorders and their differential diagnoses, as well as discussing how the terminology is best interpreted in the light of recent advances.

II. Pseudolymphoma

In 1962, Salzstein distinguished pulmonary lymphoma from "pseudolymphoma," regarding the latter as a reactive condition analogous to pseudolymphomas seen at other sites. This was based on specific histological features, a lack of nodal involvement, and localization to the lung (1). However, immunohistochemistry, gene amplification, and Southern blot analysis have all shown evidence of monoclonality within pseudolymphomas (2–5), and although some still regard pseudolymphoma as a rare rather than nonexistent reactive disorder (6), most people believe them to be low-grade B-cell non-Hodgkin's lymphomas (3–5).

III. B-Cell Non-Hodgkin's Lymphoma of Pulmonary MALT Origin

A. History

Early series of pulmonary lymphomas were categorized according to lymph node classifications (7–10), but since acceptance of the concept of lymphomas arising from MALT, recent series have classified most primary tumors under this heading (3–5,11,12). The low-grade tumors have the characteristic histology of MALT lymphomas seen at other sites, and although high-grade variants usually lack these distinctive features, it is thought that a significant number of these also arise from MALT, a view that is supported by the occasional presence of low-grade areas in high-grade tumors (4,5,13).

B. Etiology and Pathogenesis

The bronchial MALT from which these tumors originate was first described by Bienenstock in rabbits (14,15), but although bronchial MALT is always present in rabbits, it is less common in higher animals (16) and is not thought to be a normal constituent of the human bronchus. In the stomach, there is evidence that gastric lymphomas arise from MALT acquired as a result of *Helicobacter pylori* infection (17) and that antigen stimulation plays a role in clonal expansion (18). The bronchial MALT from which pulmonary lymphomas arise is also likely to develop as a response to various antigenic stimuli (19–22), but the situation in the lung is less well defined than in the stomach. However, it is known that smoking causes an increased incidence of bronchial MALT (21) and that pulmonary lymphomas are described in patients with autoimmune disorders (23), some of whom have associated fibrosing alveolitis (24). It has been suggested that prolonged high turnover of B cells in patients with autoimmune diseases may contribute to lymphomagenesis, with immunosuppressive therapy being a possible additional factor (25,26).

   Their origin at extranodal sites is reflected in the behavior of these tumors, which preferentially spread to other mucosal sites rather than to lymph nodes; likewise other MALT lymphomas may spread to the lung (5,11). This apparent "homing-in" relates to the existence of a common mucosal immune system, in line with experiments in animals which have shown IgA responses in the lung following intestinal stimulation by antigen and preferential repopulation of the lung by lymphocytes removed from this site and then reintroduced into the body (27,28). However, nodal involvement does occur, with the features then analagous to those of marginal zone or monocytoid B-cell lymphomas (29,30).

Cytogenetic studies on MALT lymphomas, including cases from the lung, have shown t(1;14) translocations in a small proportion of cases and most recently a t(11;12;18) translocation, although the most common abnormality has been trisomy of chromosome 3. Trisomy of chromosomes 7, 12, and 18 has also been identified. How these abnormalities relate to lymphomagenesis remains obscure, but the high incidence of trisomy 3 in both MALT lymphomas and marginal zone lymphomas supports the view that they are distinct from other types of non-Hodgkin's lymphomas (31–34).

C. Clinical Features

Patients with MALT lymphomas tend to be in their fifth, sixth, or seventh decades, with a slight male preponderance. Patients presenting below the age of 30 are extremely rare without underlying immunosuppression. In low-grade disease, the most common presentation is an asymptomatic mass on routine chest x-ray, with symptomatic patients most commonly presenting with cough, dyspnea, chest pain, and hemoptysis. High-grade lymphomas are nearly always symptomatic. Previous or synchronous MALT lymphoma at other extranodal sites is not uncommon, and there is often a gammopathy. One case of an associated autoantibody-mediated hemolytic anemia has been described (35). Some patients complain of systemic (B) symptoms. Imaging shows either unilateral or bilateral disease, with isolated or multiple opacities, diffuse infiltration, reticulonodular shadowing, and pleural effusions all being described. Air bronchograms are a characteristic feature, although not specific. Spirometry shows both obstructive and restrictive ventilatory defects, but in the majority of cases is normal (4,5,11).

D. Diagnostic Techniques

Bronchoalveolar lavage and fine-needle aspiration have occasionally been successful diagnostically, both for primary lung disease (36,37) and secondary involvement by other types of lymphoma (38), but a confirmatory biopsy is usually required. In general, open lung biopsies and resections have been the most common diagnostic procedures as these provide architectural as well as cytological data for the histopathologist. However, identification of gene rearrangements using the polymerase chain reaction has successfully proven monoclonality in bronchoalveolar lavage fluid (39), and both bronchoscopic and transbronchial biopsies in situations where previous diagnoses had been classified as equivocal (5,40), therefore providing a diagnosis through less invasive techniques.

E. Pathology

Pulmonary lymphomas of MALT origin can range from solitary nodules to diffuse bilateral disease, with nodules often becoming confluent. Microscopically, low-grade tumors are composed of centrocyte-like, lymphocyte-like, or monocytoid

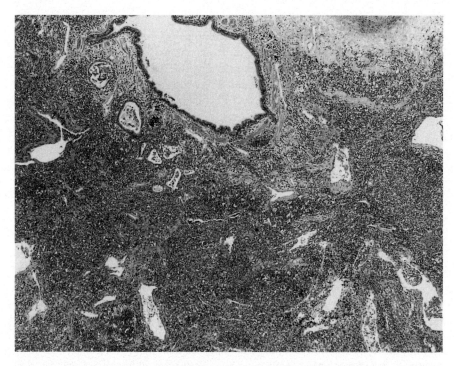

Figure 1 Low-grade MALT lymphoma showing infiltration and destruction of the pulmonary architecture with relative preservation of the airways. (H&E ×40)

cells, all of which are thought to be variations of the same neoplastic cell (13). In resection specimens, and to a lesser extent in open lung biopsies, a characteristic pattern of spread along bronchovascular bundles and interlobular septa is seen. Subsequent expansion and destruction of the alveolar walls and filling of the alveolar spaces give rise to nodules that coalesce centrally, often with hyaline sclerosis towards their centers. Vessels and airways tend to be spared from destruction, the latter in keeping with the radiological presence of air bronchograms (Fig. 1). Other features of MALT lymphomas, such as colonization of germinal centers and the development of lymphoepithelial lesions, are also seen. This pattern of spread is not seen in high-grade tumors, in which the infiltrate is more diffuse and destructive. Vascular infiltration, pleural involvement, and granuloma formation are not uncommon in both low- and high-grade disease, but have no prognostic significance. Necrosis is nearly always limited to high-grade tumors. The neoplastic cells are of B-cell phenotype with a variable reactive T-cell population in the background. Light chain restriction is observed in 30–70% of cases. Recognition of both lymphoepithelial lesions and the destructive nature of the infiltrate is facilitated by cytokeratin staining (4,5,12). Amplification of the immunoglobulin heavy chain gene with the polymerase chain reaction has shown monoclonality in 60% of low-grade lymphomas, but only occasionally in high-grade disease (5).

F. Staging, Treatment, and Survival

Staging as either Ie (unilateral or bilateral pulmonary involvement) or IIe (Ie plus hilar/mediastinal involvement) is recommended, although it is almost impossible to relate stage to therapy as cases are sporadic, treatment has varied over the years, and the diagnosis has often been made after potentially curative resection. In patients with resectable disease, surgery has resulted in prolonged remission (41), but for those with either bilateral or unresectable unilateral low-grade disease, treatment has been governed by the principles that apply to more advanced nodal lymphomas. At present, if the diagnosis can be made without resection, a "wait-and-watch" policy is perhaps best for patients with low-grade disease. When patients develop symptoms (either local or systemic), chemotherapy may be started with either single drug treatment or combination chemotherapy (42,43). Even in disseminated disease, continued single-agent chemotherapy has been shown to be effective in low-grade MALT lymphomas (44).

In contrast, most patients with high-grade lymphoma require combination chemotherapy from the outset, often with high response rates to CHOP-based regimens (45,46). Overall, 5-year survival is quoted at 84–94% for low-grade lymphomas and 0–60% for high-grade tumors (4,5,12).

G. Differential Diagnosis

In practice, there is rarely a problem with identifying lymphoma in resection specimens. Difficulties arise in the assessment of biopsies where lymphoid hyperplasia can be indistinguishable from lymphoma. The clinical history may provide information favoring one diagnosis or the other, but there are no absolute differences. Histologically, lymphoma infiltrates and destroys the alveolar architecture more than lymphoid interstitial pneumonitis, with greater widening of alveolar septa by the lymphoid infiltrate. In addition, lymphoepithelial lesions are less frequent. Using immunohistochemistry, the B cells tend to infiltrate widely in lymphomas (Fig. 2), a useful distinguishing factor, while the pattern of a reactive infiltrate is of aggregated B cells that are usually peribronchial or septal in distribution, with a predominantly T-cell infiltrate and only scattered B cells in the alveolar interstitium. Further evidence of lymphoma can be found by identifying light chain restriction using immunohistochemistry or monoclonality using the polymerase chain reaction, the latter of particular use in transbronchial or endobronchial biopsies (5,40).

The differential diagnosis of high-grade lymphoma is usually carcinoma, and differentiation can be effected using standard epithelial and lymphoid markers. Hodgkin's lymphoma can be primary in the lung, but these cases are very rare and have characteristic histology that is distinguishable from MALT lymphomas (47). Secondary involvement of the lung by Hodgkin's disease is far more common (48).

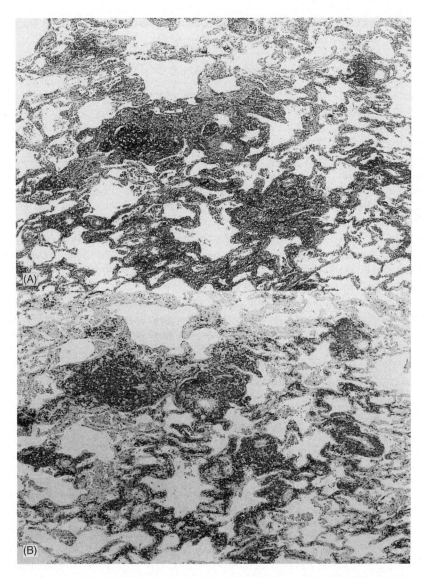

Figure 2   (A) Open lung biopsy showing an interstitial lymphoid infiltrate with features on routine staining that are not dissimilar to those seen in Figure 3 (a case of lymphoid interstitial pneumonitis). (H&E ×40) (B) Using immunohistochemistry, the interstitial infiltrate within the alveolar walls is identified as diffuse and predominantly B cells, providing strong evidence that this is infiltration by lymphoma. (CD20 immunostain ×40)

IV. Lymphoid Interstitial Pneumonitis and Follicular Bronchitis/Bronchiolitis

A. History

The term lymphoid interstitial pneumonitis was introduced by Liebow and Carrington in 1969 to describe a diffuse lymphocytic interstitial infiltrate that was to be distinguished from the usual form of interstitial pneumonitis (49), although some patients with lymphocytic interstitial pneumonitis have been shown to develop progressive interstitial fibrosis (50). The term follicular bronchitis/bronchiolitis was introduced to describe a predominantly peribronchial lymphocytic infiltrate with abundant germinal centers, often associated with various systemic disorders. Follicular bronchiolitis was to be distinguished from cases with accompanying airway dilatation, as seen in patients with conditions such as cystic fibrosis (sometimes termed follicular bronchiectasis) (51).

B. Etiology and Pathogenesis

Although often regarded as distinct, it seems likely that lymphocytic interstitial pneumonitis and follicular bronchiolitis are overlapping histological patterns which represent a response of the pulmonary immune system to a variety of unknown factors (51–53), with lymphoid hyperplasia the underlying pathogenetic mechanism in both (54). Clinically, they are similar in their age ranges and association with gammopathies, connective tissue disorders and immunodeficiency (50,51,53,55,56), although lymphocytic interstitial pneumonitis alone is reported to carry a low risk of lymphomatous transformation (57,58). (This was thought to be a more common occurrence, but it is probable that many cases so described were neoplastic from the outset.) Histopathologically, follicular bronchiolitis and lymphocytic interstitial pneumonitis appear to represent ends of the spectrum of lymphoid hyperplasia, the former being characterized by the prominent development of peribronchial lymphoid follicles with a minor interstitial inflammatory component and the latter by a heavy interstitial lymphoid infiltrate with minor peribronchial involvement. Amplification of the immunoglobulin heavy chain gene using the polymerase chain reaction shows a polyclonal pattern in both, confirming their status as reactive conditions (56). The cause of lymphoid hyperplasia is unknown and is most likely multifactorial. However, there is some evidence that Epstein-Barr virus infection may have a role in pathogenesis in some patients (59,60).

C. Clinical Features

Patients classified as lymphocytic interstitial pneumonitis are usually female, with an average age at presentation of about 50 years. Presenting symptoms tend to be dyspnea, cough, and chest pain, with hemoptysis occasionally being described. The disease is associated with disorders such as Sjögren's syndrome (52,61), Hashimoto's disease (62), pernicious anemia (63), chronic active hepatitis (64), systemic lupus erythematosus (65), autoimmune hemolytic anemia (52,66), primary biliary cirrhosis (53), myasthenia gravis (52), and, particularly in children, AIDS (67–69). Many patients with lymphocytic interstitial pneumonitis show abnormalities of immunoglobulin production, typically hyper- or hypogammaglobulinemia, or a monoclonal gammopathy (52,70,71). There is usually a restrictive ventilatory defect. Patients classified as follicular bronchiolitis commonly present in middle age and are often associated with connective tissue diseases, a subgroup in which females predominate. They present with progressive shortness of breath, fever, cough, and recurrent upper respiratory tract infections. One series divides patients into three groups: those with connective tissue disorders, those with immune deficiency syndromes, and those of uncertain etiology—this last group possibly related to hypersensitivity states (51).

Imaging in both follicular bronchiolitis and lymphocytic interstitial pneumonitis is characteristically described as reticular, coarse reticulonodular, or fine reticulonodular shadowing (50–53,55,56). In one paper correlating radiographic patterns with the histology of pulmonary lymphoid hyperplasia/lymphocytic interstitial pneumonitis in HIV-positive children, the presence of prominent linear patterns on the films was suggested as reflecting peribronchiolar lymphoid infiltrates in the biopsies (72). Lymphoid hyperplasia may also be associated with

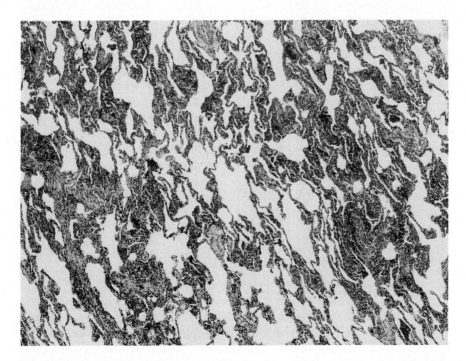

Figure 3 Lymphoid interstitial pneumonitis showing mild-to-moderate expansion of the interstitium by a lymphoid infiltrate. (H&E ×25)

amyloidosis, sometimes with the formation of cystic dilated airspaces identifiable on CT scanning (73).

D. Pathology

In lymphocytic interstitial pneumonitis, the dominant histological feature is an interstitial infiltrate of small lymphocytes, plasma cells, and histiocytes, with germinal centers identified in nearly 50% of cases in one series (Fig. 3). Granuloma formation is sometimes noted (50,53,56). Immunohistochemistry shows that B cells are mainly limited to the germinal centers, often highlighting more follicles than are seen on routine sections. The interstitial lymphocytes are predominantly T cells mixed with scattered B cells (56). In follicular bronchiolitis, there is abundant peribronchiolar germinal center formation with lymphocytes infiltrating the overlying epithelium and the airway lumen often compressed. However, most cases show ex-

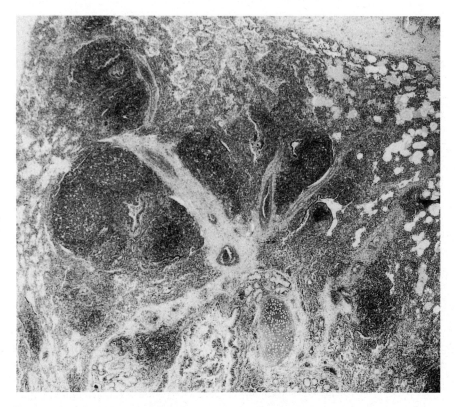

Figure 4 Follicular bronchiolitis with germinal centers compressing airway lumens. However, there is also a mild interstitial lymphoid component. (H&E ×25)

tension of a mixed lymphoid infiltrate into the interstitium, again emphasizing the overlap between the two conditions (Fig. 4) (51,55,56).

E. Treatment and Prognosis

Most patients classified as either lymphocytic interstitial pneumonitis or follicular bronchiolitis are treated with steroids, with cytotoxic therapy an additional option. Responses are variable with some people showing clearing of their chest x-ray, some remaining stable, and some progressing to death (50,53,56).

F. Differential Diagnosis

Distinguishing reactive pulmonary lymphoid hyperplasia from lymphoma has been discussed earlier in this chapter, but other reactive conditions also need to be considered. Some cases of lymphoid interstitial pneumonitis may be histologically indistinguishable from extrinsic allergic alveolitis; it is only the absence of an environmental allergen that leads to a diagnosis of lymphoid interstitial pneumonitis. It is often clinical and radiographic correlation that provides the diagnosis (74). Also, the term nonspecific interstitial pneumonitis has recently been added to the spectrum of interstitial pneumonitides, described as "a moderate to severe interstitial infiltrate of small lymphocytes and plasma cells" that is distinguished from lymphoid interstitial pneumonitis by "the lack of a densely cellular infiltrate of lymphocytes and plasma cells which disorts the architecture." Clinically, associations for lymphocytic interstitial pneumonitis and nonspecific interstitial pneumonitis are not dissimilar, and it is also interesting that one case classified as nonspecific interstitial pneumonitis was confirmed clinically to be due to hypersensitivity (75). Therefore, it seems that histological classification in this area is rather subjective, and consistency between pathologists probably difficult to obtain. As such, a combination of clinical, radiological, and histological information is especially important if correct classification and appropriate management of a patient's disease is to be achieved.

V.   Lymphomatoid Granulomatosis/Angiocentric Immunoproliferative Lesions

A. History

Lymphomatoid granulomatosis was first described by Liebow in 1972 as an angiocentric and angiodestructive lymphoreticular proliferation (76), with subsequent reports suggesting that some cases went on to develop T-cell lymphomas (77–79). In the 1980s it was suggested that lymphomatoid granulomatosis be classified under the heading of angiocentric immunoproliferative lesions (AILs), introduced to include both lymphomatoid granulomatosis and polymorphic reticulosis (also known as lethal midline granuloma), the latter a lesion with morphological and clinical similarities to lymphomatoid granulomatosis but affecting the upper airways (80).

Lipford et al. introduced a grading system (1 to 3) for AILs based on the

degree of lymphocytic atypia, the presence of necrosis, and the polymorphic/
monomorphic nature of the infiltrate, grade 3 lesions being synonymous with angiocentric lymphomas (81). In their series, these infiltrates contained lymphocytes of
T-cell phenotype, and some cases were thought to be analogous to T-cell lymphomas, although in a further series also documenting a T-cell phenotype, rearrangements of the T-cell receptor genes could only be found in one case (82). However,
in 1994 Guinee et al. showed that the atypical lymphoid cells of pulmonary lymphomatoid granulomatosis were of B-cell phenotype: this paper also showed monoclonal patterns using the polymerase chain reaction to look for immunoglobulin heavy
chain gene rearrangement (83). More recently, a series of pulmonary lymphomatoid
granulomatosis showed both B-cell and T-cell non-Hodgkin's lymphomas, indicating immunophenotypic diversity (84), and a series from our institution also supports
the view that some cases of pulmonary lymphomatoid granulomatosis are B-cell
non-Hodgkin's lymphomas (85). Also, CD56-positive hematolymphoid malignancies, CD56 being a cluster differentiation group of antibodies that stains nearly all
natural killer (NK) cells, may involve the lung, and it has been suggested that these
also fall into the AIL spectrum (86).

 This body of evidence suggests that various types of lymphoma can produce
the characteristic histological pattern of AIL/lymphomatoid granulomatosis when
they involve the lung. It seems likely, therefore, that, as a group, lymphomatoid
granulomatosis/polymorphic reticulosis/AIL are histolological manifestations of
more than one type of non-Hodgkin's lymphoma rather than a single specific primary pulmonary/sinonasal disease (84,87). The current view is that lymphomatoid
granulomatosis and polymorphic reticulosis should no longer be included together
under a group heading of AILs (88).

B. Etiology and Pathogenesis

Several studies have connected lymphomatoid granulomatosis with the Epstein-Barr
virus (EBV) (83,84,89–92). In one series, more than 70% of cases of lymphomatoid
granulomatosis were found to be positive for EBV, while other pulmonary lymphomas were consistently negative (89). A Southern blot analysis showed clonal EBV
in two of eight cases of AIL (82). EBV has also been detected in a case of lymphomatoid granulomatosis associated with AIDS, again involving cells showing a
B-cell phenotype (93). As EBV latent membrane protein is known to have oncogenic properties, EBV infection may well be a factor in lymphomagenesis.

 Other than a close association with EBV, the etiology of this disorder is obscure, although patients with AIL/lymphomatoid granulomatosis may have underlying defects in their cell-mediated immunity. These may be congenital, for example,
in association with Wiskott-Aldrich syndrome (94), or acquired; in particular AILs
in the brain have been reported in association with AIDS (95). AIL has also been reported in association with treatment for acute lymphoblastic lymphoma (96), in agnogenic myeloid metaplasia (97), and after treatment for follicular lymphoma (98).
There is also similarity between AILs and post-transplant lymphoproliferative dis-

orders, both showing angiocentricity when involving the lung, containing the EBV genome and exhibiting a range of monoclonality, oligoclonality and polyclonality (84,99,100). Overall, it appears that there is an association between AILs and immunosuppressive states, but whether the risk is greater than for lymphomas in general is unknown.

As stated earlier, it is thought that most cases of pulmonary lymphomatoid granulomatosis constitute EBV-related B-cell lymphoproliferative disorders (83,88), bearing in mind that some cases with the histological features of pulmonary lymphomatoid granulomatosis have proven to be angiocentric T-cell lymphomas (84). This author wonders whether we are seeing a heterogeneous group of neoplasms, with a particular angiocentric pattern of spread, rather than a specific cell type, and the large vascular bed of the lung in part responsible for frequent pulmonary presentation.

C. Clinical Features

Most recent series report an average age of about 50 years (range: 4–80), a male preponderance, and presentations of cough, dyspnea, hemoptysis, and chest pain. Some patients have additional B symptoms (82–84). Imaging generally shows multiple bilateral nodules, but unilateral disease is also described. Although lymphomatoid granulomatosis typically presents in the lung or the skin (77,101), it has also been described as presenting in the gastrointestinal tract (102), brain (95,103), striated muscle (104), and bladder (105).

D. Pathology

Typically, there is a polymorphous, angiocentric, and angiodestructive lymphoid infiltrate consisting of lymphocytes, plasma cells, histiocytes, and sometimes eosinophils. Some of the lymphoid cells are atypical, the degree of atypia being the principal variable in previous grading systems. Necrosis and granuloma formation are additional features. As discussed above, immunohistochemistry tends to show a rich T-cell infiltrate with the scattered atypical cells of B-cell phenotype, though some cases with atypical T cells are also seen. Although grading as AILs provides prognostic data, it is more important to use immunohistochemistry and molecular analysis in order to document the type of lymphoma underlying the lymphomatoid granulomatosis-histological pattern. In this way the disease can be classified according to a lymphoma classification system and appropriate treatment can be instigated.

E. Treatment and Survival

Lymphomatoid granulomatosis is both aggressive and associated with a high mortality if untreated, and there is evidence to suggest that conservative treatment may compromise the ability to achieve complete remission later (81). One report of six cases undergoing combination chemotherapy showed four going into remission and two failing to respond (84). Four of six patients at our hospital died within 2 years, the other two being alive with progressing disease after chemotherapy (85). Most recently, a good response to treatment using interferon-alpha 2b has been described (88). There has also been a report of successful treatment with bone marrow transplantation (106).

F. Differential Diagnosis

Differentiation from other disorders with an angiocentric/vasculitic component should not be difficult; in particular, there is no atypical lymphoid population within the inflammatory cell infiltrate. Differentiation from primary pulmonary high-grade MALT non-Hodgkin's lymphoma rests on the presence or absence of angiocentricity, which is prone to observer variation. However, as opposed to lymphomatoid granulomatosis, it seems that primary pulmonary lymphomas in the absence of immunosuppression do not show evidence of EBV infection (107).

VI. Other Entities

A. Pleural Lymphoma

Primary pleural lymphomas are extremely rare, having a consistent association with chronic inflammation of the pleura resulting from either therapeutic artificial pneumothorax or tuberculous pleuritis (108,109). Most cases have been described in Japan, suggesting the involvement of an environmental factor, although occasional series in Western countries and Taiwan are also described (110,111). There is a strong association with Epstein-Barr virus, and localized immunosuppression secondary to the chronic inflammation has been suggested as a possible cause of an EBV-driven B-cell proliferation (110,112,113). Histologically, these are high-grade lymphomas and most have a B-cell phenotype, although null-cell phenotype and T-cell phenotype have both been described (113,114). Differentiation from other forms of high-grade pulmonary non-Hodgkin's lymphoma appears to rest on localization to the pleura and a characteristic history of long-standing chronic inflammation. Some patients have gone into remission following chemotherapy, but the majority have died of their disease.

B. Intravascular Lymphomatosis

Intravascular lymphoma is a very rare but aggressive type of non-Hodgkin's lymphoma in which the neoplastic population lies within capillaries, small veins, and arteries, with little or no adjacent parenchymal involvement (115). There has been a single case of presentation with diffuse interstitial shadowing, which was diagnosed on a transbronchial biopsy (116).

C. Castleman's Disease

Castleman's disease, or angiofollicular lymph node hyperplasia, is a reactive lymphoid condition typically presenting in the mediastinum. However, it rarely presents

Table 1 Classification of Pulmonary Lymphoproliferative Disorders

---

1. B-cell non-Hodgkin's MALT lymphomas
   Low grade
   High grade
2. Reactive pulmonary lymphoid hyperplasia
   Lymphocytic interstitial pneumonitis
   Follicular bronchitis/iolitis
3. Lymphomatoid granulomatosis
   B-cell non-Hodgkin's lymphoma, often EBV-associated
   ? other types of lymphoma/lymphoproliferative disease
4. Secondary involvement by other types of lymphomas and reactive lymphoid conditions

---

at extranodal sites, including lung (117,118). Clinically, it may be solitary or multicentric, the latter having a much poorer prognosis. Recently, multicentric Castleman's disease associated with HIV infection has been shown to have a high prevalence of pulmonary symptoms (119). Histologically, there are two variants: hyaline vascular type and plasma cell type. Both should be distinguishable from lymphoma.

VII. Summary

It is clear from the above that, over the past 30 years, there has been a wealth of terminology to cover pulmonary lymphoproliferative diseases, based on information gathered as molecular studies have progressed. It has been difficult to accept that some infiltrates were neoplastic as, in the case of MALT lymphomas, they were often indolent tumors with the infiltrates sometimes histologically indistinguishable from reactive lymphoid hyperplasia. However, based on information to date, most cases should be classifiable as either B-cell non-Hodgkin's lymphomas of MALT origin, pulmonary lymphoid hyperplasia (lymphocytic interstitial pneumonitis or follicular bronchiolitis), or lymphomatoid granulomatosis/AILs (Table 1). Cases with the histological features of lymphomatoid granulomatosis/AILs are probably non-Hodgkin's lymphomas, mainly of B-cell type and distinct from lymphomas of MALT origin. Every effort should be made to prove their neoplastic nature and recategorize them as lymphomas, perhaps leaving the term lymphomatoid granulomatosis for those cases where proof of monoclonality remains elusive.

References

1. Saltzstein SL. Pulmonary malignant lymphomas and pseudolymphomas: classification, therapy and prognosis. Cancer 1963; 1:928–955.
2. Weiss LM, Yousem SA, Warnke RA. Non-Hodgkin's lymphoma of the lung. A study of 19 cases emphasizing the utility of frozen section immunologic studies in differential diagnosis. Am J Surg Pathol 1985; 9:480–490.
3. Addis BJ, Hyjek E, Isaacson PG. Primary pulmonary lymphoma: a re-appraisal of its his-

togenesis and its relationship to pseudolymphoma and lymphoid interstitial pneumonia. Histopathology 1988; 13:1–17.

4. Li G, Hansmann ML, Zwingers T, Lennert K. Primary lymphomas of the lung: morphological, immunohistochemical and clinical features. Histopathology 1990; 16:519–531.

5. Nicholson AG, Wotherspoon AC, Diss TC, Butcher DN, Sheppard MN, Isaacson PG, et al. Pulmonary B-cell non-Hodgkin's lymphomas. The value of immunohistochemistry and gene analysis in diagnosis. Histopathology 1995; 26:395–404.

6. Koss MN. Pulmonary lymphoid disorders. Sem Diagn Pathol 1995; 12:158–171.

7. Koss MN, Hochholzer L, Nichols PW, Wehunt WD, Lazarus AA. Primary non-Hodgkin's lymphoma and pseudolymphoma of lung: a study of 161 patients. Hum Pathol 1983; 14:1024–1038.

8. Turner RR, Colby TV, Dogget RS. Well-differentiated lymphocytic lymphoma. A study of 47 patients with primary manifestation in the lung. Cancer 1984; 54:2088–2096.

9. L'Hoste RJ, Filippa DA, Lieberman PH, Bretsky S. Primary pulmonary lymphomas. A clinicopathological analysis of 36 cases. Cancer 1984; 54:1397–1406.

10. Kennedy JL, Nathwani BN, Burke JS, Hill LR, Rappaport H. Pulmonary lymphomas and other pulmonary lymphoid lesions. A clinicopathologic and immunologic study of 64 patients. Cancer 1985; 56:539–552.

11. Cordier JF, Chailleux E, Lauque D, Reynaud-Gaubert M, Dietemann-Molard A, Dalphin JC, et al. Primary pulmonary lymphomas. A clinical study of 70 cases in non immunocompromised patients. Chest 1993; 103:201–208.

12. Fiche M, Capron F, Berger F, Galateau F, Cordier J, Loire R, et al. Primary pulmonary non-Hodgkin's lymphomas. Histopathology 1995; 26:529–537.

13. Isaacson PG. Lymphomas of mucosa-associated lymphoid tissue (MALT). Histopathology 1990; 16:617–619.

14. Bienenstock J, Johnston N, Perey DY. Bronchial lymphoid tissue. II Functional characteristics. Lab Invest 1973; 28:693–698.

15. Bienenstock J, Johnston N, Perey DY. Bronchial lymphoid tissue. I. Morphologic characteristics. Lab Invest 1973; 28:686–692.

16. Pabst R, Gehrke I. Is the bronchus-associated lymphoid tissue (BALT) an integral structure of the lung in normal mammals, including humans? Am J Respir Cell Mol Biol 1990; 3:131–135.

17. Wotherspoon AC, Ortiz-Hidalgo C, Falzon MR, Isaacson PG. Helicobacter pylori-associated gastritis and primary B-cell gastric lymphoma. Lancet 1991; 338:1175–1176.

18. Du M, Diss TC, Xu C, Peng H, Isaacson PG, Pan L. Ongoing mutation in MALT lymphoma immunoglobulin gene suggests that antigen stimulation plays a role in the clonal expansion. Leukemia 1996; 10:1190–1197.

19. Gould SJ, Isaacson PG. Bronchus-associated lymphoid tissue (BALT) in human fetal and infant lung. J Pathol 1993; 169:229–234.

20. Holt PG. Development of bronchus associated lymphoid tissue (BALT) in human lung disease: A normal host defence mechanism awaiting therapeutic exploitation? Thorax 1993; 48:1097–1098.

21. Richmond I, Pritchard GE, Ashcroft T, Avery A, Corris PA, Walters EH. Bronchus associated lymphoid tissue (BALT) in human lung: its distribution in smokers and non-smokers. Thorax 1993; 48:1130–1134.

22. Pabst R. Is BALT a major component of the human lung immune system? Immunol Today 1992; 13:119–122.

23. Kamel OW, van de Rijn M, Le Brun DP, Weiss LM, Warnke RA, Dorfman RF. Lymphoid neoplasms in patients with rheumatoid arthritis and dermatomyositis; frequency of Epstein-Barr virus and other features associated with immunosuppression. Hum Pathol 1994; 25:638–643.

24. Nicholson AG, Wotherspoon AC, Jones AL, Sheppard MN, Isaacson PG, Corrin B. Pulmonary B-cell non-Hodgkin's lymphoma associated with autoimmune disorders: a clinicopathological review of six cases. Eur Respir J 1996; 9:2022–2025.

25. Symmons DP. Neoplasms of the immune system in rheumatoid arthritis. Am J Med 1985; 78(1A):22–28.
26. Frizzera G. Immunosuppression, autoimmunity and lymphoproliferative disorders. Hum Pathol 1994; 25:627–629.
27. Rudzik R, Clancy RL, Perey DY, Day RP, Bienenstock J. Repopulation with IgA-containing cells of bronchial and intestinal lamina propria after transfer of homologous Peyer's patch and bronchial lymphocytes. J Immunol 1975; 114:1599–1604.
28. McDermott MR, Bienenstock J. Evidence for a common mucosal immunologic system. Migration of B immunoblasts into intestinal, respiratory, and genital tissues. J Immunol 1979; 122:1892–1898.
29. Ortiz-Hidalgo C, Wright DH. The morphological spectrum of monocytoid B-cell lymphoma and its relationship to lymphomas of mucosa-associated lymphoid tissue. Histopathology 1992; 21:555–561.
30. Ngan BY, Warnke RA, Wilson M, Takagi K, Cleary ML, Dorfman RF. Monocytoid B-cell lymphoma: a study of 36 cases. Hum Pathol 1991; 22:409–421.
31. Wotherspoon AC, Soosay GN, Diss TC, Isaacson PG. Low grade primary B-cell lymphoma of the lung. An immunohistochemical, molecular and cytogenetic study of a single case. Am J Clin Pathol 1990; 94:655–660.
32. Wotherspoon AC, Pan L, Diss TC, Isaacson PG. Cytogenetic study of B-cell lymphoma of mucosa-associated lymphoid tissue. Cancer Genet Cytogenet 1992; 58:35–38.
33. Wotherspoon AC, Finn TM, Isaacson PG. Trisomy 3 in low-grade B-cell lymphomas of mucosa-associated lymphoid tissue. Blood 1995; 85:2000–2004.
34. Kubonishi I, Sugito S, Kobayashi M, Asahi Y, Tsuchiya T, Yamashiro T, Miyoshi I. A unique chromosome translocation, t(11;12;18)(q13;q13;q12), in primary lung lymphoma. Cancer Genet Cytogenet 1995; 82:54–56.
35. Liaw YS, Yang PC, Su IJ, Kuo SH, Wang CH, Luh KT. Mucosa-associated lymphoid tissue lymphoma of the lung with cold-reacting autoantibody-mediated hemolytic anemia. Chest 1994; 105:288–290.
36. Davis WB, Gadek JE. Detection of pulmonary lymphoma by bronchoalveolar lavage. Chest 1987; 91:787–790.
37. Sprague RI, Deblois GG. Small lymphocytic pulmonary lymphoma. Diagnosis by transthoracic fine needle aspiration. Chest 1989; 96:929–930.
38. Bardales RH, Powers CN, Frierson HF, Jr., Suhrland MJ, Covell JL, Stanley, et al. Exfoliative respiratory cytology in the diagnosis of leukemias and lymphomas in the lung. Diagnos Cytopathol 1996; 14:108–113.
39. Betsuyaku T, Munakata M, Yamaguchi E, Ohe S, Hizawa N, Sukoh N, Yamashiro K, et al. Establishing diagnosis of pulmonary malignant lymphoma by gene rearrangement analysis of lymphocytes in bronchoalveolar lavage fluid. Am J Respir Crit Care Med 1994; 149:526–529.
40. Kurosu K, Yumoto N, Mikata A, Taniguchi M, Kuriyama T. Monoclonality of B-cell lineage in primary pulmonary lymphoma demonstrated by immunoglobulin heavy chain gene sequence analysis of histologically nondefinitive transbronchial biopsy specimens. J Pathol 1996; 178:316–322.
41. Uppal R, Goldstraw P. Primary pulmonary lymphoma. Lung Cancer 1992; 8:95–100.
42. Horning SJ, Rosenberg SA. The natural history of initially untreated low-grade non-Hodgkin's lymphomas. N Engl J Med 1984; 311:1471–1475.
43. Portlock CS. Deferral of initial therapy for advanced indolent lymphomas. Cancer Treat Rep 1982; 66:417–419.
44. Hammel P, Haioun C, Chaumette MT, Gaulard P, Divine M, Reyes F, Delchier JC. Efficacy of single-agent chemotherapy in low-grade B-cell mucosa-associated lymphoid tissue lymphoma with prominent gastric expression. J Clin Oncol 1995; 13:2524–2529.
45. Miller TP, Jones SE. Initial chemotherapy for clinically localized lymphomas of unfavorable histology. Blood 1983; 62:413–418.
46. Longo DL, Glatstein E, Duffey PL, Ihde JC, Hubbard SM, Fisher RI, et al. Treatment of lo-

calized aggressive lymphomas with combination chemotherapy followed by involved-field radiation therapy. J Clin Oncol 1989; 7:1295–1302.

47. Radin AI. Primary pulmonary Hodgkin's disease. Cancer 1990; 65:550–563.
48. Berkman N, Breuer R. Pulmonary involvement in lymphoma. Respir Med 1993; 87:85–92.
49. Liebow AA, Carrington CB. The interstitial pneumonias. In: Simon M, ed. Frontiers in Pulmonary Radiology. New York: Grune and Stratton, 1969:102–141.
50. Strimlan CV, Rosenow EC, Weiland LH, Brown LR. Lymphocytic interstitial pneumonitis. Review of 13 cases. Ann Intern Med 1978; 88:616–621.
51. Yousem SA, Colby TV, Carrington CB. Follicular bronchitis/bronchiolitis. Hum Pathol 1985; 16:700–706.
52. Liebow AA, Carrington CB. Diffuse pulmonary lymphoreticular infiltrations associated with dysproteinaemia. Med Clin North Am 1973; 57:809–843.
53. Koss MN, Hochholzer L, Langloss JM, Wehunt WD, Lazarus AA. Lymphoid interstitial pneumonia: clinicopathological and immunopathological findings in 18 cases. Pathology 1987; 19:178–185.
54. Kradin RL, Mark EJ. Benign lymphoid disorders of the lung, with a theory regarding their development. Hum Pathol 1983; 14:857–867.
55. Fortoul TI, Cano-Valle F, Oliva E, Barrios R. Follicular bronchiolitis in association with connective tissue diseases. Lung 1985; 163:305–314.
56. Nicholson AG, Wotherspoon AC, Diss TC, Hansell DM, DuBois R, Sheppard MN, et al. Reactive pulmonary lymphoid disorders. Histopathology 1995; 26:405–412.
57. Kradin RL, Young RH, Kradin LA, Mark EJ. Immunoblastic lymphoma arising in chronic lymphoid hyperplasia of the pulmonary interstitium. Cancer 1982; 50:1339–1343.
58. Teruya-Feldstein J, Temeck BK, Sloas MM, Kingma DW, Raffeld M, Pass HI, et al. Pulmonary malignant lymphoma of mucosa-associated lymphoid tissue (MALT) arising in a pediatric HIV-positive patient. Am J Surg Pathol 1995; 19:357–363.
59. Barbera JA, Hayashi S, Hegele RG, Hogg JC. Detection of Epstein-Barr virus in lymphocytic interstitial pneumonia by in situ hybridisation. Am Rev Respir Dis 1992; 145:940–946.
60. Kaan PM, Hegele RG, Hayashi S, Hogg JC. Expression of bcl-2 and Epstein-Barr virus LMP1 in lymphocytic interstitial pneumonia. Thorax 1997; 52:12–16.
61. Strimlan CV, Rosenov EC, Divertie MB, Harrison EG. Pulmonary manifestations of Sjögren's syndrome. Chest 1976; 70:354–361.
62. Julsrud PR, Brown LR, Li CY, Rosenow EC, Crowe JK. Pulmonary processes of mature-appearing lymphocytes: pseudolymphoma, well-differentiated lymphocytic lymphoma and lymphocytic interstitial pneumonitis. Radiology 1978; 127:289–296.
63. Levinson AI, Hopewell PC, Stites DP, Spitler LE, Fudenburg HH. Coexistent lymphoid interstitial pneumonia, pernicious anaemia and agammaglobulinaemia. Arch Intern Med 1976; 136:213–216.
64. Helman CA, Keeton GR, Benatar SR. Lymphoid interstitial pneumonia with associated chronic active hepatitis and renal tubular acidosis. Am Rev Respir Dis 1977; 115:161–164.
65. Yood RA, Steigman DM, Gill LR. Lymphocytic interstitial pneumonitis in a patient with systemic lupus erythematosus. Lupus 1995; 4:161–163.
66. DeCoteau WE, Tourville D, Ambrus JL, Montes M, Adler R, Tomasi TB. Lymphoid interstitial pneumonia and autoerythrocyte sensitization syndrome. A case with deposition of immunoglobulins on the alveolar basement membrane. Arch Intern Med 1974; 134:519–522.
67. Solal-Celigny P, Couderc LJ, Herman D, Schaffer-Deshayes L, Brun-Vezinet F, Tricot G, et al. Lymphoid interstitial pneumonitis in acquired immunodeficiency syndrome-related complex. Am Rev Respir Dis 1985; 131:956–960.
68. Grieco MH, Chinoy-Acharya P. Lymphocytic interstitial pneumonia associated with the acquired immune deficiency syndrome. Am Rev Respir Dis 1985; 131:952–955.
69. Morris JC, Rosen MJ, Marchevsky A, Teirstein AS. Lymphocytic interstitial pneumonia in patients at risk from the acquired immune deficiency syndrome. Chest 1987; 91:63–67.
70. Church JA, Isaacs H, Saxon A, Keens TG, Richards W. Lymphoid interstitial pneumonitis and hypogammoglobulinaemia in children. Am Rev Respir Dis 1981; 124:491–496.

71. Montes M, Tomasi TB, Noehreun TH, Culver GJ. Lymphoid interstitial pneumonia with monoclonal gammopathy. Am Rev Respir Dis 1968; 98:277–280.
72. Marquis JR, Berman CZ, DiCarlo F, Oleske JM. Radiographic patterns of PLH/LIP in HIV positive children. Pediatr Radiol 1993; 23:328–330.
73. Desai SR, Nicholson AG, Stewart S, Twentyman OR, Flower CDR, Hansell DM. Benign pulmonary lymphocytic infiltration and amyloidosis: computed tomographic and pathological features in three cases. J Thor Imag 1997; 12:215–220.
74. Colby TV. Lymphoproliferative diseases. In: Dail DH, Hammar SP, eds. Pulmonary Pathology. New York: Springer-Verlag, 1988:713.
75. Katzenstein AA, Fiorelli RF. Nonspecific interstitial pneumonia/fibrosis. Histologic features and clinical significance. Am J Surg Pathol 1994; 18:136–147.
76. Liebow AA, Carrington CR, Friedman PJ. Lymphomatoid granulomatosis. Hum Pathol 1972; 3:457–458.
77. Katzenstein AA, Carrington CB, Leibow AA. Lymphomatoid granulomatosis: a clinicopathologic study of 152 cases. Cancer 1979; 43:360–373.
78. Pisani RJ, DeRemee RA. Clinical implications of the histopathologic diagnosis of pulmonary lymphomatoid granulomatosis. Mayo Clin Proc 1990; 65:151–163.
79. Colby TV, Carrington CB. Malignant lymphoma simulating lymphomatoid granulomatosis. Am J Surg Pathol 1982; 6:19–32.
80. Jaffe ES. Pathologic and clinical spectrum of post-thymic T-cell malignancies. Cancer Invest 1984; 3:413–426.
81. Lipford EH, Margolick JB, Longo DL, Fauci AS, Jaffe ES. Angiocentric immunoproliferative lesions: a clinicopathologic spectrum of post-thymic T-cell proliferations. Blood 1988; 72:1674–1681.
82. Medeiros LJ, Peiper SC, Elwood L, Yano T, Raffeld M, Jaffe ES. Angiocentric immunoproliferative lesions: a molecular analysis of eight cases. Hum Pathol 1991; 22:1150–1157.
83. Guinee DJ, Jaffe E, Kingma D, Fishback N, Wallberg K, Krishnan J, et al. Pulmonary lymphomatoid granulomatosis. Evidence for a proliferation of Epstein-Barr virus infected B-lymphocytes with a predominant T-cell component and vasculitis. Am J Surg Pathol 1994; 18:753–764.
84. Myers JL, Kurtin PJ, Katzenstein AA, Tazelaar H, D., Colby TV, Strickler JG, et al. Lymphomatoid granulomatosis. Evidence of immunophenotypic diversity and relationship to Epstein-Barr virus infection. Am J Surg Pathol 1995; 19:1300–1312.
85. Nicholson AG, Wotherspoon AC, Diss TC, Singh N, Butcher DN, Pan LX, et al. Lymphomatoid granulomatosis: evidence that some cases represent Epstein-Barr virus-associated B-cell lymphoma. Histopathology 1996; 29:317–324.
86. Wong KF, Chan JK, Ng CG, Lee KC, Tsang WY, Cheung MM. CD56 (NKH1)-positive hematolymphoid malignancies: an aggressive neoplasm featuring frequent cutaneous/mucosal involvement, cytoplasmic azurophilic granules, and angiocentricity. Hum Pathol 1992; 23:798–804.
87. Strickler JG, Meneses MF, Haberman TM, Ilstrup DM, Earle JD, McDonald TJ, et al. Polymorphic reticulosis: a reappraisal. Hum Pathol 1994; 25:659–665.
88. Wilson WH, Kingma DW, Raffeld M, Wittes RE, Jaffe ES. Association of lymphomatoid granulomatosis with Epstein-Barr viral infection of B lymphocytes and response to interferon-alpha 2b. Blood 1996; 87:4531–4537.
89. Katzenstein AA, Peiper SC. Detection of Epstein-Barr virus genomes in lymphomatoid granulomatosis: analysis of 29 cases by the polymerase chain reaction technique. Mod Pathol 1990; 3:435–441.
90. Veltri RW, Raich PC, McClung JE, Shah SH, Sprinkle PM. Lymphomatoid granulomatosis and Epstein-Barr virus. Cancer 1982; 50:1513–1517.
91. Tanaka Y, Sasaki Y, Kurozumi H, Hyodo Y, Nishi T, Nakatani Y, et al. Angiocentric immunoproliferative lesion associated with chronic active Epstein-Barr virus infection in an 11 year old boy. Clonotropic proliferation of Epstein-Barr virus-bearing CD4+ T lymphocytes. Am J Surg Pathol 1994; 18:623–631.

92. Medeiros LJ, Jaffe ES, Chen Y, Weiss LM. Localisation of Epstein-Barr viral genomes in angiocentric immunoproliferative lesions. Am J Surg Pathol 1992; 16:439–447.
93. Mittal K, Neri A, Feiner H, Schinella R, Alfonso F. Lymphomatoid granulomatosis in the acquired immunodeficiency syndrome. Evidence of Epstein-Barr virus infection and B-cell clonal selection without myc rearrangement. Cancer 1990; 65:1345–1349.
94. Ilowite NT, Fligner CL, Ochs HD, Brichacek B, Harada S, Haas JE, et al. Pulmonary angiitis with atypical lymphoreticular infiltrates in Wiskott-Aldrich syndrome: possible relationship to lymphomatoid granulomatosis and EBV infection. Clin Immunol Immunopathol 1986; 41:479–484.
95. Colby TV. Central nervous system lymphomatoid granulomatosis in AIDS? Hum Pathol 1989; 20:301–302.
96. Bekassy AN, Cameron R, Garwicz S, Laurin S, Wiebe T. Lymphomatoid granulomatosis during treatment of acute lymphoblastic lymphoma in a 6 year old girl. Am J Paed Hematol-Oncol 1985; 7:377–380.
97. Naschitz JE, Yeshurun D, Grishkan A, Boss JH. Lymphomatoid granulomatosis of the lung in a patient with agnogenic myeloid metaplasia. Respiration 1984; 45:316–320.
98. Imai Y, Yamamoto K, Suzuki K, Tohda S, Miki T, Nakamura Y, et al. Lymphomatoid granulomatosis (LYG) occurring a patient with follicular lymphoma during remission. Jpn J Clin Hematol 1992; 33:507–513.
99. Swerdlow SH. Post-transplant lymphoproliferative disorders: a morphologic, phenotypic and genotypic spectrum of disease. Histopathology 1992; 20:373–385.
100. Burke MM. Complications of heart and lung transplantation and of cardiac surgery. In: Anthony PP, MacSween RNM, eds. Recent Advances in Histopathology. 16th ed. London: Churchill Livingstone, 1994:95–122.
101. Angel CA, Slater DN, Royds JA, Nelson SN, Bleehen SS. Epstein-Barr virus in cutaneous lymphomatoid granulomatosis. Histopathology 1994; 25:545–548.
102. Rubin LA, Little AH, Kolin A, Keystone EC. Lymphomatoid granulomatosis involving the gastrointestinal tract. Two case reports and a review of the literature. Gastroenterology 1983; 84:829–833.
103. Kleinschmidt-DeMasters BK, Filley CM, Bitter MA. Central nervous system angiocentric, angiodestructive T-cell lymphoma (lymphomatoid granulomatosis). Surg Neurol 1992; 37:130–137.
104. Schmalzl F, Gasser RW, Weiser G, Zur Nedden D. Lymphomatoid granulomatosis with primary manifestation in the skeletal muscular system. Klin Wochenschr 1982; 60:311–316.
105. Feinberg SM, Leslie KO, Colby TV. Bladder outlet obstruction by so-called lymphomatoid granulomatosis (angiocentric lymphoma). J Urol 1987; 137:989–990.
106. Bernstein ML, Reece E, de Chadarevian JP, Koch PA. Bone marrow transplantation in lymphomatoid granulomatosis. Report of a case. Cancer 1986; 58:969–972.
107. Sabourin JC, Kanavaros P, Briere J, Lescs M, Petrella T, Zafrani ES, et al. Epstein-Barr virus (EBV) genomes and EBV-encoded latent membrane protein (LMP) in pulmonary lymphomas occurring in nonimmunocompromised patients. Am J Surg Pathol 1993; 17:995–1002.
108. Iuchi K, Ichimiya A, Akashi A, Mizuta t, Lee YE, Tada H, et al. Non-Hodgkin's lymphoma of the pleural cavity developing from long standing pyothorax. Cancer 1987; 60:1771–1775.
109. Iuchi K, Aozasa K, Yamato S. Non-Hodgkin's lymphomas of the pleural cavity developing from long-standing pyothorax. Summary of clinical and pathological findings in thirty-seven cases. Jpn J Clin Oncol 1989; 19:249–257.
110. Martin A, Capron F, Liguory-Brunard M, DeFrejacques C, Pluot M, Diebold J. Epstein-Barr virus-associated primary malignant lymphomas of the pleural cavity occurring in longstanding pleural chronic inflammation. Hum Pathol 1994; 25:1314–1318.
111. Hsu NY, Chen CY, Pan ST, Hsu CP. Pleural non-Hodgkin's lymphoma arising in a patient with a chronic pyothorax. Thorax 1996; 51:103–104.
112. Fukayama M, Ibuka T, Hayashi Y. Epstein-Barr virus in pyothorax-associated pleural lymphoma. Am J Pathol 1993; 143:1044–1049.

113. Ohsawa M, Tomita Y, Kanno H, Iuchi K, Kawbata Y, Hikotara H, et al. Role of Epstein-Barr virus in pleural lymphomagenesis. Mod Pathol 1995; 8:848–853.
114. Nakamura S, Sasajima Y, Koshikawa T, Kitoh K, Kato M, Ueda R, et al. Ki-1 (CD30) positive anaplastic large cell lymphoma of T-cell phenotype developing in association with long-standing tuberculous pyothorax: report of a case with detection of Epstein-Barr genome in the tumour cells. Hum Pathol 1995; 26:1382–1385.
115. Demirer T, Dail DH, Aboulafia DM. Four varied cases of intravascular lymphomatosis and a literature review. Cancer 1994; 73:1738–1745.
116. Takamura K, Nasuhara Y, Mishina T, Matsuda T, Nishimura M, Kawakami Y, et al. Intravascular lymphomatosis diagnosed by transbronchial lung biopsy. Eur Respir J 1997; 10:955–957.
117. Keller AR, Hochholzer L, Castleman B. Hyaline-vascular and plasma-cell types of giant lymph node hyperplasia of the mediastinum and other locations. Cancer 1972; 29:670–683.
118. Barrie JR, English JC, Müller N. Castleman's disease of the lung: radiographic, high-resolution CT, and pathologic findings. Am J Roentgenol 1996; 166:1055–1056.
119. Oksenhendler E, Duarte M, Soulier J, Cacoub P, Welker Y, Cadranel J, Cazals-Hatem D, et al. Multicentric Castleman's disease in HIV infection: a clinical and pathological study of 20 patients. AIDS 1996; 10:61–67.

6

Rare Pulmonary Tumors and Borderline Malignancies

CESAR A. MORAN

Armed Forces Institute of Pathology
Washington, D.C.

SAUL SUSTER

Baptist Hospital of Miami
University of Miami School of Medicine
Miami, Florida

In addition to unusual morphologic variants of bronchogenic carcinoma, a number of rare primary pulmonary neoplasms have also been described. These may be separated into four general categories: (1) unusual epithelial neoplasms, (2) tumors derived from ectopic or embryologically misplaced tissues, (3) tumors of unknown histogenesis, and (4) mixed epithelial/mesenchymal neoplasms.

I. Unusual Epithelial Tumors of the Lung

The tumors grouped under this designation include mucinous (so-called "colloid") carcinoma of the lung and salivary gland–type tumors of the lung.

A. Mucin-Rich (So-Called "Colloid") Carcinoma

This family of tumors appears to represent a separate entity not yet fully recognized in any of the World Health Organization (WHO) classification of lung tumors. Therefore, controversies regarding their proper designation still exist (1–9). Lung tumors that were characterized by abundant mucinous material and the presence of columnar epithelium lining the alveolar walls were described in the literature under the designation of mucinous cystadenoma or mucinous cystic tumors (1,3–5). However, because of apparently indolent follow-up, the term carcinoma was not used. In 1991, in a report of 11 cases, Graeme-Cook and Mark (7) described tumors essentially similar to those previously reported; however, the authors designated those tumors as of "borderline malignancy." We have more recently described 24 patients with a tumor showing histologically similar features (8). In our cases, however, some of the patients developed metastatic lesions to bone, lymph node, and/or brain. Because of their demonstrated malignant potential and capability for metastasis, we currently prefer to designate these lesions as mucin-rich carcinomas, akin to similar lesions originating from the gastrointestinal tract, ovaries, and breast that have been commonly designated as "colloid" carcinoma. The tumors are characterized histologically by destruction of the pulmonary architecture with large lakes of mucin and, in some areas, clusters or singly scattered malignant epithelial cells floating in the mucin (Fig. 1). Most of these tumors are peripheral in location and amenable to surgical resection, which, when complete, appears to be curative.

The main differential diagnosis is with metastatic carcinoma from the ovary, gastrointestinal tract, or breast. In this regard, a complete and detailed clinical history and thorough clinical investigation are critical for diagnosis.

B. Salivary Gland–Type Tumors

Salivary gland–type tumors of the lung represent a group of unusual lesions bearing histological features that are virtually indistinguishable from their salivary gland counterparts (10–19). The majority of these tumors occur in adult individuals. However, cases in children have also been described.

Adenoid Cystic Carcinoma

Adenoid cystic carcinoma of the lung will show similar histologic features to their salivary gland counterparts (10). In a recent study, we identified three growth patterns in these tumors: cribriform (cylindromatous), tubular, and solid (11). The cylindromatous growth pattern, which is the one most frequently encountered is characterized by nests or islands of tumor cells containing sharply outlined luminal spaces often filled with mucinous material and separated by collagen bands of variable thickness (Fig. 2). On higher magnification, the gland-like areas are composed of a double layer of cells, which show round nuclei with clear nuclear outlines and scant eosinophilic cytoplasm and are devoid of mitotic activity. In the tubular growth pattern, there is a proliferation of small tubular structures also composed of two cell layers with round nuclei and clear cytoplasm. In the solid pattern, the tumor forms monotonous sheets of cells similar to those previously described. However, mitotic figures are more often seen and the cells may display cellular atypia. The cells in these tumors display a myoepithelial immunophenotype; i.e., they coexpress keratin and actin antibodies. The most important feature for assessing clinical outcome in these patients is the clinical staging of the tumor at the time of diagnosis. The main differential diagnosis is with a late metastasis from a salivary gland pri-

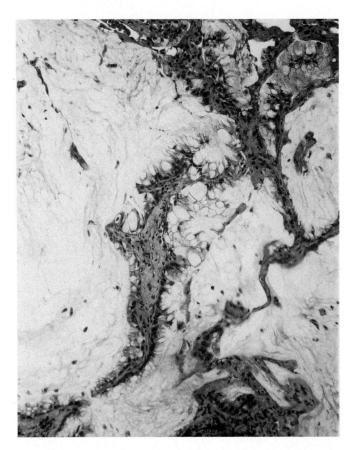

Figure 1 Mucinous ("colloid") carcinoma of the lung showing cystic spaces lined by mucin-secreting epithelium and few scattered epithelial cells floating in the mucin.

mary. Thorough clinical history and physical examination are therefore mandatory prior to making a diagnosis of primary adenoid cystic carcinoma of the lung.

Acinic Cell Carcinoma (Fechner Tumor)

Acinic cell carcinoma of lung is a rare tumor type that may also show different growth patterns including acinar, papillocystic, and oncocytic (12). The acinar growth pattern is the most common and is characterized by sheets of round to oval cells with prominent clear granular cytoplasm and small nuclei that are generally displaced towards the periphery. In the papillocystic variant the tumor cells form cytic structures occasionally containing small intraluminal papillary tufts. In the oncocytic variant the cells show a more eosinophilic granular cytoplasm with prominent nesting pattern reminiscent of a neuroendocrine neoplasm. Histochemical

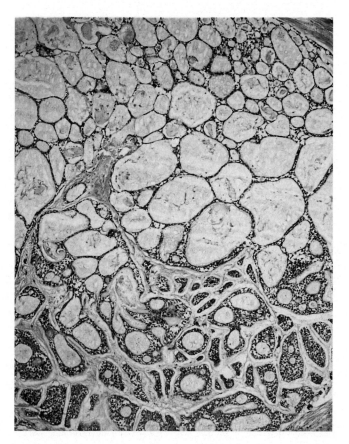

Figure 2 Cylindromatous pattern in adenoid cystic carcinoma of the bronchus.

stains for periodic acid-Schiff (PAS) show strong positive cytoplasmic staining. Antibodies that will show a positive reaction in acinic cell carcinoma include keratin, alpha-1-antichymotrypsin, and amylase. Electron microscopic studies represent the most definitive means for diagnosis and will demonstrate intracellular-zymogen granules (12,15,16). The differential diagnosis for these tumors includes a metastasis from a signet ring cell carcinoma and oncocytic carcinoid. The tumors appear to follow an indolent course. Complete surgical resection is the treatment of choice.

Salivary Gland–Type Mixed Tumor

These tumors by definition are characterized by a biphasic cellular proliferation composed of an epithelial/myoepithelial component admixed with a chondromyxoid stromal component (13). Three growth patterns have been described for these tumors: (1) the classical pattern, which shows the characteristic chondromyxoid stroma with epithelial proliferation in the form of glandular structures; (2) the solid

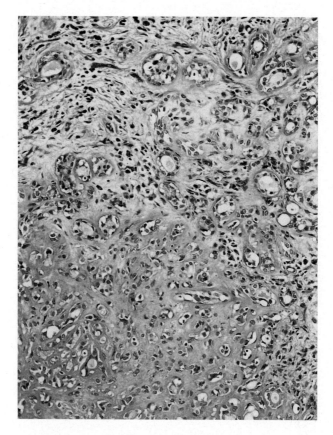

Figure 3 Solid variant of salivary gland–type mixed tumor showing proliferation of small ductular structures surrounded by myoepithelial cells.

variant, characterized by a more solid myoepithelial proliferation; and (3) the malignant variant, in which the cellular proliferation shows atypical features (Fig. 3). Interestingly, the presence of mature cartilage in mixed tumors of the lung is not as common as in mixed tumors of the salivary glands. The cases in which there is malignant transformation are characterized by necrosis, cellular atypia with increased mitotic activity, and vascular invasion. The tumor cells characteristically show features of myoepithelial differentiation, with coexpression of keratin and muscle-specific actin. Other immunohistochemical stains that may be positive include vimentin, S-100 protein, and glial fibrillary acid protein (GFAP) (17). The main differential diagnosis includes adenoid cystic carcinoma or a carcinosarcoma. In the benign cases complete surgical resection is curative, while in those cases that are deemed malignant, the tumors may follow an aggressive course with metastasis outside of the thoracic cavity leading to death.

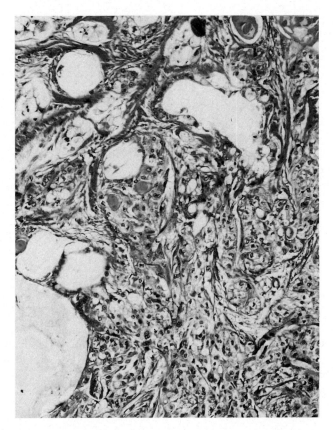

Figure 4   Mucoepidermoid carcinoma of bronchus showing sheets of squamoid cells admixed with glandular structures lined by mucin-secreting cells.

Mucoepidermoid Carcinoma

Mucoepidermoid carcinoma represents the most common type of salivary gland–type tumor of the lung (18). They can be subdivided into two prognostic categories: low- and high-grade malignancy. The low-grade malignant tumors are characterized by a solid proliferation of oval to polygonal cells with distinct cell borders, round to oval nuclei, and prominent nucleoli. These cells may show a distinct clear cytoplasm or appear squamoid with intercellular bridges. Admixed with these elements are scattered goblet cells that may be seen lining glandular structures (Fig. 4). Tumors of high-grade malignancy are those characterized by areas of necrosis, cellular atypia, and increase mitotic activity. The most important differential diagnosis includes either adenocarcinoma, squamous cell carcinoma, or adenosquamous carcinoma.

The prognosis for the tumors of low-grade malignancy is good, and complete surgical resection is the treatment of choice. However, for tumors of high-grade malignancy, the course may be more aggressive with recurrence and metastasis.

Epithelial-Myoepithelial Carcinoma

This is an extremely rare form of salivary gland–type lung tumor characterized by a glandular proliferation composed of oval cells with distinct cell borders, round to oval nuclei, and abundant clear cytoplasm (14,19). Mitotic activity, cellular atypia, necrosis, and hemorrhage are absent. This is yet another tumor that shows a myoepithelial phenotype, i.e., coexpression of keratin and actin filaments in the tumor cells.

The prognosis for these tumors is difficult to determine since only a few cases have been described in the literature. The few cases reported so far appear to indicate that complete surgical resection may be the only treatment necessary.

II. Tumors Derived from Ectopic or Embryologically Displaced Tissues

This group of unusual lung neoplasms is composed of tumors showing features of differentiation along cell lines that are not normally expected to be present in the lung, such as glomus cells, meningothelial cells, thymic epithelium, melanocytes, and ganglionic cells (20–38).

A. Pulmonary Meningioma

Primary pulmonary meningiomas are unusual neoplasms that have been rarely documented in the lung and have been the object only of sporadic case reports (20–26). We recently analyzed 10 such cases (26) in 6 men and 4 women between the ages of 30 and 72 years. Clinically, the majority of these patients were asymptomatic. Histologically, the tumors were characterized by the proliferation of plump, oval to spindle-shaped cells arranged in lobules with the characteristic whorled pattern (Fig. 5). The cells showed indistinct cell borders, pale eosinophilic cytoplasm, and round to oval nuclei with inconspicuous nucleoli. Psammoma bodies were seen in most cases. The coexpression of vimentin and epithelial membrane antigen (EMA) was the most distinctive feature. Interestingly, CD-34 may also show focal positivity in pulmonary fibrous meningiomas.

The most important differential diagnosis to consider outside of a metastatic meningioma is intrapulmonary solitary fibrous tumor. The presence of transitional areas towards the periphery of the lesion, a prominent whorled pattern, psammoma bodies, and strong EMA positivity will lead to the correct diagnosis. Our experience with these tumors appears to indicate that surgical excision alone may be curative in most cases.

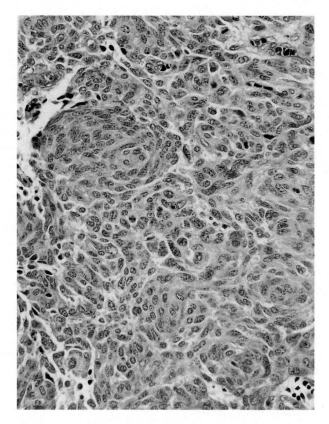

Figure 5 Pulmonary meningioma showing bland oval to spindle cells adopting a whorled pattern.

B. Intrapulmonary Thymoma

These tumors are relatively uncommon within the pulmonary parenchyma and are presumably derived from foci of ectopic thymic tissue sequestered within the lung (27–29). For the most part, such tumors have been the subject of isolated case reports. We recently reported our experience with a series of eight primary intrapulmonary thymomas (29). Radiologically, the tumors often presented as well-circumscribed, intraparenchymatous nodules that measured up to 10 cm in greatest diameter. Histologically, all varieties of thymoma can be observed, including epithelial-rich, lymphocyte-rich, and spindle cell types (Fig. 6). The tumors characteristically exhibit a lobulated low-power appearance with a biphasic cell population composed of epithelial cells admixed with lymphocytes. The differential diagnosis for these tumors includes malignant lymphoma, monophasic synovial sarcoma, solitary fibrous tumor, hemangiopericytoma, and metastases from epithelial malignancies.

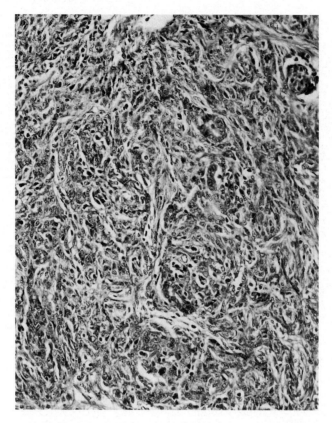

Figure 6 Intrapulmonary thymoma showing admixture of small lymphocytes with scattered thymic epithelial cells.

Keratin stains will highlight the presence of scattered thymic epithelial cells and allow for recognition of the lymphocyte-rich variant. The most important consideration in the differential diagnosis is the possibility of a metastasis from an undetected mediastinal thymoma. The diagnosis of primary intrapulmonary thymoma therefore can only be established after thorough review of radiological and clinical information to rule out the presence of a mediastinal mass. Pulmonary thymomas are usually slow-growing tumors that can be cured by surgical excision alone.

C. Glomus Tumor

Only a few cases of primary glomus tumor of the lung have been described so far (30–32). All cases involved adult patients who presented with nonspecific symptoms and were found to have pulmonary nodules on chest x-rays.

Recently we were able to review two additional cases of primary pulmonary glomus tumor (32). The patients were middle aged, asymptomatic, and presented

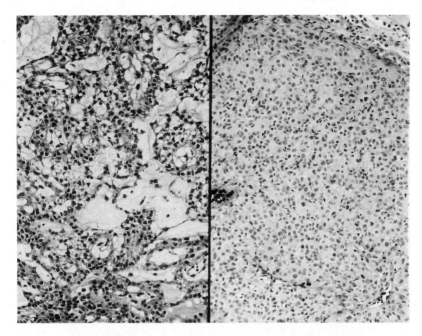

Figure 7   Intrapulmonary glomus tumor: lace-like growth pattern admixed with ectatic vessels (left); higher magnification showing uniform round cell population (right).

with a solitary intrapulmonary nodule. The tumors were characterized by a monotonous proliferation of round cells with round to oval, centrally placed nuclei surrounded by abundant amphophilic cytoplasm. The tumor cells showed a tendency to grow in sheets and were separated by multiple dilated, often cavernous thick-walled vessels (Fig. 7). Immunostains demonstrate a smooth muscle phenotype, with strong positivity of the tumor cells for vimentin and actin. Other markers including keratin or vascular markers are negative. It appears that complete surgical resection is the only treatment required in the management of these tumors.

D. Malignant Melanoma

The existence of malignant melanoma in the lung, although rare, has been reported in the literature (33–36). The tumors usually occur in adults between the ages of 29 and 80 years. Clinically, the patients may be asymptomatic or present with symptoms of bronchial obstruction. Most tumors are located centrally, in relation to the bronchus or trachea, and generally exhibit a polypoid, exophytic growth into the lumen. Recently, we reported our experience with eight cases of primary malignant melanoma of the lung in adult patients (36). The histologic features of these tumors are similar to those arising elsewhere. The tumor cells may be epithelioid, spindle, or pleomorphic, and may grow forming sheets or nests (Fig. 8). The tumor cells are

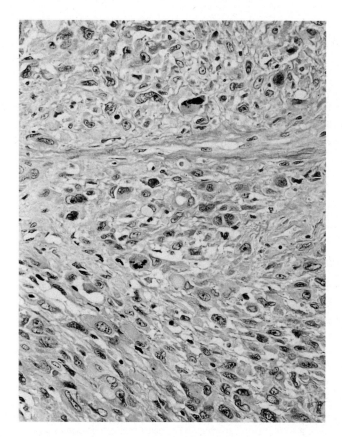

Figure 8 Malignant melanoma of bronchus. The tumor is composed of a pleomorphic spindle cell proliferation displaying cytologic atypia and mitotic activity.

frequently pigmented, a feature that obviously facilitates the diagnosis. The differential diagnosis includes other more common primary lung tumors such as pleomorphic carcinoma or carcinoid tumor, or a metastasis from other pleomorphic or spindle cell neoplasms. Demonstration of immunoreactivity for S-100 protein and HMB45 will serve to support the diagnosis in equivocal cases. In general the prognosis for these tumors is very poor. In our series the median survival was 14 months, and the patients developed widespread metastases.

E. Ganglioneuroblastoma

This is an exceedingly rare tumor, which to our knowledge had been reported only once in the literature (37). We recently were able to study two additional cases of primary ganglioneuroblastoma of the lung (38). Our cases occurred in two adult females, one asymptomatic and the other with symptoms and signs most consistent with a MEN syndrome, including gastric ulceration and hypercalcemia. In both cases the tumors extended from the bronchi, were well circumscribed, firm and homogenous, measuring between 3 and 5 cm in greatest dimension. Histologically the tumors were characterized by the presence of neurophil and neuroblastomatous components in association with mature ganglion cells. Stains for neurofilaments, S-100 protein, and NSE generally showed a positive reaction. Surgical resection appears to be the only treatment necessary for those patients whose tumors are in early stages and amenable to complete resection.

III.   Tumors of Uncertain Histogenesis

This group of tumors includes sclerosing hemangioma, alveolar adenoma, and clear cell ("sugar") tumor of the lung.

A.   Sclerosing Hemangioma

The currently accepted designation for this tumor is that of alveolar pneumocytoma (39–47). Although the tumor generally presents as an asymptomatic solitary pulmonary lesion, in rare occasions multiple lesions and extension of the tumor to regional lymph nodes have been described. The tumor is characterized by a dual cell population: one cell type is composed of round to polygonal, clear cells with abundant cytoplasm and round to oval nuclei with inconspicuous nucleoli and without marked cellular atypia; the second cell population is composed of smaller, round-to-oval cells with hyperchromatic nuclei and scant cytoplasm (Fig. 9). The tumor cells may adopt a variety of growth patterns, including papillary, angiomatous, solid, and sclerotic. Immunohistochemical studies have demonstrated consistent expression of EMA and vimentin in the tumor cells. Surfactant apoprotein is another marker that has been demonstrated in the tumor cells, supporting their pneumocytic lineage. These tumors are benign, and complete surgical resection is the treatment of choice.

B.   Alveolar Adenoma

This term was introduced to describe a tumor that in the past may have been regarded as a form of pulmonary lymphangioma (48). The tumor is exceedingly rare, and only a few reports have been published. The tumors are generally asymptomatic and present grossly as well-circumscribed nodules with hemorrhagic and cystic areas that measure from 1 to 2.5 cm in greatest dimension. Histologically the tumors are composed of cystic structures lined by alveolar pneumocytes, some of them showing a hobnail-shaped appearance. Collections of foamy macrophages may be seen within these cystic structures. No mitotic activity or cellular atypia is seen in any of these cases. The tumor cells may show positive staining for CEA and keratin antibodies.

The most important differential diagnosis is with a vascular neoplasm such as lymphangioma or epithelioid hemangioendothelioma. In this regard the use of vas-

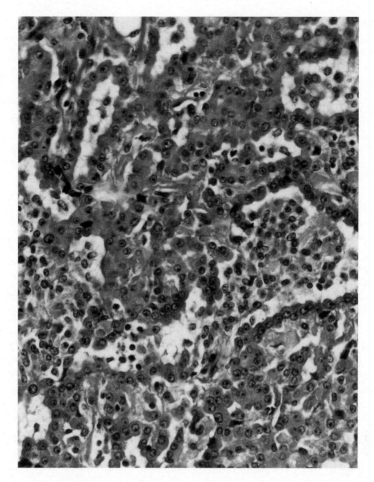

Figure 9   Sclerosing hemangioma (pneumocytoma) of lung showing dual cell population: large round cells with vesicular nuclei and abundant cytoplasm in the center, surrounded by smaller cells with hyperchromatic nuclei and scant cytoplasm in the periphery.

cular markers such as factor VIII or CD-34 may be of help since alveolar adenomas are negative for such markers. Complete surgical resection is the treatment of choice.

C.   Clear Cell ("Sugar") Tumor

This is an unusual neoplasm that affects adult individuals without predilection for any sex or lung segment. Most of the patients are asymptomatic, and the tumor is usually found on routine physical examination. The tumors are usually well-circumscribed with a homogeneous appearance (49–55). Histologically they are characterized by a solid proliferation of medium- to large-sized cells with eccentric nuclei and prominent clear cytoplasm admixed with numerous dilated vascular spaces. The tumor does not show mitotic activity and/or necrosis. Histochemical stains for PAS demonstrates abundant cytoplasmic glycogen. These tumors are characteristically positive for vimentin and HMB-45 and will be negative for S-100 protein and epithelial markers. Because of the presence of clear cells, the possibility of a metastasis from a clear cell tumor from another site should be considered in the differential diagnosis.

IV. Mixed Mesenchymal/Epithelial Neoplasms

These represent a group of relatively unusual tumors characterized by a biphasic cellular composition. These tumors represent less than 2% of all primary pulmonary neoplasms. The two main types include pulmonary blastomas and carcinosarcomas.

A. Pulmonary Blastoma

This is an uncommon neoplasm that has been reported in the literature under several names (56–60). In a large study from the AFIP, the tumors were found to affect mainly adult individuals in the fourth decade of life. However, the tumor has also been reported in children younger than 5 years. Clinically, the symptoms may vary depending on the location of the lesion. For those located centrally, the patients may present with bronchial obstruction, cough, hemoptysis, etc., while those presenting with peripheral tumors may be either asymptomatic or have symptoms of chest pain. Histologically the tumors may show two distinct growth patterns. One is composed exclusively of a glandular type of proliferation in which the tumor resembles fetal lung at approximately 9–11 weeks of gestation, also known as fetal type well-differentiated adenocarcinoma or monophasic blastoma (Fig. 10), and another one is characterized by a proliferation of immature glands admixed with an immature spindle cell stromal component, or biphasic blastoma. The glandular proliferation is composed of pseudostratified, nonciliated columnar cells with clear cytoplasm. An important diagnostic feature is the presence of squamous morules admixed with the glandular proliferation. The tumor characteristically does not show marked cellular pleomorphism and/or mitotic activity in the glandular elements. The spindle cell proliferation in the biphasic tumors may show prominent cellular atypia and mitotic activity. The tumor will show positive staining for epithelial markers such as keratin, EMA, and CEA. Interestingly, chromogranin may show positive staining in the squamous morules.

The differential diagnosis for the predominantly monophasic tumors is that of a well-differentiated adenocarcinoma of the conventional type or a metastasis from another source such as prostate or endometrium. When the tumor is biphasic, they may be mistaken for a spindle cell sarcoma or carcinosarcoma. However, neither of those tumors shows the characteristic glandular proliferation resembling fetal lung or the squamous morules characteristic of blastomas.

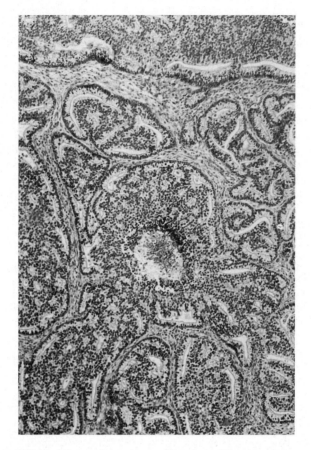

Figure 10 Pulmonary blastoma showing proliferation of glandular structures resembling fetal lung at 9–11 weeks of gestation.

Complete surgical resection possibly followed by chemotherapy and radiation therapy has been advocated as treatment for these tumors. It is believed that monophasic blastomas behave less aggressively than biphasic ones.

B. Pulmonary Carcinosarcoma

We define carcinosarcoma as a tumor showing light microscopic evidence of mesenchymal as well as epithelial differentiation. Clinically, the tumor may present either centrally as an endobronchial mass or in the periphery of the lung. There is a male:female ratio of 3:1. The tumor affects mainly adult individuals in the seventh decade of life. Grossly, the tumors are solitary and can measure from 1 to >20 cm in greatest dimension, and may show areas of necrosis and/or hemorrhage (61–64). The tumors may show different components, however, classically, there will be areas of conventional squamous cell carcinoma or adenocarcinoma in association with a sarcomatous element in the form of chondrosarcoma, osteosarcoma, rhabdomyosarcoma, leiomyosarcoma, etc.

The most important differential diagnosis is with pleomorphic carcinoma or spindle cell carcinoma of the lung (65,66). This latter tumor may show a predominantly spindle cell proliferation with multinucleated giant cells. However, pleomorphic carcinoma will not show conventional areas of rhabdomyosarcoma, chondro, or osteosarcoma. In addition, the spindle cell proliferation in pleomorphic carcinoma usually shows positive staining for epithelial markers such as keratin or EMA. There is no specific treatment for this malignant tumor. Surgical resection with combined chemotherapy and radiation therapy has been advocated, however, the patients follow a fatal course with death within one year after diagnosis in the majority of cases.

References

1. Kragel PJ, Devaney KO, Meth BM, Linnoila I, Frierson HF, Travis WD. Mucinous cystadenoma of the lung: a report of two cases with immunohistochemical and ultrastructural analysis. Arch Pathol Lab Med 1991; 114:1053–1056.
2. Traub B. Mucinous cystadenoma of the lung [letter]. Arch Pathol Lab Med 1991; 115:740.
3. Dison AY, Moran JF, Wesselius LJ, McGregor DH. Pulmonary mucinous cystic tumor: case report with review of the literature. Am J Surg Pathol 1993; 17:722–728.
4. Higashima M, Doi O, Kodama K, Yokouchi H, Tateishi R. Cystic mucinous adenocarcinoma of the lung: two cases of cystic variant of mucinous-producing lung adenocarcinoma. Chest 1992; 101:763–766.
5. Davison AM, Lowe JW, Da Costa P. Adenocarcinoma arising in a mucinous cystadenoma of the lung. Thorax 1992; 47:129–130.
6. Devaney K, Kragel P, Travis WD. Mucinous cystadenocarcinoma of the lung: a tumor of low malignant potential [abstract]. Am J Clin Pathol 1989; 92:524.
7. Graeme-Cook F, Mark EJ. Pulmonary mucinous cystic tumors of borderline malignancy. Hum Pathol 1991; 22:185–190.
8. Moran CA, Hochholzer L, Fishback N, Koss MN. Mucinous (so-called colloid) carcinomas of the lung. Mod Pathol 1992; 5:634–638.
9. Moran CA. Mucin-rich tumors of the lung. Adv Anat Pathol 1995; 2(5):299–305.
10. Moran CA. Primary salivary gland-type tumors of the lung. Sem Diag Pathol 1995; 12:106–122.
11. Moran CA, Suster S, Koss MN. Primary adenoid cystic carcinoma of the lung: a clinicopathologic and immunohistochemical study of 16 cases. Cancer 1994; 73:1390–1397.
12. Moran CA, Suster S, Koss MN. Acinic cell carcinoma of the lung (Fechner tumor): a clinicopathologic, immunohistochemical, and ultrastructural study of five cases. Am J Surg Pathol 1992; 16:1039–1050.
13. Moran CA, Suster S, Askin FB, Koss MN. Benign and malignant salivary gland-type mixed tumors of the lung: a clinicopathologic and immunohistochemical study of eight cases. Cancer 1994; 73:2481–2490.
14. Wilson RW, Moran CA. Epithelial-myoepithelial carcinoma of the lung: immunohistochemical and ultrastructural observations and review of the literature. Hum Pathol 1997; 28:631–635.
15. Fechner RE, Bentnick BR, Askew JB, Jr. Acinic cell tumor of the lung: a histologic and ultrastructural study. Cancer 1972; 29:501–508.
16. Katz DR, Bubis JJ. Acinic cell tumor of the bronchus. Cancer 1976; 38:830–832.
17. Sakamoto H, Uda H, Tanaka T, et al. Pleomorphic adenoma in the periphery of the lung: report of a case and review of the literature. Arch Pathol Lab Med 1991; 115:393–396.

18. Yousem S, Hochholzer L. Mucoepidermoid tumours of the lung. Cancer 1983; 51:1505–1509.
19. Nistal M, Garcia-Viera M, Martinez-Garcia C, Paniagua R. Epithelial-myoepithelial tumor of the bronchus. Am J Surg Pathol 1994; 18:421–425.
20. Unger PD, Geller SA, Anderson PJ. Pulmonary lesions in a patient with neurofibromatosis. Arch Pathol Lab Med 1984; 108:654–657.
21. Kemnitz P, Sporman H, Heinrich P. Meningioma of lung: first report with light and electron microscopic findings. Ultrast Pathol 1982; 3:359–365.
22. Kodama K, Osamu D, Higashiyama H, Horai T, Tateishi R, Nakagawa H. Primary and metastatic pulmonary meningioma. Am J Surg Pathol 1991; 67:1412–1417.
23. Chumas JC, Lorelle CA. Pulmonary meningioma. Am J Surg Pathol 1982; 6:795–801.
24. Drlicek M, Grisold W, Lorber J, Hackl H, Wuketich S, Jellinger K. Pulmonary meningioma. Am J Surg Pathol 1991; 15:455–459.
25. Shuanghoti S, Panyaathanya R. Ectopic meningioma. Arch Otolaryngol Head Neck Surg 1973; 98:102–105.
26. Moran CA, Hochholzer L, Rush W, Koss MN. Primary intrapulmonary meningiomas: a clinicopathologic and immunohistochemical study of ten cases. Cancer 1996; 78:2328–2333.
27. Kung M, Locke SL, So SY, et al. Intrapulmonary thymoma. Report of two cases. Thorax 1985; 40:471–474.
28. Green WR, Pressoir R, Gumbs RV, et al. Intrapulmonary thymoma. Arch Pathol Lab Med 1997; 111:1074–1076.
29. Moran CA, Suster S, Fishback NF, Koss MN. Intrapulmonary thymomas: a clinicopathologic and immunohistochemical study of eight cases. Am J Surg Pathol 1995; 19:304–312.
30. Brooks JJ, Miettinen M, Virtanen I. Desmin immunoreactivity in glomus tumors. Am J Clin Pathol 1987; 87:292–294.
31. Tang C, Toker C, Foris NP, et al. Glomangioma of the lung. Am J Surg Pathol 1978; 2:103–109.
32. Koss MN, Hochholzer L, Moran CA. Pulmonary glomus tumors: a clinicopathologic and immunohistochemical study of two cases. Mod Pathol 1998; 11:253–258.
33. Jennings TA, Axiotis CA, Kress Y, et al. Primary malignant melanoma of the lower respiratory tract. Am J Clin Pathol 1990; 94:649–655.
34. Gephardt GN. Malignant melanoma of the bronchus. Hum Pathol 1981; 12:671–73.
35. Jensen OA, Egedorf J. Primary malignant melanoma of the lung. Scand J Respir Dis 1967; 48:127–135.
36. Wilson RW, Moran CA. Primary malignant melanoma of the lung: a clinicopathologic and immunohistochemical study of eight cases. Am J Surg Pathol 1997; 21:1196–1202.
37. Cooney TP. Primary pulmonary ganglioneuroblastoma in an adult: maturation, involution, and the immune response. Histopathology 1981; 5:451–63.
38. Hochholzer L, Moran CA, Koss MN. Primary pulmonary ganglioneuroblastoma: a clinicopathologic and immunohistochemical study of two cases. Ann Diag Pathol 1998; in press.
39. Liebow AA, Hubbell DS. Sclerosing hemangioma (histiocytoma, xanthoma) of the lung. Cancer 1956; 9:53–75.
40. Katzenstein AL, Gmelich JT, Carrington CB. Sclerosing hemangioma of the lung: a clinicopathologic study of 51 cases. Am J Surg Pathol 1980; 4:343–356.
41. Shimosato Y. Lung tumors of uncertain histogenesis. Sem Diag Pathol 1995; 12:185–192.
42. Yousem SA, Wick MR, Singh G, et al. So-called sclerosing hemangioma of the lung. An epithelial tumor composed of immunohistochemically heterogeneous cells. Am J Surg Pathol 1988; 12:582–590.
43. Leong AS-Y, Chan KW, Senevirate HSK. A morphological and immunohistochemical study of 25 cases of so-called sclerosing hemangioma of lung. Histopathology 1995; 27:121–128.
44. Haimoto H, Tsutsumi Y, Nagaura H, et al. Immunohistochemical study of so-called sclerosing hemangioma of the lung. Virchows Arch A [Pathol Anat] 1985; 407:419–430.
45. Huszar M, Suster S, Herczeg E, Geiger B. Sclerosing hemangioma of the lung: Immunohistochemical demonstration of mesenchymal origin using antibodies to tissue specific intermediate filaments. Cancer 1986; 58:2422–2427.

46. Tanaka I, Inoue M, Matsui Y, et al. A case of pneumocytoma (so-called sclerosing hemangioma) with lymph node metastasis. Jpn J Clin Oncol 1986; 16:77–86.
47. Moran CA, Zeren H, Koss MN. Sclerosing hemangioma: granulomatous variant. Arch Pathol Lab Med 1994; 118:1028–1030.
48. Yousem SA, Hochholzer L. Alveolar adenoma. Hum Pathol 1986; 17:1066–1070.
49. Liebow AA, Castleman B. Benign clear cell tumors of the lung. Am J Pathol 1963; 43:13 [Abstract].
50. Gal AA, Koss MN, Hochholzer L, Chejfec G. An immunohistochemical study of benign clear cell (sugar) tumor of the lung. Arch Pathol Lab Med 1991; 105:1034–1038.
51. Gaffey MJ, Mills SE, Askin FB, et al. Clear cell tumor of the lung: a clinicopathologic, immunohistochemical, and ultrastructural study of eight cases. Am J Surg Pathol 1990; 14:248–259.
52. Sale GE, Kulander BG. Benign clear cell tumor of lung with necrosis. Cancer 1976; 37:2355–2358.
53. Hoch WS, Patchefsky AS, Takeda M, et al. Benign clear cell tumor of the lung. An ultrastructural study. Cancer 1974; 33:1328–1336.
54. Becher NH, Soifer I. Benign clear cell (sugar tumor) of the lung. Cancer 1971; 27:712–719.
55. Gaffey MJ, Mills SE, Askin FB, et al. Clear cell tumor of the lung. Immunohistochemical and ultrastructural evidence of melanogenesis. Am J Surg Pathol 1991; 15:644–653.
56. Berho M, Moran CA, Suster S. Malignant mixed epithelial/mesenchymal neoplasms of the lung. Sem Diag Pathol 1995; 12(2):123–139.
57. Nakatani Y, Dickersin R, Mark E. Pulmonary endodermal tumor resembling fetal lung: a clinicopathologic study of five cases with immunohistochemical and ultrastructural characterization. Hum Pathol 1990; 21:1095–1104.
58. Koss MN, Hochholzer L, O'Leary T. Pulmonary blastomas. Cancer 1991; 67:2368–2381.
59. Yousem SA, Wick MR, Randhawa P, et al. Pulmonary blastoma. An immunohistochemical analysis with comparison with fetal lung in its pseudoglandular stage. Am J Clin Pathol 1990; 94:167–175.
60. Manivel JC, Priest JR, Watterson J, et al. Pleuropulmonary blastoma. The so-called pulmonary blastoma of childhood. Cancer 1988; 62:1516–1526.
61. Saphir O, Vass A. Carcinosarcoma. Am J Cancer 1938; 33:331–361.
62. Bergman M, Ackerman LV, Kemler RL. Carcinosarcoma of the lung. Cancer 1951; 4:919–929.
63. Moore TC. Carcinosarcoma of the lung. Surgery 1961; 50:886–893.
64. Davis MP, Eagan RT, Weiland LH, et al. Carcinosarcoma of the lung: Mayo Clinic experience and response to chemotherapy. Mayo Clin Proc 1984; 59:598–603.
65. Fishback NF, Travis WD, Moran CA, et al. Pleomorphic (spindle/giant cell) carcinoma of the lung. Cancer 1994; 73:2936–2945.
66. Suster S, Huszar M, Herczeg E. Spindle cell squamous carcinoma of the lung. A light microscopic, immunohistochemical and ultrastructural study of a case. Histopathology 1987; 11:871–878.

7

Differential Diagnosis Between Primary and Metastatic Carcinomas

PHILIP T. CAGLE

Baylor College of Medicine
Houston, Texas

The radiographic and clinical presentation of nonpulmonary metastases to the lung may imitate the findings of a primary lung carcinoma (Table 1) (1–4). The primary risk factor for lung cancer—tobacco—is also the primary risk factor for many other solid organ neoplasms, including pancreas, kidney, bladder, and head and neck carcinomas. Therefore, especially in the case of a solitary nodule or an endobronchial mass (2,3), biopsy of the tumor may be warranted to determine the primary site, even if a previous nonpulmonary primary is known. Many metastatic malignancies may mimic lung primaries histopathologically as well, and, especially if there is no clinical history of another known primary, the surgical pathologist is the one who must suggest the possibility of a metastasis.

During a 7½-year-period at The Methodist Hospital in Houston, Texas, we found that 90 of 844 resections of malignancies in the lung or about 11% of the total were metastases from other sites. Of these, 78% were metastatic carcinomas, 14% were sarcomas, and 8% were melanomas. In the great majority of cases, a clinical history of a primary outside the lung was known and the surgery was performed to rule out a second primary in the lung. However, six tumors (7%) were the first manifestation of a nonpulmonary occult primary. Our observations are in agreement with the frequency of solitary pulmonary nodules found to be metastases from occult nonpulmonary primaries in previous series. Of course, pulmonary metastases

Table 1 Approach to Primary Lung Cancer Versus Nonpulmonary Metastasis

Clinical history of previous primary
Gross pattern
Histology: compare with previous primary if available
Histochemistry and immunohistochemistry

from a primary lung tumor also occur and may present as multiple nodules or lymphangitic spread.

Due to its rich vascular and lymphatic supply and the flow of the body's entire blood content through the lungs, the lungs are one of the most frequent sites of metastases from other solid organs. In most cases, metastases to the lungs represent end-stage disease of a known primary cancer and therapeutic intervention is not warranted. Therefore, the frequency with which nonpulmonary metastases occur is not reflected in the surgical archives and the frequency of different types of metastatic cancer removed surgically is different from the frequency of different types of metastatic cancer found at autopsy. The most frequent reasons for biopsy or surgical excision of a nonpulmonary metastasis is to determine if there is a second primary in the lung or to improve survival when metastases are solitary or limited in number in patients with a known nonpulmonary primary. On occasion, the biopsy or surgical excision may be done when the primary cancer is occult.

In our experience, the most frequent primary sites of nonpulmonary metastases to the lung removed at surgery are from breast, colorectal, and renal primaries. Five-year survival after resection of solitary nonpulmonary metastases averages about 30% in most series (5–7). This survival applies to solitary or limited multiple metastases from carcinomas, particularly renal, colorectal, and breast primaries. In our experience, the postsurgical survival of solitary metastases from sarcomas is somewhat better than it is for the carcinomas, but metastases from melanomas have only 14% survival at 3 years postresection. Therefore, if nonpulmonary metastases are solitary or limited in a patient who otherwise has had a successful treatment of his primary tumor, and there is no evidence of metastases to additional sites, resection of the metastasis may be beneficial.

The steps the pathologist should follow in differentiating between a primary lung cancer and a nonpulmonary metastasis are shown in Table 1. Comparison to the histopathology of a known primary is a key step if the slides from the previous primary are available. Immunohistochemistry can play an important role in the differentiation of primary lung carcinomas from nonpulmonary metastases (8–13). Primary lung carcinomas are immunopositive for keratin and, because they are derived from the endoderm, immunopositive for carcinoembryonic antigen (CEA) in most, but not all, cases. This includes small-cell carcinomas that may be difficult to interpret because of their scanty cytoplasm. Immunohistochemical stains that are positive in primary lung cancers are listed in Table 2 (14,15).

Table 2 Immunostains Characteristic of Primary Lung Carcinomas

Typically positive	Sometimes positive
Pan-keratin	Vimentin
Cytokeratin-7	Neuron-specific enolase (NSE)
Epithelial membrane antigen (EMA)	CA 19–9
Carcinoembryonic antigen (CEA)	CA-125
B72.3	BCA225
Leu M-1	DF3
Ber-EP4	

Some antibodies used to identify particular tumors are essentially specific. However, the likelihood in many cases is that immunohistochemistry will not differentiate between a primary lung cancer and a nonpulmonary metastasis due to overlap of immunostaining patterns. Therefore, there is some overlap for many positive immunostains and immunonegative stains contribute limited information except in certain circumstances. A panel of antibodies is often useful, but, even then, may not provide the diagnosis. In these cases, it may be necessary for the pathologist to suggest a differential to the clinician based on the microscopic appearance. The remainder of this chapter examines the various histopathological patterns of nonpulmonary metastases, which may mimic lung primaries and features that may help to distinguish them.

I.   Adenocarcinomas with Acinar or Solid Patterns

The most frequent nonpulmonary metastases by cell type are adenocarcinomas. Metastatic adenocarcinomas may have acinar or solid patterns that may be similar to those of primary lung carcinomas. The use of immunostains for antigens specific to adenocarcinomas from particular primary sites may be helpful in certain situations, for example, prostate or breast carcinoma (16–21). Histopathological and immunohistochemical stains that may be of use in the differentiation of primary lung carcinomas from metastatic carcinomas are shown in Table 3.

II.   Columnar Cells with Lepidic Growth Pattern

Metastatic carcinomas may grow in a lepidic pattern along intact alveolar septa similar to the pattern of growth of primary bronchioloalveolar carcinomas. Most metastases that grow in a lepidic pattern are from colon primaries and, because these tumors are composed of mucin-producing columnar cells, these tumors potentially may recapitulate the appearance of primary bronchioloalveolar carcinomas (Fig. 1) (22). Since both types of carcinoma are derived from endoderm, both colon and lung cancers are typically immunopositive for the same markers, including CEA and

Table 3 Differentiation of Primary Versus Metastatic Adenocarcinomas in the Lung

Favors Primary: Mixed patterns with solid, acinar, and/or bronchioloalveolar components, cytokeratin-7+ and cytokeratin-20−.
Favors Metastasis: Complex or cribriform architecture, nests of very uniform or bland cells, signet ring cells, specific immunostains.
Prostate: Prostate-specific antigen (PSA), Prostate acid phosphatase (PAP).
Breast: Gross cystic disease fluid protein-15 (GCDFP-15), Estrogen receptor (ER), Progesterone receptor (PR).

See also other Tables.

B72.3. Histological features and immunostains that may differentiate between metastatic colon cancer and primary bronchioloalveolar carcinoma are listed in Table 4.

III. Papillary Adenocarcinomas

Primary papillary adenocarcinomas occur in the lung and their classification has been subject to some controversy. Whether these tumors are papillary variants of bronchioloalveolar carcinomas or whether these tumors include a separate subtype

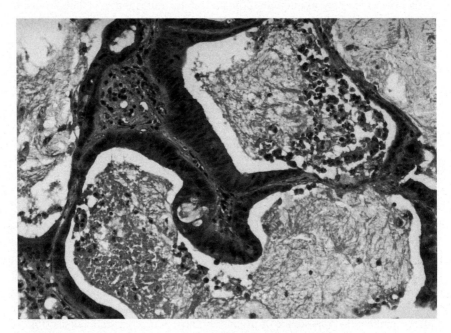

Figure 1 Metastatic adenocarcinoma of the colon growing in a lepidic pattern along intact alveolar septa. (×600)

Table 4 Differentiation of Metastatic Colon Cancer from Bronchioloalveolar Carcinoma

Favors colon metastasis: "Dirty" necrosis (Fig. 2), complex or cribriform pattern
Favors bronchioloalveolar primary: Cytological uniformity, intranuclear inclusions,
  papillary features, immunopositivity for TTF-1, surfactant B

of papillary adenocarcinomas as well as papillary bronchioloalveolar carcinomas, the differential diagnosis remains the same. Papillary adenocarcinomas from many organs can metastasize to the lungs and mimic a primary papillary lung cancer (Fig. 3). Histopathological and immunohistochemical features to distinguish between primary and metastatic papillary carcinomas is given in Table 5 (23–25). Like lung primaries, most papillary transitional cell carcinomas of the bladder are immunopositive for CEA.

IV. Cancers with Clear Cells

Metastatic clear cell carcinoma of the kidney (renal cell carcinoma) is one of the most frequent metastases surgically excised from the lungs and, when solitary, sur-

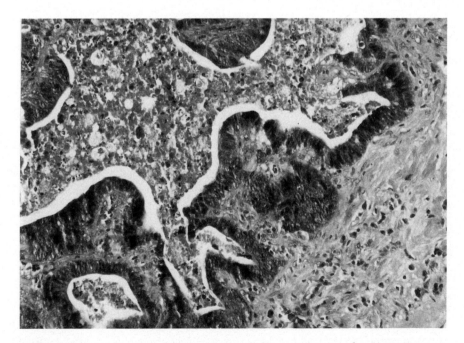

Figure 2 Metastatic adenocarcinoma of the colon showing characteristic "dirty" necrosis with nuclear and cytoplasmic debris. (×600)

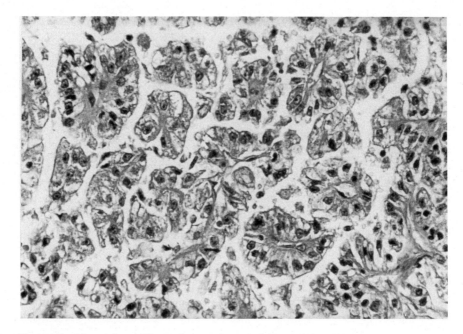

Figure 3 Metastatic papillary adenocarcinoma of the ovary. (×800)

vival may be improved by surgical resection. The clearing of the cytoplasm may be due to glycogen, water, or lipid (Fig. 4).

Primary clear cell carcinomas of the lung are variants of adenocarcinoma or squamous cell carcinoma in which some or all of the malignant cells have clear or foamy cytoplasm (Fig. 5). The clearing of the cytoplasm may be due to glycogen or water, but is not due to lipid. In one large series, 0.3% of 348 primary lung carcinomas were composed purely of clear cells, 4.3% of non-small-cell carcinomas were composed more than 50% of clear cells and 30% of non-small-cell carcinomas had foci of clear cells. Table 6 shows the differentiation of renal cell carcinoma metastases from primary clear cell lung carcinomas by histopathology, histochemical stains, and immunohistochemical stains. Renal cell carcinomas may also have spindle cell, papillary, or granular patterns which makes renal cell carcinoma a differential diagnosis for many histopathological patterns.

Table 5 Papillary Metastatic Versus Papillary Primary Adenocarcinomas in the Lung

Favors primary: Immunopositive for CEA and other markers of primary lung cancer.
Favors metastasis: Immunopositive for thyroglobulin (thyroid primary), CA-125 favors
  ovarian primary but does not rule out lung or gastrointestinal primary, CA19-9 favors
  gastrointestinal primary but does not rule out lung primary.

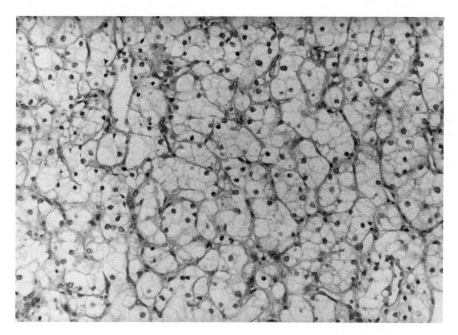

Figure 4 Metastatic renal cell carcinoma composed of comparatively bland clear cells. (×600)

V. Squamous Cell Carcinomas

Squamous cell carcinomas of the head and neck tend to be well-differentiated keratinizing tumors. Most primary squamous cell carcinomas of the lung are less well differentiated and often poorly differentiated. Nevertheless, primary squamous cell carcinomas of the lung may be well differentiated and keratinizing and cannot be differentiated from metastatic squamous cell carcinomas of the head and neck on histopathological grounds. Other metastases, such as metastatic breast carcinoma, may grow as solid nets of cells with abundant cytoplasm and be mistaken for poorly differentiated squamous cell carcinoma (Fig. 6).

VI. Spindle-Cell Tumors

Spindle-cell tumors include sarcomas (primary and metastatic), spindle-cell carcinomas (primary and metastatic), metastatic melanomas, and primary spindle-cell carcinoids. Differences in histopathology may allow differentiation between these tumors and immunohistochemistry may add critical information as shown in Table 7.

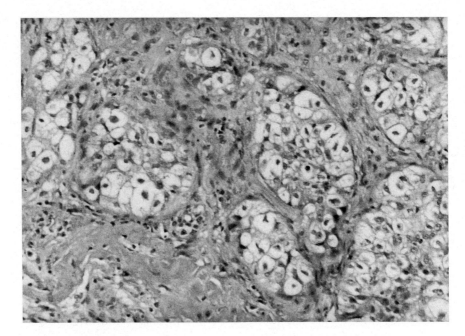

Figure 5   Clear-cell component of primary adenocarcinoma of the lung (×600)

VII. Melanoma

Like renal cell carcinoma, melanoma is notorious for its ability to mimic a variety
of histopathological patterns of other malignancies (26). The primary site of the
melanoma may spontaneously regress or may have been surgically excised years
previously. The presence of obvious cytoplasmic melanin pigment may indicate the
diagnosis, but with amelanotic melanomas immunohistochemistry is often required.
Melanomas are immunopositive for vimentin, HMB-45 and S-100 and immunonegative for keratin.

Table 6   Clear-Cell Carcinomas

Metastatic renal cell carcinoma	Primary clear-cell carcinoma of lung
Keratin + (variable)	+ (strong)
EMA + (strong)	+
Vimentin + (strong)	− (usually)
CEA − (usually)	+ (usually)
RCC antibody +	−
Lipid +	−

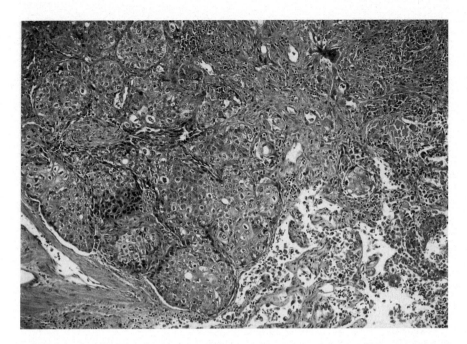

Figure 6 Metastatic breast carcinoma which superficially resembles primary squamous cell carcinoma of the lung. (×350)

VIII. Germ-Cell Tumors

Metastatic germ-cell tumors, including seminoma and choriocarcinoma, can potentially resemble primary large-cell lung carcinomas. Choriocarcinoma, in particular, may suggest a giant-cell carcinoma component of a primary lung carcinoma. Again, in the equivocal case, immunohistochemistry may be of benefit (27). Since primary

Table 7 Differentiation of Spindle-Cell Neoplasms by Immunohistochemistry

Spindle-cell carcinoma (lung primary): Immunopositive for keratin and vimentin and typically immunopositive for one or more of the following: CEA, B72.3, Leu M-1.

Spindle-cell carcinoma (kidney primary): Immunopositive for keratin and vimentin and not immunopositive for CEA, B72.3, or Leu M-1.

Sarcoma: Immunopositive for vimentin and immunonegative for keratin, may be immunopositive for keratin. Depending on differentiation, may be immunopositive for S-100, alpha-1-antitrypsin, desmin, smooth muscle actin, myoglobin, factor VIII.

Spindle-cell melanoma: Immunopositive for vimentin and immunonegative for keratin, immunopositive for HMB-45, S-100.

Spindle-cell carcinoids: Immunopositive for keratin, chromogranin, synaptophysin, other neuroendocrine markers.

lung carcinomas may sometimes be immunopositive for human chorionic gonado-tropin, a panel of immunostains for germ-cell tumors and lung primaries may be most helpful.

References

1. Baumgartner WA, Mark JBD. Metastatic malignancies from distant sites to the tracheobron-chial tree. J Thorac Cardiovasc Surg 1980; 79:499–503.
2. Toomes H, Delphendahl A, Manke H-G, Vogt-Moykoff I. The coin lesion of the lung: A re-view of 955 resected coin lesions. Cancer 1983; 51:534–537.
3. Bourke SJ, Henderson AF, Stevenson RD, Banham SW. Endobronchial metastases simulat-ing primary carcinoma of the lung. Respir Med 1989; 83:151–152.
4. Askin FB. Something old? Something new? Secondary primary or pulmonary metastasis in the patient with known extrathoracic carcinoma (editorial). Am J Clin Pathol 1993; 100(1):4–5.
5. Pogrebniak HW, Haas G, Linehan WM, Rosenberg SA, Pass HI. Renal cell carcinoma: Re-section of solitary and multiple metastases. Ann Thorac Surg 1992; 54:33–38.
6. Lanza LA, Natarajan G, Roth JA, Putnam JB. Long-term survival after resection of pulmo-nary metastases from carcinoma of the breast. Ann Thorac Surg 1992; 54:244–248.
7. Daugaard G. Unknown primary tumours. Cancer Treatment Rev 1994; 20:119–147.
8. Ramaekers F, van Niekerk C, Poels L, Schaafsma E, Huijsmans A, Robben H, Schaart G, Vooijs P. Use of monoclonal antibodies to keratin 7 in the differential diagnosis of adenocar-cinomas. Am J Pathol 1990; 136:641–655.
9. Moll R, Löwe, Laufer J, Franke WW. Cytokeratin 20 in human carcinomas: A new histodi-agnostic marker detected by monoclonal antibodies. Am J Pathol 1992; 140:427–447.
10. Ma CK, Zarbo RJ, Frierson HF Jr, Lee MW. Comparative immunohistochemical study of pri-mary and metastatic carcinomas of the liver. Am J Clin Pathol 1993; 99:551–557.
11. Gamble AR, Bell JA, Ronan JE, Pearson D, Ellis IO. Use of tumour marker immunoreactiv-ity to identify primary site of metastatic cancer. Br Med J 1993; 306:295–298.
12. Leers MPG, Theunissen PHMH, Koudstaal J, Schutte B, Ramaekers FCS. Trivariate flow cy-tometric analysis of paraffin-embedded lung cancer specimens: Application of cytokeratin subtype specific antibodies to distinguish between differentiation pathways. Cytometry 1997; 27:179–188.
13. Brown RW, Campagna LB, Dunn K, Cagle PT. Immunohistochemical identification of tumor markers in metastatic adenocarcinoma: A diagnostic adjunct in the determination of primary site. Am J Clin Pathol 1997; 107:12–19.
14. Mesa-Tejada R, Palakodety RB, Leon JA, Khatcherian AO, Greaton CJ. Immunocytochemi-cal distribution of a breast carcinoma associated glycoprotein identified by monoclonal anti-bodies. Am J Pathol 1988; 130:305–314.
15. Loy TS, Nashelsky MB. Reactivity of B72.3 with adenocarcinomas: An immunohistochemi-cal study of 476 cases. Cancer 1993; 72:2495–2498.
16. Nadji M, Tabei SZ, Castro A, Chu TM, Morales AR. Prostatic origin of tumors: An immu-nohistochemical study. Am J Clin Pathol 1980; 73:735–739.
17. Papsidero LD, Croghan GA, Asirwatham J, Gaeta J, Abenoza P, Englander L, Valenzuela L. Immunohistochemical demonstration of prostate-specific antigen in metastases with the use of monoclonal antibody F5. Am J Pathol 1985; 121:451–454.
18. Wick MR, Swanson PE, Manivel JC. Placental-like alkaline phosphatase reactivity in human tumors: An immunohistochemical study of 520 cases. Journal 1987; 18:946–954.
19. Loy TS, Quesenberry JT, Sharp SC. Distribution of CA125 in adenocarcinomas: An immu-nohistochemical study of 481 cases. Am J Clin Pathol 1992; 98:175–179.
20. Akasofu M, Kawahara E, Kurumaya H, Nakanishi I. Immunohistochemical detection of breast specific antigens and cytokeratins in metastatic breast carcinoma in the liver. Acta Pathol Jpn 1993; 43:736–744.

21. Raab SS, Berg LC, Swanson PE, Wick MR. Adenocarcinoma in the lung in patients with breast cancer: A prospective analysis of the discriminatory value of immunohistology. Am J Clin Pathol 1993; 100:27–35.
22. Flint A, Lloyd RV. Pulmonary metastases of colonic carcinoma. Arch Pathol Lab Med 1992; 116:39–42.
23. Koelma IA, Nap M, Rodenburg CJ, Fleuren GJ. The value of tumour marker CA 125 in surgical pathology. Histopathology 1987; 11:287–294.
24. DeMicco C, Ruf J, Carayon P, Chrestian M-A, Henry J-F, Toga M. Immunohistochemical study of thyroglobulin in thyroid carcinomas with monoclonal antibodies. Cancer 1987; 59:471–476.
25. Loy TS, Sharp SC, Andershock CJ, Craig SB. Distribution of CA 19–9 in adenocarcinomas and transitional cell carcinomas: An immunohistochemical study of 527 cases. Am J Clin Pathol 1993; 99:726–728.
26. Harpole DH Jr, Johnson CM, Wolfe WG, George SL, Seigler HF. Analysis of 945 cases of pulmonary metastatic melanoma. J Thorac Cardiovasc Surg 1992; 103:743–750.
27. Wick MR, Lillemoe TJ, Copland GT, Swanson PE, Manivel JC, Kiang DT. Gross cystic disease fluid protein-15 as a marker for breast cancer: Immunohistochemical analysis of 690 human neoplasms and comparison with alpha-lactalbumin. Hum Pathol 1989; 20:281–287.

8

ras Mutations in Lung Cancer

DANIEL R. JACOBSON

New York University School of Medicine
and Department of Veterans Affairs Medical Center
New York, New York

I. Introduction

Malignancies result from an accumulation of abnormalities in genes affecting cell growth and differentiation. These genes include (1) protooncogenes, such as the *ras* genes, which are components of signal transduction pathways, i.e., pathways that transmit signals from the cell surface to the nucleus (protooncogene abnormalities lead to dysregulated cell growth, i.e., abnormalities convert protooncogenes into oncogenes); (2) tumor suppressor genes, which arrest cell cycle progression; (3) genes involved in cell cycle regulation; (4) genes involved in DNA repair. According to current concepts of carcinogenesis, individual genetic abnormalities do not cause cancer, but can lead to dysregulated growth, increasing the chances for the development of additional genetic changes, which eventually can lead to malignancy. The identification of genetic abnormalities in lung cancer is improving our understanding of the molecular processes underlying lung carcinogenesis.

Molecular genetic markers are today primarily research tools in lung cancer, but are beginning to move toward clinical application. In general, molecular genetic tumor markers may be of potential use in at least six clinical settings:

1. For diagnostic purposes, when a malignancy is suspected, and molecular studies are performed on biopsy specimens or biologic fluids such as bronchoalveolar lavage (BAL) fluid or sputum (1–3).

139

2. For cancer screening, in asymptomatic populations (4).
3. For improved pathologic staging of malignancy, where the application of sensitive tumor markers may improve the ability to detect micro-metastases (5,6).
4. For prognostic purposes, based on the presence or absence of specific genetic abnormalities such as *ras* mutations in the tumor cells (7–15).
5. For the early diagnosis of disease relapse following therapy for malignancy (16).
6. For identifying candidates for new treatments directed at cancer-specific molecular abnormalities such as mutant *ras* proteins.

DNA- and RNA-based tumor markers may eventually come to play a role in all six of these areas in lung cancer.

Abnormalities have been described in lung cancer cells in many oncogenes and tumor suppressor genes, including the *ras* genes, *p53, rb, myc,* HER2/*neu* (reviewed in Refs. 17–19), plus tumor suppressor genes on chromosomes 3p, 5q, and 9p (20,21). Of these, *ras* oncogene mutations seem most suitable as clinical tumor markers and potential therapeutic targets, because of their high prevalence in non–small-cell lung cancer (NSCLC) and because most mutations occur in a single codon.

II. Biology of *ras* and the Role of Activating *ras* Mutations

The K-*ras* gene and the related genes N-*ras* and H-*ras* encode proteins, each termed p21, which are attached to the inner surface of the cell membrane, possess GTPase activity, and function in signal transduction. When bound to GDP, normal *ras* proteins are inactive; exchange of GDP for GTP leads to *ras* activation. Signal transduction is initiated by the binding of extracellular growth factors to their receptors, leading to receptor dimerization, which initiates a cascade of protein activation. Just upstream of the *ras* proteins in this cascade lies a protein called *sos,* which interacts with inactive *ras,* leading to GDP-GTP exchange and p21-ras activation. Both normal and oncogenic *ras* activity depend upon localization of the protein at the inner surface of the plasma membrane, which is mediated by posttranslational covalent binding of a farnesyl moiety to a cysteine near the p21-ras carboxy terminus. The enzyme that catalyzes this reaction, ras farnesyltransferase, is an inviting target for novel antitumor agents.

When activated, *ras* proteins can interact with multiple substrates, leading to activation of the mitogen activated protein (MAP) kinase pathway, which eventually leads to phosphorylation of nuclear proteins and DNA synthesis. Active p21-ras is converted back to its inactive, GDP-binding form by GTPase activity intrinsic to the p21-ras protein. This process is accelerated by GTPase-activating proteins (GAPs) in a tightly regulated manner (reviewed in Refs. 22,23). Activating (oncogenic) point mutations in the *ras* genes act in a dominant fashion, inactivating their GTPase activity and promoting cell growth. Abnormalities in other proteins in the *ras* pathway (including Her-2/neu, c-*myc*, and MEK-2) have also been found in human tumors, including lung cancer, but less often than have *ras* mutations (24–26). Most activating *ras* mutations in human tumors occur in codons 12, 13, and 61, with the pattern of activation varying among different tumor types.

From many studies on *ras* mutations in lung cancer (see Table 1), a few conclusions can be drawn:

1. *ras* mutations are found most often in K-*ras* codon 12, less often in K-*ras* codons 13 and 61, and rarely in N- and H-*ras*.
2. *ras* mutations are most common in adenocarcinomas and large-cell carcinomas; sensitive assays detect K-*ras* codon 12 mutations in about 50% of adenocarcinomas (4,27,28). Less sensitive assays such as PCR followed by allele-specific oligonucleotide hybridization (PCR/ASO-h) detect mutations in about 25% of adenocarcinomas.
3. In squamous cell carcinomas, most investigators have reported very few *ras* mutation–positive cases, but a few studies have found rates comparable to adenocarcinoma (10,12,14,15,29). *ras* mutations occur very rarely in lung cancers of other histologies, such as small-cell or carcinoid tumors (7,15,30–33).
4. For early-stage disease (potentially curable by surgery), the presence of a *ras* mutation identifies a poor-prognosis subgroup, which is more likely to relapse following surgery (7–15).
5. *ras* mutations are more common in lung cancers of smokers than nonsmokers (7,34–37).

Published studies contain discrepancies beyond what would be expected, which appear to arise largely from differences in the methods used to identify mutations in clinical specimens. Analysis of these studies thus requires careful evaluation of the various mutation detection assays used.

III. Interpreting *ras* Mutation Studies: The Interface Between Biology and Technology

A. "Traditional" *ras* Mutation Assays

Prior to the advent of the polymerase chain reaction (PCR), the most common assays for activating *ras* mutations were functional; DNA from a tumor was introduced into mouse fibroblast cells (NIH 3T3 cells), which were then examined for transformation in culture or for the ability to form tumors in immunoincompetent mice. Further studies could determine the specific abnormality present in a sample (28). These assays, particularly tumor formation, appear to be highly sensitive for detecting *ras* mutations (28). Beginning in the late 1980s, simpler, faster PCR-based assays for *ras* mutations emerged. These assays are generally straightforward, but can lead to false negatives and false positives; thus, the methodology must be closely examined in order to evaluate studies of *ras* mutations in human tumors.

Table 1 Studies of *ras* Mutation Frequencies in Lung Cancer[a]

Adenocarcinoma		Squamous cell carcinoma		Large-cell carcinoma		Mutation-detection method	Notes	Patient population	Ref.
K-ras 12	Other ras	K-ras 12	other ras	K-ras 12	other ras				
5/9 (56%)	1/9	0/3	1/3	1/1	0/1	Nude mouse assay		United States	28,79
14/25 (56%)	0/14					Enriched PCR	1	United States	27
7/14 (50%)				1/1	0/1	Cloning	2	United States	4
4/8 (50%)	0/8	0/5	0/5	1/1	0/1	PCR/SSCP	2, 3	United States	37
9/21 (43%)	3/21	2/21	0/21	0/2	0/2	PCR/ASO-h	4	Finland	35
3/7 (43%)	0/7	1/9	0/9			PCR/sequencing	2, 3	United States	66
6/16 (38%)		6/35		1/3		PCR/SSCP, sequencing	5, 6	South Korea	12
35/97 (36%)		0/42				PCR/sequencing	2, 7	United States	44
34/98 (35%)						PCR/ASO-h	1, 8	Italy	80
6/17 (35%)	0/17	9/39	0/39	5/15	0/15	PCR/ASO-h	9	Spain	14
3/10 (30%)	0/10	0/5	0/5	1/3	0/3	PCR/SSCP, sequencing	10	Japan	32
33/109 (30%)	5/109					PCR/DGGE	2, 6	Italy	11
10/33 (30%)	1/33	0/25	0/25			PCR/SSCP, sequencing, ASO-h	2	United States	41
3/11 (27%)	0/11	3/17	0/17			PCR/RFLP	11, 12	Greece	40
6/24 (25%)		3/27				Enriched PCR	1, 13	Canada	29
28/111 (25%)						PCR/ASO-h	1, 3, 14	United States	34
7/29 (24%)						PCR/ASO-h	1	United States	81
43/181 (24%)	1/131	0/48	0/29	1/24	0/18	PCR/ASO-h	3, 5	Holland	7
15/69 (22%)	1/69					PCR/ASO-h	5	Holland	55
6/29 (21%)						PCR/RFLP, ASO-h	1	Japan	39

% (K-ras codon 12)						Method	Notes	Region	Ref.
10/48 (21%)					0/20	Enriched PCR	1, 11, 15	Europe	54
9/43 (21%)		7/41		7/41		PCR/RFLP	1, 6, 11	Greece	15
8/41 (20%)	0/41					PCR/ASO-h	2	United States	82
2/10 (20%)	0/10	0/5	2/10	0/5	0/2	PCR/sequencing	2, 11	Switzerland	33
6/33 (18%)	4/33	2/6	0/6	4/13	5/13	PCR/RFLP	11, 16	United States	31
15/115 (13%)	3/115					PCR/ASO-h	6	Japan	9
12/104 (12%)						PCR/ASO-h	1, 3	Japan	36
6/63 (10%)	0/63	1/63	0/63	0/2	0/2	PCR/ASO-h	17	China	61
2/20 (10%)	0/20	0/20				PCR/ASO-h	1, 18	United States	83
2/22 (9%)	1/22	5/38	3/38	2/6	0/6	PCR/ASO-h	5, 6, 19	Spain	10
6/71 (8%)	8/71	0/36	2/36	2/14	0/14	PCR/SSCP	11, 16, 20	Japan	30
1/12 (8%)	4/12	0/13	7/13			PCR/SSCP	5, 20, 21	China	60
1/23 (4%)	1/23	0/13	0/13	0/1	0/1	PCR/sequencing	2	China	45
0/2 (0%)	0/2	0/6	0/6	0/2	0/2	PCR/sequencing	2	United States	43

aStudies of K-*ras* mutations in NSCLC, listed by the percentage of cases found to have a K-*ras* codon 12 mutation. A few studies with incomplete histologic or mutation information have been omitted.

ASO-h: Allele-specific oligonucleotide hybridization; DGGE: denaturing gradient gel electrophoresis; PCR, polymerase chain reaction; RFLP, restriction fragment length polymorphism; SSCP, single strand conformation polymorphism. One other large study which did not specify the histological breakdown of cases found K-*ras* codon 12 mutations in 22 of 92 NSCLC specimens (24%) (84).

Notes: (1) Studied only K-*ras* codon 12; (2) studied only K-*ras* exon 1 (or codons 12 and 13); (3) one of several studies showing an association of cigarette smoking with *ras* mutations; (4) studied K-, N-, and H-*ras* mutations; (5) studied K-*ras* codons 12, 13, and 61; (6) one of several studies showing *ras* mutations to be of prognostic significance; (7) didn't specify breakdown between codons 12 and 13; (8) included a large proportion of bronchioloalveolar carcinomas; 10/10 mucinous bronchioloalveolar carcinomas contained a mutation; (9) studied only at K-*ras* codons 12 and 61; (10) studied K- and H-*ras* exons 1 and 2; (11) included some samples with both adenocarcinoma and squamous cell carcinoma regions ("adenosquamous carcinoma"); (12) studied K-, N-, and H-*ras* codon 12; (13) included 6 bronchioloalveolar carcinomas, one with a mutation; (14) included a large proportion of former smokers; (15) 1 of 10 mutations not detectable by a less sensitive method (PCR/RFLP analysis, without enrichment); (16) studied K, N, and H-*ras* exons 1 and 2 (or codons 12, 13, and 61); (17) studied K- and H-*ras* codon 12 and N-*ras* codon 61; (18) all of the bronchioloalveolar subtype; (19) in 3 cases, multiple K-*ras* codon 12 mutations were found within the same tumor; (20) one K-*ras* codon 18 mutation found; (21) several samples had multiple mutations—unique results, in that *ras* mutations were distributed throughout K-*ras* exon 1.

In the largest published series of *ras* mutations in human lung cancer, from the Netherlands Cancer Institute, K-*ras* codon 12 mutations were found in 43 of 181 (24%) of lung adenocarcinomas, and mutations in other *ras* codons were much less common (7). This is the most widely quoted study on the subject, and several other studies have reported similar results (table). A crucial technical issue, however, is that the reported prevalence of *ras* mutations in any study depends not only upon their true prevalence, but also upon the relationship in each specimen between the percentage of cells carrying a mutation and the sensitivity of the mutation-detection assay used; if a *ras* mutation is present in only a fraction of the malignant cells, or if the DNA studied is isolated from a clinical sample containing both normal and malignant cells, the number of copies of mutant alleles in the sample may be much less than the number of normal-sequence alleles, and if an insensitive mutation assay is used, false-negative results may occur.

In recent years, most studies of *ras* mutations (including the Netherlands Cancer Institute study) have used assays based on PCR of *ras* exon 1 (containing codons 12 and 13) and exon 2 (containing codon 61) followed by ASO-h; for this assay, a mutation must be present in at least 10% of the corresponding *ras* alleles to be detected (9,38). Other groups have followed PCR of *ras* exons 1 and/or 2 by restriction fragment length polymorphism (RFLP) analysis, single strand conformation polymorphism (SSCP) analysis, denaturing gradient gel electrophoresis (DGGE), or sequencing of PCR products (Table 1) (11,12,30,31,39–45); these methods are no more sensitive than PCR/ASO-h for detecting mutant alleles contained in a background of a larger number of normal alleles (38,46,47).

Since tumors are clonal, one might expect all cells of *ras* mutation–positive cases to contain the mutation. If so, an assay that can detect 10% mutant alleles should be sensitive enough for many studies; however, whether *ras* mutations can be present in a minority of cells from a lung tumor has evidently not been formally examined. This question has been studied in acute myelogenous leukemia, and N-*ras* mutations are often contained in only a fraction of the leukemic cells (38). If lung carcinogenesis is similar, and *ras* mutations are not among the first genetic changes acquired by pulmonary cells during their evolution into cancer cells, but are only acquired after clonal growth is established, as some data suggest (48), then these mutations might be present in only a fraction of the tumor cells.

Another issue complicating attempts to detect oncogene mutations in clinical samples is that clinical specimens generally contain both tumor cells and normal pulmonary cells; DNA isolated from such specimens is derived from both populations. For example, the Netherlands Cancer Institute series included specimens containing as few as 25% malignant cells (49), while another study included samples containing as few as 20% cancer cells (9). As long as the minimum percentage of mutant alleles detectable by an assay is larger than the percentage of mutant alleles present in some DNA samples, false-negative results must arise.

B. Enriched PCR-Based Assays

Many investigators have recognized a need for assays able to detect mutations in a small minority of the alleles present in a specimen, particularly for application of mutation detection to cancer diagnosis or screening. One approach, taken by several groups, including our own, has been to use a technique often called "enriched PCR" (in our lab, termed PCR-primer-introduced restriction with enrichment of mutant alleles) (27,38,50–53); PCR is performed using a primer that introduces a restriction site (usually for the enzyme *BstN*I) into PCR products derived from the normal, but not mutant, allele. The product is digested with *BstN*I, after which only PCR products containing a mutation remain uncleaved. Additional PCR then selectively amplifies the mutant allele (the normal, digested allele is not further amplified), and the product is then analyzed for mutations, either by further PCR and restriction analysis or by other methods such as sequencing or ASO-h.

With these concerns in mind, we reexamined the prevalence of K-*ras* codon 12 mutations in a subset of the DNA samples from the Netherlands Cancer Institute series using an enriched PCR assay. We detected several mutations that had been undetectable by PCR/ASO-h, and estimated that mutations were actually present in 48% of the cases, or twice as many as had been detectable using PCR/ASO-h (27). Consistent with these results, we also found K-*ras* codon 12 mutations in 56% of lung adenocarcinomas at our institution (27). Two other small studies which used highly sensitive mutation assays have also reported *ras* mutations in over 50% of lung adenocarcinoma cases (4,28), although not all studies have confirmed these results (54,55), while, curiously, one study which did not use a sensitive mutation assay did find *ras* mutations in >50% of lung adenocarcinomas (35). Whether the discrepancies among laboratories arise from unknown differences in the assays or from the study populations is not clear (Table 1).

Despite its theoretical power, enriched PCR has technical pitfalls; the major obstacle arises from the high misincorporation rate of *Taq* polymerase. The enrichment process enriches both for PCR products derived from authentic mutant alleles and for PCR products containing "mutations" actually introduced as errors during PCR, which change the PCR product from normal (*BstN*I-sensitive) to mutant (*BstN*I-resistant) at codon 12. These products are then further amplified in subsequent PCR reactions, along with authentic mutations present in the starting material. The best method of ruling out false positives is to identify the specific mutation present in each sample, and then to demonstrate that the same mutation is present in a sample on repeat testing. Some studies without sufficient attention to these concerns have reported high prevalences of mutations, even in DNA from histologically normal tissues, and appear to include many false positives. Technical manipulations can improve PCR fidelity (27,56), but in any assay where PCR is followed by steps to identify a tiny subpopulation of PCR products containing a mutation, false-positive results remain a concern, as reviewed (27,50,53,56–58).

All other PCR-based methods, too, have limitations, e.g., SSCP analysis can lead to both false negatives and false positives (12,59), while PCR product carryover can lead to false positives and negatives in any PCR-based assay. Finally, different studies have used technologies with varying ability to detect less common mutations. Because it is established that most activating *ras* mutations in human malignancy occur in *ras* codons 12, 13, and 61, most of the studies in Table 1 used methodologies such as PCR/ASO-h, designed to detect mutations at these "hot spot" codons or a subset thereof, in some cases only K-*ras* codon 12. In contrast, the investigators who used techniques that detect mutations anywhere in a PCR product, such as SSCP analysis or sequencing, found occasional mutations in other codons, as well; for example, two groups have found a K-*ras* codon 18 mutation (30,60). Thus, experimental details must be examined closely, particularly when a study reports data that are biologically implausible or at variance with previously published data.

IV. Carcinogen Exposure: Implications for Understanding Lung Carcinogenesis

A. Cigarette Smoking and Occupational Exposures

It has been postulated that environmental carcinogens (primarily those in cigarette smoke) are likely to induce carcinogenic mutations. Several studies therefore compared the prevalence of *ras* mutations in tumors from smokers and nonsmokers and showed that *ras* mutations are found much more commonly in tumors from smokers than from nonsmokers (9,34,35,61). In addition, the *ras* mutation prevalence in adenocarcinomas from former smokers, even those who have not smoked for over 10 years, is similar to that in current smokers (34,37); these data support the theory that *ras* mutations occur early in the multistep process of lung carcinogenesis, in some cases many years before clinical evidence of disease.

Little hard data yet support an association between *ras* mutations and other environmental carcinogens. One study found a suggestion (not quite statistically significant) of a higher rate of *ras* mutations in patients with occupational asbestos exposure, while in another small study, uranium miners with heavy radiation exposure had many *p53* mutation-positive tumors, but no *ras* mutations were found (43).

B. Animal Studies

Animal studies, too, have clarified the role of *ras* mutations in lung carcinogenesis, particularly in response to chemical carcinogen exposure. In a study of a mouse strain that is susceptible to both spontaneous and carcinogen-induced lung tumors, spontaneous lung adenomas and carcinomas usually contained a K-*ras* mutation; the specific mutations were similar to those common in human tumors. When the animals were exposed to benzo[*a*]pyrene (a carcinogen in cigarette smoke) or methylnitrosourea, their tumors contained K-*ras* codon 12 mutations, while ethyl carbamate induced lung tumors with K-*ras* codon 61 mutations. The mutant and normal alleles were present in approximately equal amounts in the tumors, suggesting that the mutated allele was present in most or all tumor cells. The mutation found most often in benzo[*a*]pyrene-induced adenomas, K-*ras* codon 12 GGT → TGT, is the most common mutation in lung adenocarcinomas from human smokers. These data suggest that the chemicals directly induce K-*ras* mutations and that the induction of these mutations were early, perhaps initiating, events in tumor formation (62).

Another group found that mice exposed to polycyclic aromatic hydrocarbons in utero developed lung tumors containing K-*ras* codon 12 and 13 mutations, also similar to the types of mutations seen in human lung cancer (63). Mice exposed to urethane, in contrast, develop lung adenocarcinomas, adenomas, and hyperplasia containing mainly K-*ras* codon 61 mutations (64). In contrast, *p53* mutations were found only in late adenomas, suggesting that they are a later event in this model of lung carcinogenesis. Another disease model is provided by spontaneously occurring NSCLC in dogs; in one study, 5 of 20 spontaneously occurring NSCLC in dogs contained a K-*ras* mutation (65).

V. *ras* Mutations as Tumor Markers: Application to Early Diagnosis and Screening

We have studied whether detection of K-*ras* codon 12 mutations in BAL fluid obtained from patients undergoing evaluation for suspected lung cancer is of potential clinical value. An assay that enriches for mutant alleles is essential, because cancer cells, when present in BAL fluid, are mixed with genetically normal nucleated cells (alveolar macrophages, white blood cells, and bronchial epithelial cells). In our series of 87 BAL fluid samples, detection of a K-*ras* mutation in BAL fluid was both 100% sensitive and 100% specific for diagnosing mutation-positive cancer (1). In several cases, we have detected mutations in BAL fluid obtained during otherwise nondiagnostic procedures, i.e., when the BAL fluid and all biopsies obtained were read as cytologically and histologically negative, and cancer was not diagnosed until later in the patient's course, and in all cases, mutation analysis was at least as sensitive as cytologic examination of BAL fluid. These results suggest that molecular analysis of BAL fluid offers potential for clinical application and may lead to earlier lung cancer diagnoses; routine application of mutation detection to clinical samples, however, awaits further studies on the specificity of mutations for cancer (see below). An obvious next step is to investigate whether this assay also will enable detection of K-*ras* mutations in sputum specimens; if so, it may offer a tool not only for earlier diagnosis in patients clinically suspected of having lung cancer, but also for lung cancer–screening programs of asymptomatic populations.

The potential of identifying cancer-associated mutations in sputum prior to the diagnosis of lung cancer was demonstrated by a study in which 15 patients who provided sputum specimens as part of a randomized trial of lung cancer screening later developed lung cancer. The primary tumors of 10 of the patients contained a mutation in K-*ras* codon 12 or in *p53*. In 8 patients, the identical mutation was detected in at least one sputum sample a month or more prior to the clinical diagnosis, demonstrating the potential of screening sputum samples for mutations. The only apparent caveat with this study was that it utilized a mutation-detection method, involving cloning of PCR products, which may be too labor-intensive and expensive for routine application to clinical samples (4).

VI. Specificity of *ras* Mutations for Malignancy: Potential Limiting Factor to Clinical Application

Before *ras* mutations can be used in clinical settings, important questions about their specificity for cancer cells must be answered. A germline activating *ras* mutation has never been reported, and somatic *ras* mutations are considered oncogenic. A key question, however, is whether the presence of a K-*ras* codon 12 point mutation in DNA isolated from pulmonary-derived tissue *always* indicates that lung cancer must be present. If so, then such mutations should have strong potential for clinical utility as tumor markers. On the other hand, if *ras* mutations can occur in normal pulmonary tissue, or in premalignant tissue not irrevocably destined to develop cancer, then the clinical interpretation of finding a mutation in BAL fluid or sputum becomes problematic.

A. Studies of *ras* Mutations in Histologically Nonmalignant Lung Tissue

Recent data have begun to address this issue. One group studied DNA samples isolated from paired malignant and histologically normal lung tissue specimens obtained from the same patient at bronchoscopy (66) or thoracotomy (37). Many of the adenocarcinomas contained K-*ras* codon 12 mutations, and in several cases, a codon 12 mutation was found also in the histologically normal tissue not adjacent to the tumor. The mutation in the tumor was not always the same as the mutation in the normal tissue, and a mutation was also found in normal tissue from one patient whose primary tumor was mutation-negative. In addition, two specimens from patients with no evidence of malignancy had mutations in histologically normal tissue.

The results in these studies, if confirmed elsewhere, would have important implications for the use of K-*ras* oncogenes as clinical tumor markers, for they bring into question the specificity of *ras* mutations for fully developed cancer. However, these are examples of studies where the methodology and results need to be examined with particular care: in these two studies, mutations in histologically normal tissue were, surprisingly, detectable by PCR/SSCP analysis, i.e., no enrichment for mutant alleles was performed; thus, these results imply that histologically normal lung tissue contained large clonal populations of mutation-containing cells. Also surprising is that these studies reported in K-*ras* codon 12 one GTC sequence and several GGT → GCT mutations (37,66); the former would require two mutations and has evidently never been reported elsewhere, while the latter mutation has almost never been found in other studies. These results therefore await confirmation before they can be accepted.

In contrast, another group performed a similar study, and, more in keeping with what might be expected, they found mutations only in adenocarcinoma cells. Nonmalignant tissue from elsewhere in the pulmonary tree was always mutation-negative, even though an enriched PCR assay able to detect 1 mutant K-*ras* allele in a background of 1000 normal alleles was used (54).

B. *ras* Mutations in Premalignant Lung Tissue

Another group looked for K-*ras* mutations in histologically normal tissue, adenocarcinoma, and atypical alveolar hyperplasia (AAH), which may be a preneoplastic precursor to lung adenocarcinoma (67), from 28 patients (68). Samples of AAH (also termed atypical bronchioloalveolar cell hyperplasia, ABH, and other names) (39) were identified as microscopic growths of cytologically atypical cuboidal to columnar cells along the alveolar septa in the absence of significant inflammation and fibrosis of the surrounding lung parenchyma, and were not studied if they were directly adjacent to a primary tumor. Eight of 19 primary adenocarcinoma specimens contained a K-*ras* codon 12 mutation, as did 16 of 41 AAH specimens from the same patients. The mutation status of the carcinoma and AAH specimens from the same patient usually did not correlate, suggesting that many AAH were independent lesions and raising the question whether mutation-containing AAH can occur in patients without evidence of adenocarcinoma. Of three AAH specimens from patients without malignancy, none contained a mutation. Thus, although K-*ras* mutations were found in regions of the lung not appearing to harbor cancer, no mutation was found in tissue from a patient without lung cancer somewhere in the pulmonary tree. Another study also found K-*ras* codon 12 mutations in two of six cases of AAH from patients with adenocarcinoma elsewhere in the pulmonary tree (39).

These studies on AAH, as well as the studies of K-*ras* mutations in adenocarcinomas of former smokers (34,37) and the animal studies discussed above, all suggest that *ras* mutations occur early—perhaps even as an initiating event—in lung carcinogenesis. On the other hand, another group analyzed microdissected adenocarcinoma cells and adjacent preneoplastic cells and found that *ras* mutations occurred in neoplastic cells, but not in adjacent dysplastic, hyperplastic, or histologically normal cells; they concluded that *ras* mutations arise relatively late during lung carcinogenesis. In addition, our finding that many lung adenocarcinomas have *ras* mutations in only a small percentage of the cancer cells (as implied by their detection by enriched PCR but not by PCR/ASO-h) also suggests that *ras* mutations are not an early event, but more likely arise in a subdone of the tumor, as in acute myelogenous leukemia (38).

Analogous questions have been addressed in other malignancies, particularly colon cancer. Thus, K-*ras* codon 12 mutations have been found in about 50% of colon adenocarcinoma cases and have also been reported in small hyperplastic or dysplastic lesions (69,70). In analogy with the situation in lung cancer, many, but not all such samples studied had been removed from patients with adenocarcinoma elsewhere in the colon. These studies may not be directly applicable to lung cancer, but they indicate that *ras* mutations need not be specific for fully developed cancer. Further investigation in these areas is needed before clinicians will be able to use *ras* mutation status in making patient care decisions.

VII. Prognosis and Therapy

A. Mutation Status and Prognosis

As noted, in early (resectable) NSCLC, K-*ras* mutations portend a poor prognosis, although statistical significance has not always been reached in individual studies (8–13,15). In more advanced NSCLC, in contrast, the prognostic significance of *ras* mutations is not established: one study found *ras* mutations not of prognostic significance (55), while another study found a trend, not statistically significant, toward decreased survival in patients with mutation-positive tumors (14). The latter group did, however, find that patients with two specific codon 12 mutations (AGT and GAT) had a worse prognosis, and none responded to chemotherapy, in contrast to the patients with other mutations or mutation-negative tumors; to date, this is the only group to study whether different *ras* mutations have different biologic effects in lung cancer.

B. *ras* Overexpression and Prognosis

K-*ras* overexpression as measured immunohistochemically has also been correlated with prognosis (71,72). These studies are based on the logic that amplification of structurally normal *ras* genes can transform NIH 3T3 cells in vitro; thus, perhaps high p21-ras protein levels could provide sufficient activated protein to stimulate growth. A difficulty, however, is that differences in expression between tumor and normal cells, measured immunohistochemically, are often marginal. Also, it is not known what causes *ras* overexpression in lung cancer, or how often. In addition, unlike the situation with the *p53* gene, where most missense mutations lead directly to an increased protein half-life, and thus increased protein levels in tumor tissue, *ras* expression has never been correlated with mutation status. Finally, available anti-*ras* antibodies cannot distinguish between normal and mutated p21-ras. Thus, considerable work in this area needs to be done before *ras* overexpression can be considered a reliable tool.

C. *ras* Mutations and Sensitivity to Chemotherapy

In the studies of *ras* mutations and prognosis in early-stage lung cancer, standard treatment consisted of surgical resection, occasionally accompanied by local radiation therapy, but usually without systemic chemotherapy. The higher prevalence of relapse among patients with mutation-positive tumors suggests that *ras* mutations confer an ability for early metastasis on tumor cells; thus, patients with mutation-positive tumors may be ideal candidates for studies of adjuvant chemotherapy.

Of note is that the finding that *ras* mutations portend a poor prognosis does not imply that mutation-positive tumors are less sensitive to chemotherapy than mutation-negative tumors; indeed, the reverse may be true. In one randomized study of treatment of stage IIIA lung cancer, half of the patients received neoadjuvant chemotherapy prior to surgery, while the other half went straight to surgery. The surgically removed tumors were then examined for K-*ras* mutations, and mutations were found in significantly fewer of the tumors which had been exposed to chemotherapy (73). One interpretation of these data is that mutation-positive tumors could be heterogeneous, i.e., only a fraction of tumor cells could be mutation-positive, as discussed earlier; then, if the *ras* mutation–bearing cells are the most rapidly growing subpopulation of cells in the tumor (as is logical—*ras* mutations should confer a growth advantage on cells), they might be the cells most sensitive to chemotherapy and would be selectively killed. We have demonstrated a similar situation in patients with acute leukemia in whom *ras* mutations present at diagnosis were not detected after treatment with chemotherapy and subsequent relapse (38). Also supporting this view are two in vitro studies of NSCLC cell lines, which found that *ras* mutations conferred increased sensitivity to chemotherapy (25,74). Further studies in this direction may permit chemotherapeutic regimens to be tailored to individual tumor genotypes, based on likelihood of response.

D. Future Therapies: Inhibiting *ras* Function

Another area of potential applicability of *ras* genotyping lies in the possibility of treatment using drugs that inhibit *ras* activity for cancer chemoprevention and/or therapy. One approach to this problem is to inhibit *ras* farnesyltransferase. Many naturally occurring compounds and synthetic molecules have shown in vitro activity against the enzyme, in vitro killing of tumor cell lines, and in vivo activity against tumor growth in animal models, with few toxic side effects to normal cells in culture or in animals. Synthetic inhibitors have mimicked the structure of the two natural substrates of farnesyltransferase, farnesyl pyrophosphate and the carboxy terminal tetranucleotide motif of *ras* proteins. These investigations raise hopes that farnesyltransferase inhibitors may prove to be of clinical use (reviewed in Refs. 75,76). Another potential application lies in therapy directed against specific *ras* mutations: in in vitro studies, antisense K-*ras* constructs have inhibited growth of cell lines containing K-*ras* mutations, both for lung adenocarcinomas and for other tumor cell lines (77,78).

Acknowledgments

I thank Charles Fishman, Nancy Mills, Tibor Moskovits, Peter Leonardi, Sibyl Anderson, Ingrid Smith, and Julia Xu, John Scholes, Michael Ittman, Jaishree Jagirdar, Jane Denuto, William Rom, Sjoerd Rodenhuis, and Bert Top for their invaluable contributions to the work on lung cancer performed in this laboratory. I thank Angel Pellicer, Franco Muggia, and Joel Buxbaum for their useful critiques of the manuscript. This work was supported in part by American Cancer Society Research Grant #CN-155.

References

1. Mills NE, Fishman CL, Scholes J, Anderson SE, Rom WN, Jacobson DR. Detection of K-*ras* oncogene mutations in bronchoalveolar lavage fluid for lung cancer diagnosis. J Natl Cancer Inst 1995; 87:1056–1060.
2. Mao L, Schoenberg MP, Scicchitano M, Erozan YS, Merlo A, Schwab D, Sidransky D. Molecular detection of primary bladder cancer by microsatellite analysis. Science 1996; 271:659–662.
3. Ronai Z, Yakubovskaya M. PCR in clinical diagnosis. J Clin Lab Anal 1995; 9:269–283.
4. Mao L, Hruban RH, Boyle JO, Tockman M, Sidransky D. Detection of oncogene mutations in sputum precedes diagnosis of lung cancer. Cancer Res 1994; 54:1634–1637.
5. Brennan JA, Mao L, Hruban RH, Boyle JO, Eby YJ, Koch WM, Goodman SN, Sidransky D. Molecular assessment of histopathological staging in squamous-cell carcinoma of the head and neck. N Engl J Med 1995; 332:429–435.
6. Hayashi N, Ito I, Yanagisawa A, Kato Y, Nakamori S, Imakoka S, Watanabe H. Genetic diagnosis of lymph-node metastasis in colorectal cancer. Lancet 1995; 345:1257–1259.
7. Rodenhuis S, Slebos RJC. Clinical significance of *ras* oncogene activation in human lung cancer. Cancer Res 1992; 52(suppl):2665s–2669s.
8. Slebos RJC, Kibbelaar RE, Dalesio O, Kooistra A, Stam J, Meijer CJLM, Wagenaar SS, Vanderschueren RGJRA, van Zandwijk N, Mooi WJ, Bos JL, Rodenhuis S. K-*ras* oncogene activation as a prognostic marker in adenocarcinoma of the lung. N Engl J Med 1990; 323:561–565.
9. Sugio K, Ishida T, Yokoyama H, Inoue T, Sugimachi K, Sasazuki T. *ras* gene mutations as a prognostic marker in adenocarcinoma of the human lung without lymph node metastasis. Cancer Res 1992; 52:2903–2906.
10. Rosell R, Li S, Skacel Z, Mate JL, Maestre J, Canela M, Tolosa E, Armengol P, Barnadas A, Ariza A. Prognostic impact of mutated K-ras gene in surgically resected non-small cell lung cancer patients. Oncogene 1993; 8:2407–2412.
11. Silini EM, Bosi F, Pellegata NS, Volpato G, Romano A, Nazari S, Tinelli C, Ranzani GN, Solcia E, Fiocca R. K-ras gene mutations: an unfavorable prognostic marker in stage I lung adenocarcinoma. Virchows Archiv 1994; 424:367–373.
12. Cho JY, Kim JH, Lee YH, Chung KY, Kim SK, Gong SJ, You NC, Chung HC, Roh JK, Kim BS. Correlation between K-*ras* gene mutation and prognosis of patients with nonsmall cell lung carcinoma. Cancer 1997; 79:462–467.
13. Mitsudomi T, Steinberg SM, Oie HK, Mulshine JL, Phelps R, Viallet J, Pass H, Minna JD, Gazdar AF. *ras* gene mutations in non-small cell lung cancers are associated with shortened survival irrespective of treatment intent. Cancer Res 1991; 51:4999–5002.
14. Rosell R, Li S, Anton A, Moreno I, Martinez E, Vadell C, Mate JL, Ariza A, Monzo M, Font A, Molina F, De Anta JM, Pifarré A. Prognostic value of K-*ras* genotypes in patients with advanced non-small cell lung cancer receiving carboplatin with either intravenous or chronic oral dose etoposide. Int J Oncol 1994; 5:169–176.
15. Noutsou A, Koffa M, Ergazaki M, Siafakas NM, Spandidos DA. Detection of human papilloma virus (HPV) and K-*ras* mutations in human lung carcinomas. Int J Oncol 1996; 8:1089–1093.
16. Schilder RJ. Molecular markers and stem-cell transplants: are they made for each other? J Clin Oncol 1995; 13:1052–1054.
17. Jacobson DR, Fishman CL, Mills NE. Molecular genetic tumor markers in the early diagnosis and screening of non-small-cell lung cancer. Ann Oncol 1995; 6(suppl 3):S3–S8.
18. Smit EF, Groen HJM, Splinter TAW, Ebels T, Postmus PE. New prognostic factors in resectable non-small cell lung cancer. Thorax 1996; 51:638–646.

19. Duffy MJ. Can molecular markers now be used for early diagnosis of malignancy? Clin Chem 1995; 41:1410–1413.

20. Wei MH, Latif F, Bader S, Kashuba V, Chen JY, Duh FM, Sekido Y, Lee CC, Geil L, Kuzmin I, Zabarovsky E, Klein G, Zbar B, Minna JD, Lerman MI. Construction of a 600-kilobase cosmid clone contig and generation of a transcriptional map surrounding the lung cancer tumor suppressor gene (TSG) locus on human chromosome 3p21.3: progress toward the isolation of a lung cancer TSG. Cancer Res 1996; 56:1487–1492.

21. Sozzi G, Veronese ML, Negrini M, Baffa R, Coticelli MG, Inoue H, Tornielli S, Pilotti S, De Gregorio L, Pastorino U, Pierotti MA, Ohta M, Huebner K, Croce CM. The *FHIT* gene at 3p14.2 is abnormal in lung cancer. Cell 1996; 85:17–26.

22. Kiaris H, Spandidos DA. Mutations of *ras* genes in human tumours (review). Int J Oncol 1995; 7:413–421.

23. Katz ME, McCormick F. Signal transduction from multiple Ras effectors. Curr Opin Genet Dev 1997; 7:75–79.

24. Kern JA, Schwartz DA, Nordberg JE, Weiner DB, Greene MI, Torney L, Robinson RA. p185[neu] expression in human lung adenocarcinomas predicts shortened survival. Cancer Res 1990; 50:5184–5191.

25. Tsai CM, Chang KT, Perng RP, Mitsudomi T, Chen MH, Kadoyama C, Gazdar A. Correlation of intrinsic chemoresistance of non-small-cell lung cancer cell lines with HER-2/neu gene expression but not with ras gene mutations. J Natl Cancer Inst 1993; 85:897–901.

26. Bansal A, Ramirez RD, Minna JD. Mutation analysis of the coding sequences of MEK-1 and MEK-2 genes in human lung cancer cell lines. Oncogene 1997; 14:1231–1234.

27. Mills NE, Fishman Cl, Rom WN, Dubin N, Jacobson DR. Increased prevalence of K-*ras* oncogene mutations in lung adenocarcinoma. Cancer Res 1995; 55:1444–1447.

28. Reynolds SH, Anna CK, Brown KC, Wiest JS, Beattie EJ, Pero RW, Iglehart D, Anderson MW. Activated protooncogenes in human lung tumors from smokers. Proc Natl Acad Sci USA 1991; 88:1085–1089.

29. Kitigawa Y, Wong F, Lo P, Elliott M, Verburgt LM, Hogg JC, Daya M. Overexpression of Bcl-2 and mutations in p53 and K-*ras* in resected human non-small cell lung cancers. Am J Respir Cell Mol Biol 1996; 15:45–54.

30. Suzuki Y, Orita M, Shiraishi M, Hayashi K, Sekiya T. Detection of *ras* gene mutations in human lung cancers by single-strand conformation polymorphism analysis of polymerase chain reaction products. Oncogene 1990; 5:1037–1043.

31. Mitsudomi T, Viallet J, Mulshine JL, Linnoila RI, Minna JD, Gazdar AF. Mutations of *ras* genes distinguish a subset of non-small-cell lung cancer cell lines from small-cell lung cancer cell lines. Oncogene 1991; 6:1353–1362.

32. Kashii T, Mizushima Y, Monno S, Nakagawa K, Kobayashi M. Gene analysis of K-, H-ras, p53, and retinoblastoma susceptibility genes in human lung cancer cell lines by the polymerase chain reaction/single-strand conformation polymorphism method. J Cancer Res Clin Oncol 1994; 120:143–148.

33. Reichel MB, Ohgaki H, Petersen I, Kleihues P. *p53* mutations in primary human lung tumors and their metastases. Mol Carcinogen 1994; 9:105–109.

34. Westra WH, Slebos RJC, Offerhaus GJA, Goodman SN, Evers SG, Kensler TW, Askin FB, Rodenhuis S, Hruban RH. K-*ras* oncogene activation in lung adenocarcinomas from former smokers: evidence that K-*ras* mutations are an early and irreversible event in the development of adenocarcinoma of the lung Cancer 1993; 72:433–438.

35. Husgafvel-Pursiainen K, Hackman P, Ridanpää M, Anttila S, Karjalainen A, Partanen T, Taikina-Aho O, Heikkila L, Vainio H. K-ras mutations in human adenocarcinoma of the lung association with smoking and occupational exposure to asbestos. Int J Cancer 1993; 53:250–256.

36. Shiono S, Omoe K, Endo A. K-*ras* gene mutation in sputum samples containing atypical cells and adenocarcinoma cells in the lung. Carcinogenesis 1997;

37. Clements NCJr, Nelson MA, Wymer JA, Savage C, Aguirre M, Garewal H. Analysis of K-*ras* gene mutations in malignant and nonmalignant endobronchial tissue obtained by fiberoptic bronchoscopy. Am J Respir Crit Care Med 1995; 152:1374–1378.

38. Jacobson DR, Mills NE. A highly sensitive assay for mutant *ras* genes and its application to the study of presentation and relapse genotypes in acute leukemia. Oncogene 1994; 9:553–563.

39. Ohshima S, Shimizu Y, Takahama M. Detection of c-Ki-ras gene mutation in paraffin sections of adenocarcinoma and atypical bronchioloalveolar cell hyperplasia of human lung Virchows Archiv 1994; 424:129–134.

40. Kiaris H, Ergazaki M, Sakkas S, Athanasiadou E, Spandidos DA. Detection of activating mutations in the *ras* family genes in cytological specimens from lung tumours. Oncol Rep 1995; 2:769–771.

41. Sarkar FH, Valdivieso M, Borders J, Yao KL, Raval MMT, Madan SK, Sreepathi P, Shimoyama R, Steiger Z, Visscher EW, Crissman JD. A universal method for the mutational analysis of K-*ras* and p53 gene in non-small-cell lung cancer using formalin-fixed paraffin-embedded tissue. Diag Mol Pathol 1995; 4:266–273.

42. Lehman TA, Bennett WP, Metcalf RA, Welsh JA, Ecker J, Modali RV, Ullrich S, Romano JW, Appella E, Testa JR, Gerwin BI, Harris CC. p53 mutations, *ras* mutations, and p53-heat shock 70 protein complexes in human lung carcinoma cell lines. Cancer Res 1991; 51:4090–4096.

43. Vähäkangas KH, Samet JM, Metcalf RA, Welsh JA, Bennett WP, Lane DP, Harris CC. Mutations of p53 and *ras* genes in radon-associated lung cancer from uranium miners. Lancet 1992; 339:576–580.

44. Przygodzki RM, Koss MN, Moran CA, Langer JC, Swalsky PA, Fishback N, Bakker A, Finkelstein SD. Pleomorphic (giant and spindle cell) carcinoma is genetically distinct from adenocarcinoma and squamous cell carcinoma by K-*ras*-2 and p53 analysis. Am J Clin Pathol 1996; 106:487–492.

45. Hsu NY, Chen CY, Wu CH, Liu TJ, Kwan PC, Hsu CP, Hsia JY, Chang WT. Detection of K-*ras* point mutations in codons 12 and 13 in non-small cell lung cancers. J Formosan Med Assoc 1996; 95:741–745.

46. Mitsudomi T, Steinberg SM, Nau MM, Carbone D, D'Amico D, Bodner S, Oie HK, Linnoila RI, Mulshine JL, Minna JD, Gazdar AF. *p53* gene mutations in non-small-cell lung cancer cell lines and their correlation with the presence of *ras* mutations and clinical features. Oncogene 1992; 7:171–180.

47. Ridanpää M, Husgafvel-Pursiainen K. Denaturing gradient gel electrophoresis (DGGE) assay for K-*ras* and N-*ras* genes: detection of K-*ras* point mutations in human lung tumour DNA. Hum Molec Genet 1993; 2:639–644.

48. Sugio K, Kishimoto Y, Virmani AK, Hung JY, Gazdar AF. K-*ras* mutations are a relatively late event in the pathogenesis of lung carcinomas. Cancer Res 1994; 54:5811–5815.

49. Rodenhuis S, Slebos RJC, Boot AJM, Evers SG, Mooi WJ, Wagenaar SS, van Bodegom PC, Bos JL. Incidence and possible clinical significance of K-*ras* oncogene activation in adenocarcinoma of the human lung. Cancer Res 1988; 48:5738–5741.

50. Chen J, Viola MV. A method to detect *ras* point mutations in small subpopulations of cells. Anal Biochem 1991; 195:51–56.

51. Kahn SM, Jiang W, Culbertson TA, Weinstein IB, Williams GM, Tomita N, Ronai Z. Rapid and sensitive nonradioactive detection of mutant K-*ras* genes via 'enriched' PCR amplification. Oncogene 1991; 6:1079–1083.

52. Levi S, Urbano-Ispizua A, Gill R, Thomas DM, Gilbertson J, Foster C, Marshall CJ. Multiple K-*ras* codon 12 mutations in cholangiocarcinomas demonstrated with a sensitive polymerase chain reaction technique. Cancer Res 1991; 51:3497–3502.

53. Kahn SM, Jiang W, Weinstein IB, Perucho M. Diagnostic detection of mutant *ras* genes in minor cell populations. Meth Enzymol 1995; 255:452–464.

54. Urban T, Ricci S, Lacave R, Antoine M, Kambouchner M, Capron F, Bernaudin JF. Codon 12 Ki-ras mutation in non-small-call lung cancer: comparative evaluation in tumoral and non-tumoral lung. Br J Cancer 1996; 74:1051–1055.

55. Rodenhuis S, Boerringter L, Top B, Slebos RJC, Mooi WJ, van't Verr L, van Zandwijk N. Mutational activation of the K-*ras* oncogene and the effect of chemotherapy in advanced adenocarcinoma of the lung a prospective study. J Clin Oncol 1997; 15:285–291.

56. Loktionov A, O'Neill IK. Early detection of cancer-associated gene alterations in DNA isolated from rat feces during intestinal tumor induction with 1,2-dimethylhydrazine. Int J Oncol 1995; 6:437–445.

57. Jacobson DR. K-ras mutations as molecular markers of lung cancer. In: Martinet Y, Hirsch FR, Martinet N, Vignaud JM, Mulshine JL, eds. Clinical and Biological Basis of Lung Cancer Prevention. Basel: Birkhäuser Verlag AG, 1997.

58. Carpenter KM, Durrant LG, Morgan K, Bennett D, Hardcastle JD, Kalsheker NA. Greater frequency of K-ras Val-12 mutation in colorectal cancer as detected with sensitive methods. Clin Chem 1996; 42:904–909.

59. Hayashi K, Yandell DW. How sensitive is PCR-SSCP? Hum Mutation 1993; 2:338–346.

60. Gao HG, Chen JK, Stewart J, Song B, Rayappa C, Whong WZ, Ong T. Distribution of *p53* and K-*ras* mutations in human lung cancer tissues. Cancer Res 1997; 18:473–478.

61. Lung ML, Wong M, Lam WK, Lau KS, Kwan S, Fu KH, Cheung H, Yew WW. Incidence of *ras* oncogene activation in lung carcinomas in Hong Kong. Cancer 1992; 70:760–763.

62. You M, Candrian U, Maronpot RR, Stoner GD, Anderson MW. Activation of the Ki-*ras* protooncogene in spontaneously occurring and chemically induced lung tumors of the strain A mouse. Proc Natl Acad Sci USA 1989; 86:3070–3074.

63. Wessner LL, Fan M, Schaeffer DO, McEntee MF, Miller MS. Mouse lung tumors exhibit specific Ki-*ras* mutations following transplacental exposure to 3-methylcholanthrene. Cancer Res 1996; 17:1519–1526.

64. Horio Y, Chen A, Rice P, Roth JA, Malkinson AM, Schrump DS. Ki-*ras* and *p53* mutations are early and late events, respectively, in urethane-induced pulmonary carcinogenesis in A/J mice. Molec Carcinogen 1996; 17:217–223.

65. Kraegel SA, Gumerlock PH, Dungworth DL, Oreffo VIC, Madewell BR. K-*ras* activation in non-small cell lung cancer in the dog. Cancer Res 1992; 52:4724–4727.

66. Nelson MA, Wymer J, Clements N Jr. Detection of K-ras gene mutations in non-neoplastic lung tissue and lung cancers. Cancer Lett 1996; 103:115–121.

67. Kerr KM, Carey FZ, King G, Lamb D. Atypical alveolar hyperplasia: relationship with pulmonary adenocarcinoma, p53, and c-*erb*B-2 expression. J Pathol 1994; 174:249–256.

68. Westra WH, Baas IO, Hruban RH, Askin FB, Wilson K, Offerhaus JA, Slebos RJ. K-*ras* oncogene activation in atypical alveolar hyperplasias of the human lung Cancer Res 1996; 56:2224–2228.

69. Yamashita N, Minamoto T, Ochiai A, Onda M, Esumi H. Frequent and characteristic K-ras activation in aberrant crypt foci of colon. Is there preference among K-ras mutants for malignant progression? Cancer 1995; 75(6 suppl):1527–1533.

70. Pretlow TP. Aberrant crypt foci and K-*ras* mutations: earliest recognized players or innocent bystanders in colon carcinogenesis? Gastroenterology 1995; 108:600–603.

71. Fujino M, Dosaka-Akita H, Harada M, Hiroumi H, Kinoshita I, Akie K, Kawakami Y. Prognostic significance of p53 and *ras* p21 expression in nonsmall cell lung cancer. Cancer 1995; 76:2457–2463.

72. Dosaka-Akita H, Hu SX, Fujino M, Harada M, Kinoshita I, Xu HJ, Kuzumaki N, Kawakami Y, Benedict WF. Altered retinoblastoma protein expression in nonsmall cell lung cancer. Cancer 1997; 79:1329–1337.

73. Rosell R, Gómez-Codina J, Camps C, Maestre J, Padille J, Cantó A, Mate JL, Li S, Roig J, Olazábal A, Canela M, Ariza A, Skácel Z, Morera-Prat J, Abad A. A randomized trial comparing preoperative chemotherapy plus surgery with surgery alone in patients with non-small-cell lung cancer. N Engl J Med 1994; 330:153–158.

74. Koo HM, Monks A, Mikheev A, Rubinstein LV, Gray-Goodrich M, McWilliams MJ, Alvord WG, Oie HK, Gazdar AF, Paull KD, Zarbl H, Vande Woude GF. Enhanced sensitivity to 1-b-D-arabinofuranosylcytosine and topoisomerase II inhibitors in tumor cell lines harboring activated *ras* genes. Cancer Res 1996; 56:5211–5216.

75. Kelloff GJ, Lubet RA, Fay JR, Steele VE, Boone CW, Crowell JA, Sigman CC. Farnesyl protein transferase inhibitors as potential cancer chemopreventives. Cancer Epidemiol Biomarkers Prevent 1997; 6:267–282.

76. Gibbs JB, Oliff A. The potential of farnesyltransferase inhibitors as cancer chemotherapeutics. Ann Rev Pharmacol Toxicol 1997; 37:143–166.
77. Alemany R, Ruan S, Kataoka M, Koch PE, Mukhopadhyay T, Cristiano RJ, Roth JA, Zhang WW. Growth inhibitory effect of anti-K-*ras* adenovirus on lung cancer cells. Cancer Gene Ther 1996; 3:296–301.
78. Sakakura C, Hagiwara A, Tsujimoto H, Ozaki K, Sakakibara T, Oyama T, Ogaki M, Imanishi T, Yamazaki J, Takahashi T. Inhibition of colon cancer cell proliferation by antisense oligonucleotides targeting the messenger RNA of the Ki-*ras* gene. Anti-Cancer Drugs 1995; 6:553–561.
79. Reynolds SH, Anderson MW. Activation of proto-oncogenes in human and mouse lung tumors. Environ Health Persect 1991; 93:145–148.
80. Marchetti A, Buttitta F, Pellegrini S, Chella A, Bertacca G, Filardo A, Tognoni V, Ferreli F, Signorinie, Angeletti CA, Bevilacqua G. Bronchioloalveolar lung carcinomas: K-*ras* mutations are constant events in the mucinous subtype. Cancer Res 1996; 179:254–259.
81. Bongiorno PF, Whyte RI, Lesser EJ, Moore JH, Orringer MB, Beer DG. Alterations of K-ras, p53, and erbB-2/neu in human lung adenocarcinomas. J Thorac Cardiovasc Surg 1994; 107:590–595.
82. Li ZH, Zheng J, Weiss LM, Shibata D. c-k-ras and p53 mutations occur very early in adenocarcinoma of the lung. Am J Pathol 1994; 144:303–309.
83. Rusch V, Reuter VE, Kris MG, Kurie J, Miller WH, Nanus DM, Albino AP, Dmitrovsky E. *Ras* oncogene point mutation: an infrequent event in bronchioloalveolar cancer. J Thorac Cardiovasc Surg 1993; 104:1465–1469.
84. Capella G, Cronauer-Mitra S, Peinado MA, Perucho M. Frequency and spectrum of mutations at codons 12 and 13 of the C-K-*ras* gene in human tumors. Environ Health Perspect 1991; 93:125–131.

9

Deletions of the Short Arm of Chromosome 3 and the FHIT Gene in Lung Cancer

GABRIELLA SOZZI

Istituto Nazionale Tumori
Milan, Italy

I. Deletions of the Short Arm of Chromosome 3

Inactivation or loss of function of a tumor suppressor gene can occur by a variety of genetic mechanisms such as point mutations, translocation, or deletion. Since both deletions and translocations are often cytogenetically visible, they have served as landmarks for genes encoding regulatory signals. Both deletions and translocations involving the short arm of chromosome 3 (3p) have been detected in a number of human malignancies, including lung cancer. These findings, together with the identification of homozygous deletions in cancer cell lines, have led to the hypothesis that regions on 3p are the sites of tumor suppressor genes (TSG), whose inactivation is achieved by the loss of one allele and the presence of inactivating mutations or lack of expression of the remaining allele. These genetic changes ultimately result in the loss of the wild-type (wt) protein expression or function.

Deletions of the short arm of chromosome 3 are considered critical events in the pathogenesis of lung cancer. In 1982 Whang-Peng et al. (1) first reported a deletion of 3p in all 16 small-cell lung carcinoma (SCLC) cell lines analyzed. The most common pattern of deletion was an interstitial deletion of 3p(14-23). In contrast, Wurster-Hill et al. (2) reported a chromosome 3p deletion in only 3 of 15 cases studied. Subsequently, other groups have reported data on cell lines and primary tumors confirming that a cytogenetic deletion of 3p was present in the majority of the SCLCs (3–7). The cytogenetic analysis of the other histological types of lung tumors, grouped together as non–small-cell lung cancer (NSCLC), has revealed complex karyotypes with frequent loss and rearrangements of chromosome 3p (8–13). In addition to cytogenetically visible deletions, loss of heterozygosity (LOH) has been observed in nearly 100% of SCLC (14–16).

In contrast with the first restriction length polymorphism fragment (RFLP) analysis of allelic losses in NSCLC, showing that LOH of 3p were present in only 4 out of 15 informative patients (15), a subsequent study indicated that LOH at a locus located in 3p21 (DNF15S2) occurred in 100% of NSCLC (16). The analysis of a much larger number of primary tumors definitely demonstrated that loss of alleles on 3p is also a common event (>70%) in NSCL tumors (17,18).

These findings were further supported by a molecular mapping of deletion sites on 3p in 24 SCLC tumors, where a significant reduction in the frequency of LOH was found at some but not all of the 3p loci tested (19). In fact, a different pattern of LOH at 3p loci was observed between SCLC and NSCLC, the latter being characterized by a preferential loss of alleles at loci located in 3p21 compared to the loss of loci in a more distal 3p region observed in SCLC. However, the hypothesis of a common regulatory element located on 3p, whose loss could lead to tumors in different tissues, was also considered.

As an initial step towards positional cloning of the TSGs on 3p, a detailed analysis of the minimum deleted region(s) on 3p was performed with a large number of RFLP probes (13) and lung cancer samples (48 informative cases) (20). Three distinct regions (3p25, 3p21.3, and 3p14-cen) appeared to be frequent targets for deletions (100% of SCLCs and 80% of NSCLC). Of note, Whang-Peng et al. (21) have reached a similar conclusion by classic cytogenetic analysis of 31 NSCLC.

The first homozygous deletion in SCLC was identified in cell line U2020 (22). As mentioned before, homozygous deletions in DNA of cell lines complement LOH results and facilitate determination of deletion boundaries. This submicroscopic homozygous deletion involved the D3S3 locus on 3p14-13 and was estimated to involve 4–7 Mb of DNA (23,24). Further studies have shown that the U2020 deletion spans approximately 8 Mb and is located in 3p12-13 (25). Positional cloning strategies are ongoing to isolate a specific TSG in this proximal region of 3p.

Several groups have subsequently described homozygous deletions involving 3p21 in SCLC cell lines. Yamakawa et al. (26) found a homozygous deletion involving a single cosmid marker in 3p21.3-22 in five SCLC cell lines, and a gene related to the integrin α subunit (α_{RLC}) isolated from this deletion was identified although no mutation was observed in SCLC (27). However, this gene was aberrantly upregulated in SCLC tumors and cell lines, suggesting a possibility of misregulation of the gene by different mechanisms. A homozygous deletion in 3p21.3-p21.2 was found in SCLC cell line NCIH740 (28) involving markers that were located in a chromosomal 3p fragment previously shown to exhibit tumor suppressor activity in a mouse fibrosarcoma cell line (29). Incidentally, tumor suppressor activity for the entire chromosome 3 in a lung adenocarcinoma cell line was also demonstrated (30).

Several genes in the 3p21 homozygous deletion were isolated. They included the aminoacylase gene (ACY1), which showed reduced expression in about 20% of SCLC cell lines (31,32); the acylpeptide hydrolase gene (APEH), corresponding to the D3F15S2 polymorphic locus most frequently deleted in SCLC, found overexpressed in one of four SCLC cell lines in a single study (31) but not in subsequent analyses (33); the ubiquitin-activating enzyme E1 (UBE1L) (formerly D8), which showed a reduced expression in SCLC cell lines (33,34); the guanine nucleotide binding protein (GNAI2), which was revealed to be universally expressed in SCLC cell lines (28); and two human zinc finger genes, ZnF16 and ZnF3 (35). However, no convincing evidence of alteration at genomic, transcriptional, and translational levels in lung cancer was provided for any of these genes, and they were thus excluded as candidate TSGs. The hMLHI DNA mismatch repair gene, which is located immediately adjacent to the homozygously deleted region in 3p21.3, showed no involvement in the deletions identified in lung tumors (36). More recently, a new semaphorin gene in the common deletion region of 3p21.3 of three SCLC cell lines has been identified (36). Even though reduced expression levels of this gene were reported in two SCLC cell lines, no further evidence has been provided in order to demonstrate a tumor suppressor activity. Recently, an 80 kb clone from this same chromosomal region (3p21.3) was shown to suppress tumor growth in vivo in a mouse fibrosarcoma cell line (37). Thus, no solid candidate for the tumor suppressor gene(s) in the 3p21 region has yet been identified.

So far, the only definite 3p-linked TSG is the von Hippel-Lindau (VHL) gene, at 3p25. Von Hippel-Lindau disease is a familial cancer syndrome, dominantly inherited, that predisposes affected individuals to a variety of tumors, among them renal cell carcinoma. The VHL gene was shown to be mutated in the germline of VHL disease families (38). The gene is also inactivated in a considerable fraction of sporadic renal cancer (39) but only rarely mutated in lung tumors (40).

The region 3p14 is frequently lost not only in lung tumors (20) but also in tumors of different type such as renal (41,42), breast (43,44), and oral cancer (45,46) and is the site of homozygous deletions in a range of cancer-derived cell lines (47–49). It also contains the 3p break of a hereditary renal carcinoma–associated translocation, t(3;8) (p14.2;q24), which has been shown to segregate in a family with early onset of bilateral and multifocal clear cell renal carcinoma (50). This translocation region has been studied by several groups (51–54), the translocation break was cloned, and a cDNA mapping just telomeric to the 3p14.2 translocation has been suggested as a human renal carcinoma gene (55). The receptor protein tyrosine phosphatase γ (PTPγ) gene has been mapped at 3p21-14 and suggested as a candidate tumor suppressor gene (53). Although one PTPγ allele was lost in 50% of lung and renal carcinoma tumor samples analyzed, the gene was normally expressed in lung tumor cell lines (53). The localization of PTPγ was subsequently refined to 3p14.2 centromeric to the t(3;8) breakpoint (54), but the 6 kb coding sequence was not disrupted by the translocation.

The critical role of 3p deletions in lung cancer has been highlighted by the demonstration that allelic losses occur at the very earliest preneoplastic stages of lung cancer. In fact, molecular studies of preinvasive bronchial lesions have found a high frequency of 3p deletions in carcinoma in situ and dysplasia (56–58) and as early as in epithelial hyperplasia (59). Moreover, cytogenetic deletions of the short arm of chromosome 3 have been detected in normal-appearing bronchial mucosa distant from the tumor (60,61). These deletions were present in multiple lesions throughout the respiratory epithelium including bronchi, bronchioles, and alveoli, and the persistence of these molecular changes has been correlated with the evolution of the disease (58). The observation of 3p alterations in preinvasive lesions of the bronchus suggests that one or more tumor suppressor gene(s) may act as gate-keepers for lung cancer carcinogenesis. These observations are also consistent with the multistep model of carcinogenesis and a "field-cancerization" effect due to the chronic exposure of the bronchial mucosa to carcinogenic damage, such as tobacco smoke, resulting in an increased risk to develop multiple, separate foci of neoplasia.

Novel approaches to the detection of early stages of malignant diseases can thus be envisaged. In fact, the attraction of using somatic genetic changes, such as allele loss of 3p, as targets for early disease screening is that they may be detected using highly sensitive molecular techniques, which potentially can also be applied in exfoliated material.

II. The FRA3B

Another cytogenetic landmark in chromosome region 3p14.2 is the most common of the constitutive aphidicolin-inducible fragile sites in the human genome, FRA3B (62). Common fragile sites represent a cytogenetic puzzle. The biologic role, if any, and the molecular basis for chromosomal fragility at common fragile sites are not known. The apparent association between common fragile site localization, cancer breakpoints, and genes involved in tumorigenesis (63,64) led to the hypothesis that fragile site breakage is involved in the chromosomal rearrangements and allele losses observed in malignant diseases. Common fragile sites are highly conserved during evolution (65), are induced by agents that perturb DNA replication, are located in the euchromatic and late-replicating genome regions, and are induced by agents known to attack chromatin DNaseI-hypersensitive sites, i.e., sequences associated with expressed genes (66,67). In fact, common fragile site Xp22.1 is expressed only on the active X chromosome. Thus, common fragile sites could be associated with transcriptional activity. Consequently, the potential role of a fragile site located at the 5' end of a tumor suppressor gene could be the abrogation of the transcription of a such hypothetical gene as a result of fragile site expression. It is of interest that the rate of expression of common fragile sites can vary from person to person, and occasionally individuals could be encountered who have high levels of expression of one of these fragile sites (68).

The most active of the inducible common fragile sites of the human genome is FRA3B, contained in the 3p14.2 chromosomal band. FRA3B expression is observed after exposure of cultured cells to diverse mutagens and carcinogens, including benzo(*a*)pyrene diol-epoxide, the ultimate carcinogen of benzo(*a*)pyrene (a major constituent of tobacco smoke) (66), and ethanol (69). A significantly increased frequency of FRA3B expression has been reported in peripheral lymphocytes of smokers (70).

Aphidicolin induction of breakage and rearrangement of FRA3B in somatic cell hybrids resulted in generation of hybrid clones with human/hamster translocations involving breakpoints at FRA3B (71,72). Subsequent studies of position of hybrid clone breakpoints (73,74) have shown that the genomic region involved was up to 100 kb. This suggested that FRA3B may represent a region of fragility, rather than a single site. Recently it has been shown that an area of frequent breaks within FRA3B coincides with the spontaneous HPV16 integration site, offering direct evidence for the coincidence of viral integration genomic regions and fragile sites (75).

III. Cloning and Structural Features of the FHIT Gene

The observations summarized above indicated that the region 3p14.2 probably harbors one of the long-sought tumor suppressor genes on the short arm of chromosome 3. The isolation of a YAC contig covering the t(3;8) break and FRA3B (48,73,74,76) and the development of STS markers allowed the definition of homozygous deletions in a range of cancer-derived cell lines (48). Ohta et al. (77) then developed a cosmid contig covering the common homozygously deleted region and identified and characterized a gene that is partially deleted in uncultured tumors of the aerodigestive tract and other organs. This gene has been designated the fragile histidine triad (FHIT) gene.

The cosmid contig was assembled from cosmids subcloned from the library prepared from YAC648D4, the shorter YAC clone covering the commonly deleted region (Fig. 1). Individual cosmids were used in exon-trapping experiments aimed at identifying genes within the deleted region. An oligonucleotide primer designed from the initial trapped exon was used in primer extension to obtain a 5′ extended

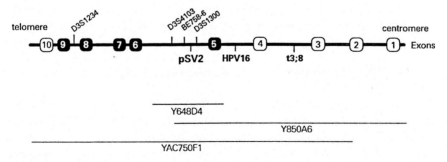

Figure 1 Organization of the FHIT gene. Approximate location of the yac clones, the relevant STSs, plasmid and HPV16 integration sites, and the t(3;8) translocation breakpoint are indicated.

product of the cDNA by a rapid amplification of cDNA ends (RACE) reaction. The longest product from the RACE reaction detected a ubiquitously expressed 1.1 kb mRNA by Northern blot analysis of mRNA from various normal tissues. Since cDNA sequences 5' and 3' of the first trapped exon (exon 5 in Fig. 1) were not within the cosmid contig, cosmid libraries from YACs 850A6 and 750F1, which extend centromeric and telomeric to the fragile region deletions, respectively, were screened with the 5' and 3' cDNA probes flanking exon 5. Cosmids containing the remaining exons were then used to derive intron sequences using cDNA primers, and the structure of the gene was determined as shown in Figure 1. The 1.1 kb FHIT cDNA consists of 10 small exons and is distributed over a genomic locus of about a megabase. Only exon 5 falls within the region of homozygous deletion originally observed in tumor-derived cell lines. The coding region of the open reading frame begins in exon 5 and ends in exon 9. Interestingly, the first three exons (E1, E2, E3 of Fig. 1) of the gene are centromeric to the t(3;8) break. Thus this gene has become a strong candidate for an involvement in the initiation of the clear cell renal carcinoma of the t(3;8)-bearing family, because one copy of the gene is disrupted by this translocation. In addition, the location of several markers, such as BE758-6 (47) and D3S1300, previously found deleted at high frequency in tumors and cell lines (48), within the FHIT gene locus, close to the first coding exon 5, suggested that FHIT is the target of these deletions. Analysis of FHIT expression in normal and tumor tissues by Northern blot revealed a low level of expression in all normal human tissues tested, whereas varying levels of FHIT transcripts, from barely detectable to almost normal levels, were found in tumor-derived cell lines (77). Reverse transcriptase PCR was used to detect abnormalities in FHIT transcripts in primary gastrointestinal tumors: a pattern of products ranging from one apparently normal-sized amplified transcript to numerous aberrant bands without a normal-sized band was observed. Sequence analysis of the usually shorter aberrant products revealed absence of various regions between exons 4 and 9, while normal tissue mRNA from the same organ did not exhibit alteration in the amplified sequences (77). Since the aberrant transcripts frequently lacked exon 5, which begins the open reading frame of FHIT, or exon 8, the highly conserved histidine triad-containing domain, it is likely that these aberrant products could not encode functional proteins. Insertions of various lengths of DNA, either between or replacing exons, were also observed (77).

IV. The Fhit Protein and Its Biochemical Activity

The FHIT gene encodes a polypeptide of 16.8 kD, which is composed of 147 amino acids that show 52% identity and 69% similarity to a core region of 109 amino acids of the diadenosine 5',5'''-P1,P4-tetraphosphate (Ap$_4$A) hydrolase from the fission yeast *Schizosaccaromyces pombe* (77–79). The latter enzyme is a 182 amino acid protein that catalyses the in vitro hydrolysis of dinucleoside polyphosphates, with Ap$_4$A as the preferred substrate. Both the Fhit protein and *S. pombe* Ap$_4$A hydrolase are related by sequence to the HIT proteins, a group of molecules of unknown function characterized by four conserved histidines, three of which make up a histidine triad (HIT) sequence, H X H X H, where X is most frequently valine (77,78). Subsequent biochemical studies (80) clearly demonstrated that the human Fhit protein could be classified as an Ap_3A hydrolase on the basis of its in vitro enzymatic activity. Ap_3A is the preferred substrate among Ap_nAs, and AMP is always one of the reaction products. By site-directed mutagenesis each of the four conserved histidine residues of FHIT was changed to an asparagine. Each change resulted in a decrease in Ap_3A hydrolase activity, demonstrating that all four conserved histidines are required for full activity, but the central histidine of the triad (H96) is absolutely essential for Ap_3A hydrolase activity (80). Consequently, alterations of exon 8 could be critical for the biological activity of the Fhit protein.

Recently, the crystal structure of histidine triad nucleotide binding protein (HINT) showed that histidine triad proteins (HIT) are nucleotide-binding proteins (81). HINT-nucleotide complexes demonstrated that the most conserved residues in the superfamily mediate nucleotide binding and that the HIT motif forms part of the phosphate-binding loop. Thus, FHIT is an enzyme of the HIT family, a family of genes involved in nucleotide metabolism. FHIT substrates Ap_4A and Ap_3A have been considered alarmones in bacterial systems, which are produced in times of cellular stress (82). Accumulation of Ap_3A is induced in human cultured cells by interferon (83), and an Ap_4A increase is reported as a consequence of contact-inhibition of growth and toxic stress (84). FHIT-substrate or substrate-enzyme complexes may thus be involved in signaling responses to cellular stress resulting in cell-cycle arrest.

V. FHIT Abnormalities in Lung Cancer

To determine the role of the FHIT gene in lung cancer, more than 100 primary lung tumors were analyzed for abnormalities of FHIT expression by reverse transcriptase PCR analyses and sequencing, LOH and Southern blot, as well as by immunocytochemistry (85 and unpublished data). Abnormalities in products amplified from FHIT transcripts were found in 80% of SCLC tumors and in 42% of NSCLC. Sequence analysis of the aberrant products showed that the absence of exons 4 or 5 through 8 was the most common abnormality. Most of the tumors also displayed a normal size-amplified product, possibly due to normal tissue mixed with the tumor. LOH at three microsatellite markers internal to the FHIT gene, located either in the fragile region (D3S1300, D3S4103) or in the more telomeric distal 3'end of the gene (D3S1234), was detected in 63% of the tumor specimens. Tumors exhibiting aberrant FHIT amplification products also lost one FHIT allele, suggesting loss of function of the FHIT gene. In order to correlate specific FHIT locus DNA lesions with their effects on transcription products and protein expression, 11 lung cancer cell lines of different type were studied by Southern blot analysis, reverse transcriptase PCR, Western blot analysis, and immunocytochemistry. Three cell lines, after hybridization with the cDNA and specific cosmid probes covering large intronic regions of FHIT, showed abnormal restriction patterns, consisting in deletions or re-arrangements involving exon 3, exon 4, and intron 5 as well as a more distal region surrounding exon 6 and 7. In addition, one cell line showed a homozygous deletion in intron 5. The RT-PCR analysis of RNAs revealed complete absence of normal FHIT transcript in three cell lines: one showed lack of exon 4 only, whereas in the other two only multiple abnormal transcripts lacking exons 3 or 4 through 8 and 9 were present. In six cell lines, FHIT mRNA products of both normal and abnormal sizes were found, while two cell lines showed the wild-type transcript only. Cloning and sequencing of the apparently normal-sized transcripts in several cell lines re-vealed a mixture of different transcripts lacking crucial coding exons such as exons 5 through 8 and often exhibiting insertions of sequences of various lengths, either between or replacing exons. The inserted sequences derived from human DNA and show identical size and sequence in some cell lines and primary tumors, suggesting that they could derive from FHIT introns. Thus, potential proteins resulting from the aberrant transcript would lack relevant portions of the wild-type protein; the inser-tion of new nucleotides would result in either adding new amino acids or altering the reading frame of the gene. This multiplicity of genetic lesions may be explained by the fact that the FHIT gene encompasses the fragile 3B region, which by definition is highly susceptible to breakage induced by carcinogens such as those in tobacco smoke. Western blot analysis, using a rabbit polyclonal antibody against the GST-FHIT fusion protein, revealed that indeed 9 of the 11 lung cancer cell lines did not produce Fhit protein. Immunocytochemistry studies using the same antibody showed that the two cell lines positive for Fhit by Western blot displayed clear cy-toplasmatic immunostaining. These data indicate that, due to the complexity of FHIT rearrangements, immunocytochemistry may be the best way to assess the level of involvement of FHIT in lung tumors since the Fhit protein was absent or greatly reduced in tumor cell lines for which DNA or RNA alterations of the FHIT locus were not observed.

Other investigators have recently confirmed that FHIT is altered in a signifi-cant proportion of NSCLC cell lines. Yanagisawa et al. (86a) observed either lack of expression or aberrant splicing in 7 out of 24 (29%) cell lines, often accompanied by intragenic homozygous deletions. Very recently, a thorough analysis of molecu-lar abnormalities of the FHIT gene in primary lung tumors, cell lines, and preneo-plastic bronchial lesions confirmed that FHIT and FRA3B abnormalities are associ-ated with lung cancer pathogenesis (86b). The results showed that the FHIT/FRA3B region undergoes allele loss in the vast majority of lung cancers (occurring first at the stage of carcinoma in situ), which may exhibit homozygous deletions (including intragenic deletions), and very frequently express aberrant FHIT transcripts, although in most cases an intact wild-type transcript was co-expressed, as assessed by RT-PCR analyses. FHIT mRNA was undetectable or barely detectable by North-ern blot analysis in tumor-derived cell lines, suggesting that most cells in the popu-lation were expressing very little wild-type or altered FHIT transcripts.

Taken together, the genetic lesions within the FHIT gene may be explained by the location of a fragile region within the gene, rendering the latter highly susceptible to breakage induced by carcinogens (71). Tumors associated with carcinogen exposure, such as cancers of the aerodigestive and respiratory tract, could be particularly susceptible to alterations of the FHIT gene. Owing to its etiology, lung cancer is likely to be strongly and directly associated with the effects of agents that interfere with DNA replication, such as chemicals in tobacco smoke. Accordingly, tumors exhibiting the highest frequency of FHIT abnormalities, such as lung, head and neck (87) and gastric cancer of the intestinal type (Baffa et al., unpublished), have been recognized to be caused by etiological agents such as tobacco and alcohol.

Accordingly, a molecular analysis of microsatellite alterations within the FHIT gene and FRA3B in lung tumors from heavy smokers and in tumors developed in never-smokers was undertaken to seek genetic damage attributable to tobacco smoking (88). LOH at D3S1300 and D3S4103 microsatellite markers, located in the epicenter of the fragile region encompassing exon 5 and intron 5 of the FHIT gene (Fig. 1) and at D3S1234 in the more distal 3' end of the gene, was analyzed in tumor tissue. LOH affecting at least one locus of the FHIT gene was observed in 41 out of 51 tumors in the smokers group (80%) but in only 9 out of 40 tumors in nonsmokers (22%). The comparison between the frequency of losses in smokers and nonsmokers was statistically significant (80% vs. 22%, $p = 0.0001$). All the tumors with loss of one FHIT marker had lost all the informative markers, suggesting that the tumor cells had lost an entire FHIT allele. No difference in loss of heterozygosity rate was observed at another locus located on chromosome 10 (D10S197) indicating that the preferential involvement of the FHIT gene in smokers is a specific event and not a result of a more general genotoxic effect of tobacco smoke. A more recent analysis of the same samples for LOH at locus D3S1339 at 3p21 showed a less striking difference in the rate of LOH in smokers' (63%) versus nonsmokers' tumors (43%), which did not reach statistical significance (unpublished data). These findings suggest that FHIT is a preferential target of carcinogens in tobacco smoke at a molecular level and indicate the possibility of using LOH at FHIT and FRA3B as early molecular indicators of damage related to tobacco smoke in screening high-risk individuals such as those belonging to the heavy smokers category.

VI. Conclusions and Perspectives

The discovery of FHIT gene abnormalities in tumors is the first molecular evidence linking the instability of fragile sites to cancer (89). Because of the frequent abnormalities in the FHIT gene in a variety of cancer-derived cell lines, as well as in primary tumors of the digestive tract, lung, and breast—three of the most common neoplasms in humans—abnormalities in this gene are becoming one of the most frequent genetic changes occurring in the tumorigenic process. Furthermore, indirect evidence suggests that this gene is also involved in other types of human neoplasms, for example, in cervical carcinoma, where one of the most frequently lost regions is 3p14 and where an insertion site for the human papillomavirus type 16 was found to be very close to the FRA3B fragile site (75).

Due to its binding capability and hydrolase activity on diadenosine tri- and tetraphosphate molecules, which may accumulate in response to cellular stress, lack of the Fhit protein could result in abnormal adaptation of cells to stress. This effect may be an early event in neoplasia of some organs, since preneoplastic cells of various tissues (oral, bronchial, breast) show abnormalities of the FHIT gene. Ongoing functional studies aimed at restoration of FHIT function and prevention of tumor growth in vivo will prove whether or not FHIT is a tumor suppressor gene. These studies could permit the development of novel therapeutic approaches, such as transfer of the wild-type FHIT gene to precancerous lesions or tumors of cancer patients carrying a disrupted FHIT gene, a gene therapy approach recently attempted for p53 by gene transfer to tumors of patients with lung cancer (90).

Acknowledgments

The author is grateful to Dr. Marco A. Pierotti for critical reading of the manuscript, to Mr. Mario Azzini for professionally preparing the illustration, and to Mrs. Anna Grassi and Mrs. Cristina Mazzadi for kindly preparing the manuscript.

References

1. Whang-Peng J, Bunn PA, Jr., Kao-Shan CS, Lee EC, Carney DN, Gazdar A, Minna JD. A nonrandom chromosomal abnormality, del 3p(14-23), in human small cell lung cancer (SCLC). Cancer Genet Cytogenet 1982; 6:119–134.
2. Wurster-Hill DH, Cannizzaro LA, Pettengill OS, Sorenson GD, Cate CC, Maurer LH. Cytogenetics of small cell carcinoma of the lung. Cancer Genet Cytogenet 1984; 13:303–330.
3. Yunis JJ. The chromosomal basis of human neoplasia. Science 1983; 221:227–236.
4. Falor WH, Ward-Skinner R, Wegryn S. A 3p deletion in small cell lung carcinoma. Cancer Genet Cytogenet 1985; 16:175–177.
5. Sozzi G, Bertoglio MG, Borrello MG, Giani' S, Pilotti S, Pierotti MA, Della Porta G. Chromosomal abnormalities in a primary small cell lung cancer. Cancer Genet Cytogenet 1987; 27:45–50.
6. Ibson JM, Waters JJ, Twentyman PR, Bleehen NM, Rabbitts PH. Oncogene amplification and chromosomal abnormalities in small cell lung cancer. J Cell Biochem 1987; 33:267–288.
7. Waters JJ, Ibson JM, Twentyman PR, Bleehen NM, Rabbitts PH. Cytogenetic abnormalities in human small cell lung carcinoma: cell lines characterized for myc gene amplification. Cancer Genet Cytogenet 1988; 30:213–223.
8. Zech L, Bergh J, Nilsson K. Karyotypic characterization of established cell lines and short-term cultures of human lung cancers. Cancer Genet Cytogenet 1985; 15:335–347.
9. Rey JA, Bello MJ, de Campos JM, Kusak ME, Moreno S, Benitez J. Deletion 3p in two lung adenocarcinomas metastatic to the brain. Cancer Genet Cytogenet 1987; 25:355–360.
10. Bello MJ, Moreno S, Rey JA. Involvement of chromosomes 1, 3, and i(8q) in lung adenocarcinoma. Cancer Genet Cytogenet 1989; 38:133–135.
11. Lukeis R, Irving L, Garson M, Hasthorpe S. Cytogenetics of non-small cell lung cancer: analysis of consistent non-random abnormalities. Genes Chrom Cancer 1990; 2:116–124.
12. Miura I, Siegfried JM, Resau J, Keller SM, Zhou JY, Testa JR. Chromosome alterations in 21 non-small cell lung carcinomas. Genes Chrom Cancer 1990; 2:328–338.
13. Testa JR, Siegfried JM, Liu Z, Hunt JD, Feder MM, Litwin S, Zhou J-y, Taguchi T, Keller SM. Cytogenetic analysis of 63 non-small cell lung carcinomas: recurrent chromosome al-

terations amid frequent and widespread genomic upheaval. Genes Chrom Cancer 1994; 11:178–194.

14. Naylor SL, Johnson BE, Minna JD, Sakaguchi AY. Loss of heterozygosity of chromosome 3p markers in small-cell lung cancer. Nature 1987; 329:451–454.

15. Brauch H, Johnson B, Hovis J, Yano T, Gazdar A, Pettengill OS, Graziano S, Sorenson GD, Poiesz BJ, Minna JD. Molecular analysis of the short arm of chromosome 3 in small cell and non-small cell carcinoma of the lung. N Engl J Med 1987; 317:1109–1113.

16. Kok H, Osinga J, Carritt B, Davis MB, van der Hout AH, van der Veen AY, Landsvater RM, de Leij LFMH, Berendsen HH, Postmus PE, Poppema S, Buys CHCM. Deletion of a DNA sequence at the chromosomal region 3p21 in all major types of lung cancer. Nature 1987; 330:578–581.

17. Yokota J, Wada M, Shimosato Y, Terada M, Sugimura T. Loss of heterozygosity on chromosomes 3, 13, and 17 in small-cell carcinoma and on chromosome 3 in adenocarcinoma of the lung. Proc Natl Acad Sci USA 1987; 84:9252–9256.

18. Rabbits P, Douglas J, Daly M, Sundaresan V, Fox B, Haselton P, Wells F, Albertson D, Waters J, Bergh J. Frequency and extent of allelic loss in the short arm of chromosome 3 in non small-cell lung cancer. Genes Chrom Cancer 1989; 1:95–105.

19. Brauch H, Tory K, Kotler F, Gazdar AF, Pettengill OS, Johnson B, Graziano S, Winton T, Buys CH, Sorenson GD, et al. Molecular mapping of deletion sites in the short arm of chromosome 3 in human lung cancer. Genes Chrom Cancer 1990; 1:240–246.

20. Hibi K, Takahashi T, Yamakawa K, Ueda R, Sekido Y, Ariyoshi Y, Suyama M, Takagi H, Nakamura Y. Three distinct regions involved in 3p deletion in human lung cancer. Oncogene 1992; 7:445–449.

21. Whang-Peng J, Knutsen T, Gazdar A, Steinberg SM, Oie H, Linnoila I, Mulshine J, Nau M, Minna JD. Nonrandom structural and numerical chromosome changes in non-small-cell lung cancer. Genes Chrom Cancer 1991; 3:168–188.

22. Rabbitts P, Bergh J, Douglas J, Collins F, Waters J. A submicroscopic homozygous deletion at the D3S3 locus in a cell line isolated from a small cell lung carcinoma. Genes Chrom Cancer 1990; 2:231–238.

23. Drabkin HA, Mendez MJ, Rabbitts PH, Varkony T, Bergh J, Schlessinger, J, Erickson P, Gemmill RM. Characterization of the submicroscopic deletion in the small-cell lung carcinoma (SCLC) cell line U2020. Genes Chrom Cancer 1992; 5:67–74.

24. Latif F, Tory K, Modi WS, Graziano SL, Gamble G, Douglas J, Heppell-Parton AC, Rabbitts PH, Zbar B, Lerman MI. Molecular characterization of a large homozygous deletion in the small cell lung cancer cell line U2020: a strategy for cloning the putative tumor suppressor gene. Genes Chrom Cancer 1992; 5:119–127.

25. Todd S, Roche J, Hahner L, Bolin R, Drabkin HA, Gemmill RM. YAC contigs covering an 8-megabase region of 3p deleted in the small-cell lung cancer cell line U2020. Genomics 1995; 25:19–28.

26. Yamakawa K, Takahashi T, Horio Y, Murata Y, Takahashi E, Hibi K, Yokoyama S, Ueda R, Nakamura Y. Frequent homozygous deletions in lung cancer cell lines detected by a DNA marker located at 3p21.3-p22. Oncogene 1993; 8:327–330.

27. Hibi K, Yamakawa K, Ueda R, Horio Y, Murata Y, Tamari M, Uchida K, Takahashi T, Nakamura Y. Aberrant upregulation of a novel integrin alpha subunit gene at 3p21.3 in small cell lung cancer. Oncogene 1994; 9:611–619.

28. Daly MC, Xiang RH, Buchhagen D, Hensel CH, Garcia DK, Killary AM, Minna JD, Naylor SL. A homozygous deletion on chromosome 3 in a small cell lung cancer cell line correlates with a region of tumor suppressor activity. Oncogene 1993; 8:1721–1729.

29. Killary AM, Wolf ME, Giambernardi TA, Naylor SL. Definition of a tumor suppressor locus within human chromosome 3p21-p22. Proc Natl Acad Sci USA 1992; 89:10877–10881.

30. Satoh H, Lamb PW, Dong JT, Everitt J, Boreiko C, Oshimura M, Barrett JC. Suppression of tumorigenicity of A549 lung adenocarcinoma cells by human chromosomes 3 and 11 introduced via microcell-mediated chromosome transfer. Mol Carcinogen 1993; 7:157–164.

31. Naylor SL, Marshall A, Hensel C, Martinez PF, Holley B, Sakaguchi AY. The DNF15S2 locus at 3p21 is transcribed in normal lung and small cell lung cancer. Genomics 1989; 4:355–361.

32. Miller YE, Daniels GL, Jones C, Palmer DK. Identification of a cell-surface antigen produced by a gene on human chromosome 3 (cen-q22) and not expressed by Rhnull cells. Am J Hum Genet 1987; 41:1061–1070.

33. Carritt B, Kok K, van den Berg A, Osinga J, Pilz A, Hofstra RM, Davis MB, van der Veen AY, Rabbitts PH, Gulati K, et al. A gene from human chromosome region 3p21 with reduced expression in small cell lung cancer. Cancer Res 1992; 52:1536–1541.

34. Kok K, Hofstra R, Pilz A, van den Berg A, Terpstra P, Buys CH, Carritt B. A gene in the chromosomal region 3p21 with greatly reduced expression in lung cancer is similar to the gene for ubiquitin-activating enzyme. Proc Natl Acad Sci USA 1993; 90:6071–6075.

35. Hoovers JM, Mannens M, John R, Bliek J, van Heyningen V, Porteous DJ, Leschot NJ, Westerveld A, Little PF. High-resolution localization of 69 potential human zinc finger protein genes: a number are clustered. Genomics 1992; 12:254–263.

36. Roche J, Boldog F, Robinson M, Robinson L, Varella-Garcia M, Swanton, M, Waggoner B, Fishel R, Franklin W, Gemmill R, Drabkin H. Distinct 3p21.3 deletions in lung cancer and identification of a new human semaphorin. Oncogene 1996; 12:1289–1297.

37. Todd MC, Xiang RH, Garcia DK, Kerbacher KE, Moore SL, Hensel CH, Liu, P, Siciliano MJ, Kok K, van den Berg A, Veldhuis P, Buys CH, Killary, AM, Naylor SL. An 80 Kb P1 clone from chromosome 3p21.3 suppresses tumor growth in vivo. Oncogene 1996; 13:2387–2396.

38. Latif F, Tory K, Gnarra J, Yao M, Duh FM, Orcutt ML, Stackhouse T, Kuzmin I, Modi W, Geil L, et al. Identification of the von Hippel-Lindau disease tumor suppressor gene. Science 1993; 260:1317–1320.

39. Gnarra JR, Tory K, Weng Y, Schmidt L, Wei MH, Li H, Latif F, Liu S, Chen F, Duh FM, et al. Mutations of the VHL tumour suppressor gene in renal carcinoma. Nature Genet 1994; 7:85–90.

40. Sekido Y, Bader S, Latif F, Gnarra JR, Gazdar AF, Linehan WM, Zbar B, Lerman MI, Minna JD. Molecular analysis of the von Hippel-Lindau disease tumor suppressor gene in human lung cancer cell lines. Oncogene 1994; 9:1599–1604.

41. Lubinski J, Hadaczek P, Podolski J, Toloczko A, Sikorski A, McCue P, Druck T, Huebner K. Common regions of deletion in chromosome regions 3p12 and 3p14.2 in primary clear cell renal carcinomas. Cancer Res 1994; 54:3710–3713.

42. Druck T, Kastury K, Hadaczek P, Podolski J, Toloczko A, Sikorski A, Ohta M, LaForgia S, Lasota J, McCue P, et al. Loss of heterozygosity at the familial RCC t(3;8) locus in most clear cell renal carcinomas. Cancer Res 1995; 55:5348–5353.

43. Pandis N, Idvall I, Bardi G, Jin Y, Gorunova L, Mertens F, Olsson H, Ingvar C, Beroukas K, Mitelman F, Heim S. Correlation between karyotypic pattern and clinicopathologic features in 125 breast cancer cases. Int J Cancer 1996; 66:191–196.

44. Teixeira MR, Pandis N, Bardi G, Andersen JA, Heim S. Karyotypic comparisons of multiple tumorous and macroscopically normal surrounding tissue samples from patients with breast cancer. Cancer Res 1996; 56:855–859.

45. Mao L, Lee JS, Fan YH, Ro JY, Batsakis JG, Lippman S, Hittelman W, Hong WK. Frequent microsatellite alterations at chromosomes 9p21 and 3p14 in oral premalignant lesions and their value in cancer risk assessment. Nature Med 1996; 2:682–685.

46. Roz L, Wu CL, Porter S, Scully C, Speight P, Read A, Sloan P, Thakker N. Allelic imbalance on chromosome 3p in oral dysplastic lesions: an early event in oral carcinogenesis. Cancer Res 1996; 56:1228–1231.

47. Lisitsyn N, Wigler M. Representational difference analysis in detection of genetic lesions in cancer. Methods Enzymol 1995; 254:291–304.

48. Kastury K, Baffa R, Druck T, Ohta M, Cotticelli MG, Inoue H, Negrini M, Rugge M, Huang D, Croce CM, Palazzo J, Huebner K. Potential gastrointestinal tumor suppressor locus at the 3p14.2 FRA3B site identified by homozygous deletions in tumor cell lines. Cancer Res 1996; 56:978–983.

49. Boldog F, Gemmill RM, West J, Robinson M, Robinson L, Li E, Roche J, Todd S, Waggoner B, Lundstrom R, Jacobson J, Mullokandov MR, Klinger H, Drabkin HA. Chromosome 3p14 homozygous deletions and sequence analysis of FRA3B. Hum Mol Genet 1997; 6, No.2:193–203.

50. Cohen AJ, Li FP, Berg S, Marchetto DJ, Tsai S, Jacobs SC, Brown RS. Hereditary renal-cell carcinoma associated with a chromosomal translocation. N Engl J Med 1979; 301:592–595.
51. Harris P, Morton CC, Guglielmi P, Li F, Kelly K, Latt SA. Mapping by chromosome sorting of several gene probes, including c-myc, to the derivative chromosomes of a 3;8 transloca-tion associated with familial renal cancer. Cytometry 1986; 7:589–594.
52. Gemmill RM, Coyle-Morris J, Ware-Uribe L, Pearson N, Hecht F, Brown RS, Li FP, Drab-kin HA. A 1.5-megabase restriction map surrounding MYC does not include the transloca-tion breakpoint in familial renal cell carcinoma. Genomics 1989; 4:28–35.
53. LaForgia S, Morse B, Levy J, Barnea G, Cannizzaro LA, Li F, Nowell PC, Boghosian-Sell L, Glick J, Weston A, et al. Receptor protein-tyrosine phosphatase gamma is a candidate tu-mor suppressor gene at human chromosome region 3p21. Proc Natl Acad Sci USA 1991; 88:5036–5040.
54. LaForgia S, Lasota J, Latif F, Boghosian-Sell L, Kastury K, Ohta M, Druck T, Atchison L, Cannizzaro LA, Barnea G, et al. Detailed genetic and physical map of the 3p chromosome region surrounding the familial renal cell carcinoma chromosome translocation, t(3;8)(p14.2;q24.1). Cancer Res 1993; 53:3118–3124.
55. Boldog FL, Gemmill RM, Wilke CM, Glover TW, Nilsson AS, Chandrasekharappa SC, Brown RS, Li FP, Drabkin HA. Positional cloning of the hereditary renal carcinoma 3;8 chromosome translocation breakpoint. Proc Natl Acad Sci USA 1993; 90:8509–8513.
56. Sundaresan V, Ganly P, Haselton P, Rudd R, Sinha G, Bleehen NM, Rabbits P. p53 and chromosome 3 abnormalities, characteristic of malignant lung tumours, are detectable in preinvasive lesions of the bronchus. Oncogene 1992; 7:1989–1997.
57. Sozzi G, Miozzo M, Pastorino U, Pilotti S, Donghi R, Giarola M, De Gregorio L, Manenti G, Radice P, Minoletti F, Della Porta G, Pierotti MA. Genetic evidence of field canceriza-tion in patients with multiple synchronous tumors of the lung. Cancer Res 1995; 55:135–140.
58. Thiberville L, Payne P, Vielkinds J, LeRiche J, Horsman D, Nouvet G, Palcic B, Lam S. Evidence of cumulative gene losses with progression of premalignant epithelial lesions to carcinoma of the bronchus. Cancer Res 1995; 55:5133–5139.
59. Hung J, Kishimoto Y, Sugio K, Virmani A, McIntire DD, Minna JD, Gazdar AF. Allele-specific chromosome 3p deletions occur at an early stage in the pathogenesis of lung carci-noma. JAMA 1995; 273:558–563.
60. Sozzi G, Miozzo M, Tagliabue E, Calderone C, Lombardi L, Pilotti S, Pastorino U, Pierotti MA, Della Porta G. Cytogenetic abnormalities and overexpression of receptors for growth factors in normal bronchial epithelium and tumor samples of lung cancer patients. Cancer Res 1991; 51:400–404.
61. Sundaresan V, Heppell-Parton A, Coleman N, Miozzo M, Sozzi G, Ball R, Cary N, Hasleton P, Fowler W, Rabbits P. Somatic genetic changes in lung cancer and precancerous lesions. Ann Oncol 1995; 6(suppl. 1):S27–S32.
62. Glover TW, Berger C, Coyle J, Echo B. DNA polymerase alpha inhibition by aphidicolin in-duces gaps and breaks at common fragile sites in human chromosomes. Hum Genet 1984; 67:136–142.
63. Yunis JJ, Soreng AL. Constitutive fragile sites and cancer. Science 1984; 226:1199–1204.
64. Le Beau MM. Chromosomal fragile sites and cancer-specific rearrangements. Blood 1986; 67:849–858.
65. Schmid M, Ott G, Haaf T, Scheres JM. Evolutionary conservation of fragile sites induced by 5-azacytidine and 5-azadeoxycytidine in man, gorilla, and chimpanzee. Hum Genet 1985; 71:342–350.
66. Yunis JJ, Soreng AL, Bowe AE. Fragile sites are targets of diverse mutagens and carcino-gens. Oncogene 1987; 1:59–69.
67. Musio A, Sbrana I. Common and rare fragile sites on human chromosomes. The cytogenetic expression of active and inactive genes? Cancer Genet Cytogenet 1996; 88:184–185.
68. Sutherland GR, Richards RI. The molecular basis of fragile sites in human chromosomes. Curr Opin Genet Develop 1995; 5:323–327.
69. Kuwano A, Kajii T. Synergistic effect of aphidicolin and ethanol on the induction of com-mon fragile sites. Hum Genet 1987; 75:75–78.

70. Kao-Shan CS, Fine RL, Whang-Peng J, Lee EC, Chabner BA. Increased fragile sites and
     sister chromatid exchanges in bone marrow and peripheral blood of young cigarette smok-
     ers. Cancer Res 1987; 47:6278–6282.
71. Glover TW, Stein CK. Chromosome breakage and recombination at fragile sites. Am J Hum
     Genet 1988; 43:265–273.
72. Paradee JD, Mullins C, He Z, Glover T, Wilke C, Opalka B, Schutte J, Smith D. Precise lo-
     calization of aphidicolin-induced breakpoints on the short arm of human chromosome 3.
     Genomics 1995; 27:358–361.
73. Wilke CM, Guo SW, Hall BK, Boldog F, Gemmill RM, Chandrasekharappa, SC, Barcroft
     CL, Drabkin HA, Glover TW. Multicolor FISH mapping of YAC clones in 3p14 and iden-
     tification of a YAC spanning both FRA3B and the t(3;8) associated with hereditary renal cell
     carcinoma. Genomics 1994; 22:319–326.
74. Boldog FL, Waggoner B, Glover TW, Chumakov I, Le Paslier D, Cohen D, Gemmill RM,
     Drabkin HA. Integrated YAC contig containing the 3p14.2 hereditary renal carcinoma 3;8
     translocation breakpoint and the fragile site FRA3B. Genes Chrom Cancer 1994; 11:216–
     221.
75. Wilke CM, Hall BK, Hoge A, Paradee W, Smith DI, Glover TW. FRA3B extends over a
     broad region and contains a spontaneous HPV16 integration site: direct evidence for the co-
     incidence of viral integration sites and fragile sites. Hum Mol Genet 1996; 5:187–195.
76. Michaelis SC, Bardenheuer W, Lux A, Schramm A, Gockel A, Siebert R, Willers C,
     Schmidtke K, Todt B, van der Hout AH, et al. Characterization and chromosomal assign-
     ment of yeast artificial chromosomes containing human 3p13-p21-specific sequence tagged
     sites. Cancer Genet cytogenet 1995; 81:1–12.
77. Ohta M, Inoue H, Cotticelli MG, Kastury K, Baffa R, Palazzo J, Siprashvili Z, Mori M, Mc-
     Cue P, Druck T, Croce CM, Huebner K. The FHIT gene, spanning the chromosome 3p14.2
     fragile site and renal carcinoma-associated t(3;8) breakpoint, is abnormal in digestive tract
     cancer. Cell 1996; 84:587–597.
78. Huang Y, Garrison PN, Barnes LD. Cloning of the Schizosaccharomyces pombe gene en-
     coding diadenosine 5′,5‴-P1,P4-tetraphosphate (Ap4A) asymmetrical hydrolase: sequence
     similarity with the histidine triad (HIT) protein family. Biochem J 1995; 312:925–932.
79. Robinson AK, de la Pena CE, Barnes LD. Isolation and characterization of diadenosine tet-
     raphosphate (Ap4A) hydrolase from Schizosaccharomyces pombe. Biochim Biophys Acta
     1993; 1161:139–148.
80. Barnes LD, Garrison PN, Siprashvill Z, Guranowski A, Robinson AK, Ingram SW, Croce
     CM, Otha M, Huebner K. Fhit, a putative tumor suppressor in humans, is a dinucleoside
     5′,5‴-P1,P3-triphosphate hydrolase. Biochemistry 1996; 35 (36):11529–11535.
81. Brenner C, Garrison P, Gilmour J, Peisach D, Ringe D, Petsko GA, Lowenstein JM. Crystal
     structures of HINT demonstrate that histidine triad proteins are GalT-related nucleotide-
     binding proteins. Nature Struct Biol 1997; 4, No. 3:231–238.
82. Kitzler JW, Farr SB, Ames BN. Intracellular functions of ApnN: prokaryotes. In: McLennan
     AG, ed. Ap4A and other dinucleoside polyphosphates. Boca Raton, FL: CRC Press, 1992:
83. Vartanian A, Narovlyansky A, Amchenkova A, Turpaev K, Kisselev L. Interferons induce
     accumulation of diadenosine triphosphate (Ap3A) in human cultured cells. FEBS Lett 1996;
     381:32–34.
84. Segal E, Le Pecq JB. Relationship between cellular diadenosine 5′,5‴-P1,P4-tetraphosphate
     level, cell density, cell growth stimulation and toxic stresses. Exp Cell Res 1986; 167:119–
     126.
85. Sozzi G, Veronese ML, Negrini M, Baffa R, Cotticelli MG, Inoue H, Tornielli S, Pilotti S,
     De Gregorio L, Pastorino U, Pierotti MA, Otha M, Huebner K, Croce CM. The *FHIT* gene
     at 3p14.2 is abnormal in lung cancer. Cell 1996; 85:17–26.
86a. Yanagisawa K, Kondo M, Osada H, Uchida K, Takagi K, Masuda A, Takahashi T. Molecu-
     lar analysis of the FHIT gene at 3p14.2 in lung cancer cell lines. Cancer Res 1996; 56:5579–
     5582.
86b. Fong KH, Biesterveed EJ, Virmani A, Wistuba I, Sckido Y, Bader SA, Ahmadian M, Ong
     ST, Rassool FV, Zimmerman PV, Giaccone G, Gazdar AF, Minna JD. FHIT and

FRA3B3p14.2 Allele loss are common in lung cancer and preneoplastic bronchial lesions and are associated with cancer-related FHIT CDNA spicing abberations. Cancer Res 1997; 57:2256-2267.

87. Virgilio L, Shuster M, Gollin SM, Veronese ML, Ohta M, Huebner K, Croce CM. FHIT gene alterations in head and neck squamous cell carcinomas. Proc Natl Acad Sci USA 1996; 93:9770-9775.

88. Sozzi G, Sard L, De Gregorio L, Marchetti A, Musso K, Buttitta F, Tornielli S, Pellegrini S, Veronese ML, Manenti G, Incarbone M, Chella A, Angeletti CA, Pastorino U, Huebner K, Bevilaqua G, Pilotti S, Croce CM, Pierotti MA. Association between cigarette smoking and *FHIT* gene alterations in lung cancer. Cancer Res 1997; 57:5207-5212.

89. Pennisi E. New gene forges link between fragile site and many cancers. Science 1996; 272:649.

90. Roth JA, Nguyen D, Lawrence DD, Kemp BL, Carrasco CH, Ferson DZ, Hong WK, Komaki R, Lee JJ, Nesbitt JC, Pisters KM, Putnam JB, Schea R, Shin DM, Walsh GL, Dolormente MM, Han CI, Martin FD, Yen N, Xu K, Stephens LC, McDonnell TJ, Mukhopadhyay T, Cai D. Retrovirus-mediated wild-type p53 gene transfer to tumors of patients with lung cancer. Nature Med 1996; 2:985-991.

10

P53 Pathway and Lung Cancer

ELISABETH BRAMBILLA and SYLVIE GAZZERI

Institut Albert Bonniot
Centre Hospitalier Universitaire de Grenoble
Grenoble, France

I. Introduction

Lung cancer is a major health problem worldwide due to its high frequency, especially in developed countries. It is the first cause of death in males (in all countries) and in females (in the United States). It has been established that lung cancer is the result of a sequential accumulation of multiple genetic alterations (10–20 mutations) involving key genes, whose protein products control proliferation and apoptosis. The malignant transformation of lung epithelial cells involve mutation of oncogenes and resultant dysregulation of their encoded proteins including ras mutation, myc amplification, EGF, and C-erb-B2 growth factor/receptor autocrine loops, which result in increasing rate of proliferation (1). It has become clear that inactivation of tumor suppressor genes through inhibition of their protein product (P53, retinoblastoma gene, CdK-I-P16) removes important regulatory constraints on the cell cycle at the G1 restriction point. P53 transcription factor on a common pathway with Rb regulates G1 arrest, and on a pathway independant from Rb regulates apoptosis. P53 inactivation could thus contribute to accelerated growth of lung cancer tissue by both increasing the rate of cell division and allowing escape from apoptosis (Fig. 1). Both the P53 and Rb genes have been consistently found to be inactivated in both small-cell lung cancer

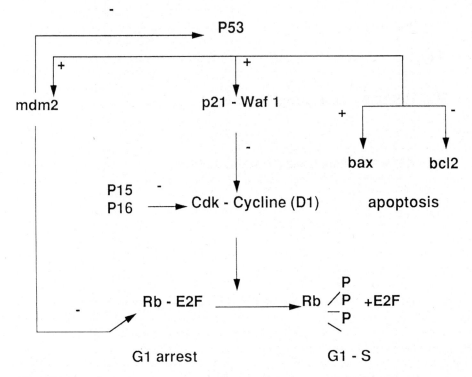

Figure 1

(SCLC) and non–small-cell lung cancer (NSCLC) (2–4). These two types of tumor biologically represent two different pathways of differentiation: the neuroendocrine (NE) lung tumors including SCLC and other NE lung tumors (carcinoids, large-cell neuroendocrine carcinoma), and nonneuroendocrine lung tumors (also called NSCLC) including squamous carcinoma, adenocarcinoma and large-cell carcinoma. Differences in pathways of carcinogenesis among different histological classes and in NE versus non-NE tumors have been shown, although in vitro and in vivo studies support the existence of a pluripotent common stem cell as an origin for all histological tumor types (except for bronchioloalveolar adenocarcinoma). Cigarette smoking is responsible for 90% of lung carcinoma in men and 78% in women (5), and there is epidemiological evidence for a dose-response relationship with the duration and amount of smoking in U.S. studies (6). P53 mutational spectrum analysis could further define this association (see Chapter 28).

   Potential mechanisms for P53 inactivation in lung cancer are not restricted to P53 mutation. Moreover, mutation or deregulation of the downstream gene or protein pathway of P53, interrupting its wild-type function, could well mimic and overcome P53 mutation.

Table 1 Products of Genes Transcriptionally Activated by P53[a]

p21, Waf1, Cip1	Inhibit several cyclin-dependent kinases; bind cdks, cyclins, and PCNA; arrest the cell cycle
MDM2	Product of an oncogene; inactivates P53-mediated transcription and so forms an autoregulatory loop with P53 activity
GADD45	Induced upon DNA damage; binds to PCNA and can arrest the cell cycle; involved directly in DNA nucleotide excision repair
Cyclin G	A novel cyclin (it does not cycle with cell division) of unknown function and no known cyclin-dependent kinase
Bax	A member of the Bcl2 family that promotes apoptosis; not induced by P53 in all cells
IGF-BP3	The insulin-like growth factor binding protein-3; blocks signaling of a mitogenic growth factor.

[a]While a large number of other genes have been suggested to be regulated by P53, those listed above all have been shown to contain P53-dependent, *cis*-acting, DNA-responsive elements.
Source: Ref. 83.

II. P53, The Gatekeeper for Clonal Growth

From the discovery of the P53 gene as a frequent target in lung (2) and many other cancers, the functions of the P53 gene and its protein product have been the center of intensive study. Yet slightly more than 50% of human, especially lung, cancers contain mutations in this gene. However, the remarkable functions of P53 in life or death in cells under stress conditions makes P53 a pivotal factor in lung carcinogenesis (7). We will focus in this chapter on the function of P53 as a sensor of cellular stress, which could be disrupted in lung cancer, whether by P53 mutation or through deregulation of its downstream gene targets, in order to abrogate efficiency of growth arrest and/or apoptosis. P53 is a transcription factor that enhances the rate of transcription of a set of genes that carry out most of the P53-dependent functions (Table 1) (8) on G1 arrest, apoptosis, and DNA repair recognition. P53 and the P53 pathway are induced in response to DNA damage and to stress conditions very common in tumors such as hypoxia, lack of paracrine growth factors from normal cells, or death induced by immune system. It is therefore not surprising that P53 and genes of its downstream pathway are so strongly selected against during clonal expansion. Moreover, many carcinogens from tobacco smoke directly affect the P53 DNA sequence, indicating that P53 mutation is a rather early event in lung cancer.

In normal cells, P53 protein is kept at low concentration by a short 20-minute half-life due to rapid ubiquitin-mediated proteolysis. The upstream events that induce P53 activation are stressful situations including DNA damage (double strand breaks of gamma irradiation, excision repairs, or chemical damage) and hypoxia (9). Both events increase P53 levels and activate it from its latent form to become transcriptionally active. Hypoxia in tumors, in addition to DNA damage, represents a way for P53 to act as a gatekeeper. Since many tumors reach a critical size where blood supply becomes rate limiting, the resultant hypoxia might trigger P53 activation and cell suicide in the absence of blood supply through neoangiogenesis. Downstream events in response to P53 activation take place in two major pathways: one for cell cycle arrest (*p16-cyclin D1-CdK4-Rb* pathway) and the other for apoptosis (*P53-bax/bcl2* pathway) (Fig. 1). The Rb pathway is essential for cell cycle regulation at the G1 restriction point. One of the genes of this pathway should be altered or mutant in almost all cancer (see Chapters 11 and 12). Rb protein regulates the G1 restriction point (the point of no return) depending on its phosphorylation by cyclin–cyclin-dependent-kinase (CdK). Underphosphorylated Rb complexes E2F, whereas phosphorylated Rb releases E2F, allowing its transcription effects on G1-to-S transition. In response to DNA damage, P53 activates p21-Waf1 transcription, which binds to and activates several cyclin-CdK complexes and prevents Rb phosphorylation. P21 is the mediator of P53-induced G1 arrest. Of course, this model of P53-Rb pathway predicts that Rb is essential for P53-induced G1 arrest. At least in human cells, where Rb1 is dominant over other Rb gene family members, Rb loss of protein functions would inhibit P53-dependent G1 arrest. Accordingly, Rb loss of function will bypass P53 wild-type functions. However, a supplementary role for P53 in triggering apoptosis under many physiological conditions indicates that P53 and Rb loss of function are not redundant and can be found in the same tumors.

Although not all apoptotic events are P53 mediated, P53 initiates apoptosis in response to DNA damage and stress conditions, as well as in response to oncogene expression or the lack of Rb function. E1A adenoviral protein and E7 of HPV bind to Rb and allow the release of E2F from the Rb-E2F1 complex, which induces a P53-dependent apoptosis. Moreover, cyclin D1 upregulation or myc activation will induce a P53-dependent apoptosis. Thus, many proliferative signals in cells are coupled with P53-dependent apoptosis. Accordingly, P53 acts to reduce the incidence of cancers by mediating apoptosis in cells with activated oncogenes (E1A, E7, cyclin D1, myc). This is the most obvious reason for many cancer cells to select clones against wild-type P53 functions. Two of the genes transcriptionally activated by P53 are bax (10) and IGF BP3 (IGF-binding protein 3) (11). Bax, in the form of a homodimer, can be considered as the main effector of apoptosis executed by the Caspace pathway. The Bax-Bax homodimer is opposed by heterodimerization with Bcl2 (Bax-Bcl2) or another Bcl2 anti-apoptotic member of the Bcl2 family such as BclXL, MCL1, or A1. Bax could be considered a tumor suppressor gene, but Bax mutations have been shown only in colon carcinoma cell lines (12). Bcl2, in contrast, can be considered an oncogene, since Bcl2 can block any kind of P53-mediated apoptosis as well as many P53-independent apoptoses. Bcl2 was shown to be negatively regulated by P53 (10). Thus, the ratio of Bax to Bcl2 in cells dictates the susceptibility to apoptosis. Conversely, IGF BP3 blocks IGF1 mitotic signaling by preventing its interaction with its tyrosine-kinase receptor, thus enhancing apoptosis and lowering IGF1 mitogenic responses.

Consequently, P53 mutation by itself or any constitutive deregulation of its apoptotic pathway, such as Bcl2 : Bax ratio or IGF BP3 depletion, would prevent apoptosis in cells with DNA damage or living under stress conditions, which is the case with most tumor cells. Moreover, P53 plays a role in cell senescence, increasing cell life span in culture, the effect which is abrogated by a transdominant acting mutant P53 (13). P53 and its downstream pathway are thus placed in the remarkable position of performing most relevant cellular functions and preventing abnormal clonal expansion.

III. P53 Genetic Inactivation in Lung Cancer

P53 mutation is the most frequent alteration in lung cancer beyond 3p loss of heterozygosity, and the highest frequency of P53 alterations is found in lung cancer (14). The spectrum of P53 mutation in lung cancer and its relationship to tobacco smoke is discussed in a previous chapter. P53 mutations can be detected at the genetic level using sequencing of genomic DNA or sequencing of RT-PCR product, allowing detection of exon mutations. Intronic mutations and splicing site abnormalities are best analyzed by genomic DNA PCR using specific primers. Because DNA sequencing is time and labor consuming, screening tests on large series have mainly used immunohistochemistry, SSCP (single strand conformation polymorphism), and DGGE (denaturant gradient gel electophoresis).

Immunohistochemistry (IH) can detect, with high efficiency, missense mutations on exons 5–8, which represent 85% of P53 mutations, and most often increase the half-life of the protein by stabilizing it, thus allowing nuclear staining in routine IH. In this respect, several antibodies can be used, most of which are directed against N-terminal epitopes. The increased quality of these antibodies and of antigen-retrieving methods (15) allows P53 detection in lung cancer. Using IH, the choice of cut-off value for "P53 positivity" has led to differences in results and prognostic value evaluation. It should be stated that PAB 240, which has a conformation-dependent linear epitope, is always used in denaturing conditions in immunohistochemistry where proteins have been (partially or completely) denatured by fixation (before embedding or on frozen sections). It would thus be misleading to regard it as an antibody specific for mutant conformation in IH. Any specific and reactive antibodies (more than one is recommended) are equally valid for detection of P53 stabilization in lung cancer with a low risk of false positives. Comparing PCR-based sequence analysis and immunohistochemistry in 30 cases we and others found that 90% of P53-positive cases had a missense mutation provided that at least 20% of cells were positive (3), and 10% for others (16) with at least two different antibodies. When we compared the results of SSCP (exons 4–9) with that of RT-PCR-sequencing, we found a 90% correlation (one mutation in exon 7 giving no shift), whereas SSCP (exons 4–9) showed an 80% shift in the P53 IH-positive cases. This signifies that IH is a sensitive method for the detection of missense-stabilizing mutation in lung cancer. Fifteen to 20% of the mutations belong to the class of splicing abnormalities (intronic insertion or deletion) with frameshift or stop codon. This second type of mutation results in a null P53 phenotype (no mRNA, no protein)

(3,17) and generates 15–20% false-negatives in immunohistochemistry. This raises the total frequency of P53 mutation in lung cancer to 70%.

Surprisingly, the frequency of reported mutations and P53 stabilization in lung cancer does not much vary according to the method used. It is likely that 15–20% of false-negatives occurred using each technique and underevaluated the real rate of P53 mutation in lung cancer. From series actually published, mutations have been detected in 50% of lung cancer of all histological types: they were found in 70–100% of SCLC (18–21) and in 45–75% of NSCLC (22,23). In all series, P53 mutant immunophenotype was more frequent in squamous carcinoma (55–65%) than in adenocarcinoma (30–40%), a prevalence that approximates that of other adenocarcinomas better than that of other lung cancer histologies. Strikingly, Japanese and recent American studies report a high frequency (70–90%) of mutations and positive IH in SCLC (24,25). The mean frequency in European countries is lower (45%) (26–30). Whether this is related to methods is not certain since the cited studies have all used IH in addition to sequencing analysis. An epidemiological difference remains possible.

Like any tumor suppressor gene, P53 should be inactivated through two successive events: mutation of one allele and loss or mutation of a second allele. Double allelic mutation or homozygous deletion are rare in lung cancer. Loss of heterozygosity (LOH), which means loss of one allele, at the 17p13 locus where P53 gene maps is frequently observed but diversely appreciated, again probably because of technical differences (number and type of microsatellite probes and contamination of tumor tissue by genetically normal stromal cells in RFLP analysis). Overall 80% of tumors with LOH had a P53 missense mutation of the remaining allele (19,22,31,32). In a recent study (33), 37% of tumors showed LOH at the primary tumor site and 88% in the metastatis. Whereas cases with mutation had all LOH at the metastatic site, only 70% of cases with mutations (exons 5–8) had LOH at the primary site. This suggests that mutation or LOH can be isolated and that double allele inactivation is not obligatory. Mutation of one allele could confer dominance (dominant negative gene). LOH without mutation of the remaining allele (20%) suggests that P53 allelic loss alone endows growth advantage to cancer cells, or that another tumor suppressor gene maps on 17p13 as already reported (34). Few reports have documented the relationship between LOH and P53 mutation in lung cancer in vivo.

IV. P53 Stabilization and Epigenetic Inactivation in Lung Cancer

It is likely that P53 stabilization reflects a stabilizing missense mutation if more than 10–20% of lung cancer cells show P53 immunostaining. However, there are nonmalignant situations where a focal staining of epithelial cells has been noted. In diffuse alveolar damage, which is a form of acute inflammatory disease, P53 is stabilized in its wild-type form (35), in response to DNA damage, and in pneumonocytes, fibroblasts, and endothelial cells.

P53 stabilization or inactivation in lung cancer could be the result of mechanisms other than mutation. Epigenetic and posttranslational P53 inactivation include stabilization by binding to a viral protein (SV40 or E1b of adenovirus), inactivation by E6 protein of the human papilloma virus (HPV), or by mdm2. Mdm2, induced by wild-type P53 only, interacts with wild-type P53 and inactivates its transcription functions, as an autoregularory feedback loop to limit the P53 responses. As a result, any constitutive deregulation of mdm2, like mdm2 amplification, could inactivate P53 by sequestration in an inactive p53-mdm2 complex (36,37). Two recent reports have found mdm2 overexpression in lung cancer (38,39) to be due to mdm2 increased transcription more than to mdm2 amplification. More than 80% of cases showed mdm2 overexpression in NSCLC. Both P53 and mdm2 were simultaneously detected in 54% of tumors. Eighty-four percent of these tumors had a P53 mobility shift, which suggests a P53-independent pathway of mdm2 overexpression. The role of mdm2 overproduction in inhibiting wild-type P53 transactivating functions in lung cancer is questionable. Interestingly, most lung adenocarcinomas are $mdm2^+ P53^-$, suggesting than the low rate of P53 mutation is offset by a high rate of mdm2 activation in this tumor type. Indeed mdm2 inhibits Rb growth-regulatory functions. Therefore, both P53 and Rb are subjected to negative regulation by mdm2 (40).

Finally, HPV 6, 11, 16, 18, 31, and 33 were identified in 30% of lung adenocarcinoma (41) with an inverse relationship between the presence of papilloma viral DNA and abnormal P53 protein accumulation, but their association with squamous carcinoma is more controversial. HPV may contribute in inactivating wild-type P53 by binding of HPV-E6 protein to P53, leading to its degradation by ubiquitins. Neither SV40 nor adenovirus has been demonstrated in lung cancer.

In addition to these epigenetic and posttranslational types of inactivation, it has become clear that the P53 downstream pathway is involved in the inactivation of G1 arrest and/or apoptosis in lung cancer. This is likely the reason that neither P53 immunohistochemical status nor the P53 genetic status was convincingly shown to correlate with prognosis.

V. P53 as a Marker for Tumor Progression and Prognosis in Non–Small-Cell Lung Carcinoma

It is a matter of controversy how P53 gene alterations affect the clinical outcome of patients with NSCLC (Table 2) (42–56). The discrepancies cannot be attributed only to technical differences: as shown in Table 1, IH as well as molecular studies have provided conflicting results for the same type of analysis and for patients selected at the same stage of the disease. The superiority of one method or the other (IH or molecular) was not confirmed in regard to evaluation of the prognostic influence of P53 alterations. It was expected that molecular biology would more accurately evaluate the real frequency of genetic P53 mutation, but most studies rely on screening tests

Table 2 Clinical Significance of P53 Alteration in Reported Series of NSCLC

Authors (ref.)	Year	No. of patients	Stage	% positive	Survival	p^a
Protein expression using immunohistochemistry:						
Quinlan et al. (42)	1992	114	I–II	43	↘	<0.001
McLaren et al. (27)	1992	125	I–IV	54	NS	
Fontanini et al. (43)	1993	103	I–II	36–68	Node spread	
Morkve et al. (44)	1993	112	I–IIIB	77	NS	0.16
Brambilla et al. (29)	1993	95	I–IV	50	NS	0.3
Marchetti et al. (45)	1993	53	I–IV	75	NS	
Volm et al. (46)	1994	209	I–IV	49	↗	0.002
Carbone et al. (47)	1994	85	I–III	64	↘	0.05
Passlick et al. (48)	1995	73	II–IV	45	NS	0.1
		34	I–II		↗	0.004
Sauter et al. (49)	1995	68	I–IV	56	NS	
					SCC ↗	0.03
Harpole et al. (50)	1995	271		38	↘	0.007
Lee et al. (51)	1995	156	I–III	66	↗	0.002
Dalquen et al. (52)	1996	247	I–III	48	NS	
		113	I–II	40	↘	0.03
Törmänen et al. (53)	1996	75	I–III	50	↘	0.005
Nishio et al. (16)	1996	208	I–III	46	NS	
			I–II ADC	37	↘	0.04
DNA mutation using SCCP ± sequencing:						
Mitsudomi et al. (54)	1992	66	I–IV	74	NS	
Mitsudomi et al. (55)	1993	120	I–IV	43	↘	0.01
Horio et al. (56)	1993	71	I–III	49	↘	0.014
Marchetti et al. (45)	1993	53	I–IV	75	Node spread	

[a]Probability for difference in survival (Kaplan Meier analysis).
SCC: Squamous cell carcinoma; ADC: adenocarcinoma; ↘: shorter survival; ↗: longer survival.

such as SSCP, which support 20% false-negatives and false-positives—as much as IH. One report even stressed the possibility that the stabilization of P53 was related to shortened survival, whereas mutational status was not (57). Again the cut-off value for "P53 positivity" from 1 to 20% appears to influence dramatically the prognostic evaluation (24,44,51,58). There was no demonstration of P53 influence on the survival of SCLC.

The main conclusion is that if P53 is a prognostic factor in the subgroup of patients at early stage or in histological subgroups (like atypical carcinoids) (24), it could only be very weak, and P53 does not support qualify as prognostic for lung cancer. A tendency for association of P53 abnormalities with node spread or extended stage was noted (29,43,45,52,59). A much higher association of LOH with

P53 mutations was shown in metastasis than at the primary site (33). P53 mutations are, however, definitely acquired before metastasis, since 30% of dysplasia displayed mutant P53. Finally, although P53 may be of considerable importance in the initiation of malignancy, as shown below, it is probably of little prognostic significance once the tumor has developed.

P53 stabilization, when associated with other oncogene or tumor suppressor gene dysregulation, could show prognostic influence, particularly in association with c-erb-B2 overexpression ($p = 0.001$) (50) or with Rb inactivation ($p = 0.005$) (60). A previous study showed synergistic effects between altered Rb or P16 and altered P53 protein in proliferative activity of NSCLC (61).

In regard to chemosensitivity, transfected wild-type P53 was shown to repress MDR1 transcription, whereas mutant P53 transfected in lung cancer cell lines could activate MDR1 transcription (62), and paradoxically more recently wild-type P53 transfer was shown to stimulate MDR1 promoter in H358 null P53 cell line (63). However, no correlation between P53 and MDR1 expression (using JSB1 antibody) in NSCLC was found, and an influence of P53 mutation or overexpression on the chemosensitivity of SCLC could not be confirmed. A recent study (64,65) showed that high P53 expression before chemotherapy in stage III NSCLC predicted resistance to cisplatin. This is in keeping with in vitro demonstration that transfer of wild-type P53 could achieve complete treatment sensitization of SCLC tumor cells expressing endogenous mutant P53 (66).

VI. P53 Stabilization in Neuroendocrine Tumors

In the spectrum of NE lung tumors, four histological types of increasing malignancy are described: the rather benign carcinoid, the atypical carcinoid with intermediate prognosis, and the highly malignant small-cell lung carcinoma (SCLC) and large-cell neuroendocrine carcinoma (LCNEC) (67). P53 mutation or stabilization is absent in typical carcinoids (24,29,30,68). Some atypical carcinoids, which showed focal (less than 10%) or patchy (10–50%) P53 positivity, were more aggressive and had significantly shorter survival ($p < 0.05$) than those without P53 staining. However, all had wild-type P53 (exons 5–8). Moreover, only high-grade NE lung tumors show diffuse mutant P53 staining and harbor P53 mutations. Thus, P53 immunochemistry could delineate cases of higher risk for aggressive behavior in this category of tumor (24).

VII. P53 Downstream Pathway in Lung Cancer

As mentioned earlier, instead of P53 inactivation by genetic (mutation of gene sequence) or epigenetic (inactivation by a protein partner) phenomena, P53 pathway inhibition could be initiated in tumors through constitutive deregulation of one or several of the downstream effector targets genes of P53-dependent transcription (Fig. 2).

Any mutation or inactivation on the P53-Rb pathway of G1 arrest control, especially mdm2, P21, or Rb (by direct or indirect inactivation), would result in growth arrest inhibition, even in the presence of a wild-type P53. P21-Waf1, which is the mediator of P53 for G1 arrest, has not been shown to reflect P53 inactivation, since lung cancer cells with obvious P53 mutation could express P21, due to induction of this gene by other P53-independent mechanisms in bronchial cancer cells (differentiation, senescence). Moreover, P21 gene mutations were not shown in lung cancer. G1 arrest deficiency in lung cancer relies directly on Rb gene inactivation, achieved by two ways: Rb genetic mutation with loss of mRNA and protein expression, which occurs in most SCLC and only 10–20% of NSCLC, or inappropriate phosphorylation as the result of CdK-inhibitor (P16^{INK4}) inactivation, which occurs in 65% of NSCLC. The protein product of the CdK4-inhibitor P16, which can block CdK-dependent Rb phosphorylation, is the first concurrent tumor suppressor gene of P53 in lung cancer (see Chapter 11).

P53 is an important regulator of apoptosis. According to the model proposed by John Reed in 1994, P53 mediator of apoptosis Bax could be inactivated by heterodimerization with Bcl2, which occurs in case of constitutive Bcl2 deregulation, thus abolishing the effect of P53 on apoptosis. A reverse image of Bcl2 to Bax phenotypes and their prognostic relevance, as well as the variable role of P53 mutation in the Bcl2:Bax dysbalance, has been demonstrated, not only in different tissues, but between NSCLC (nonneuroendocrine tumors) and NE lung tumors. The relationship between P53 immunoreactivity, indicative of P53 mutation, and the level of Bcl2 and Bax has been analyzed in the spectrum of neuroendocrine lung tumors (30). A direct relation between P53 immunopositivity and Bcl2 level of expression ($p = 0.005$) and an inverse correlation between P53 immunopositivity and Bax level of expression ($p = 0.01$) were found, accordingly to J. Reed's model. Low-grade neuroendocrine tumors such as carcinoids are characterized by a wild-type P53 (P53 negative), an intense and frequent expression of Bax, and a rare overexpression of Bcl2 in 15% of the cases. In contrast, in high-grade neuroendocrine lung tumors, P53 is mutant and immunoreactive in 50% of the cases, whereas Bax expression is low and Bcl2 overexpressed in 90% of the cases. Bax and Bcl2 levels are inversely correlated in neuroendocrine lung tumors of any grade ($p < 0.0001$). The relationship observed between P53 and Bcl2/Bax levels in neuroendocrine lung tumors is consistent with the idea that P53 contributes to the regulation of Bax and Bcl2 in these tumors. However, this regulation is probably highly dependent on tissue type and differentiation.

P53 is not the unique factor contributing to the regulation of Bax and Bcl2 genes, as inferred from results obtained on NSCLC. Overexpression of Bcl2 was shown in about 25% of NSCLC and in 70–90% of SCLC (30,69–71). Although Bcl2 expression and its P53 partial dependence could be demonstrated in neuroendocrine lung tumors, an inverse correlation was found between Bcl2 and P53 immunostaining NSCLC (with no neuroendocrine differentiation) (72,73). Moreover, overexpression of Bcl2 was associated with a better survival and disease-free interval (72,73) in NSCLC, although no consensus was reached.

In contrast, the prognostic significance of Bax and Bcl2 and their ratio was very impressive in neuroendocrine lung tumors where high Bax level, low Bcl2 expression, and Bcl2:Bax ratio lower than the unit (in favor of Bax), were significantly associated with longer survival ($p = 0.005$). Therefore, the prognostic relevance of Bcl2 and its relation to P53 mutation differs greatly between NSCLC and NE lung tumors. Moreover, when the prognostic significance of Bcl2 and Bax were investigated in breast adenocarcinoma, Bcl2 > Bax expression was lightly associated with longer survival in node-positive breast adenocarcinoma. This suggests a possible role of Bcl2 in proliferation and cell cycle entry. In stimulated B and T lymphocytes in colon carcinoma cells, Bcl2 transgene reduces proliferation and delays cell cycle entry, and these two functions of Bcl2 were demonstrated to be independent and antagonized by Bax (74). The influence of Bcl2 on survival probability in breast cancer and NSCLC suggests that Bcl2 in these cancers not only reduces the level of apoptosis, but also represses cell growth. In some tissues, regulation of cell survival could be coupled to control of cell growth by Bcl2.

We therefore question the role of apoptosis deregulation using TUNEL analysis in the prognostical differences between high-grade and low-grade neuroendocrine lung tumors with reverse Bax/Bcl2 phenotypes. In both high-grade tumors LCNEC and SCLC, apoptotic index was directly related to the level of Bax and to Bcl2:Bax ratio lower than 1 ($p = 0.02$), but it was not related to the Bcl2 level. However, apoptotic index was strikingly low ($<0.1\%$) in SCLC, where Bcl2 is quite constantly high (30). To some extent at least, this is in direct line with the finding of Bcl2 overexpression related to low apoptosis in breast cancer (75), where high Bcl2 expression was strongly associated with both apoptosis loss and presence of lymph node metastasis ($p < 0.0001$). Neither in breast cancer nor in neuroendocrine lung tumors was P53 directly correlated with apoptosis magnitude. Bax and Bcl2 thus appear to be more direct downstream regulators of cell death than P53 itself.

This suggests that Bcl2 and Bax function and their regulation by P53 could be very selective and highly dependent on differentiation type. Bcl2 and Bax may play concordant roles in apoptosis in different tissues, but the regulation of cell survival could be variously coupled to the control of cell growth in different tumor and tissue types and in neuroendocrine versus nonneuroendocrine cells. Moreover, one member of the Bcl2 protein family may not be sufficient to understand the dysregulation of apoptosis during oncogenesis.

Since P53 appears as part of both the G1 arrest and apoptotic pathway, it is predictable that P53 inactivation adds something to the Rb inactivation pathway. One study included analysis of both P53 and Rb mutations (76) and demonstrated that patients with NSCLC tumors that had both Rb loss of expression and P53 accumulation using immunohistochemical methods had a significantly shorter survival (20% 5-year survival) than those with tumors that retain Rb expression and had no P53 accumulation (73% 5-year survival), although Rb inactivation or P53 stabilization alone had no significant influence on survival in this study. In a large series of surgically treated patients, we could not find the same influence of P53 and Rb ab-

Table 3 P53 Gene Abnormalities in Preneoplastic Bronchial Lesions

Authors (Ref.)	Year	Type	N[a]	Method
Sozzi et al. (86)	1992	dysplasia	3	IH
		CIS		
				RFLP (LOH)
Sundaresan et al. (87)	1992	dysplasia	5/6	IH
		dysplasia	0/3	RFLP (LOH)
Klein et al. (88)	1993	metaplasia	4/16	IH
Bennett et al. (89)	1993	metaplasia	1/15	IH
		dysplasia	19/46	
		CIS	15/25	
Nuorva et al. (90)	1993	dysplasia	9/17	IH
Walker et al. (91)	1994	dysplasia	4/19	IH
		CIS	24/44	
Fontanini et al. (92)	1994	metaplasia	0/16	IH
		dysplasia	1/2	
		CIS	13/18	

[a]Number of P53-immunoreactive preneoplastic lesions on total number of lesions examined. All lesions studied were adjacent to invasive carcinoma.
IH: Immunohistochemistry; RFLP: restriction fragment length polymorphism; LOH: loss of heterozygosity.

normalities. It had also been demonstrated that an abnormality of the Rb-P16 pathway synergizes with P53 mutation to accelerate proliferative activity (61).

Finally, there are several lines of evidence for wild-type P53 acting as an antiangiogenetic factor (77–80). Although P53 was shown to depress urokinase plasminogen activator expression and activate its inhibitor PAI1 (80), we could not confirm this relationship of P53 with UPA-PAI1 dysbalance since UPA was highly correlated with PAI1 in lung tumors (see Chapter 25).

VIII. Time of Occurrence of P53 Alterations and Bax-Bcl2 Ratio

There is a large body of evidence that P53 mutation precedes lung cancer invasion. Experimental and in vivo studies showed that tobacco smoke induces bronchial epithelial cell tranformation through progressive morphological changes including hyperplasia, metaplasia, dysplasia of progressive severity, and carcinoma in situ (CIS) (81–85) (see Chapter 4). In search for criteria of irreversibility of these lesions and especially in former smokers, P53 appeared to be the best candidate. P53 immunostaining of clusters of basal and suprabasal cells is observed in bronchial preneoplastic lesions (Table 3) (86–92), but not in normal or metaplastic bronchia. A significant increase of frequency of P53 reactivity is noted from mild to severe dysplasia (20–53%) to reach 60–90% in CIS, which is the frequency seen in corresponding squamous cell invasive carcinoma. All studies compared malignant and premalignant lesions adjacent to invasive carcinoma. Comparing the rate of P53 mutant immunophenotype in preneoplastic lesions of patients with or without lung cancer and adjacent or distant to invasive carcinoma, we observed a significant association of P53 stabilization [mutant immunophenotype (IP)] with synchronous cancer discovered within the same year ($p = 0.0014$). Mutant P53 IP was more frequently observed in preinvasive lesions adjacent to than distant from invasive carcinoma ($p = 0.0003$). Thus, P53 reactivity in a preneoplastic lesion is highly predictive of invasion in the vicinity of this P53-positive lesion. This is in keeping with a recent study (93) that showed that the predictive value of P53 reactivity for carcinoma of the respiratory tract was 91%, as compared with 80% for the highest grade of dysplasia (severe dysplasia or CIS). Therefore, mutant or stabilized P53 protein is a good target marker for early cancer detection and diagnosis on bronchial biopsies (93a).

There is molecular evidence, using microdissection of selected areas on paraffin sections, that not only stabilization but mutation and/or LOH occurs in dysplasia (87,94,95), somewhat later than 3p and 9p LOH, which can be detected as soon as hyperplasia or even in normal bronchial epithelium in smokers (96). Detection of P53 mutations in sputum may precede the diagnosis of lung cancer (97).

Recent studies have provided evidence for P53 mutation in alveolar adenomatous hyperplasia, which is proposed to be the preneoplastic lesion of bronchiolo-alveolar carcinoma and other peripheral adenocarcinomas. These lesions are present in 10–15% of patients with adenocarcinoma, in the normal lung surrounding the tumor. Eight to 28% of these lesions express stabilized P53 with increasing rate and intensity from low- to high-grade atypia (98–100). It can be concluded that P53 mutation precedes invasion in both squamous carcinoma and adenocarcinoma but is a relatively late event, predictive of progression of these preneoplasia, as compared with early genetic events such as 3p or 9p deletion, which are more diagnostic for tobacco induce DNA damage in the "cancerization field."

Bcl2 overexpression was demonstrated in preinvasive bronchial lesions (101). Moreover, Bcl2/Bax dysbalance with Bax downregulation and Bcl2 overexpression may occur in metaplasia, dysplasia, and CIS and contribute to clonal expansion by allowing abnormal cell survival.

IX. Conclusion

P53 mutation and/or deregulation of the P53-Rb pathways in lung cancer are so common that no lung cancer cell was shown to harbor normal P53 and Rb pathways except in carcinoids. Both pathway disruptions can act to increase the rate of cell division and inhibit apoptosis, and comprehensive studies on lung carcinogenesis should embrace all of them. The nonredundancy of these gene functions apparently placed on a common pathway is reflected by the requirement of inactivation of all three mechanisms of G1 arrest and apoptosis (P53, Rb, Bcl2) for acquisition of the more malignant phenotype of lung cancer, which is that of small-cell lung carcinoma. P53-Rb pathway offers several targets for gene therapy or gene expression modulations in the future, including P53 itself, Rb-P16, and Bax-Bcl2.

References

1. Minna J, Nau M, Takahashi T, et al. Molecular pathogenesis of lung cancer. In: Bergsagel DE, Mak TW, eds. Molecular Mechanisms and Their Clinical Applications in Malignancies. Orlando, FL: Academic Press, 1990:63–83.
2. Takahashi T, Nau M, Chiba L, et al. P53: a frequent target for genetic abnormalities in lung cancer. Science 1989; 246:491–494.
3. Gazzeri S, Brambilla E, Caron de Fromentel C, et al. P53 genetic abnormalities and myc activation in human lung carcinoma. Int J Cancer 1994; 58:24–32.
4. Gouyer V, Gazzeri S, Brambilla E, Bolon I, Moro D, Perron P, Benabid AL, Brambilla C. Loss of heterozygosity at the Rb locus correlates with loss of Rb protein in primary malignant neuroendocrine lung carcinomas. Int J Cancer 1994; 58:818–824.
5. Shopland DR, Eyre HJ, Pechacek TF. Smoking attibutable cancer mortality in 1991: Is lung cancer now the leading cause of death among smokers in the United States? J Natl Cancer Inst 1991; 83:1142–1148.
6. Greenblatt MS, Bennet WP, Hollstein M, Harris CC. Mutations in the P53 tumor suppressor gene: clues to cancer etiology and molecular pathogenesis. Cancer Res 1994; 54:4855–4878.
7. Lane D. P53, guardian of the genome. Nature 1992; 358:15–16.
8. Levine AJ. P53, the cellular gatekeeper for growth and division. Cell 1997; 88:323–331.
9. Graeber AJ, Osmanian C, Jack T, Housman DE, Koch CJ, Lowe SW, Garcia AJ. Hypoxia-mediated selection of cells with diminished apoptotic potential in solid tumors. Nature 1996; 379:88–91.
10. Miyashita T, Krajewski S, Krajewski M, Wang HG, Lin HK, Hoffman B, Lieberman D, Reed JC. Tumor suppressor p53 is a regulator of Bcl2 and Bax in gene expression in vitro and in vivo. Oncogene 1994; 9:1799–1805.
11. Buckbinder L, Talbott R, Valesco-Miguel S, Takenaka I, Faha B, Seizinger BR, Kley N. Induction of the growth inhibitor IGF-binding protein 3 by P53. Nature 1995; 377:646–649.
12. Rampino N, Yamamoto H, Ionov Y, Li Y, Sawai H, Reed JC, Perucho M. Somatic frameshift mutations in the Bax gene in colon cancers of the microsatellite mutator phenotype. Science 1997; 275:967–969.
13. Bond JA, Blaydes JP, Rowson J, Haughton MF, Smith JR, Wynford-Thomas D, Wyllie FS. Mutant P53 rescues human diploid cells from senescence without inhibiting the induction of SKI1/Waf1. Cancer Res 1995; 55:2404–2409.
14. Hollstein M, Sidransky D, Vogelstein B, Harris CC. P53 mutations in human cancers. Science 1991; 253:49–53.
15. Tenaud C, Negoescu A, Labat-Moleur F, et al. P53 immunolabeling in archival paraffin-embedded tissues: optimal protocol based on microwave heating for eight antibodies on lung carcinomas. Modern Pathol 1994; 7:853–859.
16. Nishio M, Koshikawa T, Kuroidhi T, et al. Prognostic of abnormal p53 accumuation in primary, resected non small cell lung cancers. J Clin Oncol 1996; 14:497–502.
17. Bodner SM, Minna JD, Jensen SM, et al. Expression of mutant p53 proteins in lung cancer correlates with the class of p53 gene mutation. Oncogene 1992; 7:743–749.
18. Takahashi T, Suzuki H, Hida T, et al. The p53 gene is very frequently mutated in small-cell lung cancer with a distinct nucleotide substitution pattern. Oncogene 1991; 6:1775–1778.
19. Sameshima Y, Matsuno Y, Hirohashi S, et al. Alterations of the p53 gene are common and critical events for the maintenance of malignant phenotypes in small-cell lung carcinoma. Oncogene 1992; 7:451–457.

20. D'Amico D, Carbone DP, Mitsudomi T, et al. High frequency of somatically acquired P53 mutations in small-cell lung cancer cell lines and tumors. Oncogene 1992; 7:339–346.
21. Lohman D, Putz B, Reich U, Bohm J, Prauer H, Hofler H. Mutational spectrum of the P53 gene in human small-cell lung cancer and relationship to clinicopathological data. Am J Pathol 1993; 142:907–915.
22. Chiba I, Takahashi T, Nau M, et al. Mutations in the P53 gene are frequent in primary resected non-small cell lung cancer. Oncogene 1990; 5:1603–1610.
23. Kishimoto Y, Murakami Y, Shiraishi M, Hayashi K, Sekiya T. Aberrations of the P53 tumor suppressor gene in human non-small cell carcinomas of the lung. Cancer Res 1992; 52:4799–4804.
24. Przygodski RM, Finkelstein SD, Langer JC, et al. Analysis of P53, K-ras-2, and C-raf-1 in pulmorary neuroendocrine tumors. Am J Pathol 1996; 148:1531–1541.
25. Coppola D, Clarke M, Landreneau R, et al. Bcl2, P53, CD44 and CD44v6 isoform expression in neuroendocrine tumors of the lung. Modern Pathol 1996; 9:484–490.
26. Iggo R, Gatter K, Bartek J, Lane D, Harris A. Increased expression of mutant forms of P53 oncogene in primary lung cancer. Lancet 1990; 335:675–679.
27. McLaren R, Kuzu I, Dunhill M, Harris A, Lane D, Gatter KC. The relationship of p53 immunostaining to survival in carcinoma of the lung. Br J Cancer 1992; 66:735–738.
28. Vahakangas KH, Samet JM, Metcalf RA, et al. Mutations of P53 and ras genes in radon-associated lung cancer from uranium miners. Lancet 1992; 339:576–580.
29. Brambilla E, Gazzeri S, Moro D, et al. Immunohistochemical study of P53 in human lung carcinomas. Am J Pathol 1993; 143:199–210.
30. Brambilla E, Negoescu A, Gazzeri S, et al. Apoptosis related factors P53-Bcl2-Bax in neuroendocrine lung tumors. Am J Pathol 1996; 149:1941–1952.
31. Yokota J, Wada M, Shimosato Y, Terada M, Sugimura T. Loss of heterozygosity on chromosomes 3, 13, and 17 in small-cell carcinoma and on chromosome 3 in adenocarcinoma of the lung. Proc Natl Acad Sci USA 1987; 84:9252–9256.
32. Kishimoto Y, Murakami Y, Shiraishi M, Hayashi K, Sekiya T. Aberrations of the P53 tumor suppressor gene in human non-small cell carcinomas of the lung. Cancer Res 1992; 52:4799–4804.
33. Hiyama K, Hiyama E, Ishioka S, Yamakido M, Inai K, Gazdar AF. Telomerase activity in small cell and non small cell lung cancers. J Natl Cancer Inst 1995; 87:895–902.
34. Schultz DC, Vanderveer L, Berman DB, et al. Identification of two candidate tumor suppressor genes on chromosome 17p13.3. Cancer Res 1996; 56:1997–2002.
35. Guinee D, Fleming M, Hayashi T, et al. Association of P53 and Waf1 expression with apoptosis in diffuse alveolar damage. Am J Pathol 1996; 149:531–538.
36. Barak Y, Juven T, Haffner R, Oren M. Mdm2 expression is induced by wild type P53 activity. EMBO J 1993; 12:461–468.
37. Wu X, Bayle JH, Olson D, Levine AJ. The P53-mdm2 autoregulatory feedback loop. Genes Dev 1993; 7:1126–1332.
38. Pacinda SJ, Ledet SC, Gondo MM, et al. P53 and mdm2 immunostaining in pulmonary blastomas and bronchogenic carcinomas. Human Pathol 1996; 27:542–546.
39. Gorgoulis VG, Bassidakis GZ, Karameris AM, et al. Immunohistochemical and molecular evaluation of the mdm2 gene product in bronchogenic carcinoma. Modern Pathol 1996; 9:544–554.
40. Xiao ZX, Chen J, Levine AJ, Modjtahedi N, Wing J, Sellers WR, Livingston DM. Interaction between the retinoblastoma protein and the oncoprotein mdm2. Nature 1996; 372:694–698.
41. Soini Y, Nuorva K, Kamel D, et al. Presence of human papillomavirus DNA and abnormal P53 protein accumulation in lung carcinoma. Thorax 1996; 51:887–893.
42. Quinlan DC, Davidson AG, Summers CL, Warden HE, Doshi HM. Accumulation of P53 protein correlates with a poor prognosis in human lung cancer. Cancer Res 1992; 52:4828–4831.
43. Fontanini G, Bigini D, Vignati S, et al. P53 expression in non small cell lung cancer: clinical and biological correlations. Anticancer Res 1993; 13:737–742.

44. Morkve O, Halvorsent OJ, Skjaerven R, et al. Prognostic significance of P53 protein expression and DNA ploidy in surgically treated non small cell lung carcinomas. Anticancer Res 1993; 13:571–578.
45. Marchetti A, Buttitta F, Merlo G, et al. P53 alterations in non-small cell lung cancers correlate with metastatic involvement of hilar and mediastinal lymph nodes. Cancer Res 1993; 53:2846–2851.
46. Volm M, Mattern J. Immunohistochemical detection of P53 in non small cell lung cancer. J Natl Cancer Inst 1994; 86:1249.
47. Carbone DP, Mitsudomi T, Chiba I, et al. P53 immunostaining positivity is associated with reduced survival and is imperfectly correlated with gene mutations in resected non small cell lung cancer. Chest 1994; 106(suppl):377S–380S.
48. Passlick 95 B, Izbicki JR, Haussinger K, et al. Immunohistochemical detection of P53 protein is not associated with a poor prognosis in non small cell lung cancer. J Thor Cardiovasc Surg 1995; 109:1205–1211.
49. Sauter ER, Gwin JL, Mandel J, Keller SM. P53 and disease progression in patients with non small cell lung cancer. Surg Oncol 1995; 4:157–161.
50. Harpole DH, Herndon JE, Walter G, et al. A prognostic model of reccurrence and death in stage 1 non small cell lung cancer utilizing presentations, histopathology, and oncoprotein expression. Cancer Res 1995; 55:51–56.
51. Lee JS, Yaon A, Kalapurakal SK, et al. Expression of P53 oncoprotein in non small cell lung cancer: a favorable prognostic factor. J Clin Oncol 1995; 13:1893–1903.
52. Dalquen P, Sauter G, Torhorst J, et al. Nuclear P53 overexpression is an independent prognostic parameter in node negative non small cell lung carcinoma. J Pathol 1996; 178:53–58.
53. Törmänen U, Ecrola AK, Rainio P, et al. Enhanced apoptosis predicts shortened survival in non small cell lung carcinoma. Cancer Res 1995; 55:5595–5602.
54. Mitsudomi T, Steinberg S, Nau M, et al. P53 gene mutations in non-small cell lung cancer cell lines and their correlation with the presence of ras mutations and clinical features. Oncogene 1992; 7:171–180.
55. Mitsudomi T, Oyama T, Kusano T, et al. Mutations of the P53 gene as a predictor of poor prognosis in patients with non small cell lung. J Natl Cancer Inst 1993; 85:2018–2023.
56. Horio Y, Takahashi T, Kuroishi T, et al. Prognostic significance of P53 mutations and 3p deletions in primary resected non small cell lung cancer. Cancer Res 1993; 53:1–4.
57. Carbone DP, Mitsudomi T, Rush V, et al. P53 protein overexpression, but not gene mutation, is predictive of significantly shortened survival in resected non small cell lung cancer (NSCLC) patients (meeting abstract). Proc Annu Meet Am Soc Clin Oncol 1993; 12:A1112.
58. Ebina M, Steinberg SM, Mulshine JL, Linnoila RI. Relationship of P53 overexpression and up-regulation of proliferating cell nuclear antigen with the clinical course of non small cell lung cancer. Cancer Res 1994; 54:2496–2503.
59. Caamano J, Ruggeri B, Momiki S, Sickler A, Shang SY, Klein-Szanto AJP. Detection of P53 in primary lung tumors and non small cell lung carcinoma cell lines. Am J Pathol 1991; 139:839–845.
60. Xu HJ, Cagle PT, Hu SX, Li J, Benedict WF. Altered retinoblastoma and P53 protein status in non small cell carcinoma of the lung: potential synergistic effects on prognosis. Clin Cancer Res 1996; 2:1169–1176.
61. Kinoshita I, Dosaka-Akita H, Mishina T, et al. Altered P16^{INK4} and retinoblastoma protein status in non small cell lung cacner: potential synergistic effects with altered P53 protein on proliferative activity. Cancer Res 1996; 56:5557–5562.
62. Chin KV, Ueda K, Pastan I, Gottesman MM. Modulation of activity of the promoter of the human MDR1 gene by Ras and P53. Science 1992; 255:459–462.
63. Goldsmith ME, Gudas JM, Schneider F, Cowan KH. Wild-type p53 stimulates expression from the human multidrug resistance promoter in a p53 negative cell line. J Biol Chem 1995; 270:1894–1898.
64. Kawasaki M, Nakanishi Y, Kiwano K, Yatsunami J, Takayama K, Hara N. The utility of p53 immunostaining of transbronchial biopsy specimens of lung cancer: p53 overexpression

predicts poor prognosis and chemoresistance in advanced non small cell lung cancer. Clin Cancer Res 1997; 3:1195–1200.

65. Rush V, Klimstra D, Venkatraman E, Oliver J, Martini N, Gralla R, Kris M, Dmitrovsky E. Aberrant p53 expression predicts clinical resistance to cisplatin-based chemotherapy in locally advanced non small cell lung cancer. Cancer Res 1995; 55:5038–5042.

66. Gjerset RA, Turia ST, Sobol RE et al. Use of wild type P53 to achieve complete treatment sensitization of tumor cells expressing endogenous mutant P53. Mol Carcinog 1995; 14:275–285.

67. Travis WD, Linnoila RI, Tsokos MG, et al. Neuroendocrine tumors of the lung with proposed criteria for large cell neuroendocrine carcinoma: an ultrastructural, immunohistochemical, and flow cytometric study of 35 cases. Am J Surg Pathol 1991; 15:529–553.

68. Lohman D, Fesseler B, Putz B, et al. Infrequent mutations of the P53 gene in pulmonary carcinoid tumors. Cancer Res 1993; 53:5797–5801.

69. Higashiyama M, Doi O, Kodama K, Yokouchi H, Nakamori S, Tateishi R. Bcl2 oncoprotein in surgically resected non small cell lung cancer: possibly favorable prognostic factor in association with low incidence of distant metastasis. J Surg Oncol 1997; 64:48–54.

70. Higashiyama M, Doi O, Kodama K, Yokouchi H, Tateishi R. High prevalence of bcl2 oncoprotein expression in small cell lung cancer. Anticancer Res 1995; 15:503–505.

71. Kaiser U, Schilli M, Haag U, et al. Expression of bcl2 protein in small cell lung cancer. Lung Cancer 1996; 15:31–40.

72. Pezzela F, Turley H, Kuzu I, et al. Bcl2 protein in non small cell lung carcinoma. N Engl J Med 1993; 329:690–694.

73. Fontanini G, Vignati S, Bigini D, et al. Bcl2 protein: a prognostic factor inversely correlated to P53 in non small cell lung cancer. Br J Cancer 1995; 71:1003–1007.

74. O'Reilly LA, Huang DCS, Strasser A. The cell death inhibitor Bcl2 and its homologues influence control of cell cycle entry. EMBO J 1996; 15:6979–6996.

75. Sierra A, Castellsagué X, Tortola S, et al. Apoptosis loss and Bcl2 expression: key determinants of lymph node metastases in T1 breast cancer. Clin Cancer Res 1996; 2:1887–1894.

76. Dosaka-Akita H, Hu SX, Fujino M, et al. Altered retinoblastoma protein expression in non small cell lung cancer: its synergistic effects with altered ras and p53 protein status on prognosis. Cancer 1997; 79:1329–1337.

77. Van-Meir EG, Polverini PJ, Chazin VR, Su-Huang HJ, de-Tribolet N, Cavenee WK. Release of an inhibitor of angiogenesis upon induction of wild type p53 expression in glioblastoma cells. Nature Genetics 1994; 8:171–176.

78. Dameron KM, Volpert OV, Tainsky MA, Bouck N. Control of angiogenesis in fibroblasts by p53 regulation of thrombospondin-1. Science 1994; 265:1582–1584.

79. Kieser A, Weich HA, Brandner G, Marme D, Kolch W. Mutant p53 potentiates protein kinase C induction of vascular endothelial growth factor expression. Oncogene 1994; 9:963–969.

80. Kunz C, Pebler S, Otte J, Von-der-Ahe D. Differential regulation of plasminogen activator and inhibitor gene transcription by the tumor suppressor p53. Nucleic Acid Res 1995; 23:3710–3717.

81. Becci PJ, McDowel EM, Trump BF. The respiratory epithelium IV. Histogenesis of epidermoid metaplasia and carcinoma in situ in the hamster. J Natl Cancer Inst 1978; 61:577–586.

82. Auerbach O, Hammond EC, Garfinkel I. Changes in bronchial epithelium in relation to cigarette smoking 1955–1960 vs 1970–1977. N Engl J Med 1979; 300:381–386.

83. Ono J, Auer G, Caspersson T, et al. Reversibility of 20 methylcholanthrene induced bronchial cell atypia in dogs. Cancer 1984; 54:1030–1037.

84. McDowell EM, De Santi AM, Newkirk C, et al. Effect of vitamin A-deficiency and inflammation on the conducting airway epithelium of Syrian golden hamsters. Virch Arch Biol Cell Pathol 1990; 59:231–249.

85. Peters EJ, Morice M, Benner SE, et al. Squamous metaplasia of the bronchial mucosa and its relationship to smoking. Chest 1993; 103:1429–1432.

86. Sozzi G, Miozzo M, Donghi R, et al. Deletions of 17p and P53 mutations in preneoplastic lesions of the lung. Cancer Res 1992; 52:6079–6082.

87. Sundaresan V, Ganly P, Hasleton P, et al. P53 and chromosome 3 abnormalities, characteristic of malignant lung tumours, are detectable in preinvasive lesions of the bronchus. Oncogene 1992; 7:1989–1997.

88. Klein N, Vignaud JM, Sadmi M, et al. Squamous metaplasia expression of proto-oncogenes and P53 in lung cancer patients. Lab Invest 1993; 68:26–32.

89. Bennett WP, Colby TV, Travis WD, et al. P53 protein accumulates frequently in early bronchial neoplasia. Cancer Res 1993; 53:4817–4822.

90. Nuorva K, Soini Y, Kamel D, Autio-Harmainen H, Risteli L, Risteli J. Concurrent P53 expression in bronchial dysplasias and squamous cell lung carcinomas. Am J Pathol 1993; 142:725–732.

91. Walker C, Robertson LJ, Myskow NW, Pendleton N, Dixon GR. P53 expression in normal and dysplastic bronchial epithelium and in lung carcinomas. Br J Cancer 1994; 70:297–303.

92. Fontanini G, Vignati S, Bigini D, Merlo GR, Ribecchini A, Angeletti CA, Basolo F, Pingitore R, Bevilacqua G. Human non small cell lung cancer: P53 protein accumulation is an early event and persists during metastatic progression. J Pathol 1994; 174:23–31.

93. Boers JE, Ten-Velde GPM, Thunnissen FBJM. P53 in squamous metaplasia: a marker for risk of respiratory tract carcinoma. Am J Respir Crit Care Med 1996; 153:411–416.

93a. Brambilla E. Clin Cancer Res 1998, in press.

94. Sozzi G, Miozzo M, Pastorino U, et al. Genetic evidence for an independent origin of multiple preneoplastic and neoplastic lung lesions. Cancer Res 1995; 55:135–140.

95. Chung GTY, Sundaresan V, Hasleton P, et al. Clonal evolution of lung tumors. Cancer Res 1996; 56:1609–1614.

96. Mao L, Lee JS, Kurie JM, et al. Clonal genetic alterations in the lungs of current and former smokers. J Natl Cancer Inst 1997; 89:857–862.

97. Mao L, Hruban RH, Boyle JO, Tockman M, Sidransky D. Detection of oncogene mutations in sputum precedes diagnosis of lung cancer. Cancer Res 1994; 54:1634–1637.

98. Kerr KM, Carey FA, King G, Lamb D. Atypical alveolar hyperplasia: relationship with pulmonary adenocarcinoma, P53, and c-erbB-2 expression. J Pathol 1994; 174:249–256.

99. Kitamura H, Kameda Y, Nakamura N, et al. Proliferative potential and P53 overexpression in precursor and early stage lesions of bronchioloalveolar lung carcinoma. Am J Pathol 1995; 146:876–887.

100. Kitamura H, Kameda Y, Nakamura N, et al. Atypical adenomatous hyperplasia and bronchoalveolar lung carcinoma. Am J Surg Pathol 1996; 20:553–562.

101. Walker C, Robertson L, Myskow M, Dixon G. Expression of the bcl2 protein in normal and dysplastic bronchial epithelium and in lung carcinomas. Br J Cancer 1995; 72:164–169.

11

Inactivation of RB Gene and pRB Function in Lung Cancer

SYLVIE GAZZERI and VALÉRIE GOUYER

Institut Albert Bonniot
Centre Hospitalier Universitaire de Grenoble
Grenoble, France

I. Introduction

In 1971, Knudson postulated that the development of retinoblastoma tumors resulted from the inactivation of both alleles of a recessive oncogene by two discrete mutations (the two-hit hypothesis) (1). In the familial form the affected individual inherits a mutant, loss-of-function allele from the affected parent, and then a somatic event inactivates the normal allele inherited from the other parent. In contrast, the sporadic forms of the tumor involve two somatic mutational events, the second of which must occur in the descendents of the cell that received the first mutation. This hypothesis was initially supported by the detection of a specific chromosomal deletion (13q14) in some patients with familial retinoblastoma (2) and was subsequently confirmed with careful RFLP analyses of germline and tumor material from affected patients (3–5). This was followed a few years later by the isolation and cloning of the RB gene by three different groups (6–8). Evidence for this gene functioning as a tumor suppressor gene came primarily from the observation that (a) some tumor samples contained interstitial deletions within the RB gene, suggesting that the mutation was targeting the RB locus and not adjacent loci; (b) the Rb protein product is inactivated in all retinoblastoma tumors examined to date; and (c) suppression of tumorigenicity is observed after introduction of the RB gene in retinoblastoma cell lines (9).

II. The Retinoblastoma Gene

A. Isolation, Organization, and Structure

The RB gene was cloned using a positional chromosomal walking technique (6–8).
The gene spans 200 kilobases on chromosome 13 and includes 27 exons. Exon 1
contains 5′ untranslated sequences and encodes the first methionine (10). The RB
gene is conserved between the species, and its ubiquitous expression in a variety of
tissues suggests an essential role in growth regulation in virtually all cell types (11).
The full-length human RB cDNA encompasses 4757 nucleotides (4.7 kb) and encodes a protein of 928 amino acids, predicting a molecular mass of 105 kDa. pRB
is a nuclear phosphoprotein which is able to bind double-stranded DNA (12,13).
Phosphopeptide analysis of pRB suggests more than a dozen distinct sites of phosphorylation on either serine or threonine residues (Fig. 1). Of these sites, five were
confirmed to be phosphorylated in vivo (14,15). Depending on its phosphorylation
status, the RB protein is detected by Western blot technique as multiple closely
spaced bands between 105 and 116 kDa. The 105 kDa band corresponds to the hypophosphorylated form and the others to the different phosphorylated forms of pRB.
     There is now evidence for the existence of at least four functionally distinct
protein-binding domains within pRB (Fig. 1). The amino-terminal part of pRB is involved in growth suppression and oligomerization of the protein (16), and recently
a new kinase, termed RB kinase, has been shown to associate with and phosphorylate pRB in vivo in late stages of the cell cycle (17). The central domains A and B,
which constitute the so-called A/B or RB pocket, bind specifically to the transfor-

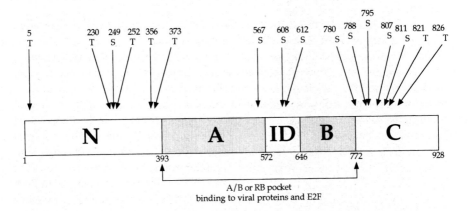

Figure 1   Distinct functional domains of pRb and phosphorylation sites. pRb exhibits four
distinct domains with protein-binding function and distinct roles in RB function. The
N-terminal domain (N) plays a role in growth suppression and oligomerization of the RB protein. The A and B domains, which are separated by an intermediate domain (ID), constitute
the RB pocket and bind to viral and cellular proteins. The C domain is required for growth
suppression and could play a role in RB-dependent apoptotic process. Potential phosphorylation sites are indicated by arrows. The single letters represent serine (S) and threonine (T).

ming proteins of at least three different classes of DNA tumor viruses (large T of SV40, E1A of adenovirus, and E7 of human papillomavirus) (18–20) and to many transcription factors including the E2F transcription factors (21). The viral oncoproteins eliminate pRB function by binding and sequestrating hypophosphorylated pRB, and it is presumably part of the strategy used by the viruses to promote cellular and hence viral DNA synthesis. The description in spontaneous tumors of several mutations in the RB pocket (22) indicates its crucial role in the function of the RB protein. Finally the carboxy-terminal domain C is required for the growth suppression function of pRB (23) and has been defined by interaction of pRB with the c-Abl tyrosine kinase (24) and MDM2 proteins (25). Furthermore, it has been recently shown that it could also play a major role in the RB-dependent apoptotic process (26,27).

pRB is a prototypic member of a protein family known as the "pocket-protein" family, which also includes p130 and p107 (28–31). Earlier studies showed that these three proteins share structural homology, bind to oncoproteins of small DNA tumor viruses, can interact with the E2F transcription factors, and can suppress proliferation when overexpressed in cultured cells (32). However, several lines of evidence, which will not be discussed here, showed that pRB significantly differ from p130 and p107. A recent study reported a possible involvement of p130 in the progression of NSCLC, which was not found with p107 (33).

B. Alternative Effector Pathways Regulated by pRB

pRB exerts its effects by cell cycle–dependent interactions with a range of transcription factors and other cellular proteins that regulate cell proliferation and differentiation (Table 1) (32,34). Prominent among them are the E2F transcription factor family (21). E2F1, 2, and 3 bind the hypophosphorylated form of pRB; phosphorylation of pRB causes the release of E2F, presumably enabling the latter to proceed with the activation of a cohort of S-phase–specific genes whose transcription it controls [most notably c-myc, N-myc, c-myb, thymidine kinase, DNA polymerase α, dihydrofolate reductase (dhfr), cdc2, and RB] (32).

Genes encoding other pRB-binding proteins have been reported over the past several years (Table 1) (34). The effector functions of most of these remain unknown. Although in most cases the significance of pRB binding is not yet clear, these interactions lead to either neutralization of the RB function by sequestration of pRB, as for MDM2 binding (25), or disruption of the pRB-bound protein function, as for transcription factors (21) or c-abl (35). However, because it has been suggested that the binding of all these proteins is also regulated by the phosphorylation of pRB, it is conceivable that the selective modification of these distinct phosphorylation sites may also play a role in these interactions.

pRB can also affect transcription without directly binding to transcription factors. Indeed pRB has been reported to repress c-myc and c-fos expression and AP-1 transcriptional activity, resulting in the negative regulation of a set of early-response genes required for cell growth (36,37). A specific region responsible for dependent

Table 1   Cellular Retinoblastoma Protein-Binding Proteins

Protein	Function	Binding site in RB
E2F-1,2,3	Transcription factor	389–892
UBF	Auxillary transcription factor	A/B
Elf-1	Transcription factor	379–928
PU-1	Transcription factor	379–928
c-Myc	Transcription factor	A/B
N-Myc	Transcription factor	A/B
Brm	Disruption of nucleosome structure	A/B
BRG1	Disruption of nucleosome structure	A/B
MyoD	Transcription factor	605–792
ATF-2	Transcription factor	A/B
Sp1-I	Negative factor	
MDM2	Oncoprotein	792–928
c-Abl	Tyrosine kinase	768–928
D1,D2,D3	Cyclin	A/B
Lamin A, C	Nuclear matrix protein	612–928
hsc73	Heat-shock protein	301–372
RBP-1	?	A/B
RBP-2	?	A/B
PP-1α2	Protein phosphatase	301–928
RbAp48	?	
RBQ-1	?	
RBQ-3	?	657–928

Source: Ref. 34.

downregulation of transcription was isolated in the c-fos promoter and called the RB-control element (RCE). pRB can also repress transcription from an E2F-binding site in its own promoter, suggesting that expression of pRB is autoregulated (38). More recently, it was demonstrated that pRB (via RB pocket region) inhibits specifically the activity of RNA polymerase I via direct interaction with the UBF (upstream binding factor) (39) and represses transcription by RNA polymerase III in vivo and in vitro (40). This repression is alleviated by tumor-associated mutations within the RB pocket domain. Recently Weintraub et al. suggested a mechanism for the active transcriptional repression by pRB, indicating that pRB is recruited to promoters through E2F, where pRB binds and inactivates neighboring transcription factors (41).

Under other circumstances, RB might act as a positive regulator of transcription. An example of positive regulation by pRB involves the transcription of transforming growth factor beta (TGF-β) 1 and 2 proteins, which induce G1 arrest in many cell types, suggesting another means for RB to constrain cell proliferation. This activation requires intact ATF-binding sites for TGF-β2 (42) and an analogous RCE for TGF-β1 (43). Taken together, these results show that pRB can function either as a positive or as a negative regulator of transcription and suggest a way in which pRB might influence cellular biosynthesis at both DNA replication and cell growth levels. Recent data reported an additional function of pRB as a negative regulator of apoptosis (44). Cells lacking a functional RB are highly susceptible to apoptosis, which can be suppressed by introduction of a fully functional RB gene (45). Also, RB$-/-$ mice are nonviable, and several tissues in their embryos show extensive cell death (45). Furthermore, several pRB-binding proteins such as c-myc, E2F, cyclin D1, E7, and E1A have been reported to induce apoptosis, and it has been suggested that these proteins do so by interfering with the protective function of pRB against apoptosis (46). More recently it was shown that pRB may serve as substrate for ICE-like protease and that RB cleavage (at its C-terminus part) is an important event in apoptosis (26,27).

C. Control of pRB Phosphorylation

pRB phosphorylation status varies during the different phases of the cell cycle and regulates the cell cycle arrest in G1. In G0 and early G1, pRB is hypophosphorylated. It becomes phosphorylated at multiple sites as cells progress through G1, being in late G1 in a so-called hyperphosphorylated state, which is maintained until the end of the cycle (32).

Phosphorylation of pRB begins in mid-to-late G1 phase approximately coinciding with the restriction point control, and most of the experimental data would be consistent with a model in which the phosphorylation of pRB is a major if not the rate-limiting step. At least three different cyclin-dependent protein kinases (CDKs) that are sequentially regulated by cyclins D, E, and A can trigger phosphorylation of pRB (Fig. 2). Cyclins of the D class (D1, D2, and D3) together with their catalytic partners CDK4 and CDK6 are responsible for the initiation of the phosphorylation of pRB in G1 phase (47). The cyclin E-CDK2 complex operates at the initiation of S phase, cyclinA-CDK2 in S and G2, and the cyclin B-CDK1 at M phase (47) (Fig. 2). The in vivo role of the cyclinE-cdk2 and cyclinA-cdk2 may be to maintain pRB in a phosphorylated state throughout the remainder of the cell cycle.

Because phosphorylation of pRB is a critical mode of inhibition of its growth-restraining activities, most recent studies have focused on the regulation of the kinases involved in pRB phosphorylation at the G1-S transition. CDK activity can be constrained by distinct CDK inhibitory proteins, which fall into two distinct categories (48,49). The proteins designated p21, p27, and p57 appear to function as broad-spectrum inhibitors capable of interacting with complexes containing cyclins D, E, and A. By contrast, the INK4 protein family (p15, p16, p18, and p19) interacts directly and specifically with CDK4 and CDK6 and therefore blocks the function of D-type cyclins only, causing G1 arrest. Members of the INK4 subfamily are particularly dependent on pRB, as their abilities to inhibit the cell cycle depend on functional pRB (32). One of these, named p16^{INK4a} (CDKN2/MTS1), is responsible for the inhibition of the cyclin D1-CDK4 (50). In normal cells, p16 negatively regulates pRB phosphorylation by blocking the cyclinD-CDK4 activity, thus leading to G1

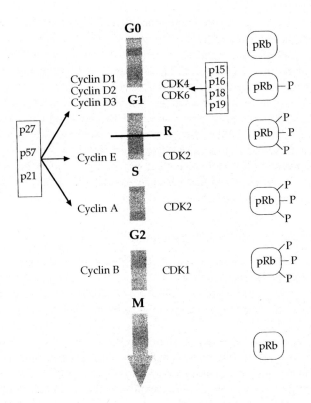

Figure 2 Proteins that regulate the mammalian cell division cycle. The different phases of the cell cycle G0, G1, S, G2, and M are in temporal order from top to bottom. The restriction point is indicated as R. Cyclin-dependent kinases (CDKs) are aligned with their corresponding regulatory subunits (cyclins) and positioned approximately according to the phase in the cycle at which their activity is most significant. The two families of CDK inhibitors are shown in boxes. The phosphorylation status of pRB in different phases of the cycle is shown on the right of the figure. The number of phosphate groups (denoted P) is intended to be symbolic and bears no relation to actual number of phosphorylation sites on the protein.

arrest. Blocking the function of p16 results in entry in S and uncontrolled cell growth. Inactivation of p16 is one of the ways to inhibit the growth-suppressive activity of pRB in tumors (see below).

As indicated by the name, CDK activity may be also influenced by the level of cyclin expression consequently regulating pRB phosphorylation. Cyclin D1 overexpression is a mechanism whereby CDK activation may induce inappropriate pRB phosphorylation and disrupt its control of G1 arrest or apoptosis.

pRB implements the decision by the cell to pass through the G1 checkpoint in mid-to-late G1. When pRB fails to undergo phosphorylation, the progress of the cell through its active growth cycle is blocked at this point. Acquired evidence indicates that a pRB-imposed block on cell cycle progression might also be a prerequisite for differentiation or senescence (32,44).

D. RB Deficiency in Animal Models

Heterozygous RB+/− mice fail to develop retinoblastoma but, instead, acquire RB−/− pituitary tumors later in life arising in cells that have sustained mutations in their second allele (45). The idea that RB may be required for the maintain of viability is suggested by the observation that a RB−/− embryo died before the 16th day of gestation (45). Prominent defects are observed in hematopoietic and neuronal development, which manifest increased mitotic index and cell death, suggesting that the role of RB may not be specifically related to control of progression through the cell cycle, but rather to control of differentiation in specific tissues.

Mice deficient in both p53 and RB develop tumors, primarily of endocrine origin, and bronchial neuroendocrine hyperplasia, but fail to show neuroendocrine lung tumors (51). Transgenic mice carrying multiple copies of human RB besides two normal alleles of mouse RB have statistically significant reduction in size and body weight, which tends to correlate with the level of pRB expression (45).

E. Involvement of the RB Gene in Human Carcinogenesis

Evidence indicates that pRB stands in the midst of a regulatory pathway that is disrupted during the pathogenesis of many human tumors. The RB gene is inactivated in both sporadic and hereditary retinoblastomas, where the absence of RB protein is found in about 100% of the cases. Inactivation of the RB gene is also observed in osteosarcomas and soft tissue sarcomas (52), which are retinoblastoma-associated tumors (second-site tumors). Furthermore, RB gene abnormalities are observed in many tumors not associated with retinoblastomas, such as osteosarcomas, soft tissue sarcomas, leukemias, glioblastomas, breast, esophagus, prostate, renal, and ovarian tumors, and small-cell lung cancers (53). In all respects, RB conforms to the "two-hit hypothesis" proposed by Knudson (1): both copies of the gene are inactivated in tumor cells. Furthermore, the role of RB in the genesis of human malignancies has been reinforced by several studies showing that replacement of a wild-type pRB in RB-negative cells from widely disparate types of tumors suppressed cell growth as well as tumorigenic activity in nude mice (45).

III. Inactivation of the RB Gene in Lung Cancer

The various changes catalogued above converge on the same endpoint of depriving the cell of the services of pRb, either through its genetic inactivation (via chromosomal mutation) or through its functional inactivation (via sequestration or deregulated phosphorylation). As a direct consequence, E2Fs are liberated from complexes with pRB and the progression of cells into late G1 and S becomes unconstrained.

The involvement in lung carcinogenesis of these two modes of inactivation of the RB gene is analyzed in the second part of this chapter.

A. Genetic Inactivation of the RB Gene

NE Lung Tumors

Inactivation of the RB gene is very frequent in lung cancers, specially in small-cell lung cancers (SCLC). Many different types of genetic lesion appear to be involved in the inactivation of the RB locus. Loss of heterozygosity (LOH) is detected in about 90% of the SCLC (54,55), and aberrant or absent pRB expression is observed in about 90% of the cases (54,56–58). Major structural abnormalities (homozygous deletion, rearrangement) are detected in 13–18% of the cases analyzed (54,56,59). Subtle structural mutations such as small deletions and point mutations leading to stop codon are also found, mainly in the RB pocket of the RB gene (60). In addition, a missense mutation leading to a nonfunctional pRB protein defective in phosphory-lation and oncoprotein binding has also been reported (61). However in the majority of the cases, the remaining allele is inactivated by a yet unknown mechanism lead-ing to loss of mRNA expression (30–75% of the SCLC cell lines analyzed) (54,56,59,62). At this time very few primary NE tumors have been analyzed, and the majority of the data presented above have been found on SCLC cell lines.

We studied RB protein expression by immunohistochemistry (IHC) with three RB antibodies on a large series of human lung tumors, including 29 NE lung tumors, and investigated the status of RB protein expression in relation with the analysis of LOH at the RB locus using three intragenic probes. We found that 87% of high-grade NE carcinomas [large-cell neuroendocrine carcinoma (LCNEC) and SCLC] exhibited an abnormal expression of pRB, with a high correlation with loss of het-erozygosity at the RB locus ($p < 0.0036$), indicating that the RB gene is the target of the LOH at the 13q14 locus in NE tumors (63). Furthermore, we found that the combination of both genetic abnormalities was significantly associated with the NE phenotype ($p < 0.0001$). We next examined in a larger series of human NE tumors (37 cases) embracing the entire spectrum of NE lung neoplasms (typical and atypi-cal carcinoids, LCNEC, and SCLC), the role and genetic mechanism of RB inacti-vation in tumor differentiation, and malignant potential (64). RB protein expression was performed with two additional RB antibodies (five antibodies in total) using IHC. Abnormal pRB expression was more frequently observed in high-grade NE lung carcinoma (82%) than in typical and atypical carcinoids (11%) ($p < 0.001$), suggesting that RB inactivation is not necessary to the development of carcinoids. We then studied the genetic events at the basis of RB silencing and found that only 4% of the tumors analyzed carried major structural abnormalities and 25% had mu-tations in the RB pocket (exons 13–18 and 20–24). All these mutations were small deletions or insertions leading to frameshift or stop codon. On the other hand, we found using RT/PCR that 58% of the NE tumors analyzed had a loss or low level of RB transcript. Since methylation had been previously described as a mean of transcriptional silencing of other tumor suppressor genes such as p16[INK4] (65) and had been reported in some sporadic retinoblastomas (66), we analyzed the possibility of hypermethylation of the CpG-rich island at the 5' end of the RB gene but did not find it. In total we detected abnormalities at the DNA or RNA level in 100% of the SCLC and 50% of the LCNEC with abnormal RB protein expression.

In summary, our studies show that inactivation of the RB gene is a prerequisite event for SCLC growth and phenotype and proceeds through Knudson's "two-hit" hypothesis: loss of one allele and mutation of the remaining allele. Complete inactivation of the RB gene results in some of the mutational events in the RB pocket, but in the majority of cases the mechanism of mRNA silencing is actually unknown. Different hypotheses are possible, such as mutations in the promotor region or outside RB pocket leading to abnormal splicing, or deregulation of transcription factor activities, and further studies are required to gain more insight into this question.

Genetic inactivation of the RB gene seems to come under other mechanisms in LCNEC, since half of these tumors with abnormal RB protein expression display neither abnormality in transcription nor mutation or major structural abnormality. Although never reported in NE tumors or cell lines, the existence of mutations outside RB pocket cannot be excluded.

The loss of pRB in carcinoids, although very rare (58), indicates that RB inactivation can be observed in well-differentiated low-grade NE proliferation since complete lack of RB transcripts was observed in one of those using semi-quantitative RT-PCR analysis (64), but considerably increased in frequency with their grade.

The frequency of RB inactivation in high-grade NE lung tumors is similar to that observed in retinoblastoma. The fact that these two types of tumors both exhibit features of neuroendocrine differentiation and that subjects carrying a RB mutant allele had a 15-fold increase risk of lung cancer, predominantly of small cell type, indicates that these tumors could be associated.

Reintroduction of a functional RB gene has been attempted in SCLC cell lines carrying multiple genetic alterations and an activated RB gene (67). The transfected clones showed either reduced growth rates in culture or suppressed tumorigenicity in nude mice. These results confirmed the major role of RB gene inactivation in the emergence and progression of NE carcinoma and suggest its utility in future genetic therapies.

Non–Small-Cell Lung Cancers

In contrast to NE lung tumors, loss of heterozygosity at the RB locus is observed in about 30% of NSCLC (63,68,69). Only 15–35% of the cases exhibit a loss of RB protein expression (63,68,70,71). In one study, altered pRB expression was reported more frequently in advanced-stage NSCLC than in low-stage tumors (70). Aberrant or absent mRNA expression has been found in about 10% of the tumors (68). Mutations have been analyzed in only one report and detected in 10% of the cases (69). This lower incidence of RB abnormalities in NSCLC more closely resembles the frequency observed in other tumor types, such as breast, prostate, and bladder cancers.

In a first study of NSCLC of all histological types (48 cases), we found a loss of pRB in 35% of cases, without any correlation with stage or survival (63). Thirty-five percent of the tumors analyzed had LOH at the RB locus, but this was not correlated with loss of pRB. Furthermore, no mutation could be detected in the RB pocket. We recently performed an extended study on 165 NSCLCs and found a loss of pRB expression in 19% of cases.

In contrast with NE tumors, RB inactivation seems to be involved only in a small subset of NSCLCs. Independance of abnormal pRB expression from RB allele status indicates that, in the majority of the cases, the LOH targets a tumor suppressor gene other than the RB gene. Our data are supported by a recent study where the authors showed a high frequency of deletion in three distinct regions on chromosome 13q14 locus (including RB gene locus) suggesting the existence of other tumor suppressor genes (72).

B. Deregulation of Phosphorylation of the RB Gene: The Role of CDK Inhibitors and Cyclins

As described above, pRb negatively controls passage from the G1 into the S phase by sequestrating transcription factors required for the G1/S transition. The ability of pRB to bind transcription factors is abolished by phosphorylation that occurs in G1 and is sustained to the end of mitosis. P16^{INK4} is a specific inhibitor of the CDK4/D kinase, which is responsible for the initiation of pRB phosphorylation in late G1 (49). Its overexpression results in G1 arrest in cells with functional RB. Other reports have provided evidence that the p16^{INK4} levels may be regulated by RB protein (73), suggesting that pRB participates in a feedback loop to limit the levels of p16^{INK4}. Genetic alterations of p16^{INK4} leading to its inactivation in tumors result in the deregulation of cell proliferation through loss of RB-dependent G1 arrest control.

Accumulating evidence implicates p16^{INK4} as a tumor suppressor gene in tumorigenesis. p16^{INK4} maps to 9p21, a chromosomal locus frequently altered in many primary tumors and cell lines (74–76). Homozygous deletions, inactivating mutations, and more recently methylation at the 5' CpG island associated with transcriptional silencing have been identified as alternative mechanisms of p16^{INK4} inactivation (65,77). Furthermore, ectopic expression of wild-type p16^{INK4} in some tumor cell lines leads to G1 arrest and growth inhibition (78). Moreover, the effects of p16^{INK4} require a functional RB, suggesting the existence of a common P16^{INK4}/RB growth suppressor pathway (32). The redundancy of RB and P16^{INK4} inactivation on this common pathway is supported by the observation of an inverse correlation between alterations in the expression of both proteins in several tumor types and especially in lung cancer (79). The notion of a feedback regulation of p16^{INK4} by RB is consistent with the accumulation of high levels of p16^{INK4} mRNA in cells lacking RB function (73).

In lung cancers, alterations of the $p16^{INK4}$ gene are mainly restricted to non–small-cell lung carcinomas (80–82). Loss of $p16^{INK4}$ protein expression is found in a large proportion of non–small-cell lung cancer cell lines (65% mean) (76,79) and primary tumors (37–67%, 50% mean) (83–86) and is strictly correlated with persistence of wild-type RB expression confirming a common $p16^{INK4}$/RB pathway (79,83–86). Absence of $p16^{INK4}$ staining was associated with more advanced pathological stage and presented as an indicator of worse prognosis in patients undergoing resection for NSCLC in one study (83). However, this was not confirmed in another study (86), and we did not observe this unfavorable influence on prognosis in 165 patients with NSCLC studied for RB and p16 staining. In fact, patients with p16-positive tumors had longer survival than those with p16-negative tumors. This suggests that impairment of RB function through CDK inhibitor inactivation could inhibit tumor cells from a stringent control of apoptosis, thus leading to apoptotic loss and retardation of tumor progression. Interestingly, in the same study loss of pRB conferred shorter rate of survival in limited stages I-II, suggesting a more thorough loss of G1 arrest control when RB is genetically mutated. Loss of heterozygosity at the 9p21 locus is detected in about 65% of NSCLC (87,88). It occurs at 9p loci at the earliest stage in the pathogenesis of lung cancer (38% of LOH in hyperplasia foci) and involves all regions of the respiratory tract (89). Homozygous deletions appear to be an important mechanism of $p16^{INK4}$ inactivation, but their frequency is variable from one study to another (9–39%) (74,76,82,88,90) depending on the tumoral material analyzed (cell lines or primary tumors) and the techniques used (Southern blotting, PCR with microsatellite markers, FISH). One study on NSCLC cell lines reported an association between homozygous deletions and advanced tumor stage but without influence on survival (82). Methylation of the 5′ CpG island associated with transcriptional silencing was found in 50% of a series of NSCLC cell lines with absent $P16^{INK4}$ (91) and in 28% of human NSCLC (65). $p16^{INK4}$ mutations are less common (0–8%) (81,90,92,93), but one study reported 30% of intragenic mutations (94). These consist, in the majority of the cases, in frameshift or nonsense mutations, but missense mutations are also reported. Some of these missense mutations have been shown to encode a functionally inactive protein with lower half-life or loss of CDK4-binding function (95). In some reports mutations have been related to metastatic diffusion to thoracic lymph node (78,90) or to advanced tumor stage (90).

We studied in 43 human NSCLCs $p16^{INK4}$ inactivation in human lung tumors, with the aim to correlate loss of $p16^{INK4}$ protein expression with the genetic mechanisms underlying them (96). Using IHC and with two $p16^{INK4}$ antibodies, we found that 49% of the tumors exhibited an absence of $p16^{INK4}$ nuclear staining. These results have since been confirmed in the lab for a larger series of human NSCLC, where 65% of the cases were found to lack $p16^{INK4}$ expression. In contrast with Kraztke's study (83), this was observed at all stages and in primary tumors as well as at metastatic sites. We detected frameshift or missense mutations in 14% of the tumors with $p16^{INK4}$-negative staining. Methylation of exon 1α was found in 33% of the cases with $p16^{INK4}$-negative staining and was never detected in the tumors with p16^{INK4}-positive staining. Using FISH, we demonstrated a major implication of the homozygous deletion in the tumors with p16^{INK4}-negative staining (48% of incidence). Furthermore, we found an apparent clonal outgrowth of cells showing three or more chromosome 9 copies, which reveals the high degree of chromosome 9 instability in these tumors as was previously described in bronchial metaplasia (97). In total, 95% of the tumors with p16^{INK4}-negative staining carried one of the three known alternative genetic alterations (mutation, methylation of exon 1α, or homozygous deletion) indicating a high correlation between IHC and genetic analysis. Furthermore, and in contrast with some previous studies, we did not find any correlation between any specific abnormality of the p16^{INK4} gene (i.e., mutation, methylation of exon 1α, and homozygous deletion) and cancer extension, including node invasion. P16 inactivation is probably an early event in non–small-cell lung cancer progression. In a large study of 90 patients with precursor bronchial lesions (preinvasic lesions), we found a loss of p16 expression in 25%, from moderate dysplasia to carcinoma in situ (Brambilla, unpublished). This is in contrast with the earlier demonstration in hyperplasia of a 38% incidence of LOH at the 9p21 locus where p16 maps, reaching 80–100% in CIS and invasive carcinoma (89). This raises the possibility that another candidate-tumor suppressor gene might be present at 9p21 locus. In contrast with p16, pRB expression was never lost before invasion (Brambilla, unpublished data).

These results demonstrate that deregulation of the p16 gene locus is an early event occurring frequently in NSCLCs through distinct mechanisms including rare point mutations, promotor methylation, and frequent homozygous deletions. Using the same approach on a small subset of neuroendocrine carcinomas with p16^{INK4} negative staining (about 20% of all NE tumors in our series), our preliminary data seem to show that p16^{INK4} inactivation could preferentially result from methylation of exon 1α rather than from homozygous deletion, which we did not detect among 10 tumors analyzed. Although these data have to be confirmed, they indicate the probable existence of specific kinds of p16^{INK4} inactivation among the two major classes of lung tumors (NE tumors and NSCLCs).

Our results also show that, with specific criteria of analysis, immunohistochemistry appears to be a rapid and reliable technique for studying the inactivation of p16^{INK4} in lung tumors. However, although negative immunostaining of p16^{INK4} is a strong indication for the presence of one of the three above-mentioned genetic abnormalities, great care must be taken in the interpretation of positive nuclear reactivity, which may not necessarily indicate the presence of a functional p16^{INK4} protein in some tumors. Indeed, we detected missense mutations in 13% of the tumors with p16^{INK4}-positive staining. Knowing that some missense mutations, especially those located in the p16^{INK4} CDK4-binding domain, were shown to encode a functionally inactive protein (95), we believe that some of the missense mutations we detected are potential p16^{INK4}-inactivating mutations.

Another possibility is the potential role of these mutations on an alternate reading frame of the p16^{INK4} gene, which leads us to consider recent data concerning the p16^{INK4} gene. The existence of an alternative transcript for p16 (p16β) has recently been shown consisting of a distinct exon 1 (exon 1β) spliced onto the remaining exons 2 and 3 of p16 (77). Because of a shift in the open reading frame (ORF), the β transcript theoretically encodes a protein that is structurally distinct from $p16^{INK4}$ protein. Indeed, the presence of a similar alternative transcript encoding a $p19^{ARF}$ protein has been reported in mouse cells (98). A human $p19^{ARF}$ protein has also been characterized in various cells including normal fibroblasts (Larsen, personal communication). Strikingly, in spite of this unrelated structure, $p19^{ARF}$ also arrests cells in G1/S and G2/M (98). Furthermore, the inhibitory role of human $p19^{ARF}$ in HeLa cells, a cell line with inactive pRB, suggests that it may act downstream from pRB or in a distinct parallel pathway. The place of $p19^{ARF}$ in tumorigenic processes is still poorly understood. To date, except for one published study, no mutation in exon 1β has been detected in several tumor types, including lung cancers (99). However, specific deletions of exon 1β with intact exons 1α, 2, and 3 have been reported in some lymphocytic leukemia and melanoma cell lines (99). In addition, both expression of $p19^{ARF}$ mRNA and absent $p19^{ARF}$ have been reported in some tumor cells, suggesting that the protein might play a still unknown function in tumorigenic processes despite the absence of point mutation in the coding sequence (Larsen, personal communication). A recent report by Sherr's group has shown that point mutations located in the part of exon 2 that is common to $p16^{INK4}$ and $p19^{ARF}$ did not result in the incapacity of the latter to exert its inhibitory role (100). In addition, the same group also showed that the amino-terminal part of $p19^{ARF}$ encoded by exon 1β is necessary and sufficient to abolish the functional activity of the protein, whereas exon 2 may help to stabilize the protein. We attempted to evaluate whether the missense mutations we found in exon 2 of tumor expressing $p16^{INK4}$-positive staining might have an effect on the alternate reading frame of human $p19^{ARF}$. While one of these mutations led to a silent mutation, the other led to another missense mutation. Further studies are required to gain more insight into the potential role of $p19^{ARF}$ in lung carcinogenesis. Other components of the p16-cyclinD/CDK-pRB-E2F pathway are susceptible to deregulate pRB phosphorylation and promote cell cycle progression. The $p15^{INK4B}$ gene, which also belongs to the CDK4 inhibitor family, has homology with $p16^{INK4}$, with which it maps in tandem at the 9p21 locus (75). Increased expression of $p15^{INK4B}$ has been observed in G1 arrest induced by treatment of TGF-β, suggesting that it may be an effector of TGF-β–mediated cell cycle arrest (49). Although homozygous deletions at 9p21 usually include the adjacent $p15^{INK4B}$ gene (32), this last one is rarely targeted by inactivating mutations and never hypermethylated in lung cancer (81,90,101), suggesting that $p16^{INK4A}$ is the main target of inactivation at 9p21.

Because some cyclins can negatively modulate RB function, it is reasonable to speculate that overexpression of cyclins will have oncogenic effects and that deregulation of these genes will be found in tumors carrying intact RB. In that way, cyclin D1 acts in conjunction with CDK4 and participates in the phosphorylation of pRB at the end of the G1 phase. In a report on lung cancer cell lines, Schauer et al. showed that cyclin D1 overexpression occurs only in pRB-positive NSCLC and not in pRB-negative SCLC, suggesting different mechanisms for escape of normal growth controls in SCLC and NSCLC (102). However, probably due to differences in the affinity and avidity of anticyclin D1 antibodies used, these data were not confirmed in human tumors where overexpression of cyclin D1 was found in both SCLC and NSCLC, which is intriguing given the lack of pRB in SCLC rendering overexpression of cyclin D1 useless (84). Nevertheless, the demonstration in the same study of frequent cyclin D1 gene amplification in resection samples tends to indicate that it is a primary transforming event (84). Finally, in a recent immunohistochemical analysis of cyclin D1 expression in human NSCLC, overexpression of cyclin D1 was not only associated with a high cell proliferation rate but also with poor tumor differentiation (103) and was even positively correlated with tunnel labeling in apoptotic cells.

IV. Conclusion

The evidence is becoming increasingly persuasive that perturbation of the RB pathway toward loss of restriction point control and apoptosis are critical factors in lung tumorigenesis. In all cases examined, at least one of the cell cycle regulators involved in the cyclin D-CDK-p16-pRB pathway is disturbed in its functions, consistent with the emerging concept of RB being an obligatory target in lung carcinogenesis. It is likely that all genetic mutational events in lung tumor cells converge at the same endpoint of depriving the cell of the services of pRB, either through its genetic inactivation, via chromosomal mutation as in SCLCs, or through its functional inactivation via deregulated phosphorylation by inactivation of p16 or activation of cyclin D1 as in NSCLCs. The histological diversity of emerging lung tumors is highly dependent on the genetic mechanisms selected by the stem cells to achieve complete inhibition of the growth-restraining functions of pRB. Understanding these different mechanisms at the level of individual tumors holds great promise in deciphering new therapeutic targets.

References

1. Knudson AG. Mutation and cancer: statistical study of retinoblastoma. Proc Natl Acad Sci USA 1971; 68:820–823.
2. Yunis JJ, Ramsey N. Retinoblastoma and subband deletion of chromosome 13. Am J Dis Child 1979; 132:161–163.
3. Benedict WF, Weissman BE, Mark C, Stanbridge EJ. Tumorigenicity of human HT1080 fibrosarcoma X normal fibroblast hybrids: chromosome dosage dependency. Cancer Res 1984; 44:3471–3479.
4. Cavenee WK, Dryja TP, Phillips RA, Bendict WF, Godbout R, Gallie BL, Murphree AL, Strong LC, White RL. Expression of recessive alleles by chromosomal mechanisms in retinoblastoma. Nature 1983; 305:779–784.
5. Godbout R, Dryja TP, Squire J, Gallie BL, Phillips RA. Somatic inactivation of genes on chromosome 13 is a common event in retinoblastoma. Nature 1983; 304:451–453.
6. Fung YKT, Murphree AL, T'Ang A, Qian J, Hinriches SH, Benedict WF. Structural evidence for the authenticity of the human retinoblastoma gene. Science 1987; 236:1657–1661.

7. Friend SH, Bernards R, Rogelj S, Weinberg RA, Rapaport JM, Albert DM, Dryja TP. A human DNA segment with properties of the gene that predisposes to retinoblastoma and osteosarcoma. Nature 1986; 323:643–646.

8. Lee WH, Bookstein R, Hong F, Young LJ, Shew JY, Lee EY. Human retinoblastoma susceptibility gene: cloning, identification and sequence. Science 1987; 235:1394–1399.

9. Huang HJS, Yee JK, Shew JY, Chen PL, Bookstein R, Friedmann T, Lee EYHP, Lee WH. Suppression of the neoplastic phenotype by the replacement of the Rb gene in human cancer cells. Science 1988; 242:1563–1566.

10. Hong FD, Huang SHJ, To H, Young LJS, Oro A, Bookstein R, Lee EYHP, Lee WH. Structure of human retinoblastoma gene. Proc Natl Acad Sci USA 1989; 86:5502–5506.

11. Bernards R, Schackleford GM, Gerber MR, Horowitz JM, Friend SH, Schartl M, Bogenmann E, Rapaport JM, McGee T, Dryja TP. Structure and expression of the murine retinoblastoma gene and characterization of its encoded protein. Proc Natl Acad Sci USA 1989; 86:6474–6478.

12. Lee WH, Shew JY, Hong F, Sery TW, Donoso LA, Young LJ, Bookstein R, Lee EYHP. The retinoblastoma gene susceptibility gene encodes a nuclear phosphoprotein associated with DNA binding activity. Nature 1987; 329:642–645.

13. Wang NP, Chen PL, Huang S, Donoso LA, Lee WH, Lee EYHP. DNA-binding activity of retinoblastoma protein is intrinsic to its carboxy terminal region. Cell Growth Diff 1990; 1:233–239.

14. Lees JA, Buchkovich KJ, Marshak DR, Anderson CW, Harlow E. The retinoblastoma protein is phosphorylated on multiple site by human cdc2. EMBO J 1991; 10:4279–4290.

15. Lin BTY, Gruenwald S, Morla AO, Lee WH, Wang JYJ. Retinoblastoma cancer suppressor gene product is a substrate of the cell cycle regulator cdc2 kinase. EMBO J 1991; 10:857–864.

16. Hensey CE, Hong F, Durfee T, Qian YW, Lee EHP, Lee WH. Identification of discrete structural domains in the retinoblastoma protein. J Biol Chem 1994; 269:1380–1387.

17. Sterner JM, Tao Y, Kennett SB, Kim HG, Horowitz JM. The amino terminus of the retinoblastoma (Rb) protein associates with a cyclin-dependent kinase-like kinase via Rb amino acids required for growth suppression. Cell Growth Diff 1996; 7:53–64.

18. DeCaprio JA, Ludlow JW, Figge J, Shew JY, Huang CH, Lee WH, Marsilio E, Paucha E, Livingston DM. SV40 large tumor antigen forms a specific complex with the product of the retinoblastoma susceptibility gene. Cell 1988; 54:275–283.

19. Dyson N, Howey PM, Münger K, Harlow E. The papilloma virus-16 E7 oncoprotein is able to bind to the retinoblastoma gene product. Science 1989; 243:934–337.

20. Whyte P, Williamson NM, Harlow E. Association between an oncogene and an anti-oncogene: the adenovirus E1A proteins bind to the retinoblastoma gene product. Nature 1988; 334:124–129.

21. Chellappan SP, Hiebert S, Mudryj M, Horowitz JM, Nevins JR. The E2F transcription factor is a cellular target for the RB protein. Cell 1991; 65:1053–1061.

22. Hu Q, Dyson N, Harlow E. Regions of retinoblastoma protein needed for the binding to adenovirus E1A or SV40 large T antigen are common sites for mutations. EMBO J 1990; 9:1147–1155.

23. Qin XQ, Chittenden T, Livingston DM, Kaelin WG. Identification of a growth suppression domain within the retinoblastoma gene product. Genes Dev 1992; 6:953–964.

24. Welch PJ, Wang JYJ. A C-terminal protein binding domain in RB regulated the nuclear c-Abl tyrosine kinase in the cell cycle. Cell 1993; 75:779–790.

25. Xiao ZX, Chen J, Levine AJ, Modjtahedi N, Xing J, Sellers WR, Livingston DM. Interaction between the retinoblastoma protein and the oncoprotein MDM2. Nature 1995; 375:694–698.

26. Jänicke RU, Walker PA, Yu Lin X, Porter AG. Specific Cleavage of the retinoblastoma protein by an ICE-like protease in apoptosis. EMBO J 1996; 15:6969–6978.

27. Chen WD, Otterson GA, Lipkowitz S, N Khleif S, Coxon AB, Kaye FJ. Apoptosis is associated with cleavage of a 5 kDa fragment from Rb which mimics dephosphorylation and modulates E2F binding. Oncogene 1997; 14:1243–1248.

28. Ewen ME, Xing Y, Bentley Lawrence J, Livingston DM. Molecular cloning, chromosomal mapping and expression of the cDNA for p107, a retinoblastoma gene product-related protein. Cell 1991; 66:1155–1164.

29. Hannon GJ, Demetrick D, Beach D. Isolation of the Rb-related p130 through its interaction with CDK2 and cyclins. Genes Dev 1993; 7:2378–2391.

30. Mayol X, Grana X, Baldi A, Sang N, Hu Q, Giordano A. Cloning of a new member of the retinoblastoma gene family (pRb2) which binds to the E1A transforming domain. Oncogene 1993; 8:2561–2566.

31. Li Y, Graham C, Lacy S, Duncan AMV, Whyte P. The adenovirus E1A-associated 130-kD protein is encoded by a member of the retinoblastoma gene family and physically interacts with cyclins A and E. Genes Dev 1993; 7:2366–2377.

32. Weinberg RA. The retinoblastoma protein and cell cycle control. Cell 1995; 81:323–330.

33. Baldi A, Boccia V, Claudio PP, De Luca A, Giordano A. Genomic structure of the human retinoblastoma-related Rb2/p130 gene. Proc Natl Acad Sci USA 1996; 93:4629–4632.

34. Taya Y. RB kinases and RB-binding proteins: new points of view. TIBS 1997; 22:14–17.

35. Welch PJ, Wang JY. Disruption of retinoblastoma protein function by coexpression of its C pocket fragment. Genes Dev 1995; 9:31–46.

36. Pietenpol JA, Munger K, Howley PM, Stein RW, Moses HL. Factor-binding element in the human c-myc promoter involved in transcriptional regulation by transforming growth factor β1 and by the retinoblastoma gene product. Proc Natl Acad Sci 1991; 88:10227–10231.

37. Robbins PD, Horwitz JM, Mulligan RC. Negative regulation of human c-fos expression by the retinoblastoma gene product. Nature 1990; 346:668–671.

38. Hamel PA, Gill RM, Phillipps RA, Gallie BL. Transcriptional repression of the E2-containing promoters EIIaE, c-myc, and RB1 by the product of the RB1 gene. Mol Cell Biol 1992; 12, 8:3431–3438.

39. Cavanaugh AH, Hempel WM, Taylor LJ, Rogalsky V, Todorov G, Rothblum LI. Activity of RNA polymerase I transcription factor UBF blocked by Rb gene product. Nature 1995; 374:177–180.

40. White RJ, Trouche D, Martin K, Jackson SP, Kouzarides T. Repression of RNA polymerase III transcription by the retinoblastoma protein. Nature 1996; 382:88–91.

41. Weintraub SJ, Chow KNB, Luo R X, Zhang SH, He S, Dean DC. Mechanism of active transcriptional repression by the retinoblastoma protein. Nature 1995; 375:812–815.

42. Kim SJ, Wagner S, Lui F, O'Reilly MA, Robins PD, Green MR. Retinoblastoma gene product activates expression of the human TFG-β2 gene through transcription factor ATF-2. Nature 1992; 358:331–334.

43. Kim SJ, Lee HD, Robbins PD, Busam K, Sporn MB, Roberts AB. Regulation of transforming growth factor-β1 gene expression by the product of the retinoblastoma-susceptibility gene. Proc Natl Acad Sci USA 1991; 88:3052–3056.

44. Herwig S, Strauss M. The retinoblastoma protein: a master regulator of cell cycle, differentiation and apoptosis. Eur J Biochem 1997; 246:581–601.

45. Wang JYJ, Knudsen ES, Welch PJ. The retinoblastoma tumor suppressor protein. Adv Cancer Res 1994; 64:25–83.

46. Haas-Kogan DA, Kogan SC, Levi D, Dazin P, T'Ang A, Fung YKT, Israel MA. Inhibition of apoptosis by the retinoblastoma gene product. EMBO J 1995; 14:461–472.

47. Sherr CJ. Cancer cell cycles. Science 1996; 274:1672–1677.

48. Elledge SJ, Harper JW. Cdk inhibitors: on the threshold of checkpoints and development. Curr Opin Cell Biol 1994; 6:847–852.

49. Sherr CJ, Roberts JM. Inhibitors of mammalian G1 cyclin-dependent kinases. Genes Dev 1995; 9:1149–1163.

50. Serrano M, Hannon GJ, Beach D. A new regulatory motif in cell-cycle control causing specific inhibition of cyclin D/CDK4. Nature 1993; 366:704–707.

51. Harvey MH, Vogel E Y H P, Lee A, Bradley L A, Donehower. Mice deficient in both p53 and Rb develop tumors primarily of endocrine origin. Cancer Res 1995; 55:1146–1151.

52. Weichselbaum RR, Beckett M, Diamond A. Some retinoblastomas, osteosarcomas and

soft tissue sarcomas may share a common etiology. Proc Natl Acad Sci USA 1988; 85:2106–2109.

53. Bookstein R, Lee WH. Molecular genetics of the retinoblastoma suppressor gene. CRC Crit Rev Oncogenesis 1991; 2:211–217.

54. Hensel CH, Hsieh CL, Gazdar AF, Johnson BF, Sakaguchi AY, Naylor S, Lee WH, Lee AYHP. Altered structure and expression of the human retinoblastoma susceptibility gene in small cell lung cancer. Cancer Res 1990; 50:1067–1072.

55. Yokota J, Wada M, Shimasoto Y, Terada M, Sugimura T. Loss of heterozygosity on chromosomes 3, 13 and 17 in small cell carcinoma and on chromosome 3 in adenocarcinoma of the lung. Proc Natl Acad Sci 1987; 84:9252–9256.

56. Yokota J, Akiyama T, Fung YKT, Benedict WF, Namba Y, Hanaoka M, Wada M, Terasaki T, Shimosato Y, Sugimura T, Terada M. Altered expression of the retinoblastoma (RB) gene in small-cell carcinoma of the lung. Oncogene 1988; 3:471–475.

57. Shimizu E, Coxon A, Otterson GA, Steinberg SM, Kratzke RA, Whan Kim Y, Fedorko J, Oie H, Johnson BE, Mulshine JL, Minna JD, Gazdar AF, Kaye F J. Rb protein status and clinical correlation from 171 cell lines representing lung cancer, extrapulmonary small cell carcinoma, and mesotheliama. Oncogene 1994; 9:2441–2448.

58. Cagle PT, El-Naggar A, Xu HJ, Hu SX, Benedict WF. Differential retinoblastoma protein expression in neuroendocrine tumors of the lung. Am J Pathol 1997; 150:393–400.

59. Harbour JW, Lai SL, Whang-Peng J, Gazdar AF, Minna JD, Kaye FJ. Abnormalities in structure and expression of the human retinoblastoma gene in SCLC. Science 1988; 241:353–357.

60. Mori N, Yokota J, Akiyama T, Sameshima Y, Okamoto A, Mizoguchi H, Toyoshima K, Sugimura T, Terada M. Variable mutations of the RB gene in small-cell lung carcinoma. Oncogene 1990; 5:1713–1717.

61. Kaye FJ, Kratzke RA, Gerster JL, Horowitz JM. A single acid substitution results in a retinoblastoma protein defective in phosphorylation and oncoprotein binding. Proc Natl Acad Sci USA 1990; 87:6922–6926.

62. Ryggard K, Sorenson D, Petengill OS, Cate CC, Spang-Thomsen M. Abnormalities in structure and expression of the retinoblastoma gene in small cell lung cancer cell lines and xenografts in nude mice. Cancer Res 1990; 50:5312–5317.

63. Gouyer V, Gazzeri S, Brambilla E, Bolon I, Moro D, Perron P, Benabid AL, Brambilla C. Loss of heterozygosity at the Rb locus correlates with loss of Rb protein in primary malignant neuro-endocrine lung carcinomas. Int J Cancer 1994; 58:818–824.

64. Gouyer V, Gazzeri S, Bolon I, Drevet C, Brambilla C, Brambilla E. Mechanism of retinoblastoma gene inactivation in the spectrum of neuroendocrine lung tumors. Am J Respir Cell Mol Biol 1998; 18(2): 188-196.

65. Merlo A, Herman JG, Mao L, Lee DJ, Gabrielson E, Burger PC, Baylin SB, Sidransky D. 5' CpG island methylation is associated with transcriptional silencing of the tumor suppressor p16/CDKN2/MTS1 in human cancers. Nature Med 1995; 1:686–692.

66. Greger V, Debus N, Lohman D, Hôpping W, Passarge E, Horsthemke B. Frequency and parental origin of hypermethylated RB1 alleles in retinoblastoma. Hum Genet 1994; 94: 491–496.

67. Ookawa K, Shiseki K, Takahashi R, Yoshida Y, Terada M. Reconstitution of the RB gene suppresses the growth of small-cell lung carcinoma cells carrying multiple genetic alterations. Oncogene 1993; 8:2175–2181.

68. Reissmann PT, Koga H, Takahashi R, Figlin RA, Holmes C, Piantadosi S, Cordon-Cardo C, Slamon DJ. Inactivation of the retinoblastoma susceptibility gene in non-small-cell lung cancer. Oncogene 1993; 8:1913–1919.

69. Sachse R, Murakami Y, Shiraishi M, Hayashi K, Sekiya T. DNA aberrations at the retinoblastoma gene locus in human squamous cell carcinomas of the lung. Oncogene 1994; 9:39–47.

70. Xu HJ, Hu SX, Cagle PT, Moore GE, Benedict WF. Absence of retinoblastoma protein expression in primary non-small cell lung carcinomas. Cancer Res 1991; 51:2735–2739.

71. Higashiyama M, Doi O, Kodama K, Yokouchi H, Tateishi R. Retinoblastoma protein expression in lung cancer: an immunohistochemical analysis. Oncology 1994; 51:544–551.

72. Tamuka K, Zhang X, Murakami Y, Hirohashi S, Xu H, Hu SX, Benedict WF, Sekiya T. Deletion of three distinct regions on chromosome 13q in human non-small-cell lung cancer. Int J Cancer 1997; 74:45–49.

73. Li Y, Nichols MA, Shay JW, Xiong Y. Transcriptional repression of the D-type cyclin-dependent kinase inhibitor p16 by the retinoblastoma susceptibility gene product pRb. Cancer Res 1994; 54:6078–6082.

74. Nobori T, Miura K, Wu DJ, Lois A, Takabayashi K, Carson DA. Deletions of the cyclin-dependent kinase-4 inhibitor gene in multiple human cancers. Nature 1994; 368:753–756.

75. Kamb A, Gruis NA, Weaver-Feldhaus J, Liu Q, Harshaman K, Tavtigian SV, Stockert E, Day III RS, Johnson BE, Skolnick MH. A cell cycle regulator potentially involved in genesis of many tumor types. Science 1994; 264:436–440.

76. Okamoto A, Demetrick DJ, Spillare EA, Hagiwara K, Hussain SP, Bennett WP, Forrester K, Gerwin B, Serrano M, Beach DH, Harris CC. Mutations and altered expression of p16^{INK4} in human cancer. Proc Natl Acad Sci 1994; 91:11045–11049.

77. Larsen CJ. P16^{INK4a}: a gene with a dual capacity to encode unrelated proteins that inhibit cell cycle progression. Oncogene 1996; 12:2041–2044.

78. Spillare EA, Okamoto A, Hagiwara K, Demetrick DJ, Serrano M, Beach D, Harris CC. Suppression of growth in vitro and tumorigenicity in vivo of human carcinoma cell lines by transfected p16^{INK4}. Mol Carc 1996; 16:53–60.

79. Otterson GA, Kratzke RA, Coxon A, Kim YW, Kaye FJ. Absence of p16^{INK4} protein is restricted to the subset of lung cancer lines that retains wiltype RB. Oncogene 1994; 9:3375–3378.

80. Washimi O, Nagatake M, Osada H, Ueda R, Koshikawa T, Seki T, Takahashi T, Takahashi T. In vivo occurrence of p16 (MTS1) and p15 (MTS2) alterations preferentially in non-small cell lung cancers. Cancer Res 1995; 55:514–517.

81. Okamoto A, Perwez Hussain S, Hagiwara K, Spillare EA, Rusin MR, Demetrick DJ, Serrano M, Hannon GJ, Shiseki M, Zariwala M, Xiong Y., Beach DH, Yokota J, Harris CC. Mutations in p16^{INK4}/MTS1/CDKN2, and p18 genes in primary and metastatic lung cancer. Cancer Res 1995; 55:1448–1451.

82. Kelley MJ, Nakagawa K, Steinberg SM, Mulshine JL, Kamb A, Johnson BE. Differential inactivation of CDKN2 and Rb protein in non-small-cell and small-cell lung cancer cell lines. J Natl Cancer Inst 1995; 87:756–761.

83. Kratzke RA, Greatens TM, Rubins JB, Maddaus MA, Niewoehner DE, Niehans GA, Geradts J. Rb and p16^{INK4a} expression in resected non-small cell lung tumors. Cancer Res 1996; 56:3415–3420.

84. Shapiro GI, Edwards CD, Kobzik L, Godleski J, Richards W, Sugarbaker DJ, Rollins BJ. Reciprocal Rb inactivation and p16^{INK4} expression in primary lung cancers and cell lines. Cancer Res 1995; 55:505–509.

85. Geradts J, Kratzke RA, Niehans GA, Lincoln CE. Immunohistochemical detection of the cyclin-dependent kinase inhibitor 2/multiple tumor suppressor gene 1 (CDKN2/MTS1) product p16^{INK4A} in archival human solid tumors: correlation with retinoblastoma protein expression. Cancer Res 1995; 55:6006–6011.

86. Sakaguchi M, Fujii Y, Hirabayashi H, Yoon HE, Komoto Y, Oue T, Kusafuka T, Okada A, Matsuda H. Inversely correlated expression of p16 and Rb protein in non-small cell lung cancers: an immunohistochemical study. Int J Cancer 1996; 65:442–445.

87. Merlo A, Gabrielson E, Askin F, Sidransky D. Frequent loss of chromosome 9 in human primary non-small cell lung cancer. Cancer Res 1994; 54:640–642.

88. Cairns P, Polascik TJ, Eby Y, Tokino K, Califano J, Merlo A, Mao L, Herath J, Jenkins R, Westra W, Rutter JL, Buckler A, Gabrielson E, Tockman M, Cho KR, Hedrick L, Bova GS, Isaacs W, Koch W, Schawb D, Sidransky D. Frequency of homozygous deletion at p16/CDKN2 in primary human tumours. Nature Gen 1995; 11:210–213.

89. Kishimoto Y, Sugio K, Hung JY, Virmani AK, McIntire DD, Minna JD, Gazdar AF. Allele-

specific loss in chromosome 9p loci in preneoplastic lesions accompanying non-small-cell lung cancers. J Natl Cancer Inst 1995; 87:1224–1229.

90. Nakagawa K, Conrad NK, Williams JP, Johnson BE, Kelley MJ. Mechanism of inactivation of CDKN2 and MTS2 in non-small cell lung cancer and association with advanced stage. Oncogene 1995; 11:1843–1851.

91. Otterson GA, Khleif SN, Chen W, Coxon AB, Kaye FJ. CDKN2 gene silencing in lung cancer by DNA hypermethylation and kinetics of p16^{INK4} protein induction by 5-aza 2'deoxycytidine. Oncogene 1995; 11:1211–1216.

92. Cairns P, Mao L, Merlo A, Lee DJ, Schwab D, Eby Y, Tokino K, Van der Riet P, Blaugrund JE, Sidransky D. Rates of p16 (MTS1) mutations in primary tumors with 9p loss. Science 1994; 265:415–416.

93. Marchetti A, Buttitta F, Pellegrini S, Bertacca G, Chella A, Carnicelli V, Tognoni V, Filardo A, Angeletti CA, Bevilacqua G. Alterations of p16 (MTS 1) in node-positive non-small cell lung carcinomas. J Pathol 1997; 181:178–182.

94. Hayashi N, Sugimoto Y, Tsuchiya E, Ogawa M, Nakamura Y. Somatic mutations of the MTS (multiple tumor suppressor) 1/CDK4I (cyclin-dependent kinase-4 inhibitor) gene in human primary non-small cell lung carcinomas. Biochem Biophys Res Com 1994; 202:1426–1430.

95. Arap W, Knudsen ES, Wang JYJ, Cavenee WK, Huang HJS. Point mutations can inactivate in vitro and in vivo activities of p16^{INK4a}/CDKN2A in human glioma. Oncogene 1997; 14:603–609.

96. Gazzeri S, Gouyer V, Vour'ih C, Brambilla C, Brambilla E. Mechanisms of p16^{INK4A} inactivation in non small-cell lung cancers. Oncogene 1998; 16: 497-504.

97. Hittelman WN, Kim HJ, Lee JS, Shin DM, Lippman SM, Kim J, Ro JY, Hong WK. Detection of chromosome instability of tissue fields at risk: in situ hybridization. J Cell Biochem 1996; 258:57–62.

98. Quelle DE, Zindy F, Ashmun RA, Sherr CJ. Alternative reading frames of the INK4a tumor suppressor gene encode two unrelated proteins capable of inducting cell cycle arrest. Cell 1995; 83:993–1000.

99. Stone S, Jiang P, Dayananth P, Tavtigian SV, Katcher H, Parry D, Peters G, Kamb. A Complex structure and regulation of the p16 (MTS1) locus. Cancer Res 1995; 55:2988–2994.

100. Quelle DE, Cheng M, Ashmun RA, Sherr CJ. Cancer-associated mutations at the INK4a locus cancel cell cycle arrest by p16^{INK4} but not by the alternative reading frame protein p19^{ARF}. Proc Natl Acad Sci 1997; 94:669–673.

101. Herman JG, Jen J, Merlo A, Baylin SB. Hypermethylation-associated inactivation indicates a tumor suppressor role for p15^{INK4B1}. Cancer Res 1996; 56:722–727.

102. Schauer E, Siriwardana S, Langan TA, Sclafani RA. Cyclin D1 overexpression vs Retinoblastoma inactivation: implications for growth control evasion in non-small cell and small cell lung cancer. Proc Natl Acad Sci 1994; 91:7827–7831.

103. Mate JI, Ariza A, Aracil C, Lopez D, Isamat M, Perez-Piteira J, Navas-Palacios JJ. Cyclin D1 overexpression in non-small cell lung carcinoma: correlation with Ki67 labelling index and poor cytoplasmic differentiation. J Pathol 1995; 180:395–399.

12

Deregulation of the Cell Cycle in Lung Cancer

R. J. A. M. MICHALIDES

The Netherlands Cancer Institute
Amsterdam, The Netherlands

I. Introduction

Cancer arises as a consequence of multiple genetic alterations in the cell resulting in a continuing progression of tumor cells, which evolve from previous stages of tumor development. These genetic lesions lead to a diminished control over cellular proliferation and reduce the ability of cells to differentiate and to enter apoptosis under less favorable conditions. They involve alterations within genes that promote (oncogenes) or repress (tumor suppressor genes) cell growth and ultimately affect the regulation of the cell cycle. Cell cycle progression in eukaryotic cells is governed by a series of cyclins and cyclin-dependent kinases'cdk. Individual cyclins act at different phases of the cell cycle by binding and stimulating the activities of cdk. Because these cyclins and cdk are pivotal to cell cycle control and thereby cell proliferation, mutational changes and alterations in expression of the corresponding genes play a critical role in transformation and tumor progression (for reviews, see Refs. 1,2). In epithelial cells most of these alterations affect the requirement of cells to respond to external growth factors and to adhere onto extracellular matrix components for proliferation.

This chapter deals with deregulation of the G_1-S regulatory pathway in cancer cells, in particular in lung cancer, and the use of these deregulation(s) as markers for improved diagnosis and treatment of lung cancer patients.

II. G₁-S Control in Normal Cells

The commitment of mammalian cells in late G_1 to replicate in response to mitogenic factors depends ultimately on phosphorylation of the retinoblastoma protein, pRb, a process controlled by cyclin D1, cyclin D1–associated cyclin-dependent kinases, and their inhibitors (cdi) (Fig. 1). The activation of various mitogenic signal transduction pathways converges and strictly requires cyclin D–cdk activity to induce S phase (3). A transient accumulation of the cyclin D1 protein in response to mitogenic stimulation results in binding to, and activation of its cdk partner, predominantly cdk-4. Subsequent activation of the complex by CAK (cyclin-dependent kinase–associated kinase) and cdc25 phosphatase leads to phosphorylation of its major target, the retinoblastoma protein (pRb). Phosphorylation of pRb results in the release of E2F transcription factors, which mediate transcription of genes essential for further progression through the cell cycle (4).

Cyclin D1 does complex with cdk4 or cdk6 to regulate the early to mid G_1 transition of the cell cycle (5), whereas cyclin E–cdk2 and cyclin A–cdk2 complexes control the G_1-S and S phase transition, respectively (1,6). Cyclin E and A are both E2F-responsive genes (7,8), implying that once a cyclin D1–cdk4 activity has set the G_1 regulatory circuit into motion, cyclin E– and A–cdk2 activity is induced and acts on progression through the cell cycle.

All three G_1-S cyclins, D, E, and A, phosphorylate pRb in vitro, with cyclin D1 being the first one in action in vivo and being rate-limiting for G_1-phase progression. The effects as well as the sites of pRb phosphorylation by cyclin D_1–cdk4 are different from those by cyclin E– and cyclin A–cdk2 (6,9,10), indicating a division

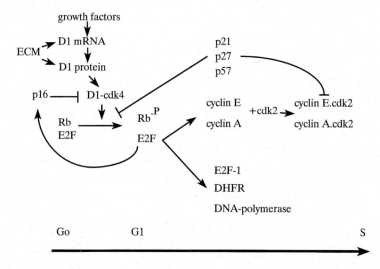

Figure 1   Regulation of transition through G_1 and S phase of the cell cycle by cyclin-cdk's and cki's. ECM: Extracellular matrix; DHFR: dihydrofolate-reductase.

of labor among the G_1 cyclins. Indeed, cyclin E–cdk2 and, more prominently, cyclin A–cdk2 activity is in late G_1 phase involved in activation of the DNA-replication machinery.

Three closely related human D-type cyclins have been identified, all of which interact with and activate cdk4 and cdk6, although cyclin D2 also activates cdk2 (11). Cyclins D2 and D3 may have specialized functions in distinct cell types. These cyclins behave similarly to cyclin D1, but appear not to be involved in tumor development (12).

The serine-threonine kinase activity of cyclin-cdk's becomes manifest when cyclin-cdk's have overcome inhibitory thresholds set by inhibitors of cyclin-dependent kinase, (cki) (13). Some of the cki's, including p16, p18, and p19 (taken together as the INK4 family), specifically inhibit cyclin D1–cdk4/6 activity by binding to either cdk4 or cdk6, thereby preventing association between cyclin D1 and its catalytic cdk partner. The free form of cyclin D1 is degraded much faster than the cdk-bound form, resulting in lower levels of cyclin D1 in cells with an overexpression of p16 (14). This situation is met in tumor cells with a functional inactivation of pRb resulting in overexpression of E2F-responsive p16 and in low levels of cyclin D1 protein (15).

The other class of cki, including p21, p27, and p57, inhibits all of the cyclin-cdk (13). Since cyclin D–cdk complexes are formed early during G_1 and are the first to bind to cki p21 and p27 (before cyclins E–cdk2 and A–cdk2), cyclin D–cdk complexes are perceived to titrate out the inhibiting effects of cki p21 and p27. Once cyclin E– and cyclin A–cdk2 complexes are formed upon cyclin D–cdk activity, p21 and p27 cki act subsequently upon these newly formed complexes, thus regulating the order of cyclin-cdk activities during G_1-S.

Cyclin D1 mRNA and subsequent protein synthesis is induced when arrested cells are released from G_0 to G_1 by growth factors (14). Protein levels of cyclin D fluctuate slightly during the cell cycle; the protein contains a PEST destruction motif, which accounts for their short half-lives (12). Accumulation of cyclin E, however, is highly periodic, with a sharp decline during S phase, which is due to autophosphorylation of cyclin E on threonine 380 site by cyclin E–cdk2, rendering cyclin E a target for ubiquitin-dependent degradation (16).

Adhesion onto extracellular matrix (ECM) components, such as laminin, fibronectin, or collagen, is mandatory for G_1 progression of normal epithelial cells. Adhesion affects induction of cyclin D1 mRNA and protein and results in degradation of p27 when this is complexed to cyclin E–cdk2 (17–19; Michalides and Muris, unpublished data). Degradation of p27 during this step releases cyclin E–cdk2 activity, which results in progression of the cell cycle in normal adherent cells.

Although the level of cyclin D1 protein, and subsequently of cyclin D1–cdk4 activity, is influenced by adhesion of cells onto extracellular matrix components, a major control over adhesion-restricted proliferation of cells is exerted by cyclin A– and E–cdk2 activity. Overexpression of cyclin A or E or reduced levels of p27 enable normal adherent cells to proliferate in suspension (20). In tumors, overexpression of cyclin E and reduced expression of p27 has recently been observed in breast and stomach cancer and was found to be associated with poor prognosis (21,22).

Overwhelming evidence in recent years on the function of cyclins has led to the qualification of cyclin D1–cdk4 as a "sensor" of cells for growth factor conditions, whereas cyclin D1–cdk4 together with cyclin E–cdk2 act as "sensors" of cellular attachment onto ECM. Deregulation of these cyclins releases the restrictions imposed by the external regulators on cell proliferation and affects the determinative phosphorylation of pRb, which permits progression of the cell cycle. In the scenario of increasing cellular autonomy, functional inactivation of pRb represents the most drastic genetic alteration leading to autonomy, whereas deregulation of cyclins and cki's does in part overcome the restrictions on proliferation imposed by external factors.

III. Deregulation of the Cyclin D/cdk4/p16/pRb Pathway in Cancer

A coordinated control by growth factors and the extracellular matrix is required for progression of the G_1 phase of the cell cycle in normal epithelial cells. This control is disturbed in tumor cells. In various tumor types, genetic alterations have been found that affect the cyclin D1/cdk4/p16/pRb regulatory circuit of G_1 progression (for review, see Ref. 15). Tumor cells with alterations in this pathway become less dependent on external growth factors. These genetic alterations involve either amplification of cyclin D1, mutation of p16 or pRb, and, although less frequently observed, amplification of cdk4 (Fig. 2).

A. Overexpression of Cyclin D1 and cdk4

Overexpression of cyclin D1 may result from various genetic alterations, including inversion of part of chromosome 11, inv(11)(p15:13), which placed cyclin D1 adjacent to the promotor of the parathyroid hormone gene in parathyroid adenomas (23).

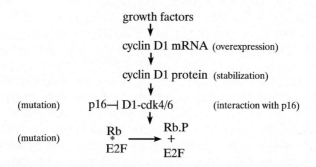

Figure 2 The cyclin D1/p16/cdk4/pRb pathway. Mode of deregulation of the pathway is placed in parentheses.

This rather infrequent alteration led to the identification of the cyclin D1 gene, which was also found to be overexpressed as a result of t(11;14) translocations in a relative low number of chronic B-cell lymphomas but in practically all mantle cell lymphomas (24,25). In a few B-cell lymphomas, overexpression of cyclin D1 is ascribed to interstitial deletion or rearrangements that affect the 3' untranslated region of exon 5, resulting in removal of the AUUUA destabilizing motifs (26). By far the most cases of overexpression of cyclin D1 are associated with amplification of the 11q13 amplicon, which encompasses cyclin D1 (for review, see Ref. 27). These tumors include carcinoma of the breast, liver, bladder, and lung, squamous cell carcinoma of the head and neck, and esophagus, sarcoma, and intestinal adenoma of patients with familial adenomatous polyposis. In the latter, concurrent overexpression of cyclin D1 and cdk4 was found in proliferative tumor areas (28).

Cyclin D1 overexpression is observed in early stages of development of breast tumor (29; Peters and Michalides, unpublished data), of squamous cell carcinoma of the head an neck (30), and of intestinal adenoma (28). Abnormal upregulation of this important G_1 regulator is, therefore, a relatively early event in progression of these tumors and may define a transition from a benign stage to commitment to carcinoma.

The clinical relevance of overexpression of cyclin D1 is different for the various tumor types, largely due to variance in the size of tumor panels analyzed, the composition of the tumor panels, the methodology used, and the negation of other genetic alterations in conjunction with cyclin D1 overexpression. In breast cancer, various studies indicated that amplification and corresponding overexpression of cyclin D1 is associated with a more advanced stage of disease, but no such association was found when overexpression of cyclin D1 was judged by immunohistochemistry alone (27,31–34). Moreover, most of the larger studies found a significant association between cyclin D1 overexpression and positivity for estrogen receptor (32,33,35). In squamous cell carcinomas of the head and neck (SCC-HN), many groups have reported on a correlation between overexpression of cyclin D1 and a more advanced stage of disease, lymph node involvement, and reduced overall survival time or time to recurrence (30,36–40).

In vitro, cyclin D1 cooperates with activated oncogenes such as *ras* and *myc* in the transformation of embryo fibroblast cells (41). Enforced overexpression of cyclin D1 alone in these and other cell types does not lead to transformation, but results in a more rapid transition through G_1 and in a reduced dependency on growth factors and on adhesion for cellular proliferation. We recently demonstrated that the combined effects of overexpression of cyclin D_1, i.e., a reduced exit from G_1 to G_0, an increased exit from G_0 to G_1, and reduced requirements for growth factors, yield a greater growth fraction of tumor cells when they are exposed to limiting amounts of growth factors, providing under these conditions a selective advantage to tumor cells with overexpression of cyclin D1 (42). Furthermore, we demonstrated that overexpression of cyclin D1 activates the estrogen receptor in estrogen receptor–positive breast tumor cells (43). These events may provide a selective advantage to tumor cells with overexpression of cyclin D1.

The effects of overexpression of cyclin D1 in vitro are also seen in cyclin D1–transgenic mice, in which overactivation of cyclin D1 resulted in development of hyperplasia in target tissues depending on the promoter-enhancer constructs being used to generate these cyclin D1–transgenic mice (44–47). Eventually, neoplasia arise within these hyperplasia, indicating that additional oncogenic alterations are apparently also in vivo mandatory to the later development of full neoplasia.

Amplification and concurrent overexpression of cdk4 is only rarely observed in glioblastomas, sarcomas, and hereditary intestinal adenomas (28,48). Since cdk4 proteins are present in excess amounts over cyclin D proteins, overexpression of cdk4 alone is a rather unusual way to disturb the cyclin D1/p16/pRb pathway.

B. Mutations of p16 and pRb

p16, the product of the CDKN2 gene, belongs to the group of tumor suppressors that specifically inhibit cdk 4 and 6. These include $p16^{INK4A}$, $p15^{INK4B}$, both located on chromosome 9p21, $p18^{INK4C}$ on 1p32, and $p19^{INK4D}$ on chromosome 19 (49). Initial studies indicated that the majority of human tumor cell lines carried homozygous deletion or mutations in the p16 gene (50,51), but these are less frequent in certain types of sporadic cancer (gliomas, melanomas, leukemias, and carcinomas of the pancreas and esophagus) (49). Germline mutations in p16 are associated with familial melanoma (52). Since the loss of p16 function occurs more frequently in cancer cell lines than in primary tumors, it was concluded that such an alteration provides a selective advantage to cells in culture.

Inactivation of the p16 suppressor gene may occur by homozygous deletion or by hemizygous deletion and inactivation of the remaining p16 allele by either point mutation or by methylation of CpG islands surrounding the first exon of p16, thereby silencing expression of p16 (53–56). Methylation of CpG sequences in the p16 gene provides another way of suppressing expression of p16 in the absence of any mutation in the DNA. Analysis of p16 inactivation in tumors should, therefore, preferably be performed by combining deletion and mutation analysis with an immunohistochemical examination of tumors for the absence of the p16 protein.

Transcription of the p16 gene is affected by the status of pRb. Human cell lines that lack functional pRb, resulting in an unrestricted expression of E2F, contain high levels of p16 mRNA and protein, which is due to the presence of an E2F-responsive element in the promoter of p16 (57).

Loss of p16 expression is associated with an extended in vitro life span of normal cells (58) and in vivo with increased susceptibility to cancer development in p16 knock-out mice, whereas p16−/−cells from those mice do not senesce in culture (59). These data indicate that loss of function of p16 results in immortalization of cells.

The INK4A locus on human chromosome 9 p21 encodes two alternative reading frames, $p16^{INK4A}$ and $p19^{ARF}$, of which only mutations in $p16^{INK4A}$ appear to contribute to cancer development (60). In lung tumors, mutations are rarely found in the other INK4A members, p15 and p18 (61). Their role in development of lung cancer is limited, which is also the case for novel regions with homozygous deletions in the vicinity of 9p21. This indicates that even more tumor suppressor genes may be located in that region (62,63).

The target of cyclin D1/p16/cdk4 activity is the pRb protein. The *RB1* gene on chromosome 13 is frequently lost in malignant disease (4,64). Analysis of Rb mutations is hampered by the large size of the Rb gene and is usually performed by immunohistochemistry, where inactivation of the Rb gene is indicated by the absence or reduced expression of the protein.

IV. Deregulation of the Cyclin D1/p16/cdk4/pRb Pathway in Lung Cancer

The cyclin D/p16/cdk4/pRb pathway functions as a single regulatory unit controlling release of E2F transcription factors, which mediate progression of the cell cycle into S phase (4,15). This notion is supported by the observation of an inverse relationship between p16 mutation and loss of function of pRb in several tumor types, including lung cancer (56,65–67). Coincident loss of function of both pRb and p16 apparently does not contribute to a greater selective advantage for tumor cells and is therefore not selected for in the process of tumor progression.

A summary of recent studies on deregulation of the cyclin D1/p16/pRb pathway in lung tumors is presented in Table 1. In these studies, mutation or deletion was determined either by Southern blotting, PCR analysis, single-strand conformation polymorphism and DNA sequencing, and/or immunostaining. Since different methodologies were applied in the various studies, the data presented in Table 1 are only given to indicate a trend in concurrence between markers. These trends are:

1. Loss of function of pRb is frequently observed in SCLC, and less frequently in NSCLC.
2. Loss of function of p16 is almost exclusively observed in NSCLC, and not in SCLC. Of the rare cases of SCLC carrying a normal pRb, most of them contained p16 mutations, whereas the few NSCLC cases with Rb mutations contained mostly wild-type p16. This confirms the inverse relationship between p16 and pRb in lung tumors.
3. Overexpression of cyclin D1 is found in tumors that lack pRb expression as well as in pRb-positive tumors.

The associations between deregulations in the cyclin D/p16/pRb pathway and clinical parameters that were found in these studies indicate:

1. An aberrant (lack of) expression of p16 is associated with advanced stages of NSCLC (65,68,69) and with worse survival (70).
2. Loss of pRb, which is infrequently found in NSCLC, was associated with poor prognosis in one study (71), but not in another (70).
3. Overexpression of cyclin D1 in NSCLC, as detected by immunohistochemistry, does not predict postoperative survival (72,73). However, am-

Table 1 Deregulation of Cyclin D1/p16/pRb Pathway in Lung Cancer

pRb	p16	cyclin D1	Ref.
	Frequency of alterations (no. cases/total) in SCLC		
9/9*		1/9*	87
	6/6 pRb+*		69
	0/5 pRb−*		
	0/20*		88
	0/24		68
	0/5*	2/5*	66
	1/5	4/5	
	6/7 pRb+*		67
	0/48 pRb−*		
	Frequency of alterations (no. cases/total) in non-SCLC		
15/100	50/85 pRb+		70
	1/15 pRb−		
		15	
	6/9*		89
	7/34		
0/9*	9/9 pRb+*	9/9*	66
	0/1 pRb−*		
	18/27	15/27	
	22/26 pRb+*		67
	1/7 pRb−*		
10/105	30/95 pRb+		75
	0/10 pRb−		
	6/20*		88
8/61*	46/53 pRb+*		69
	1/8 pRb−*		
	6/22 metastatic tumors		68
	0/25 nonmetastatic tumors		
0/12*		11/12*	87
		18/102	73
		25/53	74
		24/56	90
		55/96	72

*Studies performed on cell lines derived from lung tumors.
pRb+: pRb-positive tumors; pRb−: pRb-negative tumors.

plification of the cyclin D1 was found in 8 of 53 NSCLC and was associated with poor differentiation and reduced time to local relapse (74).

4. The relatively rare loss of pRb in NSCLC, but not the loss of p16 in pRb-positive NSCLC, is associated with heavy smoking (75).

No p16 protein was detected by immunohistochemistry in early stages (I–II) (70) of NSCLC, whereas homozygous deletions and point mutations were more frequently observed in more advanced stages of NSCLC (65,68,69). This discrepancy may well be due to silencing of p16 expression by methylation in early stages of NSCLC, whereas homozygous deletions and/or mutations in p16 occur more frequently in a later stage of development. Both events were associated with tumor dissemination.

In summary, deregulation of the cyclin D1/p16/pRb pathway is, in one way or the other, mandatory for lung tumor development, with loss of function of pRb to occur more frequently in SCLC and loss of function of p16 in NSCLC. Loss of pRb excludes loss of p16, and overexpression of cyclin D1 coincides with both. Loss of p16 in NSCLC seems to be indicative of a more aggressive tumor type.

These results clearly indicate that deregulation of the regulatory pathway leading to E2F release from pRb is involved in development of lung cancer. This pathway provides, therefore, a target for interfering with the course of disease. Whether deregulation of specific steps within this pathway is associated with clinically distinct subtypes of lung cancer should be a matter of further investigation, in particular for the association between loss of function of p16 and dissemination of NSCLC tumors. If this turns out to be the case, this marker could be used to indicate patients who require specific treatment strategies.

V. Apoptosis, Cell-Cycle Regulation, and Lung Cancer

It has become increasingly clear that tumor cells have not only become independent of regulatory signals that restrict growth of normal cells, but also have evaded programmed cell death, apoptosis, in response to DNA damage or other conditions that would induce a normal cell to commit suicide. Apoptosis is controlled by members of the bcl-2 family and by p53.

Apoptosis is also influenced by cell cycle regulators. Reintroduction of the Rb gene in Rb−/− Saos-2 cells, for instance, reduced the frequency of apoptosis after exposure of these cells to X-irradiation (76). Furthermore, normal cells undergo p53-mediated growth arrest in response to DNA damage, whereas the same cells transformed with the viral E1A oncogene, inactivating pRb, undergo apoptosis (77–79). From these studies the picture arises that apoptosis results from conflicting signaling within the cell. Such a conflict situation leading to apoptosis is also met in terminally differentiated neurons with overexpression of cyclin D1 (80), whereas overexpression of E2F1 or of cyclin D1 in normal cells under limited growth factor conditions also results in apoptosis (81,82). The induction of apoptosis by overexpression of E2F under low serum conditions is depending on a normal p53 in the cells, since co-overexpression of wild-type p53 and E2F results in rapid loss of cells through apoptosis, whereas co-overexpression of E2F in the presence of a mutated p53 results in proliferation (83,84). Apoptosis induced by overexpression of cyclin D1 is suppressed by bcl-2 and by p16 (80). p16 prevents the association between cyclin D1 and cdk4, resulting in free cyclin D1, which becomes rapidly degraded (16).

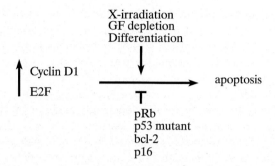

Figure 3   Cyclin D1, E2F, and apoptosis. Inhibition of E2F-induced apoptosis by p53 mutant was demonstrated by Qin et al. (83), of cyclin D1–induced apoptosis by bcl-2 Sofer-Levi et al. (81).

One study included analysis of both p53 and pRb mutations (86) and demonstrated that patients with NSCLC tumors that were mutated in both pRb and p53 (as determined by immunohistochemistry) survived for a significantly shorter period (20% 5-year survival) than patients with NSCLC tumors with a normal pRb and p53 (73% 5-year survival). Mutations in pRb or p53 alone were not informative in this study, and they were independent of postsurgical chemotherapy or stage. A previous study from the same group showed that altered pRb or p16 synergized with altered p53 in stimulating proliferation of NSCLC cells (75). The results from these studies strongly suggest that pRb and p16 mutations synergize with p53 mutations in yielding a more aggressive tumor phenotype.

In summary, multiple interacting factors appear to influence the ability of cells to undergo apoptosis, either spontaneously as a consequence of conflicting growth factor signaling or in response to DNA-damaging agents, oxygen depletion (85), or other forms of cellular stress. Apoptosis seems a mechanism for cells to respond to a combination of conflicting signals, which induce an arrest as well as proliferation (Fig. 3). A defect in growth control without arrest results in apoptosis, whereas a deficiency in both results in unrestricted proliferation.

VI.   Conclusions

Two regulatory pathways restrict tumor growth—one controlling proliferation, the other the ability to undergo apoptosis. Proliferation control is regulated by the cyclin D/p16/cdk4/pRb pathway, whereas the apoptotic pathway is controlled by the bcl-2/bax/caspase pathway. Intermediates between these two pathways are pRb and p53. The ability of tumor cells to proliferate unrestrictedly and not to undergo apoptosis depends on alterations in both of these pathways.

Studies on lung cancer have revealed that a single alteration in these pathways may already be of prognostic value. For instance, p16 mutation in NSCLC and p53 mutation in SCLC and NSCLC is associated with a more aggressive tumor phenotype. A combination of these markers, however, may be even more informative, as was demonstrated in the study of Dosaka-Akita et al. (86), where mutations in both pRb and p53 indicated a significantly worse prognosis that was not detected when either marker was examined alone in this cohort of NSCLC patients. Mutations in both of these regulators in normal cells yielded unrestricted proliferation in experimental studies (83,84) and indicated in vivo a more aggressive phenotype in NSCLC.

The studies summarized in this chapter provide only fragmentary proof of an association between deregulation of growth or apoptosis regulators and tumor progression and suggest that combination(s) of these deregulations are leading to a more aggressive tumor phenotype. If these tentative associations are confirmed in larger prospective studies, then combinations of mutations in both regulatory pathways may be used to identify lung cancer patients with different risks of recurrence.

Acknowledgments

The research of the author is supported by grants from the Dutch Cancer Society. I thank Drs. B. Kwa and S. Roodenhuis for critical reading of the manuscript.

References

1. Sherr CJ. Cancer cell cycles. Science 1996; 274:1672–1677.
2. Hunter T. Oncoprotein networks. Cell 1997; 88:333–346.
3. Lukas J, Bartkova J, Bartek J. Convergence of mitogenic signalling cascades from diverse classes of receptors at the cyclin D-cyclin-dependent kinase-pRb-controlled G1 checkpoint. Mol Cell Biol 1996; 16:6917–6925.
4. Weinberg RA. The retinoblastoma protein and cell cycle control. Cell 1995; 81:323–330.
5. Ewen ME, Sluss HK, Sherr CJ, Matsushime H, Kato J, Livingston DM. Functional interactions of the retinoblastoma protein with mammalian D-type cyclins. Cell 1993; 73:487–497.
6. Ohtsubo M, Theodoras AM, Schumacher J, Roberts JM, Pagano M. Human cyclin E, a nuclear protein essential for the G1-to-S phase transition. Mol Cell Biol 1995; 15:2612–2624.
7. Schulze A, Zerfass K, Spitkovsky D, Middendorp S, Berges J, Helin K, et al. Cell cycle regulation of the cyclin A gene promoter is mediated by a variant E2F site. Proc Natl Acad Sci USA 1995; 92:11264–11268.
8. Ohtani K, DeGregori J, Nevins JR. Regulation of the cyclin E gene by transcription factor E2F1. Proc Natl Acad Sci USA 1995; 92:12146–12150.
9. Resnitzky A, Reed SI. Different roles for cyclin D1 and E in regulation of the G1-to-S transition. Mol Cell Biol 1995; 15:3463–3469.
10. Kitagawa M, Higashi H, Jung HK, Suzuki-Takahashi I, Ikeda M, Tamai K, et al. The consensus motif for phosphorylation by cyclin D1-Cdk4 is different from that for phosphorylation by cyclin A/E-Cdk2. EMBO J 1996; 15:7060–7069.
11. Wiethege T, Voss B, Muller KM. P53 accumulation and proliferating-cell nuclear antigen expression in human lung cancer. J Cancer Res Clin Oncol 1995; 121:371–377.
12. Bates S, Peters G. Cyclin D1 as a cellular proto-oncogene. Semin Cancer Biol 1995; 6:73–82.
13. Sherr CJ, Roberts JM. Inhibitors of mammalian G1 cyclin-dependent kinases. Genes Dev 1995; 9:1149–1163.

14. Bates S, Parry D, Bonetta L, Vousden K, Dickson C, Peters G. Absence of cyclin D/cdk complexes in cells lacking functional retinoblastoma protein. Oncogene 1994; 9:1633–1640.
15. Bartek J, Bartkova J, Lukas J. The retinoblastoma protein pathway and the restriction point. Curr Opin Cell Biol 1996; 8:805–814.
16. Won KA, Reed SI. Activation of cyclin E/CDK2 is coupled to site-specific autophosphorylation and ubiquitin-dependent degradation of cyclin. EMBO J 1996; 15:4182–4193.
17. Fang F, Orend G, Watanabe N, Hunter T, Ruoslahti E. Dependence of cyclin E-CDK2 kinase activity on cell anchorage. Science 1996; 271:499–502.
18. Assoian RK. Anchorage-dependent cell cycle progression. J Cell Biol 1997; 136:1–4.
19. Shulze A, Zerfass-Thome K, Berges J, Middendorp S, Jansen-Durr P, Henglein B. Anchorage-dependent transcription of the cyclin A gene. Mol Cell Biol 1996; 16:4632–4638.
20. Guadagno TM, Ohtsubo M, Roberts JM, Assoian RK. A link between cyclin A expression and adhesion-dependent cell cycle progression. Science 1993; 262:1572–1575.
21. Porter PL, Malone KE, Heagerty PJ, et al. Expression of cell-cycle regulators p27Kip1 and cyclin E, alone and in combination, correlate with survival in young breast cancer patients. Nat Med 1997; 3:222–225.
22. Catzavelos C, Bhattacharya N, Ung YC, et al. Decreased levels of the cell-cycle inhibitor p27Kip1 protein: prognostic implications in primary breast cancer. Nat Med 1997; 3:227–230.
23. Rosenberg CL, Kim HG, Shows TB, Kronenberg HM, Arnold A. Rearrangement and overexpression of D11S287E, a candidate oncogene on chromosome 11q13 in benign parathyroid tumors. Oncogene 1991; 6:449–453.
24. de Boer CJ, Loyson S, Kluin PM, Kluin-Nelemans HC, Schuuring E, van Krieken JH. Multiple breakpoints within the BCL-1 locus in B-cell lymphoma: rearrangements of the cyclin D1 gene. Cancer Res 1993; 53:4148–4152.
25. Swerdlow SH, Yang WI, Zukerberg LR, Harris NL, Arnold A, Williams ME. Expression of cyclin D1 protein in centrocytic/mantle cell lymphomas with and without rearrangement of the BCL1/cyclin D1 gene. Hum Pathol 1995; 26:999–1004.
26. Rimokh R, Berger F, Bastard C, Klein B, French M, Archimbaud E, et al. Rearrangement of CCND1 (BCL1/PRAD1) 3′ untranslated region in mantle-cell lymphomas and t(11q13)-associated leukemias. Blood 1994; 83:3689–3696.
27. Hall M, Peters G. Genetic alterations of cyclins, cyclin-dependent kinases, and Cdk inhibitors in human cancer. Adv Cancer Res 1996; 68:67–108.
28. Zhang T, Nanney LB, Luongo C, Lamps L, Heppner KJ, DuBois RN, et al. Concurrent overexpression of cyclin D1 and cyclin-dependent kinase 4 (Cdk4) in intestinal adenomas from multiple intestinal neoplasia (Min) mice and human familial adenomatous polyposis patients. Cancer Res 1997; 57:169–175.
29. Weinstat-Saslow D, Merino MJ, Manrow RE, et al. Overexpression of cyclin D mRNA distinguishes invasive and in situ breast carcinomas from non-malignant lesions. Nat Med 1995; 1:1257–1260.
30. Michalides RJ, van Veelen R, Kristel P, Hart A, Loftus B, Hilgers FJ, et al. Overexpression of cyclin D1 indicates a poor prognosis in squamous cell carcinoma of the head and neck. Arch Otolaryngol Head Neck Surg 1997; 123:497–502.
31. Gillett C, Fantl V, Smith R, Fisher C, Bartek J, Dickson C, et al. Amplification and overexpression of cyclin D1 in breast cancer detected by immunohistochemical staining. Cancer Res 1994; 54:1812–1817.
32. Gillett C, Smith P, Gregory W, Richards M, Millis R, Peters G, et al. Cyclin D1 and prognosis in human breast cancer. Int J Cancer 1996; 69:92–99.
33. Michalides R, Hageman P, van Tinteren H, Houben L, Wientjens E, Klompmaker R, et al. A clinico-pathological study on overexpression of Cyclin D and of p53 in a series of 248 patients with operable breast cancer. Br J Cancer 1996; 73:728–734.
34. McIntosh GG, Anderson JJ, Milton I, Steward M, Parr AH, Thomas MD, et al. Determination of the prognostic value of cyclin D1 overexpression in breast cancer. Oncogene 1995; 11:885–891.
35. Barbareschi M, Girlando S, Mauri FM, Forti S, Eccher C, Mauri FA, et al. Quantitative

growth fraction evaluation with MIB1 and Ki67 antibodies in breast carcinomas. Am J Clin Pathol 1994; 102:171–175.

36. Michalides RJ, Van Veelen N, Hart A, Loftus B, Wientjens E, Balm A. Overexpression of cyclin D1 correlates with recurrence in a group of forty-seven operable squamous cell carcinomas of the head and neck. Cancer Res 1995; 55:975–978.

37. Meredith SD, Levine PA, Burns JA, Gaffey MJ, Boyd JC, Weiss LM, et al. Chromosome 11q13 amplification in head and neck squamous cell carcinoma. Association with poor prognosis. Arch Otolaryngol Head Neck Surg 1995; 121:790–794.

38. Masuda M, Hirakawa N, Nakashima T, Kuratomi Y, Komiyama S. Cyclin D1 overexpression in primary hypopharyngeal carcinomas. Cancer 1996; 78:390–395.

39. Bellacosa A, Almadori G, Cavallo S, Cadoni G, Galli J, Ferrandina G, et al. Cyclin D1 gene amplification in human laryngeal squamous cell carcinomas: prognostic significance and clinical implications. Clin Cancer Res 1996; 2:175–180.

40. Fracchiolla NS, Pruneri G, Pignataro L, Carboni N, Capaccio P, Boletini A, et al. Molecular and immunohistochemical analysis of the bcl-1/cyclin D1 gene in laryngeal squamous cell carcinomas: correlation of protein expression with lymph node metastases and advanced clinical stage. Cancer 1997; 79:1114–1121.

41. Hinds PW, Dowdy SF, Eaton EN, Arnold A, Weinberg RA. Function of a human cyclin gene as an oncogene. Proc Natl Acad Sci USA 1994; 91:709–713.

42. Zwijsen RM, Klompmaker R, Wientjens EB, Kristel PM, Van der Burg B, Michalides RJ. Cyclin D1 triggers autonomous growth of breast cancer cells by governing cell cycle exit. Mol Cell Biol 1996; 16:2554–2560.

43. Zwijsen RM, Wientjens E, Klompmaker R, Van der Sman J, Bernards R, Michalides RJ. CDK-independent activation of estrogen receptor by cyclin D_1. Cell 1997; 88:405–415.

44. Wang TC, Cardiff RD, Zukerberg L, Lees E, Arnold A, Schmidt EV. Mammary hyperplasia and carcinoma in MMTV-cyclin D1 transgenic mice. Nature 1994; 369:669–671.

45. Bodrug SE, Warner BJ, Bath ML, Lindeman GJ, Harris AW, Adams JM. Cyclin D1 transgene impedes lymphocyte maturation and collaborates in lymphomagenesis with the myc gene. EMBO J 1994; 13:2124–2130.

46. Lovec H, Grzeschiczek A, Kowalski MB, Moroy T. Cyclin D1/bcl-1 cooperates with myc genes in the generation of B-cell lymphoma in transgenic mice. EMBO J 1994; 13:3487–3495.

47. Robles AI, Larcher F, Whalin RB, Murillas R, Richie E, Gimenez-Conti IB, et al. Expression of cyclin D1 in epithelial tissues of transgenic mice results in epidermal hyperproliferation and severe thymic hyperplasia. Proc Natl Acad Sci USA 1996; 93:7634–7638.

48. He J, Allen JR, Collins VP, Allalunis-Turner MJ, Godbout R, Day RS, et al. CDK4 amplification is an alternative mechanism to p16 gene homozygous deletion in glioma cell lines. Cancer Res 1994; 54:5804–5807.

49. Shapiro GI, Rollins BJ. p16INK4A as a human tumor suppressor. Biochim Biophys Acta 1996; 1242:165–169.

50. Kamb A, Gruis NA, Weaver-Feldhaus J, Liu Q, Harshman K, Tavtigian SV, et al. A cell cycle regulator potentially involved in genesis of many tumor types. Science 1994; 264:436–440.

51. Nobori T, Miura K, Wu DJ, Lois A, Takabayashi K, Carson DA. Deletions of the cyclin-dependent kinase-4 inhibitor gene in multiple human cancers. Nature 1994; 368:753–756.

52. Hussussian CJ, Struewing JP, Goldstein AM, Higgins PA, Ally DS, Sheahan MD, et al. Germline p16 mutations in familial melanoma. Nat Genet 1994; 8:15–21.

53. Merlo A, Herman JG, Mao L, et al. 5' CpG island methylation is associated with transcriptional silencing of the tumour suppressor p16/CDKN2/MTS1 in human cancers. Nat Med 1995; 1:686–692.

54. Merlo A, Gabrielson E, Askin F, Sidransky D. Frequent loss of chromosome 9 in human primary non-small cell lung cancer. Cancer Res 1994; 54:640–642.

55. Otterson GA, Khleif SN, Chen W, Coxon AB, Kaye FJ. CDKN2 gene silencing in lung cancer by DNA hypermethylation and kinetics of p16INK4 protein induction by 5-aza 2'deoxycytidine. Oncogene 1995; 11:1211–1216.

56. Shapiro GI, Park JE, Edwards CD, Mao L, Merlo A, Sidransky D, et al. Multiple mechanisms

of p16INK4A inactivation in non-small cell lung cancer cell lines. Cancer Res 1995; 55:6200–6209.

57. Hara E, Smith R, Parry D, Tahara H, Stone S, Peters G. Regulation of p16CDKN2 expression and its implications for cell immortalization and senescence. Mol Cell Biol 1996; 16:859–867.

58. Noble JR, Rogan EM, Neumann AA, Maclean K, Bryan TM, Reddel RR. Association of extended in vitro proliferative potential with loss of p16INK4 expression. Oncogene 1996; 13:1259–1268.

59. Serrano M, Lee H, Chin L, Cordon-Cardo C, Beach D, DePinho RA. Role of the INK4a locus in tumor suppression and cell mortality. Cell 1996; 85:27–37.

60. Quelle DE, Cheng M, Ashmun RA, Sherr CJ. Cancer-associated mutations at the INK4a locus cancel cell cycle arrest by p16INK4a but not by the alternative reading frame protein p19ARF. Proc Natl Acad Sci USA 1997; 94:669–673.

61. Rusin MR, Okamoto A, Chorazy M, Czyzewski K, Harasim J, Spillare EA, et al. Intragenic mutations of the p16(INK4), p15(INK4B) and p18 genes in primary non-small-cell lung cancers. Int J Cancer 1996; 65:734–739.

62. Wiest JS, Franklin WA, Otstot JT, Forbey K, Varella-Garcia M, Rao K, et al. Identification of a novel region of homozygous deletion on chromosome 9p in squamous cell carcinoma of the lung: the location of a putative tumor suppressor gene. Cancer Res 1997; 57:1–6.

63. Kim SK, Ro JY, Kemp BL, Lee JS, Kwon TJ, Fong KM, et al. Identification of three distinct tumor suppressor loci on the short arm of chromosome 9 in small cell lung cancer. Cancer Res 1997; 57:400–403.

64. Gallie BL. Retinoblastoma gene mutations in human cancer. N Engl J Med 1994; 330: 786–787.

65. Kelley MJ, Nakagawa K, Steinberg SM, Mulshine JL, Kamb A, Johnson BE. Differential inactivation of CDKN2 and Rb protein in non-small-cell and small-cell lung cancer cell lines. J Natl Cancer Inst 1995; 87:756–761.

66. Shapiro GI, Edwards CD, Kobzik L, Godleski J, Richards W, Sugarbaker DJ, et al. Reciprocal Rb inactivation and p16INK4 expression in primary lung cancers and cell lines. Cancer Res 1995; 55:505–509.

67. Otterson GA, Kratzke RA, Coxon A, Kim YW, Kaye FJ. Absence of p16INK4 protein is restricted to the subset of lung cancer lines that retains wildtype RB. Oncogene 1994; 9:3375–3378.

68. Okamoto A, Hussain SP, Hagiwara K, Spillare EA, Rusin MR, Demetrick DJ, et al. Mutations in the p16INK4/MTS1/CDKN2, p15INK4B/MTS2, and p18 genes in primary and metastatic lung cancer. Cancer Res 1995; 55:1448–1451.

69. Nakagawa K, Conrad NK, Williams JP, Johnson BE, Kelley MJ. Mechanism of inactivation of CDKN2 and MTS2 in non-small cell lung cancer and association with advanced stage. Oncogene 1995; 11:1843–1851.

70. Kratzke RA, Greatens TM, Rubins JB, Maddaus MA, Niewoehner DE, Niehans GA, et al. Rb and p16INK4a expression in resected non-small cell lung tumors. Cancer Res 1996; 56:3415–3420.

71. Xu H, Quinlan DC, Davidson AG, Hu SX, Summers CL, Li J, et al. Altered retinoblastoma protein expression and prognosis in early-stage non-small-cell lung cancer. J Natl Cancer Inst 1994; 86:695–699.

72. Kwa HB, Michalides RJ, Dijkman JH, Mooi WJ. The prognostic value of NCAM, p53 and cyclin D1 in resected non-small cell lung cancer. Lung Cancer 1996; 14:207–217.

73. Yang WI, Chung KY, Shin DH, Kim YB. Cyclin D1 protein expression in lung cancer. Yonsei Med J 1996; 37:142–150.

74. Betticher DC, Heighway J, Hasleton PS, Altermatt HJ, Ryder WD, Cerny T, et al. Prognostic significance of CCND1 (cyclin D1) overexpression in primary resected non-small-cell lung cancer. Br J Cancer 1996; 73:294–300.

75. Kinoshita I, Dosaka-Akita H, Mishina T, Akie K, Nishi M, Hiroumi H, et al. Altered p16INK4 and retinoblastoma protein status in non-small cell lung cancer: potential synergistic effect with altered p53 protein on proliferative activity. Cancer Res 1996; 56:5557–5562.

76. Haas-Kogan DA, Kogan SC, Levi D, Dazin P, T'Ang A, Fung YK, et al. Inhibition of apoptosis by the retinoblastoma gene product. EMBO J 1995; 14:461–472.
77. Lowe SW, Bodis S, McClatchey A, Remington L, Ruley HE, Fisher DE, et al. p53 status and the efficacy of cancer therapy in vivo. Science 1994; 266:807–810.
78. Lowe SW. Cancer therapy and p53. Curr Opin Oncol 1995; 7:547–553.
79. Liebermann DA, Hoffman B, Steinman RA. Molecular controls of growth arrest and apoptosis: p53-dependent and independent pathways. Oncogene 1995; 11:199–210.
80. Kranenburg O, van der Eb AJ, Zantema A. Cyclin D1 is an essential mediator of apoptotic neuronal cell death. EMBO J 1996; 15:46–54.
81. Sofer-Levi Y, Resnitzky D. Apoptosis induced by ectopic expression of cyclin D1 but not cyclin E. Oncogene 1996; 13:2431–2437.
82. Shan B, Lee WH. Deregulated expression of E2F-1 induces S-phase entry and leads to apoptosis. Mol Cell Biol 1994; 14:8166–8173.
83. Qin XQ, Livingston DM, Kaelin WG, Jr., Adams PD. Deregulated transcription factor E2F-1 expression leads to S-phase entry and p53-mediated apoptosis. Proc Natl Acad Sci USA 1994; 91:10918–10922.
84. Wu X, Levine AJ. p53 and E2F-1 cooperate to mediate apoptosis. Proc Natl Acad Sci USA 1994; 91:3602–3606.
85. Graeber TG, Osmanian C, Jacks T, Housman DE, Koch CJ, Lowe SW, et al. Hypoxia-mediated selection of cells with diminished apoptotic potential in solid tumours. Nature 1996; 379:88–91.
86. Dosaka-Akita H, Hu SX, Fujino M, Harada M, Kinoshita I, Xu JH, et al. Altered retinoblastoma protein expression in non-small cell lung cancer: its synergistic effects with altered ras and p53 protein status on prognosis. Cancer 1997; 79:1329–1337.
87. Schauer IE, Siriwardana S, Langan TA, Sclafani RA. Cyclin D1 overexpression vs. retinoblastoma inactivation: implications for growth control evasion in non-small cell and small cell lung cancer. Proc Natl Acad Sci USA 1994; 91:7827–7831.
88. Washimi O, Nagatake M, Osada H, Ueda R, Koshikawa T, Seki T, et al. In vivo occurrence of p16 (MTS1) and p15 (MTS2) alterations preferentially in non-small cell lung cancers. Cancer Res 1995; 55:514–517.
89. de Vos S, Miller CW, Takeuchi S, Gombart AF, Cho SK, Koeffler HP. Alterations of CDKN2 (p16) in non-small cell lung cancer. Genes Chromosomes Cancer 1995; 14:164–170.
90. Mate JL, Ariza A, Aracil C, Lopez D, Isamat M, Perez-Piteira J, et al. Cyclin D1 overexpression in non-small cell lung carcinoma: correlation with Ki67 labelling index and poor cytoplasmic differentiation. J Pathol 1996; 180:395–399.

13

Relevance of DNA Methylation to Lung Cancer

SAMIR M. HANASH, BRUCE RICHARDSON, and DAVID BEER

University of Michigan Medical School
Ann Arbor, Michigan

I. DNA Methylation

The view that DNA methylation may be altered in cancer is gaining acceptance (1–3). However, a full understanding of the process through which DNA methylation may become aberrant in cancer requires a better understanding of the regulation of DNA methylation in normal cells. In eukaryotic cells, DNA methylation refers primarily to the postsynthetic methylation of deoxycytosine (dC) at the 5 position to form 5-deoxymethylcytosine (d^mC) (4). Nearly all d^mC is found in the dinucleotide CpG. The sequence CpG is underrepresented in the genome, presumably as a result of an increased mutation rate of 5-methylcytosine residues. Most unmethylated CpG pairs are found in GC-rich sequences referred to as CpG islands, while the majority of the methylated pairs are found elsewhere in the genome. The lack of methylation of CpG pairs in CpG islands accounts for the escape of CpG islands from CpG erosion. CpG islands are approximately 1 kb long and are almost always located near coding sequences of genes (5). CpG islands contain multiple binding sites for transcription factors and function as promoters for the associated genes (5). Nearly all "housekeeping" genes, and some tissue-specific genes, contain CpG islands (6). Current estimates indicate that there are approximately 45,000 CpG islands per haploid genome in humans (7). Approximately 56% of human genes are associated with CpG islands (7).

In mature cells, DNA methylation patterns are maintained through mitosis by the enzyme DNA (cytosine-5-) methyltransferase (DNA MTase) (8). During mitosis, DNA MTase recognizes hemimethylated CpG dinucleotides in the parent and daughter DNA strands and catalyzes the transfer of the methyl group from S-adenosylmethionine to the cytosine residues in the unmethylated daughter DNA strand, producing symmetrically methylated sites and maintaining methylation patterns (9). Since DNA methylation patterns may affect gene expression and are heritable through mitosis, yet do not involve sequence mutations, DNA methylation has been referred to as an "epigenetic" mechanism of gene regulation (10). De novo methylation of unmethylated DNA sequences also occurs. However, the mechanisms regulating de novo methylation are poorly understood. A few CpG islands have been investigated in aging and found to be methylated (5,11,12). However, the extent of CpG island methylation changes in aging and the relevance of this change to cancer are unknown.

II. DNA Methylation Changes During Carcinogenesis

DNA methylation has been implicated in carcinogenesis. Reduced $d^m C$ levels have been described in a variety of malignancies. Hypomethylation of proto-oncogenes has been reported in a variety of tumor types and may contribute to malignant transformation by modifying proto-oncogene expression. The methylation of normally unmethylated CpG islands has also been associated with various tumors. For example, hypermethylation of the *Rb* gene may contribute to neoplastic transformation in retinoblastoma by inactivating its tumor-suppressor function. DNA methylation can also lead to point mutations as a result of deamination of $d^m C$ to form thymine. Repair mechanisms may then repair the mismatched guanidine to adenosine, causing a point mutation. This process is further accelerated by DNA MTase overexpression, which may be an early event in transformation of certain cells (4). The estimated mutation rate of CpG dinucleotides is 10–40 times that of other dinucleotides (4), and this mutation has been implicated in 25–33% of p53 mutations in human tumors (4). Altered DNA methylation has also been linked to genomic instability (2). A clue to this relationship is the observation that treatment with 5-azacytidine induces undercondensations in human chromosomes, certain chromosomes being affected more than others (13). Regional DNA hypomethylation has also been related to sequence-specific strand breaks and deletions, which can contribute to malignant transformation (14). A correlation between genetic instability and methylation of exogenously introduced DNA has been reported in colorectal cancer cells (15).

III. DNA Methylation and Lung Cancer

Most current knowledge of methylation changes in lung cancer is of a general nature. Unique methylation changes associated with lung cancer have yet to be identified. A number of genes known to exhibit hypermethylation from other tumors have been investigated for their methylation status in lung tumors (Table 1). Genes shown to be hypermethylated in some lung tumors include tumor suppressor genes p16/CDKN2 and p15INK4B. Hypomethylated genes include c-H-ras (16,17).

A recent study suggests that in lung cancer, methylation of some CpG islands may be related to the specific type of carcinogen exposure. The estrogen receptor (ER) gene contains a CpG island, which is methylated in different cancers (18–20). In a study of ER gene methylation in lung tumors, promoter methylation was detected in 4 of 11 tumors from never-smokers and 7 of 35 tumors from smokers. A significant difference in ER methylation was also observed in a rodent lung tumor model. Lung tumors induced by a tobacco carcinogen had a low incidence of ER methylation relative to spontaneous and plutonium-induced tumors, which had a very high incidence.

The role of MTase in tumor initiation or development has been of interest, particularly in view of the demonstration that disruption of MTase in knockout mice results in partial protection from colon tumor development when crossed with *min* mice that have susceptibility to colon tumors. Additionally, overexpression of the murine MTase in NIH 3T3 cells was shown to cause transformation. In a mouse model of lung carcinogenesis, Belinsky et al. (21) examined MTase levels in mice that exhibit high or low susceptibility for lung tumor formation. They reported increased levels of MTase in the target alveolar type II cells in the high-susceptibility mice after carcinogen exposure. While it could be suggested that an increase in MTase activity is associated with tumor development and might represent an important step in carcinogenesis, it is likely that the increase in MTase activity observed is attributable in part to an increase in the proliferative activity of the target cells. For example, a recent study of colon tumors, showed limited upregulation of MTase activity in colon cancer commensurate with increased cell proliferation (22). We have also observed a marked increase in MTase activity following mitotic stimulation of resting T cells with PHA (23).

Table 1 Hypermethylated Loci in Lung Cancer

Hypermethylated loci	Ref.
p16/CDKN$_2$	Otterson et al., 1995 (33)
p15/INK4B	Herman et al., 1996 (34)
Calcitonin	Baylin et al., 1987 (35)
Carbohydrate antigen Le^y	Saitoh et al., 1995 (36)
BC12	Nagatake et al, 1996 (37)
Estrogen receptor	Issa et al., 1996 (38)
Parathyroid hormone	Ganderton et al., 1995 (39)

IV. Analysis of Methylation Changes in Lung Tumors by Means of Two-Dimensional Separations of *Not* I Genomic Digests

Several approaches have become available to uncover methylation changes across the genome. These approaches include methylation-sensitive arbitrarily primed PCR (24) and methylation-sensitive representational difference analysis (25). The effects of methylation are most consistently observed in CpG islands, where methylation has a strong correlation with transcriptional suppression (26), and lack of methylation is usually required for expression of the associated gene. These observations, together with the common localization of CpG islands in gene promoters, make CpG islands ideal landmarks for genome-scanning approaches to detect changes in DNA methylation.

We have implemented a computerized approach for the analysis of two-dimensional separations of enzyme-digested genomic DNA (27–30) based on the initial procedure described by Hatada et al. (27). By utilizing different combinations of restriction enzymes and/or different electrophoretic conditions, the number of independent fragments in a human genomic DNA sample that can be analyzed in multiple two-dimensional patterns can reach several thousand. The approach relies on radioisotope labeling of genomic fragments at cleavage sites specific for a rare cutting restriction enzyme. The labeled genomic digests are separated in a first dimension, followed by in situ digestion prior to second-dimension separation. The reliance on the rare cleaving restriction enzyme *Not*I to digest genomic DNA prior to labeling allows visualization of DNA fragments that occur preferentially in CpG islands of the genome. Because of the localization of CpG islands in proximity to transcribed sequences, the two-dimensional patterns obtained with this enzyme are highly targeted to a functional component of the genome (30,31). Thus, there is a strong likelihood that *Not* I fragments detected in two-dimensional gels represent sequences in genes.

An application of this approach is the study of genomic methylation changes by measuring fragment intensities (28,29). The two-dimensional genome-scanning approach is being implemented by our group for the study of genomic alterations in lung tumors. Our current findings pertaining to DNA methylation changes in lung adenocarcinomas are reviewed.

A. Hypomethylation of Repetitive DNA Sequences in Lung Adenocarcinoma

To date we have analyzed some 20 lung adenocarcinomas by means of two-dimensional genome scanning. Representative patterns of a tumor and of normal lung tissue from the same patients are shown in Figure 1. Multicopy fragments observed in patterns of normal DNA are largely attributed to ribosomal DNA (rDNA) genes (29). The transcribed portion of the rDNA results in some 20 labeled fragments visible on each gel as multicopy spots. We have mapped these spots to the

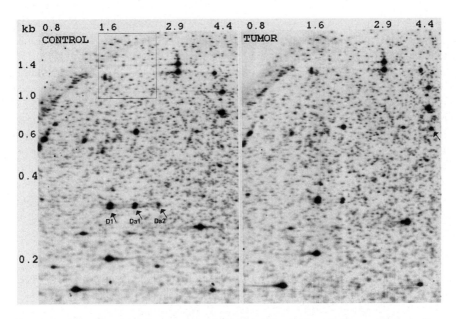

Figure 1 Two-dimensional separation of genomic digests of normal lung and tumor from the same patient. Hypomethylation of the D fragment of rDNA is evident by decreased intensity of Da1 and Da2 in the tumor. The multicopy fragment indicated with a large arrow in the tumor is a part of the ErbB2 amplicon present in this tumor. The boxed area appears as a close-up in Figure 2.

sequences responsible for their occurrence on the gels, based in part on direct sequencing of fragments. Some fragments display a shift in their position, to a larger size, attributable to methylation at specific *Not* I sites. The majority of tumors analyzed displayed diminished intensity of the shifted rDNA fragments, consistent with hypomethylation of their *Not* I sites. In addition, in two tumors, we have observed one multicopy fragment that was absent in normal tissue. In one of the two tumors, two additional multicopy fragments were observed. The three fragments, designated Nbl-1, Nbl-2, and Nbl-3 because of their initial detection in neuroblastomas, are part of repetitive units that are methylated in a variety of normal cell populations analyzed to date (32). Cloning and sequence analysis of fragment Nbl-1 revealed strong homology between this fragment and a subtelomeric sequence that was reported to occur in chimpanzees but was not detectable in humans region of many chromosomes. The appearance of all three fragments in two-dimensional gels was demonstrated to be due to demethylation of cytosine at the *Not* I sites.

B. Hypermethylated CpG Islands in Lung Adenocarcinomas

The methylation pattern of some of the genes known to be hypermethylated in tumors can be reversed following treatment with methylation inhibitors. To determine the extent and reversibility of hypermethylation of CpG islands in lung cancer cell lines, we have compared the two-dimensional patterns of cell lines before and after treatment with 5-aza-2′-deoxycytidine. For example, following such treatment of the lung adenocarcinoma cell line A549, we observed a ~5% increase in the number of CpG island containing fragments in two-dimensional patterns. The increase is presumed to result from demethylation of *Not* I sites in genomic DNA. We have further determined the status of these *Not* I-derived fragments in two-dimensional patterns of normal lung and in lung tumors. A substantial number of these fragments were detectable in normal lung and were absent in lung tumors (Fig. 2). Their inducibility with 5-aza-2′-deoxycytidine suggests that their absence in tumor two-dimensional patterns is due to hypermethylation.

It is unlikely that the methylation changes are simply the result of stochastic errors in methylation as previously suggested. A case in point is the demethylation

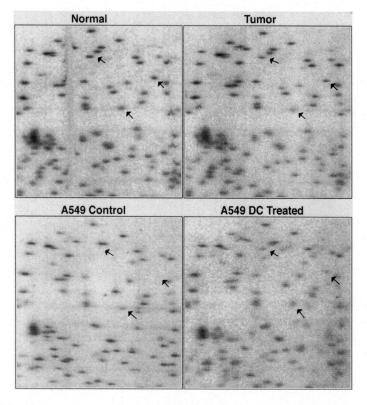

Figure 2   Close-up of two-dimensional patterns pointing to fragments that appear in reduced intensity in lung tumors (tumor) relative to normal lung (normal) and that are also absent in lung carcinoma cell line A549 (control) and detectable following 5-aza-2′-deoxycytidine treatment (dC).

of repetitive units. Our findings with respect to Nbl-1 indicate that only a fraction of the Nbl-1 repetitive units exhibit demethylation at the *Not* I sites. If the change in cytosine methylation were a random process, it would follow that the multiple copies of the repetitive sequence would be randomly demethylated. However, the data indicate that a tandem subset is demethylated. Thus it would appear that factors other than the sequence motif or random errors are responsible for the change in methylation status. Such factors may include chromatin structure, interaction with binding proteins, and methylation changes induced as a result of deregulation of cancer-related genes. A better understanding of the methylation process will be necessary in order to develop strategies to reverse methylation changes in cancer by pharmacologic or other means.

References

1. Laird PW, Jaenisch R. The role of DNA methylation in cancer genetics and epigenetics. Annu Rev Genet 1996; 30:441–464.
2. Jones PA, Gonzalgo ML. Altered DNA methylation and genome instability: A new pathway to cancer? Proc Natl Acad Sci USA 1997; 94:2103–2105.
3. Versteeg R. Aberrant methylation in cancer. Am J Hum Genet 1997; 60:751–754.
4. Adams RLP, Burdon RH. DNA methylation in the cell. In: A Rich, ed. Molecular Biology of DNA Methylation. New York: Springer-Verlag, 1985:9–18.
5. Antequera F, Bird A. CpG islands. In: JP Jost, HP Saluz, eds. DNA Methylation: Molecular Biology and Biological Significance. Basel: Birkhäuser Verlag, 1993:169–185.
6. Yeivin A, Razin A. Gene methylation patterns and expression. In: JP Jost, HP Haluz, eds. DNA Methylation: Molecular Biology and Biological Significance. Basel: Birkhäuser Verlag, 1993: 523–568.
7. Antequera F, Bird A. Number of CpG islands and genes in the human and mouse. Proc Natl Acad Sci USA 1993; 90:11995–11999.
8. Bestor T, Laudano A, Mattaliano R, Ingram V. Cloning and sequencing of a cDNA encoding DNA methyltransferase of mouse cells. J Mol Biol 1988; 203:971–983.
9. Adams RLP, Burdon RH. S-Adenosyl-L-methionine—donor of methyl groups. In: A Razin, H Cedar, AD Riggs, eds. Molecular Biology of DNA Methylation. New York: Springer-Verlag, 1985:31–41.
10. Stein WD. The epigenetic address: a model for embryological development. J Theor Biol 1980; 82:663–677.
11. Issa J-PJ, Ottaviano YL, Celano P, Hamilton SR, Davidson NE, Baylin SB. Methylation of the oestrogen receptor CpG island links ageing and neoplasia in human colon. Nat Genet 1994; 7:536–540.
12. Watanabe S, Kawai J, Hirotsune S, et al. Accessibility to tissue-specific genes from methylation profiles of mouse brain genomic DNA. Electrophoresis 1995; 16:218–226.
13. Schmid M, Haaf T, Grunert D. 5-Azacytidine-induced undercondensations in human chromosomes. Hum Genet 1984; 67:257–263.
14. Pogribny IP, Basnakian AG, Miller BJ, Lopatina NG, Poirier LA, James SJ. Breaks in genomic DNA and within the *p53* gene are associated with hypomethylation in livers of folate/methyl-deficient rats. Cancer Res 1995; 55:1894–1901.
15. Lengauer C, Kinzler KW, Vogelstein B. DNA methylation and genetic instability in colorectal cancer cells. Proc Natl Acad Sci USA 1997; 94:2545–2550.
16. Feinberg AP, Vogelstein B. Hypomethylation of *ras* oncogenes in primary human cancers. Biochem Biophys Res Commun 1983; 111:47–54.
17. Vachtenheim J, Horakova I, Novotna H. Hypomethylation of CCGG sites in the 3′ region of

H-ras protooncogene is frequent and is associated with H-ras allele loss in non-small cell lung cancer. Cancer Res 1994; 54:1145–1148.

18. Ottaviano YL, Issa J-PJ, Parl FF, Smith HS, Baylin SB, Davidson NE. Methylation of the estrogen receptor gene CpG island marks loss of estrogen receptor expression in human breast cancer cells. Cancer Res 1994; 54:2552–2555.

19. Millikin D, Meese E, Vogelstein B, Witkowski C, Trent J. Loss of heterozygosity for loci on the long arm of chromosome 6 in human malignant melanoma. Cancer Res 1991; 51:5449–5453.

20. Issa J-PJ, Zehnbauer BA, Civin CI et al. The estrogen receptor CpG island is methylated in most hematopoietic neoplasms. Cancer Res 1996; 56:973–977.

21. Belinsky SA, Nikula KJ, Baylin SB, Issa J-PJ. Increased cytosine DNA-methyltransferase activity is target-cell-specific and an early event in lung cancer. Proc Natl Acad Sci USA 1996; 93:4045–4050.

22. Lee PJ, Washer LL, Law DJ, Boland CR, Horon IL, Feinberg AP. Limited upregulation of DNA methyltransferase in human colon cancer reflecting increased cell proliferation. Proc Natl Acad Sci USA 1996; 93:10366–10370.

23. Yang J, Deng C, Hemati N, Hanash SM, Richardson BC. Effect of mitogenic stimulation and DNA methylation on human T-cell DNA methyltransferase expression and activity. J Immunol 1997; 159:1303–1309.

24. Gonzalgo ML, Liang G, Spruck III CH, Zingg J-M, Rideout III WM, Jones PA. Identification and characterization of differentially methylated regions of genomic DNA by methylation-sensitive arbitrarily primed PCR. 1997; 57:594–599.

25. Ushijima T, Morimura K, Hosoya Y, et al. Establishment of methylation-sensitive-representational difference analysis and isolation of hypo- and hypermethylated genomic fragments in mouse liver tumors. Proc Natl Acad Sci USA 1997; 94:2284–2289.

26. Triboli C, Tamanini F, Patrosso C, et al. Methylation and sequence analysis around Eagi sites: identification of 28 new CpG islands in XQ24—XQ28. Nucl Acids Res 1992; 20:727–733.

27. Hatada I, Hayashizaki Y, Hirotsune S, Komatsubara H. A genomic scanning method for higher organisms using restriction sites as landmarks. Proc Natl Acad Sci USA 1991; 88:9523–9527.

28. Asakawa J, Kuick R, Neel JV, Kodaira M, Satoh C, Hanash SM. Genetic variation detected by quantitative analysis of end-labeled genomic DNA fragments. Proc Natl Acad Sci USA 1994; 91:9052–9056.

29. Kuick R, Asakawa J, Neel JV, Satoh C, Hanash SM. High yield of restriction fragment length polymorphisms in two-dimensional separations of human genomic DNA. Genomics 1995; 25:345–353.

30. Larsen F, Gundersen G, Lopez R, Prydz H. CpG islands as gene markers in the human genome. Genomics 1992; 13:1095–1107.

31. Lindsay S, Bird AP. Use of restriction enzymes to detect potential gene sequences in mammalian DNA. Nature 1987; 327:336–338.

32. Thoraval D, Asakawa J, Kodaira M, et al. A methylated human 9 Kb repetitive sequence on acrocentric chromosomes is homologous to a subtelomeric repeat in chimpanzee. Proc Natl Acad Sci USA 1996; 93:4442–4447.

33. Otterson GA, Khleif SN, Chen W, Coxon AB, Kaye FJ. CDKN2 gene silencing in lung cancer by DNA hypermethylation and kinetics of p16INK4 protein induction by 5-aza 2′-deoxycytidine. Oncogene 1995; 11:1211–1216.

34. Herman JG, Jen J, Merlo A, Baylin SB. Hypermethylation-associated inactivation indicates a tumor suppressor role for $p15^{INK4B1}$. Cancer Res 1996; 56:722–727.

35. Baylin SB, Fearon ER, Vogelstein B, et al. Hypermethylation of the 5′ region of the calcitonin gene is a property of human lymphoid and acute myeloid malignancies. Blood 1987; 70:412–417.

36. Saitoh F, Hiraishi K, Adachi M, Hozumi M. Induction by 5-aza-2′-deoxycytidine, an inhibitor of DNA methylation, of Le^y-antigen, apoptosis and differentiation in human lung cancer cells. Anticancer Res 1995; 15:2137–2144.

37. Nagatake M, Osada H, Kondo M et al. Aberrant hypermethylation at the *bcl-2* locus at 18q21 in human lung cancers. Cancer Res 1996; 56:1886–1891.
38. Issa J-PJ, Baylin SB, Belinsky SA. Methylation of the estrogen receptor CpG island in lung tumors is related to the specific type of carcinogen exposure. Cancer Res 1996; 56:3655–3658.
39. Ganderton RH, Day IN, Briggs RS. Patterns of DNA methylation of the parathyroid hormone-related protein gene in human lung carcinoma. Eur J Cancer 1995; 31A:1697–1700.

14

Clinical Basis for Early Detection of Lung Cancer

KELL ØSTERLIND

Hillerød Sygehus
Hillerød, Denmark

FRED R. HIRSCH

Finsen Center, Rigshospitalet
Copenhagen, Denmark

I. Introduction

Lung cancer is today the leading cause of cancer death in both males and females in many countries. The incidence rates in males are slowly decreasing in some countries, reflecting the fact that the proportion of males who smoke has decreased from some 60 to some 40% (1,2), while the tendency in females is the opposite: more and more women smoke, predominantly those who have a job outside the home, and for them the incidence rates of lung cancer are increasing (3). Lung cancer is clearly the most preventable cancer in the Western world, as more than 85% of the cases occur in active tobacco smokers, an additional 3–5% are caused by passive smoke exposure, and up to 4% are caused by radon exposure. Annual mortality from tobacco including cardiovascular and other non-neoplastic diseases approaches three million deaths worldwide (4–7). This public health crisis is highly relevant to Europe as the European Union is the second largest producer of cigarettes after China (694 billion in 1993). Europe has the highest overall per capita consumption of manufactured cigarettes, as 42% of men and 28% of women are smoking, numbers which are worsening in younger age groups (8). Antitobacco campaigns seem to have little effect on adult smokers, and no means are yet available to effectively prevent teenagers—especially girls—from starting to smoke. Although much more must be done to reduce tobacco smoking, we have to face the fact that lung cancer will remain a major clinical problem for many years ahead.

The problem with lung cancer could briefly be characterized as too high incidence rates and much too high mortality rates. The high mortality rate (more than 85%) reflects the failure of systemic treatment as well as lack of effective early detection measures. In Denmark the overall 5-year survival rate is about 5%, with no significant improvement over the last 40 years (3). Introduction of chemotherapy seems to have improved 1- and 2-year survival rates for patients with small-cell lung cancer, but less than 5% of patients with small-cell lung cancer become 5-year survivors (9). In other Scandinavian countries such as Norway and Sweden, however, the 5-year survival rates have improved to about 10% (10), and a comparative analysis performed by the cancer registries in the three countries has disclosed that a larger proportion of patients in Norway and Sweden compared to Denmark have an operable stage of disease when the lung cancer is diagnosed (11). The prognostic role of clinical/pathological stage of disease at time of diagnosis is well documented for patients with lung cancer. For patients with non–small-cell lung cancer (NSCLC), the TNM staging system is generally used and is documented to give a good prognostic information. More than 90% of patients with small-cell lung cancer (SCLC) have stage III (locally advanced) or stage IV (systemic) disease at time of primary diagnosis. Thus, it is not practical to apply the TNM system to this disease. Instead patients with SCLC are generally staged according to a simple two-stage system developed by the Veterans Administration Lung Cancer Study Group. This system classifies patients as having limited disease when the tumor is confined to one hemithorax and its regional lymph nodes (including mediastinal, contralateral supraclavicular- and contralateral hilar lymph nodes) or extensive disease. The prognostic difference between limited and extensive disease is well documented (12). It is a clear goal that early diagnosis of lung cancer should result in more stage I patients and thus significant reductions of the mortality rate.

Primary prevention measures for lung cancer are dominated by efforts to decrease tobacco smoking. The International Association for the Study of Lung Cancer (IASLC) endorsed a 10-point policy statement on tobacco at the VII World Conference on Lung Cancer in Colorado Springs in 1994, including strong positions on a number of issues including tobacco taxation, public education, and advertising (13). This declaration was followed up by IASLC workshops, most recently in Elsinore, Denmark, in 1996 (14).

Secondary prevention strategies are directed at interrupting the natural history of lung cancer prior to the development of symptomatic disease. Secondary prevention measures include the use of early detection, chemoprevention, and tracking of micronutrients in the diet. Secondary prevention strategies are very important, as a growing percentage of new lung cancer cases are being discovered in former smokers (7). Screening for lung cancer has been discussed for many years. Previous screening trials included annual chest x-rays, quarterly sputum cytology examinations, and sputum occult blood testing plus serum markers. None of these procedures resulted in decreased lung cancer mortality. Controversy regarding the design and power of previous studies has prompted new randomized studies, of which a few are in progress.

Within the last decade there has been an explosion in the knowledge of the biology, molecular biology techniques, and genetics of lung cancer. Increased knowledge regarding the nature of preneoplastic and early neoplastic lesions has opened new possibilities for early detection of lung cancer. Clinical aspects of early diagnosis in lung cancer will be discussed in this chapter.

II. Early Detection/Screening of Lung Cancer

A. Chest X-Rays

For many years and through various improvements in the technique, the chest x-ray (CXR) has been the initial diagnostic tool for detecting lung cancer. More sensitive imaging methods have been hampered by inavailability, inacceptability, and insufficient skills, and the CXR is likely to remain on the front line for many years in the future. CXR fulfills many of the test characteristics required for screening. It is widely available, relatively inexpensive, acceptable to patients, and without significant radiation exposure or other morbidity. However, other attributes remain in question, namely, specificity, sensitivity, and predictive value.

The sensitivity of the CXR in lung cancer detection is variably estimated from as high as 85% to as low as 16%, depending on whether the calculation is based on prevalence data (15), longitudinal incidence data (16,17), or mathematical modeling (18). In their evaluation of a large retrospective database (about 300,000 subjects), Soda et al. (17) found an overall sensitivity of 70%. The figures varied depending on tumor histology (adenocarcinoma 85%, squamous cell carcinoma 52%, large-cell carcinoma 75%).

During the 1960s uncontrolled trials suggested that annual CXR and/or quarterly sputum cytologic examinations might be useful as screening and as early detection strategy to reduce lung cancer mortality. Four randomized studies have been conducted (19–22). The National Cancer Institute (NCI) supported three prospective randomized trials to examine the role of these screening modalities in reducing lung cancer mortality. Each of the studies included about 10,000 men, 45 years or older, with a history of heavy tobacco smoking (21,23,24). The design plus some essential data of the three NCI-supported studies (plus a Czechoslovak study) (22) are shown in Table 1.

Two of the trials, Memorial Sloan-Kettering Cancer Center (MSKCC) and John Hopkins, randomized patients to receive annual CXR (control group) versus annual CXR plus sputum cytology examination every 4 months (screened group) for 6 years. In the Mayo study, the control group received no screening examinations, but an annual CXR and sputum analysis was their standard recommendation, while the screened group received both screening procedures for 6 years. At the start of all three studies, all patients were screened with both CXR and sputum cytologic examination.

Table 1 Four Prospective Randomized Trials on Screening for Lung Cancer in Males 45 Years or Older, Smoking 20+ Cigarettes a Day

Trial	Period	Screening (yr)	Follow-up (yr)	Group	No. of persons	Prevalence cases	Incidence cases	5-year survival (%)	Mortality rate[a]
MSKLP	1974–84	5–8	2–5	Experimental	5072	30	114	35	2.7
				Control	4968	23	121	35	2.7
JHLP	1973–84	5–8	2–5	Experimental	5226	39	155	20	3.4
				Control	5161	40	162	20	3.8
MLP	1971–83	6	1–5	Initial	10933	91			
				Experimental	4618		206	40	3.2
				Control	4593		160	15	3.0
Czechoslovak trial[b]	1976–80	3	5	Initial	6364	18			
				Experimental	3172		39	23	3.6
				Control	3174		27	19	2.6

[a]Deaths per 1000 persons per year.
[b]Subjects were 40–64 years of age.
MSKLP: Memorial Sloan-Kettering Lung Project; JHLP: Johns Hopkins Lung Project; MLP: Mayo Lung Project.

Table 1 includes figures on prevalence cases at initial examination as well as incidence cases. Chest x-rays detected more cases than sputum cytology. The fraction of resectable cases and the 5-year survival rates were higher than expected from historical series. In the incidence phase of the Mayo study, the percentage of patients resected and the 5-year survival rate were higher in the screened group compared to the control group, while resection rates and 5-year survival were identical in the screened and the control groups in both the Hopkins and MSKCC series. In none of the studies was a decreased lung cancer mortality rate observed. Consequently, the American Cancer Society, NCI, and other organizations resolved that large-scale radiologic and cytologic screening for lung cancer could not be justified (25).

Reexamination of these studies (18,21,26–28) has, however, uncovered many problems. In addition, improvements have been made in the technology associated with both chest x-rays and sputum cytologic examination. To readdress the efficacy of annual chest x-ray screening, NCI has instituted a new randomized trial termed the PLCO Screening Trial (29). The PLCO study stands for prostate, lung, colorectal, and ovarian cancer screening. The lung cancer screening is an annual chest x-ray in this ongoing trial. A fourth, Czechoslovak, study comparing regular and frequent rescreening CXRs in an experimental group, with sporadic or infrequent rescreening in a control group showed, like the Mayo study, advantage for screening with respect to stage distribution, resectability, and survival (22).

It can be concluded from the four randomized studies that periodic CXRs lead to clinically meaningful improvements in stage distribution, resectability, and survival. Mortality reductions, however, have not been demonstrated. Mortality is the number of deaths due to the disease. Mortality rate and incidence rates are highly correlated to each other, in contrast to overall survival. Survival is a function of age, sex, race, social status, cancer histology, location, stage, and treatment. Cancer survival can be influenced by improvement in treatment, and early diagnosis and screening trials that use survival as endpoint are subject to bias, while mortality is not. This problem has been discussed and analyzed by Strauss et al. (28).

B. Sputum Cytology

The other tool in screening for early detection of lung cancer is sputum evaluation. This technique using cytologic examination of induced or 3-day pooled collections of spontaneously produced material was intensively studied in the NCI-sponsored trials and was found to be most sensitive and specific for squamous cell carcinoma. The sensitivity fell off considerably, however, when applied to all histologic types.

The three NCI-sponsored screening studies described above were based on the early studies of Saccomanno and coworkers, which showed that exfoliated cells in sputum samples could be fixed, processed, stained, and examined morphologically under the light microscope (30,31). Serial sputum analyses showed that before developing cancer, patients often showed progressive atypia. However, only about 10% of all cancers in the three NCI studies were detected by sputum cytology alone, and these studies clearly showed no benefit of routine cytologic examination in reducing lung cancer mortality. Several approaches have been taken to improve the results of sputum examination, including:

Selection of high-risk individuals
Use of computer-assisted morphologic measurements
Use of phenotypic markers
Use of genetic markers

Using immunocytochemistry, a study was done based on archival sputum specimens derived from a completed Johns Hopkins clinical trial where eventual lung cancer status was known. In a prospective, blinded analysis, two immunocytochemical markers showed a 90% accuracy in determining who would or would not go on to cancer (32).

The same Johns Hopkins archival material was used again to show that in morphologically normal sputum specimens, mutations of *ras* and *p53* genes could be detected up to one year before the clinical diagnosis of lung cancer (33).

III. Newer Clinical Methods

A. Computerized Technologies

Computerized tomography (CT scan) is more expensive than conventional chest x-rays and is less well tolerated by some persons, e.g., due to claustrophobia. The predictive value, specificity, and sensitivity have only been investigated in a few, small clinical series. High sensitivity in detection of any pulmonary lesion combined with insufficient specificity in differing between cancer and benign lesions weakens the applicability of the method in larger-scale screening programs.

Computerization can also be combined with fluorescence bronchoscopy, a new technique for search of early lung cancer developed by Lam et al. (34). The method exploits altered fluorescence patterns of neoplastic transformed bronchial mucosa, invisible to the human eye but easily depicted in a contrasting color on a monitor by the computer. The procedure opens interesting possibilities for detection of preinvasive lung cancer.

B. Bronchioloalveolar Lavage

Early diagnosis of lung cancer requires sampling from the bronchial epithelium. Bronchial cells could be obtained from sputum but negative sampling is too frequent by this method. Harvesting yield is improved considerably by bronchiolo alveolar lavage (BAL). BAL at fiberbronchoscopy could be combined with brush and forceps biopsy plus fluorescence bronchoscopy, if this apparatus is available. Blood samples enable genetic analyses of the host genome, and based on a standard questionnaire important data could be obtained about exposure, lifestyle, previous cancer, and cancer plus inherited diseases in the family.

Harvested bronchial cells should be examined for general genetic damage as well as for specific markers on the pathway of cancer. Both should be investigated, and material should be kept in a tissue bank for later analysis.

Fiberoptic bronchoscopy might be difficult in a mass screening program but is essential for follow-up in persons who prove positive at BAL. Bronchial biopsies could be carried out randomly and/or guided by macroscopic findings plus suspect fluorescent lesions, if the technique is available. If the theory of in-field cancerization holds, BAL as well as random biopsies are reasonable procedures, which have the advantage that they can be standardized. Yield of BAL depends much on training of the staff, and it would be advantageous if the procedure could be supported by technical means before it is introduced in large-scale screening trials.

C. DNA Analysis Microchip

The DNA analysis microchip is a small device, built on principles from computer processor chip architecture. The chip contains a biological multitest system processing 25 or more tests at one passage of a minute specimen through the chip, and the technology may therefore revise our current concepts about population-based screening (35,36). The biochip technology is new and still in development, but it can already probe large numbers of clinical specimens for multiple biomarkers without expensive instrumentation. The biomedical engineers developing this technique need cooperation of clinical collaborators to provide advice on how best to use this potent technology. Using state-of-art molecular diagnostic techniques, it is possible to analyze simple sputum, bronchial lavage, or bronchial biopsy specimens with many different probes (37).

D. Data Management

Data derives from many sources such as forms filled in by the examined person themselves or by professional interviewers, objective findings at sputum cytology or BAL, bronchoscopy, histomorphology, general biochemical tests, and investigative marker analyses. Computers and modern information transfer technology will be of major help, but it does not diminish the need for a well-planned database, a data center staffed to manage data capture and validation, a data steering group, and a data-monitoring committee.

IV. Methodologic Aspects

Preliminary studies with various cytologic or molecular markers are encouraging, prompting new large-scale screening trials to be initiated soon, but many fundamental methodological issues have to be addressed before population-based early cancer-detection programs can be established.

A. Target Population

The general lifetime probabilities of developing lung cancer in Denmark are 7.5% in males and 3% in females (3,38). Highest incidence rates are observed in persons 70–84 years of age, where they are 0.46% per year in males and 0.19% in females compared to 0.06% and 0.05% per year in males and females, respectively, aged 50–54 years (Fig. 1) (38). Defining target populations with a higher risk of developing lung cancer improves the prospect of success and reduces the cost of population-based screening approaches.

Smokers with chronic obstructive lung disease have a greater than 3 time incidence of lung cancer compared to smokers without chronic obstructive lung disease (39). A family history of lung cancer in a person who smokes also increases the risk of developing lung cancer (40,41). Inclusion of high-risk populations in trials on early diagnosis enable reduction of study size and duration, but with our current knowledge about risk factors we can only increase the a priori incidence rate 10 times compared to that of the general population, by which a clinical validation trial still requires a considerable size to be statistically valid (42).

B. Diagnostic Tests

Many new sensitive methods are now available, and although clinical data for these tests are still scarce, it seems to be increasingly important to establish a clinical basis for future screening examinations. Outcome of the big NCI trials conducted in

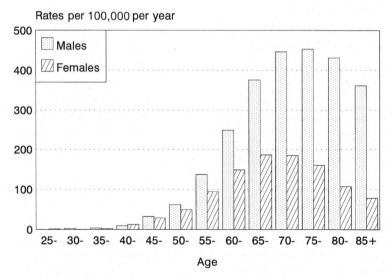

Figure 1   Age-specific incidence rates of lung cancer in Denmark, 1993.

the 1970s was disappointing, but reexamination of data has resulted in useful experience. Flehinger et al. (18) thus reanalyzed data from the Mayo Lung Cancer Project and established a mathematical simulation model for prediction of changes in mortality obtained by screening—for different values of diagnostic sensitivity, prevalence in the selected high-risk group, mean duration of early stage disease, and curability. From this simulation study it was concluded that screening based on chest radiographs and sputum examinations, as in the Mayo trial, would have a less than 20% probability of showing significant benefit, and that vastly improved methods of detection and treatment are required before mortality from lung cancer can be reduced by more than 50%.

A difficult point in the establishment of simulation models is to derive predictive test rates from the corresponding nosological rates. The nosological sensitivity and specificity are typically obtained in clinical series testing patients with newly diagnosed lung cancer and controls, which could be healthy persons or patients with nonmalignant pulmonary disease, enabling calculation of the probability of a positive test, given cancer—P(T|D) (sensitivity)—and the probability of a negative test, given no cancer (specificity)—P(nT|nD). The relevant predictive or diagnostic sensitivity and specificity can then be calculated if prevalence rates can be estimated in the population supposed to be included in the screening trial when it is first screened (the prevalence screening) and when it undergoes subsequent incidence screenings. The probability that a person has the disease given a positive test follows from Bayes theorem:

$$P(D|T) = P(T|D)/P(D)$$

in which P (D) is the likelihood of lung cancer in the risk group, i.e., the *prevalence*. Positive and negative predictive values and true and false-positive diagnostic rates may thus be calculated for individual tests, and a priori requirements for sensitivity and specificity could be set for inclusion of a test in a screening trial. To reduce the number of false-positive findings, the prevalence should be sufficiently high. In order to optimize yield of a screening program it may be necessary to be rather selective in the definition of risk group, and persons who are too young (45–55 years) or with too modest a tobacco consumption (less than 20 cigarettes a day) should probably not be included, albeit many in this marginal category may wish to be tested.

A promising new test might have both nosological sensitivity and specificity of 90%, which seems rather good. As an example, this test is supposed to be used for screening of 10,000 high-risk persons defined as persons with an incidence rate of 2% per year, which is five times higher than that occurring in Danish males 65–70 years of age (Fig. 1). The test is supposed to be positive up to 12 months before cancer usually is diagnosed. True positive tests will then be observed in 180 persons (Table 2), but as an unwanted result of the test 980 persons will erroneously be suspected of having cancer. The example illustrates that tests for early cancer leave us with major logistic as well as ethical problems.

Table 2   Outcome of Screening 10,000 High-Risk
Persons[a] Having an Average 2% Yearly Incidence
Rate of Lung Cancer Using a Test with 90%
Sensitivity and 90% Specificity

	Cancer	No cancer	
Positive test	180	980	1,160
Negative test	20	8,820	8,840
Total	200	9,800	10,000

[a]It was assumed that test was positive 12 months (mean)
before usual diagnostic threshold.

C. Lead Time

A diagnosis of cancer is based on certain histomorphological features, and cancer
treatment can currently not be instituted before these criteria are fulfilled. The time
from disclosure of abnormality of an early cancer test to cancer is proven is a black
box. When will the cancer develop? Will it develop at all? Could spontaneous nor-
malization of the test occur? Lead time is very problematic from a methodological
point of view—as for those individuals who host the changes. For example, Tockman et al. (32) investigated two monoclonal antibodies against small-cell and non–
small-cell lung cancer cells, respectively. Sixty-nine sputum specimen samples were
randomly selected from the John Hopkins Lung Project pathological archive. Neoplastic antigens were detected in 14 of 26 persons who later had lung cancer diagnosed, which—after exclusion of four unsatisfactory samples—gave a specificity of
64%. Some of the false-negative specimens were very early, however, sampled in
average 40 months before cancer was diagnosed compared to an average of 24
months in the true positive. Later specimens were available, sampled an average of
26 months before the cancer, and now six of the eight had become positive, improving sensitivity to 91%.

Lead time is a challenge for any clinical program of early cancer detection.
There seems to be an urgent need for threshold standards for calculation of sensitivity and specificity, e.g., 2 years from the test proved positive. But how should those
cases be handled that do not pass the threshold because they die or because the test
reverts to normal? It is evident that lead time must be integrated in mathematical and
statistical models for design and interpretation of multitest screening trials. Finally,
the ethical aspects of telling healthy people that they may hide an early cancer
should be thoroughly thought through.

D. Endpoints

The purpose of early detection of lung cancer is to increase the proportion of
patients who are operable and thereby to reduce mortality rates in the long term.
Stage at diagnosis and resectability rates may serve as surrogate effect vari-

ables in screening trials, but 5-year survival rate is by far the most reliable endpoint.

Other endpoints or response variables are necessary in studies of clinical applicability of new, early diagnostic tests. In clinical series it will be natural to relate the test result to subsequent diagnostic workup, with calculation of sensitivity and specificity as the goal. In larger cohort studies, where a group of high-risk persons are repeatedly screened with a number of tests, it will be possible to clarify predictive accuracy and lead time, i.e., time from positive test to overt cancer, supposing that a proportion of first-time test-positive persons will not have detectable disease. It should be investigated if lead time differs with subsequent histomorphological subtype—is lead time shorter for small-cell carcinomas, for example? A positive test may prove negative at next screening, and—precluding inappropriate sampling—investigations of factors related to reversion should be carried out. Could it be related to smoking cessation or to reduction in other lung cancer risk factors? Cohort trials could include intervention such as intensive "quit smoking" training or treatment (vitamins, gene therapy), if early changes are proven. Relevant outcome variables would then be "reversion to normal" of abnormal tests and (reduced) incidence of subsequent cancer.

E. Design

Statistical models will be a prerequisite in all future screening trials. Once procedures have been selected, all investigative variables should be clarified and endpoints defined, followed by choice of an appropriate trial design, including dimensioning based on statistical considerations.

The required number of trial subjects should be realistic in relation to the available test population, and exclusion criteria should be considered, such as medical indications against fiber bronchoscopy, if this procedure is included in the screening program.

Number and intervals between examinations must be defined as well as estimated duration of intake and follow-up. Ten to 20 years may be necessary to obtain reliable mortality rates. Duration of the trial should be long enough to enable development of cancer from early or premalignant changes. Screening trials should be randomized in order to assess the influence of screening on the mortality of the disease. Impact of contamination due to smoking cessation in screened persons, prompted by the intervention, should be minimized and the possible influence of this type of bias should be included in dimensioning calculations together with other risk factors, which might change during a study period of 10–20 years.

Large, randomized screening trials will run for several years, and new tests, which are not yet prepared for inclusion in large screening trials, may in the meantime become interesting, but must wait or, hopefully, be added to the current panel of tests, if that can be done without deleterious methodological consequences for the trial. It should be possible to simulate this situation in computer models, and guidelines based on such models should be included in protocols for future large-scale screening trials.

In general, it is important to establish a robust setting for clinical research, combining accurate, reproducible, and efficient assays. Furthermore, in the current cost-sensitive environment economical considerations are required. Chest radiography will certainly remain a key procedure, and in choosing other tests, features such as price, acceptability for test subjects, radiation exposure, or other impacts on health must be considered.

F. Multimarker Strategy

None of the currently investigated markers has the sensitivity and specificity to be *the test* of early diagnosis of lung cancer. There are many to choose among but the choice is difficult, because the markers correspond to a variety of cytogenetic defects—general as well as specific—on which data on phenotypic effects and interactions with normal gene function are incomplete and because nosologic sensitivity of early diagnostic tests based on the markers rarely exceeds 60–70%, with wide confidence intervals because the data derives from small clinical series. Confidence limits for a sensitivity of 70% based on a series of 100 patients is thus 60–79% (Table 3). Specificity should be close to 100%, which it normally is not, in order to

Table 3 Confidence Limits (95%)
for Sensitivities Ranging from 60 to 98%
of a Diagnostic Test

Sensitivity (%)	N	CI (%)	δ^a (%)
98	50	89–100	6
	100	93–100	4
	500	96–99	2
90	50	78–97	9
	100	82–95	7
	500	87–92	3
80	50	66–90	12
	100	71–87	8
	500	76–83	4
70	50	55–82	14
	100	60–79	10
	500	66–74	4
60	50	45–74	15
	100	50–70	10
	500	56–64	4

[a]One-half of range of confidence interval for each sensitivity.

reduce the "false-positive" problem in large-scale screening trials. In general, most new early diagnostic tests are still in an investigative phase and selection of a definitive panel for screening in large randomized trials is still too early. More must be known about the predictive accuracy, which can be achieved with multiple tests performed in parallel, and the most appropriate strategy at the moment is probably to carry out restricted trials in cohorts with especially high risk of lung cancer.

With a methodology similar to that applied in epidemiology and in prognostic factor studies, a panel of variables could be related to a dependent outcome variable, which could be the likelihood of a present and/or an incipient cancer. In the latter case the model might give an estimate of when overt cancer could be expected. The statistical model could be a semiparametric or a clustering model, both assigning a certain probability figure to the observed pattern of abnormal tests. The level of probability will indicate whether or not diagnostic procedures should be initiated. Technologically new procedures may improve chances to detect early cancer, still defined by histomorphological criteria, and marker test probabilities would then need adjustment.

Statistical clustering models organize tests hierarchically in a treelike structure, where positive and negative test values lead to alternative branches, finally ending in discrete probability categories. Whether clustering methods, semiparametric or other types of statistical models are applied, it will always be problematic to define a risk level below which diagnostic workup can be omitted. And should the likelihood of overt cancer be close to 100%, it is still necessary to localize it and to obtain specimens for histopathological typing. If standard diagnostic procedures do not prove cancer, future policy for the individual person could be related to the likelihood that he or she has cancer. Should new but expensive procedures such as fluorescence endoscopy or PET scan be applied, or would it be sufficient to repeat the screening program earlier than otherwise scheduled? In the interesting work with such predictive mathematical models it is urgent not to forget ethics and empathy with the study persons, and strategies should be established as to how to handle fear and anxiety in those who test positive but do not have cancer.

V. Do We Have Optimal Markers for Early Detection?

Better methods for early detection of lung cancer are fundamental to a paradigm shift allowing routine management of true early (premetastatic) lung cancer. Long-standing evidence suggests that invasive lung cancer is the end of a multistep process (30), in which progressive molecular changes accompany or even precede morphological changes (43). Due to exquisite specificity or selectivity, biomarkers may be a suitable tool to phenotype a premalignant stage of cancer. However, greater knowledge of the genetic etiology would facilitate the selection of genetic markers most appropriate for evaluation in clinical management of early cancer. With smoking, the entire bronchial epithelium is the target of carcinogens as conveyed in the concept of field cancerization (44,45). However, the steps in the clonal progression of the cancer between the pre- and postinvasion are not yet defined, and issues such as whether a random biopsy in a high-risk individual could yield information about the status of the rest of the organ epithelium need to be systematically evaluated in clinical studies.

Today, the following types of specimens are available for testing biomarkers: bronchial biopsies and brushings (obtained with or without fluorescence bronchoscopy), sputum, and BAL. Further technological development is required for new assays to get meaningful clinical information easily on a few cells such as exfoliated bronchial cells in a sputum specimen. How many cells may be enough to be representative for an abnormal clonal population in the cancerization field is currently being evaluated in ongoing clinical trials.

An emerging area of diagnostic pathology is the development of *risk-assessment markers*, since these tools may be used to identify patients at higher risk of cancer. Risk-assessment research frequently complements early-detection studies by identifying populations at high risk for developing malignant disease, and thus suitable as cohorts for early cancer screening trials. Biological considerations can be used in selecting markers for clinical applications (46).

As summarized elsewhere (14), potential markers for progression of initial clones can be classified into or according to (1) morphological changes, (2) immunocytochemical markers for differentially expressed proteins, (3) markers for genomic instability, (4) markers for epigenetic change (abnormal methylation), and (5) gene mutations. Other classifications are possible, e.g., into two types according to specificity for tumor progression. Generalized markers reflect genetic damage, which may be exclusively a pathway to cancer. The other type are characterized as specific markers, identifying genetic abnormalities definitely on an irreversible development to cancer (e.g., oncogene activation and inactivation of identified tumor suppressor genes).

Our knowledge about the chronology of these different genetic events is incomplete: 3p and 9p loss of heterogenecity (LOH) as well as aneuploidy can be considered as early markers for initiation and promotion, while mutations of *ras* oncogene or *p53* as well as the retinoblastoma gene (Rb) currently are regarded by some as late molecular abnormalities, predictive of progression and invasion (14). These hypotheses, however, need to be evaluated in larger clinical trials. In a recent IASLC workshop, criteria were defined for clinical application of new markers (Table 4).

Data on a priori diagnostic usefulness of individual tests for an investigative screening trial are scarce, and the predictive power of various combinations of positive markers has not yet been investigated, so selection of tests for a screening panel must be largely empiric, albeit selected to combine early and late markers, tests of cytogenetic as well as phenotypic abnormalities, and tests based on different methodologies.

Table 4 Considerations in Validating Prevention Markers

1. Clear definition of the particular clinical application (early diagnosis, progression marker, metastatic marker).
2. The following criteria should be fulfilled: the marker must be expressed by a large proportion of clinical specimens from individuals who eventually develop lung cancer (retrospective study on archived material); the marker must allow stratification of individuals by clinical risk; the marker must be expressed at high enough levels to allow detection, detectable in small samples by technologically feasible methods (i.e., the assay should have low cost and high throughput capacity).
3. Prospective clinical trials to rigorously define the performance characteristics of the new marker imply that comprehensive databases (clinical, epidemiological, genetic susceptibility) should be included in the trial design.

Source: Ref. 14.

VI. Concluding Remarks

Throughout the 1960s and 1970s many controlled and uncontrolled studies were performed in order to detect early lung cancer, with the goal of reducing the mortality of this disease. Most studies on chest x-ray with or without sputum cytology proved that screening resulted in an increased number of resectable patients and a positive influence on survival. However, none of the studies demonstrated significant reduction in lung cancer mortality. A number of publications, however, have addressed the methodological problems in many of these studies.

Within the last decade there has been an explosion in knowledge about biology, molecular biology techniques, and genetics. Increasing understanding of the nature of preneoplastic and early neoplastic lesions opens new possibilities for early detection of lung cancer. However, despite the fact that preliminary studies with various cytologic or molecular markers are encouraging, many fundamental methodological issues have to be addressed before population-based screening programs can be established. Further technological development is required, including new assays for samples of few exfoliated cells, disclosing possible abnormal clonal development of in-field cancerization.

Another important question is how to manage high-risk individuals and persons with signs of early malignant transformation. Chemoprevention is an option, but much more clinical research on this issue is required. Large, prospective randomized trials are necessary to prove if screening and intervention result in reduced mortality. This definitive endpoint requires very long follow-up, however, so it is important to identify and to validate other intermediate endpoints. Several biomarker tests could be potential candidates. Much has to be done, yet, in clinical validation of these tests. Studies hitherto seem promising, and many more, larger investigations certainly will be carried out in the next decade.

References

1. Todd G. Medicine—Statistics of Smoking in the Member States of the European Community. Luxembourg: Commission of the European Communities, 1986.
2. Harkin AM, Anderson P, Goos C. Smoking, Drinking and Drug Taking in the European Region. Copenhagen: World Health Organization, 1997.
3. Hirsch FR, Olsen JH, Carstensen B. Lung cancer in Denmark, 1943–1987. Incidence and survival. In: Hirsch FR, ed. Lung Cancer: Status and Future Perspectives. Copenhagen: Bristol-Myers Squibb, 1993:9–31.
4. Peto R, Lopez AD, Boreham J, et al. Mortality from tobacco in developed countries: indirect estimation from national vital statistics. Lancet 1992; 339:1268.
5. Samet JH, Nero AV. Indoor radon and lung cancer. N Engl J Med 1989; 320:591–594.
6. Janerich DT, Thompson WD, Vareta LR, et al. Lung cancer and exposure to tobacco smoke in the household. N Engl J Med 1990; 323:632–636.
7. Strauss GM, De Camp M, Dibbicaro E, et al. Lung cancer diagnosis is being made with increasing frequency in former cigarette smokers (abstr). Proc ASCO 1995; 14:362.
8. Boyle P, Maisonneuve P. Lung cancer and tobacco smoking. Lung Cancer 1995; 12:167–181.
9. Lassen U, Østerlind K, Hansen M, Dombernowsky P, Bergman B, Hansen HH. Long-term survival in small-cell lung cancer. J Clin Oncol 1995; 13:1215–1220.
10. Engeland A, Haldorsen T, Tretli S, Hakulinen T, Hørte LG, Luostarinen T, et al. Prediction of cancer mortality in the Nordic countries up to the years 2000 and 2010. APMIS 1995; 103:s66–s71.
11. Storm HH. Differences in Lung Cancer Mortality Between the Nordic Countries. 1997.
12. Østerlind K. Staging of lung cancer. In: Hirsch FR, ed. Lung Cancer: Status and Future Perspectives. Copenhagen: Bristol-Myers Squibb, 1993:41–47.
13. Tobacco policy recommendations of the International Association for the Study of Lung Cancer (IASLC): a ten point program. Lung Cancer 1994; 11:405–407.
14. Hirsch FR, Brambilla E, Gray N, Gritz E, Kelloff GJ, Linnoila RI, et al. Prevention and early detection of lung cancer—clinical aspects. Lung Cancer 1997; 17:163–174.
15. Brett GZ. Earlier diagnosis and survival in lung cancer. Br Med J 1969; 4:260–262.
16. Marfin AA, Schenker M. Screening for lung cancer: effective tests awaiting effective treatment. Occup Med State Art Rev 1991; 6:111–131.
17. Soda H, Tomita H, Kohno S, et al. Limitation of annual screening chest radiography for the diagnosis of lung cancer. Cancer 1993; 72:2341–2346.
18. Flehinger BJ, Kimmel M, Polyak T, Melamed MR. Screening for lung cancer. Cancer 1993; 72:1573–1580.
19. Frost JK, Ball WC, Levin ML, Tockman MS, Baker RR, Carter D, et al. Early lung cancer detection: results of the initial (prevalence) radiologic and cytologic screening in the Johns Hopkins study. Am Rev Respir Dis 1984; 130:549–554.
20. Flehinger BJ, Melamed MR, Zaman MB, Heelan RT, Perchick WB, Martini N. Early lung cancer detection: results of the initial (prevalence) radiologic and cytologic screening in the Memorial Sloan-Kettering study. Am Rev Respir Dis 1984; 130:555–560.
21. Fontana RS, Sanderson DR, Woolner LB, Taylor WF, Miller WE, Muhm JR, et al. Screening for lung cancer. A critique of the Mayo Lung Project. Cancer 1991; 67:1155–1164.
22. Kubik A, Polak J. Lung cancer detection. Results of a randomized prospective study in Czechoslovakia. Cancer 1986; 57:2427–2437.
23. Tockman MS. Survival and mortality from lung cancer in a screened population. The Johns Hopkins study. Chest 1986; 89 (suppl.):324–325.
24. Melamed MR, Flehinger BJ. Screening for lung cancer. Chest 1984; 86:2–3.
25. Eddy DH. Screening for lung cancer. Ann Intern Med 1989; 111:232–237.
26. Flehinger BJ, Kimmel M, Melamed MR. The effect of surgical treatment on survival from early lung cancer. Implications for screening. Chest 1992; 101:1013–1018.
27. Bunn PA, Kelly K, Cook R, Proudfoot S, Kennedy T. Prevention and early detection of lung

cancer. In: Hirsch FR, ed. Lung Cancer. Prevention, Diagnosis and Treatment. Copenhagen: Bristol-Myers Squibb, 1995:31–54.

28. Strauss GM, Gleason RE, Sugarbaker DJ. Screening for lung cancer. Another look; a different view. Chest 1997; 111:754–768.

29. Kramer BS, Gohagan J, Prorok PC, Smart CR. A National Cancer Institute sponsored screening trial for prostatic, lung, colorectal, and ovarian cancers. Cancer 1993; 71:589–593.

30. Saccomanno G, Archer VE, Auerbach O, et al. Cancer of the lung: the cytology of sputum prior to the development of carcinoma. Acta Cytol 1965; 9:413–423.

31. Saccomanno G, Archer VE, Auerbach O, et al. Development of carcinoma of the lung as reflected in exfoliated cells. Cancer 1974; 33:256–270.

32. Tockman MS, Gupta PK, Myers JD, Frost JK, Baylin SB, Gold EB, et al. Sensitive and specific monoclonal antibody recognition of human lung cancer antigen on preserved sputum cells: a new approach to early lung cancer detection. J Clin Oncol 1988; 6:1685–1693.

33. Mao L, Hruban RH, Boyle J, et al. Detection of oncogene mutation in sputum precedes the diagnosis of lung cancer. Cancer Res 1994; 54:1634–1637.

34. Lam S, MacAulay C, Hung J, LeRiche J, Profio AE, Palcic B. Detection of dysplasia and carcinoma in situ with a lung imaging fluorescence endoscope device. J Thorac Cardiovasc Surg 1993; 105:1035–1040.

35. Eggers M, Hogan M, Reich RK, et al. A microchip for quantitative detection of molecules utilizing luminescent and radioisotope reporter groups. Bio Techniques 1994; 17:515–524.

36. Lamture JB, Beattie KL, Burke BE, et al. Direct detection of nucleic acid hybridization on the surface of charged couple devise. Nucleic Acid Res 1994; 22:2121–2125.

37. Martinez A, Miller MJ, Quinn K, et al. Non-radioactive localization of nucleic acids by direct in situ PCR and in situ RT-PCR in paraffin-embedded sections. J Histochem Cytochem 1995; 43:739–747.

38. Storm HH, Pihl J, Michelsen E, Nielsen AL. Cancer incidence in Denmark 1993. Copenhagen: Danish Cancer Society, 1996.

39. Tockman MS, Antonisen N, Wright E, et al. The intermittent positive pressure breathing trial group and the John Hopkins Lung Project for the early detection of lung cancer: airway obstruction and the risk for lung cancer. Ann Intern Med 1987; 106:512–518.

40. Ambrosone C, Rao U, Michalek A, et al. Lung cancer histologic types and family history of cancer. Analysis of histological subtypes of 872 patients with primary lung cancer. Cancer 1993; 72:1192–1198.

41. Sellers T, Bailey-Wilson J, Elston R, et al. Evidence of mendelian inheritance in the pathogenesis of lung cancer. J Natl Cancer Inst 1990; 82:1272–1279.

42. Mulshine JL, Scott F, Zhou J, et al. Development of molecular approaches to early lung cancer detection. Sem Rad Oncol 1996; 6:72–75.

43. Yakubovskaya MS, Spiegelman V, Luo FC, et al. High frequency of K-ras mutations in normal appearing lung tissue and sputum of patients with lung cancer. Int J Cancer 1995; 63:810.

44. Slaughter DP, Southwick HW, Smejkal W. Field cancerization in oral stratified squamous epithelium. Cancer 1953; 6:963–968.

45. Auerbach O, Gere JB, Forman JB, et al. Changes in the bronchial epithelium in relation to smoking and cancer of the lung. N Engl J Med 1957; 256:97.

46. Harris CC, Hollstein M. Clinical implication of the p53 tumor-suppressor gene. N Engl J Med 1993; 329:1318.

15

Genetic Instability Assessments in the Lung Cancerization Field

WALTER N. HITTELMAN

University of Texas M.D. Anderson Cancer Center
Houston, Texas

I. Introduction

Early detection strategies and chemoprevention trials for lung cancer are limited by the ability to identify high-risk individuals. While tobacco exposure has been shown to be a major etiologic factor in aerodigestive tract cancer, and while there appears to be a dose-response relationship between the degree of tobacco exposure and the likelihood of cancer development, it is difficult to identify individuals at highest risk. For example, 20 pack-year smokers, while considered at relatively high risk for cancer development, have an approximately 10% risk of developing cancer over their life span (1). As a result, lung cancer prevention studies that use lung cancer development as an endpoint require large numbers of subjects and long follow-up periods. The recently completed Finland lung prevention trial, for example, involved 30,000 subjects and required 10 years in order to examine the impact of prevention strategies on lung cancer development (2). These large numbers limit the number of studies that can be carried out to determine effective agents, doses, combinations, and schedules. Thus, the fields of cancer prevention and early detection would benefit greatly by the development of assays that can be used in the assessment of individual risk as well as response to chemopreventive intervention.

One approach to assessing individual risk and response to intervention is to directly examine lung tissue for histological changes in individuals already known to be at increased risk due to factors such as prior tobacco exposure and/or evidence of lung dysfunction. However, evidence of premalignant histological change in the lungs, while associated with increased cancer risk, may not provide sufficient information to identify those individuals at highest risk. For example, in a recent study of 20 pack-year smokers where bronchial biopsies were obtained from six independent sites in the lung, evidence of bronchial metaplasia in at least one of the six sites was found in nearly 80% of the cases. However, if these subjects stopped smoking, at least 50% of the subjects reversed their metaplastic condition (3). Nevertheless, it is known that lung cancer risk continues for many years beyond smoking cessation (4). Thus, tissue biomarkers are needed to distinguish individuals with simple reactive conditions (and at low risk for lung cancer) from individuals with an active tumorigenesis process.

Since the development of cancer is thought to reflect a process involving the accumulation of specific genetic changes in the tissue at risk, it might be useful to develop assays that provide information about the number of specific genetic events that have already occurred in the lungs. Thus, an individual whose lung tissues already exhibit the majority of necessary genetic changes might be at greater lung cancer risk than an individual with few evident genetic changes. However, it has to be remembered that any tissue sampling must be considered random since one cannot predict the future location of a lung tumor. Thus, genetic biomarkers are also required that can reflect the processes that drive lung cancer development (e.g., the process of genetic instability, which drives the accumulation of specific genetic hits). One might then hypothesize that those individuals in which the rate of accumulation of genetic hits is high might be at the highest risk of developing lung cancer. However, the ability to assess genetic risk from a random biopsy requires that what is detected in one site of the lung is representative of a process that is ongoing throughout the lung tissue field at risk for cancer development. The likelihood of successfully developing such an assay requires understanding the process of genetic change in the lung associated with lung cancer risk. The purpose of this brief review is to summarize recent findings on the nature and distribution of molecular genetic changes in the lungs of individuals at increased risk for lung cancer and describe progress toward developing tissue risk markers.

II. Clinical and Histologic Evidence for a Field Cancerization Process in the Lung

Tumors of the aerodigestive tract have been proposed to reflect a "field cancerization" process whereby the whole tissue is exposed to carcinogenic insult (e.g., tobacco smoke) and is at increased risk for multistep tumor development (5,6). Several types of clinical and laboratory data support this notion. First, from a clinical perspective, the finding of synchronous primary tumors in the lung is not an unusual event, and these tumors frequently exhibit dissimilar histologies as well as distinct genetic signatures (7). Second, individuals who develop a first primary tumor in the field have a 15–20% chance of developing a secondary lung cancer at the rate of about 2–3% per year (8,9). In fact, second primaries become a major source of clinical failure beyond 3–5 years after definitive treatment of the first primary (10). In addition, patients who are definitively treated for a first head and neck primary have a 5–40% risk of developing second primaries (11). These second primaries frequently occur in the lung, especially after a laryngeal primary. Third, individuals with an increased risk for developing lung cancer (e.g., heavy smokers) will often exhibit lesions in the lungs such as bronchial metaplasia/dysplasia or sputum cell abnormalities (12).

Evidence for a cancerization field also derives from careful pathologic examination of the lungs of smokers. Studies by Auerbach and colleagues demonstrated that 90–100% of the tissue sections derived from the lungs of most light smokers, from all heavy smokers, and from individuals with lung cancer showed evidence of epithelial change, including loss of cilia, basal cell hyperplasia, to carcinoma in situ (13). These changes were evident throughout the lung field, and the degree of change correlated strongly with the extent of tobacco exposure.

Clinical and histologic evaluations of lung tissue or exfoliated lung cells also suggest that progression towards tumor may be a multistage process. For example, Saccomanno et al. evaluated serial sputum specimens from individuals at risk for lung cancer and found evidence for increasing degrees of histological abnormalities over time (14). However, it was not possible to predict the rate of progression for any individual based on cytopathological analysis of any one sputum sample.

III. Cytogenetic Evidence for a Field Cancerization Process in the Lung

In recent years, a number of groups have used a variety of cellular and molecular probes to explore the hypothesis that a field cancerization process can occur in the lungs. One approach has been to visualize the chromosome constitution of "normal" lung cells in the field of a lung cancer. While conventional cytogenetic analysis of normal lung tissue is difficult, the technique of premature chromosome condensation has been useful for visualizing the interphase chromosomes of nondividing or very slowly growing cells following fusion with mitotic inducer cells (15). Using this technique to characterize the chromosome constitutions of lung tumor cells as well as normal lung cells from the resected specimen, we showed that, as expected, the lung tumor cells showed a variety of karyotypic changes in both chromosome number per cell as well as specific chromosome gains, losses, and rearrangements. Interestingly, however, the cells derived from "normal" lung tissue of these lung cancer patients also showed chromosome changes (16). In some cases, the distribution of chromosome numbers per cell as well as the presence of specific chromosome changes in the normal cells resembled that observed in the corresponding lung tumor. In other cases, however, the normal cells also showed changes not found in the tumor, and vice versa. Interestingly, the degree of chromosome change found in the normal tissues of individuals with lung cancer varied from case to case, suggesting that the field cancerization process might be ongoing at different rates in different individuals.

Chromosome changes in normal lung cells derived from lung cancer patients were also demonstrated cytogenetically in epithelial outgrowths from normal lung tissue of individuals with lung cancer. For example, Lee et al. found an increased frequency of cells with trisomy chromosome 7 (17). Similarly, Sozzi et al. examined short-term cultures of "normal" lung cells from patients with lung tumors and found evidence for chromosomal rearrangements, including 3p and 17p deletions, and overexpression of growth factor receptors (18,19). In this situation, the frequencies of these changes appeared to be significantly higher in patients with multiple tumors of the aerodigestive tract (20). Thus, it appears that chromosome changes can be found throughout the lung tissue of the individuals with lung cancer, lending genetic support for the notion of a field of cancerization. Moreover, the finding of different amounts of chromosome change in the normal lung tissue of different individuals supports the idea the lung tumorigenesis is a multistep process, and the degree of risk for second (or first) primaries might be related to the levels of accumulated genetic changes.

IV. Molecular Evidence for a Field Cancerization Process in Lung Tissue Associated with Tumors

A number of specific molecular genetic changes involving specific oncogenes, tumor suppressor, and cell regulatory and repair genes have been observed in lung tumors. These include mutations in the genetic families of myc, myb, jun, ras, raf, fms, fur, p53, and her2/neu as well as loss of heterozygosity in other regions of the genome, frequently including sites on chromosomes 1,3,5,6,9,11,13,17, and 18 (21,22). More recently, the technique of comparative genomic hybridization demonstrated frequent increased copy numbers of chromosome regions 3q, 5p, 8q, and 17q and decreased copy numbers of chromosome regions 3p, 5q, 10q, 13q, and 17p (23,24).

While a more extensive review of the specific molecular genetic changes involved in lung cancer can be found in other contributions to this volume, the identification of specific gene involvements in lung cancers has provided specific molecular markers with which to probe the lung tumorigenesis process. For example, Rabbitts and colleagues showed that regions of bronchial dysplasia adjacent to invasive squamous cell carcinoma of the lung showed some of the same molecular changes as was found in the tumor (25). Similarly, Gazdar dissected premalignant epithelial regions from lung tissues of cancer patients and, using polymerization chain reaction technology and microsatellite primers and probes, demonstrated a variety of clonal changes in premalignant lesions including ras mutations and allelic losses (26).

While these molecular genetic studies supported the notion that clonal genetic events are present in the "normal" and premalignant lung regions of individuals with lung cancer, it was not known whether these clonal outgrowths represented precursor lesions for the associated tumors (i.e., a manifestation of a multistep tumorigenesis process) or independent sites of clonal outgrowth in a carcinogenesis field. Loss of heterozygosity of chromosome regions 9p and 3p (often involving the FHIT gene locus) are frequently found in lesions with low-grade histology in the field of lung tumors, whereas K-ras mutations are found more frequently in more advanced premalignant lesions (27–29). Several groups have reported the finding that the particular alleles lost on chromosomes 3p and 9p or the particular types of p53 or K-ras mutations may differ from one premalignant lesion to another in the same lung cancers field (30). On the other hand, Gazdar et al. found evidence for preferential loss of one allele of chromosomes 3p or 9p when looking at multiple regions of the lung; however, the deletion sizes appeared to differ from one lesion to the next (27,31). Thus either these lesions represent genetically distinct clones, or there is a progressive expansion of the deleted region with histologic progression.

V. Molecular Evidence for a Field Cancerization Process in High-Risk Lung Tissue

The model system used in the genetic studies described above involved lungs in which a tumor had already occurred. Thus, the "normal" and "premalignant" lesions examined represented epithelium in fields at 100% risk of developing lung cancer. The next question is whether a field cancerization process can be detected in individuals who are at increased risk for lung cancer. Lam and associates (32) obtained serial lung biopsies using fluorescence-assisted bronchonscopy from individuals at very high risk for lung cancer (individuals with moderate dysplasia, strong smoking or asbestos exposure history, and evidence of functional lung defects) and probed the biopsies for evidence of loss of heterozygosity (LOH) of chromosomes 3p21, 5q21, and 9p21. While hyperplasia/metaplasia lesions showed no evidence for LOH of 3p or 9p, 30–40% of the dysplastic lesions and 80–100% of the carcinoma in situ lesions showed LOH at one or more of the chromosome loci. At the same time, only 11% of the hyperplasia/metaplasia samples showed LOH for chromosome 5q (32).

A similar question was addressed by Mao et al. where bronchial biopsies from six independent lung sites were obtained from individuals with at least a 20 pack-year smoking history, and the lesions were examined for LOH of chromosome regions 3p14, 9p21, and 17p13. Of the informative cases, 76% showed evidence for LOH in at least one of the six biopsy sites (33). Taken on a per site basis, some form of LOH was observed in around 25% of the sites examined. Interestingly, different sites within the same individual often exhibited the loss of different alleles, suggesting that these lesions were of different genetic origins. In addition, current smokers appeared to exhibit higher levels of LOH than former smokers. Similar findings were reported by Gazdar and colleagues where multiple genetic loci were examined, including 3p, 9p, 5q, 17q, and 13q. Among individuals with a smoking history, 86% demonstrated LOH in one or more biopsy specimens, and among all biopsy specimens, 24% showed evidence of LOH (34). In this study, while current and former smokers showed similar frequencies of LOH, no genetic alterations were detected in nonsmokers.

These cytogenetic and molecular results provide considerable evidence that a field cancerization process underlies lung tumorigenesis. A cartoon model for this progressive process is shown in Figure 1. One might imagine that exposure of the lung to tobacco, other exogenous carcinogens, or damaging endogenous processes leads to the induction of genetic changes in individual cells throughout the lung field. If the damaged DNA is not repaired, then genetic damage can accumulate throughout the lung in the form of DNA adducts, mutations, deletions, and chromosome breaks. It is likely that this damage also leads to wound healing, and this proliferation may then fix premutational lesions (e.g., DNA adducts or base changes) into permanent genetic lesions. If the genetic hits occur in genes important for regulatory control of cellular growth, differentiation, and cell loss, clonal outgrowths with preferential growth capabilities may develop. With continued damage and continued wound healing, these clones may continue to enlarge in size as well as accumulate the genetic changes necessary for lung tumor development. At some point in the process, some lesions will progress to a stage where they exhibit clinical manifestations of premalignant disease (metaplasia/dysplasia). With continued insult and cellular response, an invasive tumor may develop in one part of the lung. Even if the first primary is definitively treated, the remaining lung is still likely to harbor multiple regions of clonal outgrowth and with time, and continued carcinogen exposure, would be at high risk for developing a second or multiple primaries.

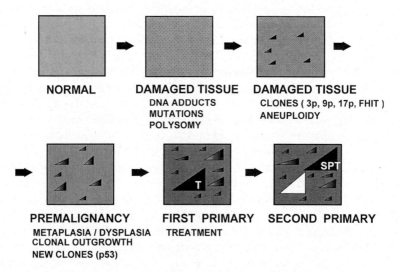

Figure 1 Lung field cancerization and multistep tumorigenesis.

VI. Quantitation of Ongoing Genetic Instability in the Lung by In Situ Hybridization

With the above model in mind, one approach to cancer risk assessment would be to determine the accumulated number of genetic changes in a particular lung biopsy. This might indicate how far along the multistep tumorigenesis process that site has progressed. However, since it is impossible to target a biopsy to the future site of a lung tumor, it is not clear that the determination of specific changes in one biopsy would provide an assessment for the whole field at risk. An alternative approach is to look for markers of the forces that drive the tumorigenesis process, e.g., measurements of both the rate of accumulation of genetic damage and the cumulative amount of generalized genetic change. Since most lung tumors and their adjacent "normal" and "premalignant" tissues have been shown to exhibit both numerical and structural chromosome changes, this could be accomplished by determining the amount of chromosome change present in the target tissue. Given the constraints of the clinical setting (i.e., small bronchial biopsies or exfoliated cells), assays are needed that can detect genetic changes in small amounts of material. While the molecular approaches described above (involving bulk examination of polymorphic microsatellite sequences) are useful for detecting clonal outgrowths that constitute a significant fraction of the sampled cells, they have limited use in the setting where one wants to measure the rate of accumulation of genetic events in the target tissue.

The technique of in situ hybridization involves the use of DNA probes that recognize either chromosome-specific repetitive target sequences, chromosome single copy gene sequences, or sequences along the whole chromosome length or chromosome segments (35). These probes can be labeled and applied to groups of cells and visualized using either fluorescence or cytochemical techniques. Probes that detect chromosome-specific repetitive target sequences result in small dots of hybridization when placed on cells. Thus, to look at chromosome copy number changes within a cell population, one would use a chromosome-specific probe and then examine each cell for the number of spots (36,37). When whole cells are examined, if the cell population were unaltered, one would expect to see all the cells having two chromosome copies for any autosomal chromosomal probe. On the other hand, if the cell population has been damaged, one might expect to detect cells with fewer or more than two chromosome copies (Fig. 2).

The in situ hybridization technique has recently been used to examine cellular outgrowths from bronchial brushings of individuals with possible lung cancer or at high risk for lung cancer. Using a chromosome 7 probe and in situ hybridization techniques, cells with trisomy 7 could be found in the "normal" or histologically altered epithelial cells from multiple lung sites, especially in samples from patients with lung cancer, former uranium miners, and in one of four smokers (38). On the other hand, significant chromosome changes were not observed in never smokers, and similar levels of trisomy were not found using a chromosome 2 probe. These results supported the field cancerization and multistep tumorigenesis concepts and

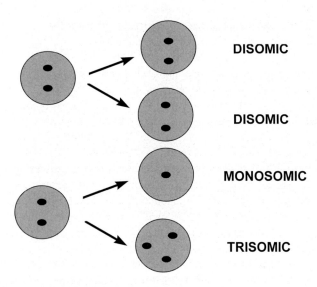

Figure 2   Development of polysomy.

also suggested that alterations of chromosome 7 might preferentially be associated with cellular outgrowth.

   In order to examine cellular changes on biopsy material, our own group has applied the technique of in situ hybridization to tissue sections of paraffin-embedded bronchial biopsies. While chromosome copy numbers can be evaluated in tissue sections, there is an underrepresentation of chromosome copy numbers due to nuclear truncation. Nevertheless, rare events such as chromosome polysomy can still be detected and used as an indicator of ongoing genetic instability (39,40). Moreover, since the tissue architecture is preserved, localized epithelial regions can be examined for evidence of clonal outgrowths and used as an indicator for the degree of progression. This approach has previously been used in a number of multistep progression models to examine the rate of genetic instability. For example, it was found that the frequency of cells with chromosome polysomy increases with histologic progression in the premalignant lesions adjacent to head and neck tumors (41). Similarly, premalignant lesions such as oral leukoplakia lesions showed evidence of genetic instability using this technique, and individuals with evidence of high levels of genetic instability (i.e., high chromosomal polysomy) were found to subsequently progress to cancer at a relatively high rate compared to individuals with low degrees of genetic instability in their biopsied lesions (42,43).

   This technique has more recently been applied to bronchial biopsies obtained from individuals at relatively high risk for lung cancer (due to a 20 pack-year smoking history) who were about to enter lung chemoprevention trials. In one study, tissue sections from each of six biopsy sites were analyzed by in situ hybridization for changes in copy number for chromosomes 7, 9, and 17. The first important finding was that some degree of chromosome polysomy was evident in all lung sites examined, supporting the notion that random chromosome changes may be occurring throughout the exposed lung field (44). The second important finding was that chromosome polysomy could be detected with each of the chromosome probes, again suggesting that random chromosome events were being detected.

In a second study, bronchial biopsies were obtained from individuals with a 20 pack-year smoking history and analyzed for chromosome 9 polysomy using in situ hybridization. Interestingly, all 29 cases (134 biopsies) who showed metaplasia at one of six biopsy sites also showed chromosome polysomy in at least one biopsy site; overall, 88% of the sites showed some evidence of chromosome 9 polysomy. Evidence for genetic instability was also detected in patients who did not show evidence of bronchial metaplasia in any of six biopsy sites despite a strong smoking history. In fact, 11 of 12 cases (91%) and 33 of 52 (63%) biopsy sites showed significant chromosome polysomy (i.e., ≥ 3 copies in $\geq 2\%$ of the cells examined). These results suggest that the lungs of long-term smokers show significant evidence of genetic instability, even after cessation of tobacco exposure and even after histologic changes have disappeared. How long these genetic changes will remain in the lung following smoking cessation remains to be determined. Nevertheless, these findings may help to explain why lung tumor risk remains relatively high for several years beyond the cessation of smoking (4).

In some of the cases of bronchial metaplasia, the chromosome index (average chromosome copy number per cell) was observed to fall somewhere between that expected for a diploid population and that expected for a trisomic population. One possible explanation for this finding was that carcinogen treatment induced chromosome polysomy but there was preferential loss of cells with an underrepresentation of chromosome copies (Fig. 3). In this case, the apparent fraction of cells with chromosome polysomy would increase, yet these cells would still be randomly distrib-

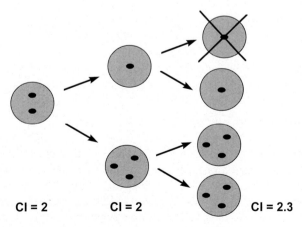

CI = 2   CI = 2   CI = 2.3

Figure 3   Development of aneuploidy.

STATEGY FOR ANALYSIS

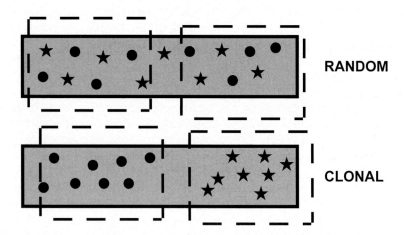

Figure 4   Random polysomy vs. focal clonality.

uted in the tissue. An alternative hypothesis is that the cells with three chromosome copies per cell are clustered together, perhaps a result of a clonal outgrowth. To distinguish between these possibilities (i.e., random distribution versus localized clonal outgrowth), the location of each cell within the epithelium and its chromosome copy number can be recorded using an image analysis system and a spatial genetic map for the epithelium generated. The average chromosome copy number for localized groups of cells could then be calculated (Fig. 4). This spatial analysis demonstrated the presence of microclones within the bronchial epithelium of individuals with a long smoking history. Interestingly, when adjacent tissue sections were probed separately for evidence of clones of cells with trisomy chromosome 7, 9, or 17, the detected clones appeared to occupy separate areas of the epithelium. These results therefore suggest that not only are the lungs of individuals exposed to tobacco undergoing a process of genetic instability, they are also experiencing the outgrowth of multiple clones throughout the exposed lung field as hypothesized by the model shown in Figure 1.

VII. Conclusion

Taken together, several types of data support the notion that lung tumorigenesis represents a field cancerization process with multiple sites undergoing localized progression along a multistep pathway. The cytogenetic and in situ hybridization data suggest that random genetic instability due to carcinogen exposure can be detected throughout the tissue field at risk. The molecular genetic and in situ hybridization data suggest that at some point, clones of cells develop a preferential growth and survival advantage and begin to take over larger regions of the lung epithelium. In some cases, these clones appear to be microscopic in size and can only be detected by examining local accumulations of cells with common genetic features (e.g., chromosome monosomy or trisomy for a particular chromosome). In other cases, the clones appear to cover large regions of epithelium since the same clonal genetic defect can be observed in biopsies far apart in space. The finding of high frequencies of genetic changes in the adjacent epithelium in the field of lung cancers, and relatively high frequencies of genetic changes in the epithelium of relatively high-risk individuals, suggest that the measurement of genetic instability may eventually be useful for individual assessment of lung cancer risk. It now remains to be determined whether the degree of genetic instability and clonal outgrowth found in tissue biopsies or exfoliated cells is related to lung cancer risk. These assays may therefore play an important role for identifying individuals at high risk for lung cancer who might benefit from participating in chemoprevention trials.

Acknowledgments

These studies were supported in part by NIH grants CA-52051, CA-16672, CA-68437, CA-68089, and CA-70907.

References

1. Garfinkel L, Silberberg E. Lung cancer and smoking trends in the United States over the past 25 years. CA Cancer J Clin 1993; 42:137–145.
2. Heinonen OP, Albanes D, the Alpha-tocopherol, Beta Carotene Cancer Prevention Study Group. The effect of vitamin E and beta carotene on the incidence of lung cancer and other cancers in male smokers. N Engl J Med 1994; 330:1029–1035.
3. Lee JS, Lippman SM, Benner SE, Lee JJ, Ro JY, Lukeman JM, Morice RC, Peters EJ, Pang AC, Fritsche, HA, Hong WK. Randomized placebo-controlled trial of isotretinoin in chemoprevention of bronchial squamous metaplasia. J Clin Oncol 1994; 12:937–945.
4. Tong L., Spitz MR, Faeger JJ, Amos CA. Lung cancer in former smokers. Cancer 1996; 78:1004–1010.
5. Slaughter DP, Southwick HW, Smejkal W. Field cancerization in oral stratified squamous epithelium: clinical implications of multicentric origin. Cancer 1953; 6:963–968.
6. Farber E. The multistep nature of cancer development. Cancer Res 1984; 44:4217–4223.
7. Gluckman JO, Crissman JD, Donegan JO. Multicentric squamous cell carcinoma of the upper aerodigestive tract. Head Neck Surg 1980; 3:90–96.
8. Fontana RS, Sanderson DR, Woolner LB, Taylor WF, Miller WE, Muhm, JR. Lung cancer screening: the Mayo program. J Occup Med 1986; 28:746–750.
9. Pastorino V, Infante M, Maioli M, Chiesa G, Buyse M, Finket P, Rosmentz N, Clerici M, Soresi E, Valente M, Belloni PA, Ravasi G. Adjuvant treatment of stage I lung cancer with high dose vitamin A. J Clin Oncol 1993; 11:1216–1222.
10. Shields, TW, Humphrey EW, Higgins, GA Jr. Long-term survivors after resection of lung carcinoma. J Thorac Cardiovasc Surg 1978; 89:1782–1788.
11. Lippman SM, Hong WK. Second malignant tumors in head and neck squamous carcinoma. The overshadowing threat for patients with early stage of disease. Int J Radiat Oncol Biol Phys 1989; 17:691–694.
12. Lee JS, Lippman SM, Benner SE, Lee JJ, Ro JY, Lukeman JM, Morice RC, Peters EJ, Pang

AC, Fritsche, HA, Hong WK. Randomized placebo-controlled trial of isotretinoin in chemoprevention of bronchial squamous metaplasia. J Clin Oncol 1994; 12:937–945.

13. Auerbach O, Stout AP, Hammond EC, Garfinkel L. Changes in bronchial epithelium in relation to cigarette smoking and in relation to lung cancer. N Engl J Med 1961; 265:253–267.

14. Saccomanno G, Archer VE, Auerbach O, Saunders RP, Brennan, LM. Development of carcinoma of the lung as reflected in exfoliated cells. Cancer 1974; 33:256–270.

15. Hittelman WN. PCC in the diagnosis of malignancy. In: Johnson R, Rao PN, Sperling K, eds. PCC: Application in Basic and Clinical Research. New York: Academic Press, 1982:309–358.

16. Hittelman WN, Lee JS, Cheong N, Shin D, Hong WK. The chromosome view of "field cancerization" and multistep carcinogenesis. Implications for chemopreventive approaches. In: Pastorino V, Hong WK, eds. Chemoimmunoprevention of Cancer. Stuttgart: Georg Thieme Verlag, 1991:41–47.

17. Lee JS, Pathak S, Hopwood V, Tomasovik B, Mullins, TD, Baker BL, Spitzer G, Neidhart JA. Involvement of chromosome 7 in primary lung tumor and nonmalignant normal lung tissue. Cancer Res 1987; 47:6349–6352.

18. Sozzi G, Miozzi M, Tagliabue E, Calderonce C, Lambardi L, Pilotti S, Pastorino V, Pierotti MA, Della Porta G. Cytogenetic abnormalities and overexpression of receptors for growth factors in normal bronchial epithelium and tumor samples of lung cancer patients. Cancer Res 1991; 51:400–404.

19. Sozzi G, Miozzo M, Donghi R, Pilotti S, Cariani CT, Pastorino V, Della Porta G, Pierotti MA. Deletions of 17p and p53 mutations in preneoplastic lesions of the lung. Cancer Res 1992; 52:6079–6082.

20. Sozzi G, Miozzi M, Pastorino V, Tagliabue E, Donghi R, Manenti G, Minoletti F, Pilotti S, Ravasi G, Pierotti M. Genetic elements in the multi-step lung carcinogenesis. Lung Cancer 1994; 11(suppl 1):20.

21. Iman DS, Harris CC. Oncogenes and tumor suppressor genes in human lung carcinogenesis. Crit Rev Oncogenesis 1991; 2:161–171.

22. Viallet J, Minna JD. Dominant oncogene and tumor suppressor genes in the pathogenesis of lung cancer. Am J Respir Cell Mol Biol 1990; 2:225–232.

23. Petersen I, Bujard M, Petersen S, Wolf G, Goeze A, Schwendel A, Langreck H, Gellert K, Reichel M, Just K, duManoir S, Cremer T, Dietel M, Ried T. Patterns of chromosomal imbalances in adenocarcinoma and squamous cell carcinoma of the lung. Cancer Res 1997; 57:2331–2335.

24. Ried T, Petersen I, Holtgreve-Grez H, Speicher MR, Schrock E, du Manoir S, Cremer T. Mapping of multiple DNA gains and losses in primary small cell lung carcinomas by comparative genomic hybridization. Cancer Res 1994; 54:1801–1806.

25. Sundaresan V, Ganly P, Hasleton P, Rudd R, Sinha G, Bleehen NM, Rabbits P. p53 and chromosome 3 abnormalities, characteristics of malignant lung tumors, are detectable in preinvasive lesions of the bronchus. Oncogene 1992; 7:1989–1997.

26. Gazdar AF. Molecular changes preceding the onset of invasive lung cancers. Lung Cancer 1994; 11(suppl 2):16–17.

27. Kishimoto Y, Sugio K, Hung JY, Virmani AK, McIntire DD, Minna JD, Gazdar AF. Allele-specific loss in chromosome 9p loci in preneoplastic lesions accompanying non-small-cell lung cancers. J Natl Cancer Inst 1995; 87:1224–1229.

28. Fong KM, Biesterveld EJ, Virmani A, Wistuba I, Sekido Y, Badder SA, Ahmadian M, Ong ST, Rassool FV, Zimmerman PV, Giaccone G, Gazdar AF, Minna JD. FHIT and FRA3B 3p14.2 allele loss are common in lung cancer and preneoplastic bronchial lesions and are associated with cancer-related FHIT cDNA splicing aberrations. Cancer Res 1997; 57:2256–2267.

29. Sugio K, Kishimoto Y, Virmanti AK, Hung JY, Gazdar AF. K-ras mutations are a relatively late event in the pathogenesis of lung carcinomas. Cancer Res 1994; 54:5811–5815.

30. Chung GTY, Sundaresan V, Hasleton P, Rudd R, Taylor R, Rabbits PH. Clonal evolution of lung tumors. Cancer Res 1996; 56:1609–1614.

31. Hung J, Kishimoto Y, Sugio K, Virmani A, McIntire DD, Minna JD, Gazdar AF. Allele-

specific chromosome 3p deletions occur at an early stage in the pathogenesis of lung carcinoma. JAMA 1995; 273:558–563.

32. Thiberville L, Payne P, Vielkinds J, LeRiche J, Horsman D, Nouvet G, Palcic B, Lam S. Evidence of cumulative gene losses with progression of premalignant epithelial lesions to carcinoma of the bronchus. Cancer Res 1995; 55:5133–5139.

33. Mao L, Lee JS, Kurie JM, Fan YH, Lippman SM, Lee JJ, Ro JY, Broxson A, Yu R, Morice RC, Kemp BL, Khuri FR, Walsh GL, Hittelman WN, Hong WK. Clonal genetic alterations in the lungs of current and former smokers. J Natl Cancer Inst 1997; 89:857–862.

34. Wistuba II, Lam S, Behrens C, Virmani AK, Fong KM, LeRiche J, Samet JM, Srivastava S, Minna JD, Gazdar AF. Molecular damage in the bronchial epithelium of current and former smokers. J Natl Cancer Inst 1997; 89:1366–1373.

35. Pinkel D, Straume T, Gray JW. Cytogenetic analysis using quantitative, high sensitivity, fluorescence hybridization. Proc Natl Acad Sci USA 1986; 83:2934–2938.

36. Cremer T, Lichter P, Borden J, Ward DC, Manuelidis L. Detection of chromosome aberrations in metaphase and interphase tumor cells by in situ hybridization using chromosome-specific library probes. Hum Genet 1988; 80:235–246.

37. Hopman AHN, Wiegant J, Raap AK, Landgent JE, Van der Ploeg M, Van Duijn P. Bicolor detection of two target DNAs by non-radioactive in situ hybridization. Histochemistry 1986; 85:1–4.

38. Crowell RE, Gilliland FD, Temes RT, Harms HJ, Neft RE, Heapy E, Auckley DH, Crooks LA, Jordan SW, Samet JM, Lechner JF, Belinsky SA. Detection of trisomy 7 in nonmalignant bronchial epithelium from lung cancer patients and individuals at risk for lung cancer. Cancer Epiderm Biomarkers Prevent 1996; 5:631–637.

39. Kim SY, Lee JS, Ro JY, Gay ML, Hong WK, Hittelman WN. Interphase cytogenetics in paraffin sections of lung tumors by non-isotopic in situ hybridization. Mapping genotype/phenotype heterogeneity. Am J Pathol 1993; 142:307–317.

40. Dhingra K, Sneige N, Pandita TK, Johnston DA, Lee JS, Emami K, Hortobagyi GN, Hittelman WN. Quantitative analysis of chromosome in situ hybridization signal in paraffin-embedded tissue sections. Cytometry 1994; 16:100–112.

41. Voravud N, Shin DM, Ro JY, Lee JS, Hong WK, Hittelman WN. Increased polysomies of chromosomes 7 and 17 during head and neck multistage tumorigenesis. Cancer Res 1993; 53:2874–2883.

42. Lee JS, Kim SY, Hong WK, Lippman SM, Ro JY, Gay ML, Hittelman WN. Detection of chromosomal polysomy in oral leukoplakia, a premalignant lesion. J Natl Cancer Inst 1993; 85:1951–1954.

43. Kim HJ, Lee JS, Shin DM, Lippman SM, Ro JY, Hong WK, Hittelman WN. Chromosomal instability, p53 expression, and retinoid response in oral premalignancy. Proc ASCO 1995; 14:81.

44. Hittelman WN, Yu R, Kurie J, Lee JS, Morice RC, Walsh GL, Ro JY, Hong WK, Lee JJ. Evidence for genomic instability and clonal outgrowth in the bronchial epithelium of smokers. Proc AACR 1997; 38:3097.

16

Telomerase and Lung Cancer

ASHA RATHI, YASHIMA KAZUO, NAOYOSHI ONUKI, ARVIND VIRMANI, and ADI F. GAZDAR

University of Texas Southwestern Medical Center
Dallas, Texas

I. Telomeres, Telomerase, and Cancer

Telomerase is currently recognized as a nearly ubiquitous tumor marker. Telomerase is a specialized ribonucleoprotein polymerase that adds TTAGGG repeats at the ends of vertebrate chromosomal DNA called telomeres (1). Human telomeres undergo progressive shortening with cell division through replication-dependent sequence loss at DNA termini (2–4). This shortening of telomeres has been proposed as a mechanism for cellular senescence (5,6). Telomerase is thought to compensate for the loss of telomeric repeats and is associated with the acquisition of the immortal phenotype. A variety of immortal cell lines, malignant tumors, and germ cells have been found to specifically express telomerase activity (7–15), whereas most normal somatic cells do not express this activity, suggesting that telomerase activation may be a critical step in cell immortalization (16) and oncogenesis.

Telomerase may be detected by its enzyme activity, using the PCR-based TRAP assay, or by expression of the RNA component (hTR). Enzyme activity requires the presence of fresh or frozen tissue, and cellular localization is not possible. Detection of hTR can be performed on paraffin-embedded archival materials and can be used to detect the cellular types expressing it. The detection of telomerase enzyme is based on its ability to act as a template and add telomeric repeats

(TTAGGG)n onto the 3′ ends of a specific primer followed by subsequent PCR amplification of the telomerase extension products. Incorporation of radioactivity (12) or fluorescein end-labeled primers (17) into a six-base-pair ladder can be detected by autoradiography or an automated sequencer and activity semiquantitated with reference to an internal standard. At the cellular level, telomerase can be detected by a radioactive-based in situ hybridization using the cloned human telomerase RNA (hTR) component as a probe (18). There is a high degree of concordance between the two tests, indicating that data of either test may be utilized to determine extent of activation.

II.   Telomerase Activity in Lung Carcinogenesis

Telomerase is activated in most lung cancers (19). The role of telomerase in lung cancer is of special significance since lung cancer is the leading cause of cancer deaths among both males and females in the United States (20). Furthermore, incidence of lung cancer has risen to epidemic proportions during the twentieth century (21). Survival rates differ significantly for the two major lung cancer types being 30% in non–small cell lung cancers (NSCLC) and 10% in the more aggressive small-cell lung cancers (SCLC). The latter account for 20–25% of bronchogenic carcinomas (22).

Measurements of telomerase activity in surgically resected lung cancer tissue have been carried out by a PCR-based telomeric repeat amplification (12). In NSCLC, telomerase-positivity is 73% (35/48) with weak to moderate activities, whereas 100% of SCLC (11/11) are positive and show strong signal activities (9). In contrast, levels of telomerase activity are similar in all SCLC and NSCLC immortal lung cancer cell lines (12). Since SCLCs have a greater malignant potential than NSCLCs, these observations are in keeping with the correlation of telomerase activity with the malignant potential of the tumor and the ratio of mortal to immortal cells in each tumor (21,23,24). High levels of telomerase may in some cases be due to an increase in copy number of the human telomerase RNA gene (25).

Most metastatic lesions from lung cancer patients are positive for telomerase. Although histologically benign lymph nodes from lung cancer patients have telomerase activity, levels are sixfold lower than invasive tumor (18). Furthermore, cell extracts from pleural effusions of patients with adenocarcinoma of the lung (9) also show activity.

While the vast majority of lung carcinomas express telomerase activity and hTR, differences in the pattern of expression were noted (Fig. 1). Whereas adenocarcinomas expressed hTR in all cells examined with little variability, expression in squamous cell carcinomas was more variable. In particular, well-differentiated squamous (and nondividing) cells had little or no expression. The outer cells of the squamous nests (which are the dividing cells of the tumor) had high expression. In contrast, all of the cells of adenocarcinomas are capable of division. Thus, even in carcinomas, downregulation was noted in nondividing differentiated cells.

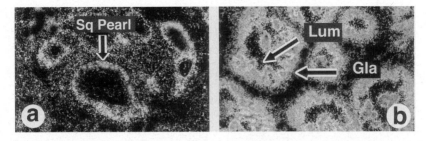

Figure 1 Dark field images of squamous cell (a) and adenocarcinoma (b). In the squamous pearls only the peripheral dividing cells express hTR, while the more differentiated cells in the center are negative for expression. In adenocarcinomas, where every tumor cell is capable of division, all cells intensely express hTR.

III. Alterations in Telomere Length

Alterations of telomere length, a representative of the number of cell divisions, are frequently associated with high telomerase activity as well as allelic loss of tumor suppressor genes p53 and Rb, which play a role in tumor progression of the lung (26,27). Alterations have been observed in the early stages in adenocarcinoma or at late stages in other histologic types and metastatic lesions of lung (28). Most (85%) of lung cancer cases with low or undetectable telomerase activity have telomere lengths similar to adjacent (29) normal tissue. In SCLC and metastatic lesions, variant patterns of telomere length (either reduction, elongation, or convergence) have been observed, and cases with elongated telomeres indicate poor prognosis.

IV. Telomerase in Neuroendocrine Tumors

Neuroendocrine tumors of the lung represent a spectrum of clinicopathological types ranging from the low grade carcinoids to the highly malignant SCLC. Two intermediate forms are now recognized: the atypical carcinoid and large-cell neuroendocrine carcinomas (LCNEC) (30). Telomerase RNA expression has been determined in these subtypes of pulmonary neuroendocrine (NE) tumors by in situ hybridization using the human telomerase RNA (hTR) component (31). Expression correlates to histologic grade of the tumor. Thus, while 55% of typical and atypical carcinoids having low-grade malignant potential characteristics are weakly positive, 100% of the rapidly growing and widely metastatic LCNEC and small cell carcinomas show high expression (Fig. 2).

V. Telomerase in Preneoplasia

Telomerase is detected in preinvasive lesions in a number of organ systems (32), including colon (15), head and neck (33), and lung cancer (34).

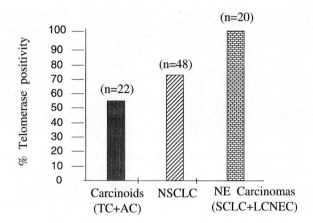

Figure 2 Telomerase positivity in carcinoids (typical and atypical), non–small cell lung cancer (NSCLC), and neuroendocrine carcinomas.

A series of morphologically distinct preoplastic changes (hyperplasia, dysplasia, and carcinoma in situ) can be observed in bronchial epithelium before the appearance of a clinically overt cancer (35,36). The sequential changes for cancers that arise in squamous and SCLC have long been recognized, whereas similar changes in adenocarcinomas and large-cell carcinomas are more recently described. A number of genetic abnormalities identical to overt cancer cells are found in these preoplastic cells.

Low levels of telomerase activity (<1 unit/μg protein) have been detected in hyperplasia, dysplasia, and CIS compared to invasive cancer (34 units/μg protein) (Fig. 3). Weak telomerase RNA (hTR) expression is seen in basal layers of normal (Fig. 4) and hyperplastic epithelium from lung cancer patients. Dysregulation of telomerase expression increases with tumor progression, with moderate to strong expression throughout the multilayers of the epithelium in metaplasia and dysplasia (Fig. 5) and foci of upregulation in CIS in the vicinity of invasive cancer (34) (Fig. 6).

A similar pattern of dysregulation in telomerase expression with increasing histologic grade was also noted in a study of 68 biopsies of smoking-damaged epithelium from current or ex-smokers with or without cancer (unpublished data). Telomerase expression was present in 20% of hyperplasia, 53% of dysplasia, 100% of microinvasion, and CIS (Fig. 7). These findings suggest that telomerase could serve as a potential marker for the early detection of lung cancer.

hTR was not detected in the few samples of atypical adenomatous hyperplasia (AAH) examined to date (34). AAH is considered to be a precursor lesion of adenocarcinomas, although conclusive evidence for this viewpoint is lacking. These findings suggest one of two possibilities: AAH is not a true precursor lesion of invasive carcinomas, or telomerase activation is a late event during the pathogenesis of peripheral adenocarcinomas.

units / µg protein

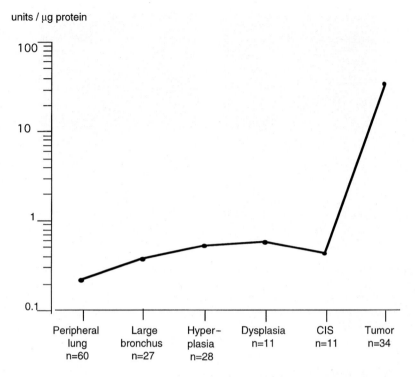

Figure 3 Telomerase activity relative to an internal standard in different preneoplastic stages of lung cancer. Values are on a log scale.

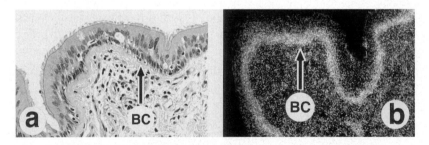

Figure 4 hTR expression in normal epithelium, H and E (a) and dark field (b) images. hTR expression is limited to the basal cells.

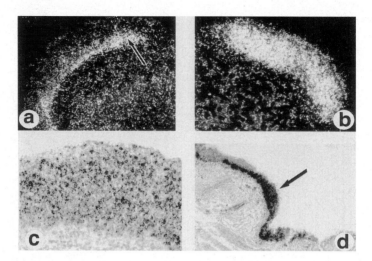

Figure 5 hTR expression in preneoplasia. Dark field image of hyperplasia (a), with expression in parabasal cells (arrow). Dark field image of metaplasia (b), with expression in all layers. Bright field image of severe dysplasia (c) with focal moderate intensity expression in all cell layers. Bright field image of severe dysplasia (d), demonstrating focal, unusually intense expression (arrow).

VI. Mechanisms of Telomerase Expression During Lung Cancer Pathogenesis

The findings reported above suggest two mechanisms of activation during carcinogenesis. Low-level activity is present in the stem cells of many regenerative tissues including bronchial epithelium. This activity is closely related to cell division and decreases or is absent in differentiated cells such as ciliated and mucus-producing cells. In many preneoplastic tissues including some cases of CIS, low-level expres-

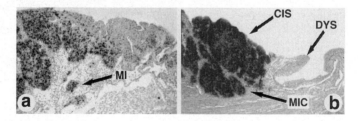

Figure 6 Bright field images of hTR expression in CIS. In (a) there is focal intense expression in part of the in situ lesion and in the foci of microinvasion (MI). In (b) there is intense expression throughout the focus of CIS and underlying microinvasive carcinoma (MIC), but not in the adjacent epithelium with moderate dysplasia.

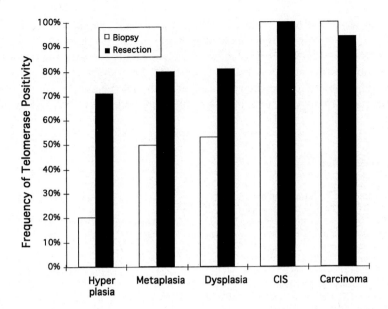

Figure 7 Telomerase positivity in bronchial biopsies and resection samples in preneoplastic lung cancer lesions.

sion is also present, although expression may be dysregulated, with expression in multiple epithelial layers of full thickness. We presume that this so-called physiological expression is maintained in many preneoplastic conditions. However, high-level, focal expression occurs in some foci of CIS, frequently adjacent to or continuous with invasive carcinomas. Telomerase expression may be due to loss of repressors located on chromosome 3p (37). Loss of genetic material on chromosome 3p is common in many carcinomas including lung cancers (38). We presume the high level expression that occurs shortly before invasion is due to loss of one or more repressors. Thus, telomerase expression in carcinomas appears to be due to dual mechanisms.

VII. Potential Clinical Implications in Lung Cancers

The majority (>90%) of invasive lung cancers express high telomerase activity, while normal tissues are negative or weakly positive. The direct relationship between the more aggressive lung cancers (SCLC) and telomerase activity may explain the correlation of telomerase activity and the malignant potential of tumors. In situ hybridizations could rule out false-positive cases by identification of reactive or regenerating cells. Telomerase activity may then prove to be very useful in cancer diagnostics. Telomerase expression increases in both frequency and intensity with increasing histopathological grade in preneoplasia, which indicates the potential of telomerase as a valuable prognostic marker.

An increasing need to identify risk factors for premalignant bronchial tissue exists. Detection of telomerase in the early stages of lung cancer at levels similar to invasive tumor suggest its role as an intermediate marker for assessing risk for malignant progression and as a marker to evaluate the efficacy of chemopreventive regimens. Inhibitors of the catalytic subunit of the telomerase protein (39) or the telomerase RNA may well be the focus of future endeavors in the treatment of cancer.

References

1. Morin GB. The human telomere terminal transferase enzyme is a ribonucleoprotein that synthesizes TTAGGG repeats. Cell 1989; 59:521–529.
2. Hastie ND, Dempster M, Dunlop MG, Thompson AM, Green DK, Allshire RC. Telomere reductase in human colorectal carcinoma and with ageing [see comments]. Nature 1990; 346:866–868.
3. Allsopp RC, Vaziri H, Patterson C, Goldstein S, Younglai EV, Futcher AB, Greider CW, Harley CB. Telomere length predicts replicative capacity of human fibroblasts. Proc Natl Acad Sci USA 1992; 89:10114–10118.
4. Harley CB, Futcher AB, Greider CW. Telomeres shorten during ageing of human fibroblasts. Nature 1990; 345:458–460.
5. Harley CB. Telomere loss: mitotic clock or genetic time bomb? Mutat Res 1991; 256:271–282.
6. Harley CB, Villeponteau B. Telomeres and telomerase in aging and cancer. Curr Opin Genet Dev 1995; 5:249–255.
7. Chadeneau C, Hay K, Hirte HW, Gallinger S, Bacchetti S. Telomerase activity associated with acquisition of malignancy in human colorectal cancer. Cancer Res 1995; 55:2533–2536.
8. Hiyama E, Yokoyama T, Tatsumoto N, Hiyama K, Imamura Y, Murakami Y, Kodama T, Piatyszek MA, Shay JW, Matsuura Y. Telomerase activity in gastric cancer. Cancer Res 1995; 55:3258–3262.
9. Hiyama K, Hiyama E, Ishioka S, Yamakido M, Inai K, Gazdar AF, Piatyszek MA, Shay JW. Telomerase activity in small-cell and non-small-cell lung cancers [see comments]. J Natl Cancer Inst 1995; 87:895–902.
10. Hiyama E, Gollahon L, Kataoka T, Kuroi K, Yokoyama T, Gazdar AF, Hiyama K, Piatyszek MA, Shay JW. Telomerase activity in human breast tumors. J Natl Cancer Inst 1996; 88:116–122.
11. Hiyama E, Hiyama K, Yokoyama T, Matsuura Y, Piatyszek MA, Shay JW. Correlating telomerase activity levels with human neuroblastoma outcomes [see comments]. Nature Med 1995; 1:249–255.
12. Kim NW, Piatyszek MA, Prowse KR, Harley CB, West MD, Ho PL, Coviello GM, Wright WE, Weinrich SL, Shay JW. Specific association of human telomerase activity with immortal cells and cancer. Science 1994; 266:2011–2015.
13. Kyo S, Kanaya T, Ishikawa H, Ueno H, Inoue M. Telomerase activity in gynecological tumors. Clin Cancer Res 1996; 2:2023–2028.
14. Lin Y, Miyamoto H, Fujinami K, Uemura H, Hosaka M, Iwasaki Y, Kubota Y. Telomerase activity in human bladder cancer. Clin Cancer Res 1996; 2:929–932.
15. Tahara H, Kaniyasu H, Yokozaki H, Yusui W, Sahy JW, Ide T, Tahara E. Telomerase activity in preneoplastic and neoplastic gastric and colorectal lesions. Clin Cancer Res 1995; 1:1245–1251.
16. Counter CM. The roles of telomeres and telomerase in cell life span (review). Mutat Res Rev Genetic Toxicol 1996; 366:45–63.
17. Aldous WK, Grabill NR. A fluorescent method for detection of telomerase activity. Diag Mol Pathol 1997; 6:102–110.
18. Yashima K, Piatyszek MA, Saboorian HM, Virmani AK, Brown D, Shay JW, Gazdar AF.

Telomerase activity and in situ telomerase RNA expression in malignant and non-malignant lymph nodes. J Clin Pathol 1997; 50:110–117.

19. Ahrendt SA, Yang SC, Wu L, Westra WH, Jen J, Califano JA, Sidransky D. Comparison of oncogene mutation detection and telomerase activity for the molecular staging of non-small cell lung cancer. Clin Cancer Res 1997; 3:1207–1214.

20. Parker SL, Tong T, Bolden S, Wingo PA. Cancer statistics, 1997. CA 1997; 47:5–27.

21. Samet JM. The epidemiology of lung cancer. Chest 1993; 103:20S–29S.

22. Gazdar AF, Carbone DP. The Biology and Genetics of Lung Cancer. Austin: R.G. Landes Company, 1994.

23. de Lange, T. Activation of telomerase in a human tumor. Proc Natl Acad Sci USA 1994; 91:2882–2885.

24. Stamps AC, Gusterson BA, O'Hare MJ. Are tumours immortal? Eur J Cancer 1992; 28A:1495–1500.

25. Soder AI, Hoare SF, Muir S, Going JJ, Parkinson EK, Keith WN. Amplification, increased dosage and in situ expression of the telomerase RNA gene in human cancer. Oncogene 1997; 14:1013–1021.

26. Horio Y, Takahashi T, Kuroishi T, Hibi K, Suyama M, Niimi T, Shimokata K, Yamakawa K, Nakamura Y, Ueda R, et al. Prognostic significance of p53 mutations and 3p deletions in primary resected non-small cell lung cancer. Cancer Res 1993; 53:1–4.

27. Sachse R, Murakami Y, Shiraishi M, Hayashi K, Sekiya T. DNA aberrations at the retinoblastoma gene locus in human squamous cell carcinomas of the lung. Oncogene 1994; 9:39–47.

28. Shirotani Y, Hiyama K, Ishioka S, Inyaku K, Awaya Y, Yonehara S, Yoshida Y, Inai K, Hiyama E, Hasegawa K, et al. Alteration in length of telomeric repeats in lung cancer. Lung Cancer 1994; 11:29–41.

29. Hiyama K, Ishioka S, Shirotani Y, Inai K, Hiyama E, Murakami I, Isobe T, Inamizu T, Yamakido M. Alterations in telomeric repeat length in lung cancer are associated with loss of heterozygosity in p53 and Rb. Oncogene 1995; 10:937–944.

30. Travis WD, Linnoila RI, Tsokos MG, Hitchcock CL, Cutler GBJ, Nieman L, Chrousos G, Pass H, Doppman J. Neuroendocrine tumors of the lung with proposed criteria for large cell neuroendocrine carcinoma. An ultrastructural, immunohistochemical, and flow cytometric study of 35 cases. Am J Surg Pathol 1991; 15:529–553.

31. Feng J, Funk WD, Wang SS, Weinrich SL, Avilion AA, Chiu CP, Adams RR, Chang E, Allsopp RC, Yu J, et al. The RNA component of human telomerase. Science 1995 269:1236–1241.

32. Shay JW, Gazdar AF. Origins of telomerase in the early detection of cancer. J Clin Pathol 1997; 50:106–109.

33. Califano J, Ahrendt SA, Meininger G, Westra WH, Koch WM, Sidransky D. Detection of telomerase activity in oral rinses from head and neck squamous cell carcinoma patients. Cancer Res 1996; 56:5720–5722.

34. Yashima K, Litzky LA, Kaiser L, Rogers T, Lam S, Wistuba II, Milchgrub S, Srivastava S, Piatyszek MA, Shay JW, Gazdar AF. Telomerase expression in respiratory epithelium during the multistage pathogenesis of lung carcinomas. Cancer Res 1997; 57:2373–2377.

35. Saccomanno G, Archer VE, Saunders RP, Auerbach O, Klein MG. Early indices of cancer risk among uranium miners with reference to modifying factors. Ann NY Acad Sci 1976; 271:377–383.

36. Auerbach O, Hammond EC, Garfinkel L. Changes in bronchial epithelium in relation to cigarette smoking, 1955–1960 vs. 1970 1977. N Engl J Med 1979; 300:381–385.

37. Ohmura H, Tahara H, Suzuki M, Ide T, Shimizu M, Yoshida MA, Tahara E, Shay JW, Barrett JC, Oshimura M. Restoration of the cellular senescence program and repression of telomerase by human chromosome 3. Jpn J Cancer Res 1995; 86:899–904.

38. Minna JD. Neoplasms of the lung. In: Braunwald E, Isselbacher K, Petersdorf R, Wilson J, Martin J, Fauci A, eds. Neoplasms of the Lung. New York: McGraw-Hill, 1997:1221–1229.

39. Nakamura TM, Morin GB, Chapman KB, Weinrich SL, Andrews WH, Lingner J, Harley CB, Cech TR. Telomerase catalytic subunit homologs from fission yeast and human. Science 1997; 277:955–959.

17

Clonal Development of Lung Cancer

GRACE CHUNG

MRC Laboratory of Molecular Biology
Cambridge, England

PAMELA RABBITTS

University of Cambridge
Cambridge, England

I. Introduction

The microscopic examination of the morphological appearance of fully developed epithelial tumors often reveals the coexistence of various cell types, sometimes representing different histological subtypes of a particular tumor. These variants could represent different stages in the evolution of a tumor which originally developed following a change in a single cell, or they could have arisen in parallel but independently. Evidence to support the clonal theory of tumor development has been provided by cytogenetic studies of many primary tumors in which all cells showed the same abnormal karyotype, suggesting a unicellular origin (1). In addition, studies of isoenzymes of glucose-6-phosphatase dehydrogenase (G-6-PD) in a number of tumors in heterozygous women showed that the same allele on the X chromosome is functional in all the cells of the tumor, indicating that they were descended from a single precursor cell (2).

Although it has been demonstrated that many human tumors are monoclonal, cancer may develop in several different sites simultaneously (multicentric). The evidence for this is again from G-6-PD studies; for example, heterozygosity has been detected in inherited neurofibromatosis (3) and in tumors due to viral infection such as condyloma acuminata (4). More recently, analysis of p53 mutations occurring in multiple lesions in head and neck cancer, both synchronously and sequentially, has indicated discordance with respect to mutation, suggesting the distinct lesions are of different clonal origin (5,6). Those cancers that show evidence of multiple-arising tumors are characterized by exposure of the whole tissue at risk to a carcinogen— the "field of cancerization" either chemical, viral or genetic in the form of inherited predisposition. Nonetheless, the development of multicentric tumors is not mandatory in these circumstances: multifocal bladder tumors, for example, arise in an epithelial sheet undergoing carcinogen exposure, but the separate foci are clonally related (7). Similarly, there are examples of virus-associated tumors and "inherited" cancers which are clonal.

II. Lung Tumors

Lung cancer is often described as multifocal, not so much because fully malignant tumors are detected synchronously, but more because preinvasive bronchial lesions, which are believed to be the preneoplastic stage of the disease, are found in association with invasive tumors (8–10). Since lung cancers of the common histologies are known to be initiated following prolonged carcinogen exposure, particularly to cigarette smoke, then the multifocal lesions could arise independently due to field cancerization or they could be clonally related, although this requires that cells from the original initiating clone can migrate throughout the lung to seed other distinct and distant bronchial lesions.

Lung tumors are characterized by consistent genetic abnormalities including activation or overexpression of oncogenes and inactivation of tumor suppressor genes. These include changes in the p53, Rb, and p16/MTS genes and several chromosomal regions including 3p12–14, 3p21.3, and 3p25 (11). Many of these genetic changes have also been detected in preinvasive lesions providing the opportunity to compare the genotype of dysplasias and tumor from the same patient and thus to predict the likely clonal relationship of physically distinct lesions. Several studies have compared loss of alleles on chromosome 3 in tumors (squamous cell carcinomas) and the corresponding adjacent preinvasive lesions and have shown the same pattern of allele loss (12–14). The study of Hung et al. is of particular importance as it compared the pattern of 3p allele loss in hyperplasias, dysplasias, and tumors (mainly adenocarcinomas) occurring in different lobes of the lung and found the same pattern of allele loss even in distant lesions (Fig. 1) (14). This observation, termed allele-specific loss, has been noted by the same group following studies of LOH on chromosome 9 (15). One explanation of these observations of damage of the same chromosomal homolog in distant lesions is that the lesions are clonally related, although other explanations, such as genome imprinting are possible.

Allele loss is not an ideal marker of clonality. However, in some dysplasia/ tumor comparisons it has been possible to follow the occurrence of a p53 mutation. At least 70 point mutations in the p53 gene have been found to occur in lung tumors, thus the finding of the same mutation in distinct tumors and dyplasias is unlikely to

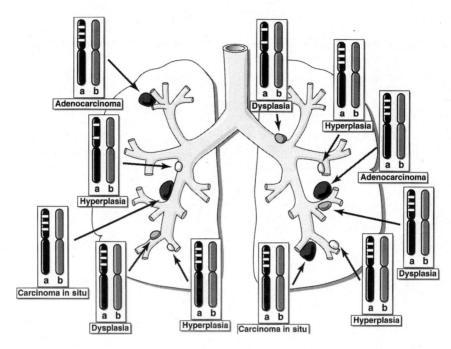

Figure 1 Deletions in the short arm of chromosome 3 in multiple lesions throughout the respiratory epithelium. Note that all lesions demonstrated allelic loss from the same homolog (a).

be a chance event and is more likely to be due to a clonal relationship. We have studied a patient with tumor, dysplasia, and squamous metaplasia and shown that a few of the cells in the squamous metaplasia carried the same p53 mutation that was prevalent throughout the dysplasia and tumor (Fig. 2) (16). Our interpretation is that within the squamous metaplasia a p53 mutation arose in one cell, which provided a growth advantage and resulted in a small clone of cells, one of which accrued further genetic changes resulting in the appearance of dysplasia and then invasive tumor. Even when preinvasive lesions throughout the lung have been examined, the same p53 mutation has been detected (W. Franklin, personal communication).

However, not all genetic analyses of physically distinct lesions has identified the same pattern of genetic damage. Multicentric development is supported by a study by Sozzi et al. of five patients with multiple lesions in their bronchial tree (17). Loss of different alleles on chromosome 3p and different mutations in the p53 and K-ras genes was observed in the lung tumors and preneoplastic lesions from the same patient. One example is shown in Figure 3. Multiclonal origin was also found in a study of bronchioloalveolar lung carcinomas (18). This was demonstrated following polymerase chain reaction amplification of a region within the first intron of the human hypoxanthine phosphoribosyltransferase gene, which contains the inac-

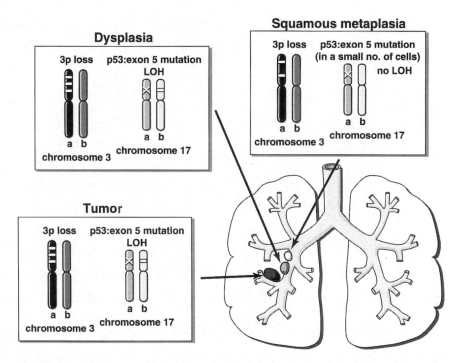

Figure 2 Loss of 3p alleles and p53 mutation were present in squamous metaplasia, dysplasia, and tumors adjacent to each other. The same allele was lost in all three lesions, indicating the same homolog (a) was involved. In addition, the same p53 mutation was identified in all three lesions. LOH of the same allele was present in dysplasia and tumor, but no LOH was observed in squamous metaplasia.

tive X chromosome obligately methylated HpaII/MspI sites. Analysis of three bronchioloalveolar lung carcinomas revealed the presence of different alleles in different loci within the same case. Lung cancers arise from cells within a large epithelial sheet chronically exposed to carcinogen. Thus the observation of different genetic changes in different lesions is not unexpected. It is much more difficult to explain the observation of the same genetic change in physically distinct lesions. Nonetheless, this pattern has been observed in studies from several independent laboratories. One possible explanation is that the physically distinct lesions are clonally related, but as mentioned above this would require an unexpected fluidity of the bronchial epithelium, or at least of those cells in which the initial genetic damage occurs.

III. Implications for the Early Detection of Lung Cancer

Understanding the relationship between preinvasive bronchial lesions and invasive tumors is crucial for early disease detection and chemoprevention. Therefore, the

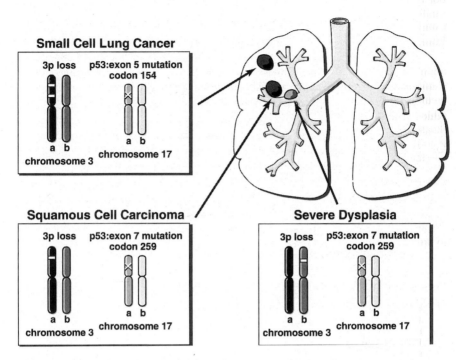

Figure 3 In a patient with small-cell lung cancer, squamous cell carcinoma, and severe dysplasia, different p53 mutation as well as loss of allele from different chromosome 3 homolog was observed. 3p loss involving homolog (b) was found in severe dysplasia while loss involving homolog (a) was observed in squamous cell carcinoma. Moreover, in the small-cell lung tumor, p53 mutation was at codon 154 while in squamous metaplasia and severe dysplasia, the mutation was at codon 259.

elucidation of the meaning of field cancerization and clonal evolution and its implications represents an important area in carcinogenesis research. Lung tumors (particularly squamous cell carcinomas) develop through a series of histological recognizable preneoplastic lesions, and the expectation is that the detection of genetic damage should identify those patients with preneoplastic foci that have not yet advanced to invasive cancer (19). Some small preliminary studies indicate that this might be possible. Retrospective studies of patients with lung cancer who had sputum samples collected before the clinical diagnosis of their tumor identified the same mutation in both the tumor sample and sputum sample obtained before the diagnosis of cancer (20). In one case, this was a year before a confirmed diagnosis. This implies that a clonal population of cancer or precancerous cells was already present in the bronchial epithelium.

The recently identified genetic abnormality, microsatellite instability, has been reported to occur in many cancers including lung cancer (21). Current evidence suggests that these alterations probably arise in transformed cells as a replication error during cell division and they are then propagated to daughter cells so that they harbor the same genetic events that provides a growth advantage. When these microsatellite alterations are used as a marker to screen patients' lung tumor and sputum samples, the same altered microsatellite pattern was found in both samples (22). Similar results were observed in histopathologically negative surgical margins.

Both the tumor and the resection margin share the same microsatellite alteration, with the alteration in the resection margin at a lower intensity, indicating only a small fraction of cells were indeed cancerous. These studies demonstrate that molecular genetic techniques can identify the presence of tumor cells in situations in which conventional pathological approaches have been ineffective and therefore indicate future strategies for the early detection of lung cancer. However, if the hope is to detect preneoplastic lesions, rather than early invasive tumors, then a full understanding of the relationship between dysplasia and tumor is required.

Acknowledgments

We are very grateful to Dr. Gabriella Sozzi and Professor Adi Gazdar for permission to construct figures based on their published results.

References

1. Sandberg AA, Hossfeld DK. Chromosomal abnormalities in human neoplasia. Ann Rev Med 1970; 21:379–408.
2. Fialkow PJ. The origin and development of human tumors studied with cell markers. N Engl J Med 1974; 291:26–35.
3. Fialkow PJ, Sagebiel RW, Gartler SM, Rimoin DL. Multiple cell of origin of hereditary neurofibromas N Engl J Med 1971; 284:298–300.
4. Friedman JM, Fialkow PJ. Viral tumorigenesis in man: cell markers in condylomata acuminata. Int J Cancer 1976; 17:57–61.
5. Chung KY, Mukhopadhyay T, Kim J, Casson A, Ro JY, Goepfert H, Hong WK, Roth JA. Discordant p53 gene mutations in primary head and neck and corresponding secondary primary cancer of the upper aerodigestive tract. Cancer Res 1993; 53:1676–1683.
6. Nees M, Homann N, Discher H, Andl T, Enders C, Herold-Mende C, Svhuhmann A, Bosch FX. Expression of mutated p53 occurs in human-distant epithelia of head and neck cancer patients: A possible molecular basis for the development of multiple tumors. Cancer Res 1993; 53:4189–4196.
7. Sidransky D, Frost P, Von Eschenbach AV, Oyasu R, Preisinger AC, Vogelstein B. Clonal origin of bladder cancer. N Engl J Med 1992; 326:737–740.
8. Auerbach O, Gere JB, Forman JB, Petrick TG, Smolin HJ, Merhsam GE, Kassouny DY, Stout AP. Changes in the bronchial epithelium in relation to smoking and cancer of the lung. N Engl J Med 1957; 256:97–104.
9. Auerbach O, Stout AP, Hammond EC, Garfinkel L. Changes in bronchial epithelium in relation to sex, age residence, smoking and pneumonia. N Engl J Med 1962; 267:111–119.
10. Auerbach O, Hammond EC, Garfinkel L. Changes in bronchial epithelium in relation to cigarette smoking. N Engl J Med 1979; 300:381–386.
11. Minna J. The molecular biology of lung cancer pathogenesis. Chest 1993; 103:449S–456S.
12. Sundaresan V, Ganly P, Hasleton P, Rudd R, Sinha G, Bleehen NM, Rabbitts P. p53 and chro-

mosome 3 abnormalities, characteristic of malignant lung tumours, are detectable in preinvasive lesions of the bronchus. Oncogene 1992; 7:1989–1997.

13. Chung GTY, Sundaresan V, Hasleton P, Rudd R, Taylor R, Rabbitts PH. Sequential molecular genetic changes in lung cancer development. Oncogene 1995; 11:2591–2598.
14. Hung J, Kishimoto Y, Sugio K, Virmani A, McIntire DD Minna JD, Gazdar AF. Allele-specific chromosome 3p deletions occur at an early stage in the pathogenesis of lung carcinoma. JAMA 1995; 273:558–563.
15. Kishimoto Y, Sugio K, Hung JY, Virmani AK, McIntire DD, Minna JD, Gazdar AF. Allele-specific loss in chromosome 9p loci in preneoplastic lesions accompanying non-small-cell lung cancers. J Natl Cancer Inst 1995; 87:1224–1229.
16. Chung GTY, Sundaresan V, Hasleton P, Rudd R, Taylor R, Rabbitts PH. Clonal evolution of lung tumors. Cancer Res 1996; 56:1609–1614.
17. Sozzi G, Miozzo M, Pastorino U, Pilotti S, Donghi D, Giarola M, De Gregorio L, Manenti G, Radice P, Minoletti F, Della Porta G, Pierotti MA. Genetic evidence for an independent origin of multiple preneoplastic and neoplastic lung lesions. Cancer Res 1995; 55:135–140.
18. Barsky SH, Grossmann DA, Ho J, Holmes EC. The multifocality of bronchioloalveolar lung carcinoma: evidence and implications of a multiclonal origin. Modern Pathol 1994; 7:633–640.
19. Sidransky D. Molecular screening-how long can we afford to wait? JNCI 1994; 86:955–956.
20. Mao L, Hruban RH, Boyle JO, Tockman M, Sidransky D. Detection of oncogene mutations in sputum precedes diagnosis of lung cancer. Cancer Res 1994; 54:1634–1637.
21. Mao L, Lee DJ, Tockman MS, Erosan YS, Askin F, Sidransky D. Microsatellite alterations as clonal markers for the detection of human cancer. Proc Natl Acad Sci 1994; 91:9871–9875.
22. Chen XQ, Stroun M, Magnenat, J-L, Nicod LP, Kurt A-M, Lyautey J, Lederrey C, Anker P. Microsatellite alterations in plasma DNA of small cell lung cancer patients. Nature Med 1996; 2:1033

18

Selection and Validation of New Lung Cancer Markers for the Molecular-Pathological Assessment of Individuals with a High Risk of Developing Lung Cancer

J. K. FIELD

Roy Castle International Centre for Lung Cancer Research
and The University of Liverpool
Liverpool, England

Lung cancer is one of the most prevalent malignancies in the world (1) but is one of the most preventable cancers if the primary prevention measure of reducing tobacco smoking were successful. However, even if smoking cessation was immediate in the population, lung cancer would remain as a major problem for at least the next two decades, as half of all lung cancers in the western world develop in former smokers (1). To date, none of the lung cancer screening and early detection procedures using cytology, radiology, or serum markers have been successful in reducing mortality (2–4).

In the last decade there has been a dramatic increase in our understanding of the molecular genetics of lung cancer, especially in our knowledge of the molecular events leading to the progression of the disease from genetically normal tissue through preneoplastic stages to neoplasia. These developments require a major paradigm shift in research endeavor toward the development of early detection and intervention strategies. Rapid and reproducible methods for the unambiguous detection of molecular lesions in lung cancer at an early stage could have great impact on the survival and treatment of lung cancer patients.

Carcinogenesis of the lung is a multistep process involving multiple genetic changes that may include genetic instability due to DNA mismatch repair defects, activation or overexpression of oncogenes, and loss or inactivation of tumor sup-

287

Table 1   Potential Markers for Early Detection of Lung Cancer

Morphological changes of cells (digital analysis)
Abnormal expression of proteins (e.g., p53, hnRNP, EGFR)
Oncogene activation, mutations in tumor suppressor genes (e.g., *p53, ras, myc,* cyclins)
Genetic instability (e.g., LOH, microsatellite alterations)
Differentiation/maturation, markers (e.g., telomerase, retinoic acid receptor)
Others (i.e., abnormal methylation, markers of apoptosis)

pressor genes. It is unclear whether these events are part of a common pathway toward cancer or if the genetic aberrations are unique to a particular carcinogen. It is unlikely that any one genetic abnormality will have sufficient sensitivity and specificity to identify individuals at risk of developing lung cancer, thus it is more appropriate that a panel of markers that represent different stages and carcinogenic pathways are used in developing a risk-assessment model. The markers currently considered to contribute to the progression of lung cancer are given in Table 1. In this chapter the most promising early detection markers will be discussed with recent supporting evidence from patients and those considered to be at high risk for developing the disease in the Liverpool region. A number of other candidate markers which may be considered as early detection markers but await evaluation in sputum and bronchial lavage are discussed in detail by other authors in this book.

The way to verify the value of these early detection markers is in a large population-based study containing archived, serially collected samples from individuals who are considered to be at risk of developing lung cancer. Concomitant to the serial collection of sputum and blood samples, an in-depth epidemiological study should be undertaken to identify the lifestyle risk factors (i.e., smoking history, occupation, exposure to carcinogens, family history of cancer, diet). In addition, this population study should be underpinned with a genotype analysis of at-risk individuals in order to identify subpopulations with a genetic susceptibility to lung cancer. All of these elements are being incorporated into the Liverpool Lung Project (LLP), which will be outlined in the final section of this chapter.

I.   *ras* Gene Mutations in Lung Cancer

The *ras* family of oncogenes include three closely related genes: H-*ras*, N-*ras*, and K-*ras*. These genes encode highly conserved 21 kDa proteins that functionally resemble G-proteins and appear to be involved in signal transduction and cell cycle control. To date, mutations in these genes have been the most frequently observed genetic lesions in a number of human malignancies (5).

In lung cancer members of the *ras* oncogene family are considered to be one of the candidate target genes. In a study of *ras* mutations in 141 adenocarcinoma samples from smokers, 41 tested positive for a point mutation in codon 12 for Ki-*ras*, whereas only two of 40 nonsmokers had a mutation at this site (6). In a study of *ras* mutations in 66 non–small-cell lung cancers (NSCLC), 20% were found to have K-*ras* mutations in codons 12 or 61 and the majority were found in squamous cell carcinomas (8/38) compared to adenocarcinomas (3/22). The most common substitution was from glycine to valine in a large study on 173 lung tumors (7), and it is of note that this showed a strong trend ($p = 0.07$) towards a poorer prognosis compared to other amino acid substitutions. In contrast, substitution of the wild-type glycine for aspartate showed a strong trend ($p = 0.06$) for a better outcome. These results indicate that the prognostic significance of *ras* mutations may be amino acid substitution dependent on the p21 protein. A number of groups have found a correlation between K-*ras* point mutations and a poor clinical outcome (8–10). Li et al. (11) consider K-*ras* mutations to be a early event in the development of adenocarcinomas, however, Sugio et al. (9) found few K-*ras* mutations in dysplastic lesions.

We have investigated mutations in the Ki-*ras* gene in bronchial carcinomas using a PCR-RFLP detection system and a PCR-based ARMS (amplification refractory mutation system) assay (12). In particular, the ARMS assay allows the specific detection of rare mutant sequences in a background of normal DNA (i.e., 1 in 1000–2000). ARMS employs the powerful discriminatory potential of PCR amplification from primers modified at the 3′ end such that extension from nonmatched templates is essentially eliminated under appropriate conditions. ARMS analysis can be used for Ki-*ras* mutation detection, and since the relevant mutational spectrum is limited, the procedure requires either a general PCR multiplex for "broad" Ki-*ras* mutations or a relatively few single tests to pinpoint exactly which mutation may be present. We have demonstrated mutations in 25% of our current database of adenocarcinomas using both PCR-RFLP and the ARMS techniques, and although both showed mutations in the same group of tumors, the ARMS assay specified the actual Ki-*ras* 12 mutations (13). Other K-*ras* mutation assays under development such as the PCR/ligase chain reaction assay (14) have the advantage of potential multiplex assay of multiple base changes in a single codon.

Ras and *p53* mutations have been identified in sputum specimens from patients well in advance of clinical malignancy in a pilot study using samples from the Johns Hopkins Lung Project (15). An identical mutation in *ras* or *p53* genes was identified initially in the primary tumor and then identified in a previous sputum from these patients taken prior to clinical diagnosis of lung cancer. These results were one of the first to demonstrate the power of molecular biology techniques in identifying genetic aberrations in individuals who are progressing to clinical lung cancer.

II. Cytogenetic Analysis

A range of genetic changes at the chromosomal level have been identified in lung tumor specimens and in cell lines derived from human lung tumors. An extensive cytogenetic analysis of 63 non–small-cell lung carcinomas was undertaken by Tesa et al. (16), who found loss of chromosomes 13 and 9 to be the most frequent changes

(71% and 65%, respectively). A gain on chromosome 7 was seen in 41% of cases. The chromosome arms that most frequently had losses were 9p (in 79% of cases), 3p, 6q, 8p, 9q, 13q, 17p, 18q, 19p, 21q, 22q, and the short arm of the acrocentric chromosomes. In addition, chromosomal rearrangements were found on 1p, 1q, 3p, 3q, 6q, 7, 9p, 11, 17p, and 19q.

III. Allelic Imbalance

Allelic imbalance or loss of heterozygosity (LOH) has been widely used to assess genetic changes and has been used primarily to identify regions on specific chromosomes that contain putative tumor suppressor genes. Loss of heterozygosity studies on NSCLC tumors have demonstrated that certain chromosomal regions, in particular 3p, 5p, 9p, and 17p, are involved in the development of these tumors (17–21), and these sites may represent novel tumor suppressor genes as well as confirming the role of a number of previously identified tumor suppressor genes in this disease. A number of allelotype analyses have been undertaken in lung and head and neck cancers (22–26). Two previous allelotype analyses of NSCLC using restriction fragment length polymorphism (RFLP) markers have demonstrated LOH on chromosome arms 3, 9, and 17 and less frequently on chromosome arms; 1q, 2q, 5q, 8q, 9q, 10q, 13q, 18p, 19q, and 21q. In an allelotype analysis we have undertaken with 45 NSCLC specimens using 92 polymorphic microsatellite markers (27), we provided evidence of genetic imbalance on the majority of the chromosome arms, which is in general agreement with the previous allelotype analysis using RFLP analysis by Tsuchiya et al. (22) and Sato et al. (23), especially on 3p, 9p, and 17p. The results of this study provided evidence for the presence of a novel tumor suppressor gene on 9p at 9p23 (D9S157), (28).

The role of allelic imbalance on the short arms of chromosomes 3, 9, and 17 in NSCLC has received a great deal of attention, and it has been proposed that these events are associated with the early stages of pathogenesis of these tumors (17–21). In these studies, a small number of dysplastic and neoplastic tissues from the same patient were investigated in great detail by performing microdissection of the specimens. All of the six paired dysplastic and tumor tissue specimens investigated by Sundaresan et al. (17) showed allelic imbalance on 3p, and, similarly, Hung et al. (19) found that six of the seven patients examined with paired preneoplastic and neoplastic lesions showed loss on 3p. Kishimoto et al. (20) also reported similar findings of LOH on 9p in the same specimens. Thiberville et al. (21) have investigated LOH with a number of microsatellite markers on 3p, 5q, and 9p in 13 patients, demonstrating progressive stages of bronchial carcinoma. Their results indicate that the corresponding genetic alterations in the dysplastic samples are often found in the invasive carcinomas in the same patients. These results raise the question as to whether all NSCLC have allelic imbalance on 3p and 9p as their initiating events. We addressed this hypothesis by examining allelic imbalance at 3p, 9p, and 17p in 45 NSCLC specimens for which a FAL value had been previously calculated.

Table 2 Loss of Heterozygosity on 3p, 9p, and 17p in NSCLC Correlates with a High FAL (HFAL) Value

	LFAL	MFAL	HFAL	Total
3p	3/14 (21%)	2/16 (13%)	12/15 (80%)[a]	17/45 (38%)
9p	2/14 (13%)	12/16 (75%)	12/15 (80%)[b]	26/45 (58%)
17p	1/14 (7%)	5/16 (35%)	11/15 (73%)[c]	17/45 (38%)

[a] $p = 0.002$ LFAL compared with HFAL.
[b] $p = 0.0006$ LFAL compared with HFAL.
[c] $p = 0.0004$ LFAL compared with HFAL.
Source: Ref. 29.

We reexamined the LOH data for the 45 NSCLC specimens on the basis of their FAL scores. FAL values were calculated for all of these tumors and found to have a median of 0.09 (range 0.00–0.45) (29). Fractional allele loss (FAL) has been calculated for each tumor:

$$FAL = \frac{\text{Number of chromosome arms showing LOH}}{\text{Number of informative chromosome arms}}$$

No clinical correlations were found in these NSCLC between the tumor stage or histopathology grading and FAL. The tumors were subdivided into low FAL (LFAL, 0.00–0.04), medium FAL (MFAL, 0.05–0.13), and high FAL (HFAL 0.14–0.45) groups (29). Thirty-eight percent LOH was observed on 3p using 9 markers, 58% on 9p using 15 markers, and 38% on 17p using 5 markers, and a median FAL value of 0.09 was obtained in the 45 NSCLC studied. Tumors with HFAL values showed a very clear polarization of the LOH data on chromosome arms 3p, 9p, and 17p such that 80% showed loss on 3p, 80% on 9p, and 73% on 17p (Table 2, Fig. 1). These incidences of LOH were significantly higher than would be expected since overall genetic instability in these HFAL tumors ranged from 14 to 45% LOH. Nine of the 14 patients in the LFAL group were found to have no LOH on 3p, 9p, or 17p, but 5 of these had LOH at other sites: 5p, 5q, 8p, 13q, 16q, and 19q. These results indicate that LFAL patients form a new subset of NSCLC tumors with distinct molecular initiating events and may represent a discrete genetic population (Fig. 2).

IV. Genomic Instability

Genomic instability is now considered to be a hallmark of cancer. Analysis of microsatellite markers in tumor tissue compared to its normal counterpart has become the most widely used method to determine genomic instability in the form of microsatellite alterations (MA) or LOH (30–34). Genomic instability has been found in 42–49% of NSCLC (27–35). We have now studied 90 bronchial lavage specimens from individuals with suspected lung cancer. Genomic instability was found in 15

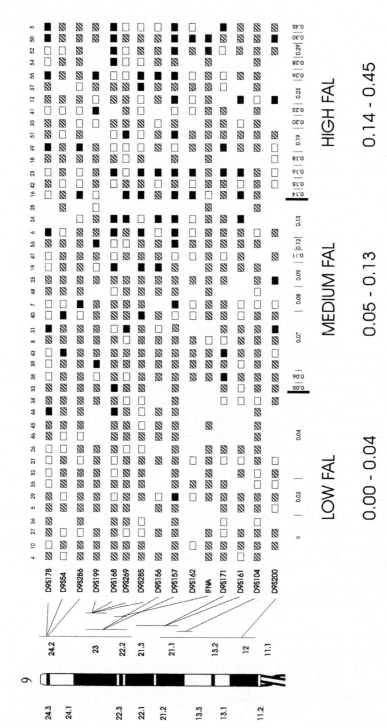

Figure 1 Loss of heterozygosity in 9p correlates with high FAL values in non–small-cell lung cancer. ■, Loss of heterozygosity; ▨, heterozygous; □ homozygous. (From Ref. 29.)

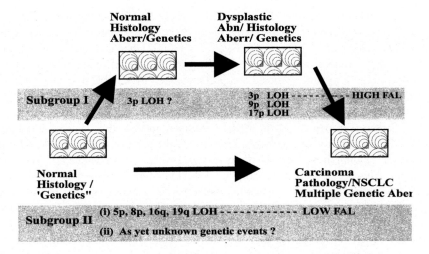

Figure 2 FAL subgroups determine development of NSCLC? The LFAL patients form a new subset of NSCLC tumors with distinct molecular initiating events and may represent a discrete genetic population from the patient's tumor with HFAL values.

of 43 (35%) patients with lung cancer, however, it was also found in 11 of 47 (23%) patients with no cytological or radiological evidence of bronchial neoplasia (Field et al., unpublished). No significant differences were found between the referring symptoms in any of the individuals with and without genomic instability. Thus, microsatellite alterations provides a powerful new technique by which to identify individuals who may potentially develop lung cancer, however, a large prospective study is required to substantiate these results.

V. *p53* Gene Mutations

The *p53* gene has been found to be mutated in a large range of human tumors (37,38). Many international research groups have contributed to the identification of *p53* mutations and in a number of cases have correlated the presence of *p53* mutations with stage, histology, prognosis, and exposure to certain environmental agents. Mutagens can produce specific base substitutions at certain sites, and a mutation spectrum analysis may provide information about the origins of mutations that give rise to human tumors. Lung tumors have been shown to contain various genetic aberrations within the *p53* gene, including point mutations, insertions, deletions, and loss of heterozygosity at the TP53 locus (39–47). With respect to point mutations, GC→TA transversions have been shown to occur more frequently in smokers than in nonsmokers with lung cancer and may be the result of specific carcinogenic agents present in tobacco smoke, like benzo(*a*)pyrene (37,49,50).

In a recent study into *p53* gene aberrations in NSCLC in patients in the Liverpool area, we found that 28% of the tumors contained mutations in the *p53* gene (51). This incidence is significantly lower ($p < 0.0002$) than that reported in a major review of *p53* mutations in 897 lung cancer patients with *p53* mutations who have smoked (37). Our results indicate that *p53* mutations in NSCLC may be caused by carcinogens other than those found in tobacco smoke. This may account for the population-specific mutation spectrum.

Sixty-seven percent of the NSCLC samples in this study demonstrated *p53* positive staining. It is of note that all but one of the patient's tumors with *p53* mutations, excluding those with insertions or deletions, also demonstrated *p53*-positive staining. This provides further evidence for the hypothesis that there is an increased *p53* gene product in tumors containing mutations in the *p53* gene. The positive *p53* staining is considered to represent stable *p53* protein overexpression which results from posttranslational modification and/or p53 protein complexing. However, there are also NSCLC tumors that demonstrated *p53*-positive staining but in which no mutations were found. These differences between molecular and immunohistochemical results may be explained by the possibility that there are mutations in the *p53* gene outside exons 4–9; within the *p53* promoter region or that overexpression of *p53* is not only due to *p53* mutations but also to some other factors (e.g., mdm2), which binds to the p53 protein and thus increases its half-life. Furthermore, it may be argued that the DO-1 antibody which was used in this study may also detect a stable conformationally altered wild-type p53 protein, which in its own right may lead to genetic instability without an initial *p53* mutation.

In contrast with most previous reports, we have found a prevalence of GC→AT transitions (37.5% of all mutations) instead of GC→TA transversions (12.5%), which would be expected from a smoking population. Comparison of the ratio GC→TA:GC→AT in this study and Greenblatt's review showed a significant difference ($p = 0.04$) (Fig. 3). Husgafvel-Pursiainen et al. (50) reviewed the mutational profile in smokers and ex-smokers among lung cancer patients and found that 34% of the *p53* mutations were G→T base substitutions. In our study of individuals in the northwest of England, only 18% of the smokers had G→T transversions. Findings similar to our own have been reported in NSCLC patients from Taiwan, where G→T mutations were found to comprise only 6% of the *p53* mutations detected in a population sample which consisted of 61% smokers (52). GC→TA transversions have been attributed to the action of benzo(*a*)pyrene, a member of the polycyclic aromatic hydrocarbons, which represent the major carcinogens found in tobacco smoke. However, other carcinogens like 4-(methylnitrosamino)-1-(3-pyridyl)-1–butanone (NNK) cause GC→AT transitions and GC→TA transversions at CpG and non-CpG sites, depending on the experimental system used (53). Tobacco smoke is a complex mixture of compounds, and the mutational spectrum it causes needs further investigation (54). So it remains unclear if the prevalence of GC→AT transitions found in the smoking population in the Liverpool area is a paradox or not. It is possible that rather than one factor acting alone, a synergism of one or many environmental components may exist.

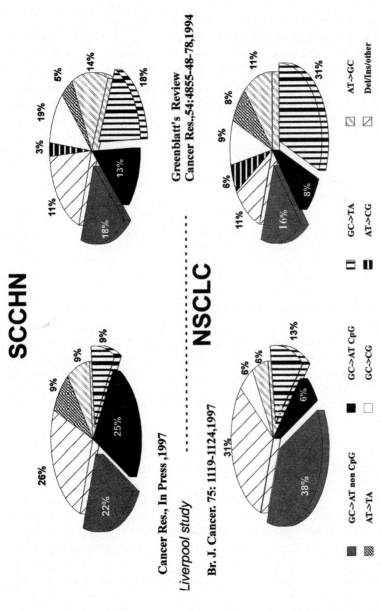

Figure 3 p53 Mutational profile in SCCHN and NSCLC patients' tumors in the northwest of England. All of these patients were smokers apart from one SCCHN individual. It is of note that both groups have a higher percentage of G∶A transition than previously reported.

It is of particular note that we have examined the *p53* mutational profile of 65 squamous cell carcinomas (SCCHN) from patients also living in northwest England (55). Twenty-three *p53* mutations were detected in 20 samples (31%), and GC→AT transitions were the predominant type of mutations (Fig. 3). Thus the *p53* mutational profile of SCCHN tumors was similar to that found in the non–small-cell lung tumors from patients within the same geographical area, supporting the concept of a common model for carcinogenesis in the upper aerorespiratory tract in the Liverpol region (Fig. 3). The incidence of *p53* mutations among present and former SCCHN smokers was significantly higher than in nonsmokers ($p < 0.02$). In the SCCHN study, we demonstrated that the *p53* mutations were found to predominate in a group of patients with low genetic damage, as indicated by the fractional allelic loss (FAL) value. These findings suggest an early initiating role for *p53* and imply that at least two separate carcinogenic pathways may be involved in the development of SCCHN.

No correlation was found between the presence of mutations and the stage of tumor, indicating that *p53* mutations may be considered to play a role in the early development of lung cancer. It is probable that these tumors may carry additional alterations in genes that function as oncogenes or tumor-suppressor genes, indeed, the allelotype study for this set of tumors showed a median FAL value of 0.09, indicating allelic imbalance throughout the genome (27). In particular, LOH at the TP53 locus, as shown in this study, was found in 25% of these tumors. It is of note that only 2 out of 10 samples with LOH at TP53 were found to contain a mutation in *p53*, implying that another candidate tumor-suppressor gene may also exist at this locus.

The role of *p53* in the early development of lung cancer is still unclear; however, there is a compelling body of evidence that indicated that this gene plays a very important role in lung cancer, and this warrants its inclusion in an early detection program. Initially it is more appropriate to assess *p53* expression immunohistochemically in sputum and bronchial lavage samples, but with the advent of biochip technology it will be feasible to undertake mutational profiling of *p53* in these specimens.

VI. hnRNP Overexpression in Sputum Specimens

The 31 kDa protein has been characterized as homologous to the pre-mRNA binding heterogeneous nuclear ribonuclear protein, hnRNP A2/B1 (56). These RNA-binding proteins are responsible for the posttranscriptional regulation of gene expression by capping, splicing, polyadenylation, and cytoplasmic transportation of mRNAs (57).

A particularly informative lung cancer screening trial was undertaken using immunohistochemical analysis of sputum samples using antibody to p31kD protein antigen of NSCLC (58–60). Immunostaining specimens from patients who had known clinical outcomes was 90% accurate in predicting those that would develop lung cancer. The earliest epitope expression was detected among serial specimens that were collected approximately 2 years before the clinical appearance of the disease. These results have been replicated in exfoliated sputum specimens from underground miners who subsequently developed lung cancer in China (Tockman et al., unpublished).

These studies support the use of quantitative monoclonal antibody binding as a supplement to cytomorphology in distinguishing precancer epithelial cells from individuals who develop lung cancer from normal specimens with an accuracy exceeding that commonly used in PSA cancer-screening tests (61).

VII. Genetic Predisposition

The development of risk-assessment markers is now being considered as a way of identifying populations who are at risk of developing cancer. We are constantly exposed to chemical carcinogens, but only a small proportion of even those with the highest exposure (i.e., smokers) develop lung cancer. Several enzymes have been put forward as being critical in determining an individual's risk of contracting lung cancer, and, as might be expected, they are associated with the metabolism of xenobiotics.

Cytochrome P450s are a superfamily of oxidizing enzymes, the majority of which are involved in the metabolism of xenobiotics (62). Their principal function is to convert xenobiotics into derivatives that can be more easily excreted from the body.

CYP2D6 is associated with the oxidation of a wide range of therapeutic drugs. A polymorphism at the CYP2D6 gene locus has been shown to have a significant effect on the rate of metabolism of many drugs. Ayesh et al. (63) showed a strong association between this CYP2D6 polymorphism and reduced lung cancer susceptibility. This work has been supported by other studies, summarized by Wolf et al. (64), who concluded that among lung cancer patients there is approximately a 4% prevalence of poor metabolizers. In the general population this figure would be around 8%. The glutathione-S-transferase (GST) family is a group of multifunctional proteins; one of their major roles is to catalyze the conjugation of electrophilic compounds to glutathione (GSH). GST1 or GSTM1, the best characterized GST, belongs to the Mu subgroup. Approximately 40–50% of the population are deficient in this enzyme (65), shown to be due to a homozygous nulled GST1 gene (66). Being deficient in a major detoxification pathway is likely to increase the risk of carcinogenesis. Kihara et al. (67) showed that the lung cancer risk of those with a GSTM1 null phenotype is dependent on the extent of tobacco exposure but that the proportion of patients with GSTM1 null phenotype increases progressively in the squamous cell carcinoma group.

The relative risk of individuals with a combination of both a homozygous rare allele of CYP1A1 and a nulled GST1 was "remarkably high" at 5.8 for lung cancer and 9.1 for squamous cell carcinoma compared with other combinations of genotypes (68). However, the role of genetic susceptibility remains somewhat controversial. (69).

VIII. Liverpool Lung Project

To test the potential markers for assessing individuals at risk in a population-based study, we set up the Liverpool Lung Project (LLP). The highest incidence rates of lung cancer for both men and women are found in the Merseyside region of the northwest of England. In the Liverpool area the cumulative rate (0–74 years) in 1989–1993 was 12.5% for males and 6.0% for females compared with a national average of 7.3% for males and 3.0% for females in 1991. Furthermore, the rate for females is increasing at a faster rate than nationally and has now exceeded the incidence rate for breast cancer in Liverpool. The incidence rate in males is also not showing the same decline as nationally. Detection of lung cancer usually occurs late in the disease when it is beyond effective treatment, consequently, there is a high mortality rate and a 5-year overall survival rate of 6% in Merseyside. The Liverpool Lung Project, funded by the Roy Castle Foundation, will use risk factors identified by molecular genetics and epidemiology to define populations and individuals most at risk of developing lung cancer.

We are proposing a 10-year prospective cohort study to investigate three specific groups of high-risk patients: (1) patients referred to the two Lung Cancer Early Diagnosis Clinics in Liverpool, (2) individuals with a high risk of developing lung cancer from "high-incidence" GP practices' in the Liverpool region, and (3) patients at a high risk of second primary lung cancer (SPLC), postsurgery for complete bronchial resection of NSCLC, stage $T_{1,2} N_0$. Individuals who have been recruited into the Liverpool Lung Project will have an in-depth epidemiological interview using a structured questionnaire, plus blood and sputum sampling. Patients will be recalled annually for sputum sampling over a 10-year follow-up period. We plan to analyze the sputum/bronchial lavage specimens using a range of the molecular pathological techniques outlined in Table 1. It is unlikely that any single molecular-pathological marker will have the predictive power to identify at-risk individuals, thus algorithms on panels of these markers will have to be developed and validated in the Liverpool Lung Project. In addition, we are undertaking a case-control study, which will include patients diagnosed as having lung cancer to study risk factors in lung cancer. Two controls per case matched for age and gender will be selected from the registers of the GP practice nearest to the case address. Cases and controls will be interviewed in the same way as patients entered into the cohort study.

The uniqueness of this study is the combined approach of using both molecular and epidemiological techniques to assess the progression of lung cancer over a 10-year period. This will enable us to develop a risk-assessment model based on the data. In conjunction with the early-detection program an intervention strategy will be developed since there is a need to develop a noninvasive intervention therapy appropriate to the preneoplastic stage at which the diagnosis was made.

In the longer term, the success of early-detection tools requires success in the parallel field of chemoprevention and in addressing the political issues around health care: i.e., who will pay for the screening and chemoprevention?

References

1. Strauss G, DeCamp M, Dibbicaro E, Richards W. Lung cancer diagnosis is being made with increased frequency in former cigarette smokers. Proc ASCO 1995; 14:362.
2. Frost JK, Ball WCJ, Levin ML, Tockman MS, Baker RR, Carter D, Egglesto JC, Erozan YS, Gupta PK, Khouri NF. Early lung cancer detection: Summary and conclusions. Am Rev Respir Dis 1984; 130:561.
3. Smart CR. Annual screening using chest X-ray examination for the diagnosis of lung cancer. Cancer 1993; 72:2295–2298.
4. Saccomanno G, Archer VE, Auerbach O, Saunders RP, Brennan LM. Cancer of the lung, the cytology of sputum prior to the development of carcinoma. Acta Cytol 1965; 9:413–423.
5. Bos JL, Fearon ER, Hamilton SR, Verlaan-de Vries M, Van Boom JH, Van der Eb AJ, Vogelstein B. Prevalence of ras gene mutations in human colorectal cancers. Nature 1987; 327:293–297.
6. Rodenhuis S, Slebos RJC. Clinical significance of ras oncogene activation in human lung cancer. Cancer Res 1992; 52:2665s–2669s.
7. Keohavong P, Demichele MAA, Melacrinos AC, Landreneau RJ, Weyany RJ, Siefgried JM. Detection of K-ras mutations in lung carcinomas—relationship to prognosis. Clin Cancer Res 1996; 2:411–418.
8. Slebos RJC, Kibbelaar RE, Dalesio O, Kooistra A, Stam J, Meijer CJLM, Wagenaar SS, Vanderschueren RGJRA, Van Zandwijk N, Moot WJ, Bos JL, Rodenhuis S. K-Ras oncogene activation as a prognostic marker in adenocarcinoma of the lung. N Engl J Med 1990; 323:561–565.
9. Sugio K, Inoue T, Inoue K, Yaita H, Inuzuka S, Ishida T, Sugimachi K. Different site mutation of the K-ras gene in a patient with metachronous double lung cancers. Anticancer Res 1993; 13:2469–2471.
10. Rosell R, Li S, Skacel Z, Mate JL, Maestre J, Canela M, Tolosa E, Armengol P, Barnadas A, Ariza A. Prognostic impact of mutated K-ras gene in surgically resected non-small cell lung cancer patients. Oncogene 1993; 8:2407–2412.
11. Li ZH, Zheng J, Weiss LM, Shibata D. c-k-ras and p53 mutations occur very early in adenocarcinoma of the lung. Am J Pathol 1994; 144:303–309.
12. Newton CR, Graham A, Heptinstall LE, Powell SJ, Summers C, Kalsheker N, Smith JC, Markham AF. Analysis of any point mutation in DNA—the amplification refractory mutation system (ARMS). Nuc Acids Res 1989; 17:2503–2516.
13. Neville EM, Ellison G, Kiaris H, Stewart MP, Spandidos DA, Fox JC, Field JK. Detection of K-ras mutations in non-small cell lung carcinoma. Int J Oncol 1995; 7:511–514.
14. Lehman TA, Scott F, Seddon M, Kelly K, Dempsey EC, Wilson VL, Mulshine JL, Modali R. Detection of K-ras mutations by polymerase chain reaction based ligase chain reaction. Anal Biochem 1996; 239:153–159.
15. Mao L, Hruban RH, Boyle JO, Tockman M, Sidransky D. Detection of oncogene mutations in sputum precedes diagnosis of lung cancer. Cancer Res 1994; 54:1634–1637.
16. Tesa JR, Siegfried JM, Liu Z, Hunt JD, Feder MM, Litwin S, Zhou J, Taguchi T, Keller S. Cytogenetic analysis of 63 non-small cell lung carcinomas: recurrent chromosomal alterations amid frequent and widespread genomic upheaval. Gene Chrom Cancer 1994; 11:178–194.

17. Sundaresan V, Ganly P, Haselton P, Rudd R, Sinha G, Bleehen NM, Rabbitts P. p53 and chromosome 3 abnormalities, characteristic of malignant lung tumours, are detectable in preinvasive lesions of the bronchus. Oncogene 1992; 7:1989–1997.
18. Gazdar AF. The molecular and cellular basis of human lung cancer. Anticancer Res 1994; 14:261–267.
19. Hung J, Kishimoto Y, Sugio K, Virmani A, Mcintire DD, Minna JD, Gazdar AF. Allele-specific chromosome 3p deletions occur at an early-stage in the pathogenesis of lung carcinoma. JAMA 1995; 273:558–563.
20. Kishimoto Y, Sugio K, Hung JY, Virmani AK, McIntire DD, Minna JD, Gazdar AF. Allele-specific loss in chromosome 9p loci in preneoplastic lesions accompanying non-small-cell lung cancers. J Natl Cancer Inst 1995; 87:1224–1229.
21. Thiberville L, Bourguignon J, Metayer J, Bost F, Diarra-Mehrpour M, Bignon J, Lam S, Martin JP, Nouvet G. Frequency and prognostic evaluation of 3p21–22 allelic losses in non-small-cell lung cancer. Int J Cancer 1995; 64:371–377.
22. Tsuchiya E, Nakamura Y, Weng SY, Nakagawa K, Tsuchiya S, Sugand H, Kitagawa T. Allelotype of non-small cell carcinoma: comparison between loss of heterozygosity in squamous cell carcinoma and adenocarcinoma. Cancer Res 1992; 52:2478–2481.
23. Sato S, Nakamura Y, Tsuchiya E. Difference of allelotype between squamous-cell carcinoma and adenocarcinoma of the lung. Cancer Res 1994; 54:5652–5655.
24. Ah-See KW, Cooke TG, Pickford IR, Soutar D, Balmain A. An allelotype of squamous carcinoma of the head and neck using microsatellite markers. Cancer Res 1994; 54:1617–1621.
25. Nawroz H, Vanderriet P, Hruban RH, Koch W, Ruppert JM, Sidransky D. Allelotype of head and neck squamous cell carcinoma. Cancer Res 1994; 54:1152–1155.
26. Field JK, Kiaris H, Risk JM, Tsiriyotis C, Adamson R, Zoumpourlis V, Rowley H, Taylor K, Whittaker J, Howard P, Beirnie JC, Gosney JR, Woolgar J, Vaughan ED, Spandidsos DA, Jones AS. Allelotype of squamous cell carcinoma of the head and neck: fractional allele loss correlates with survival. Br J Cancer 1995; 72:1180–1188.
27. Neville EM, Stewart MP, Swift A, Risk JM, Liloglou T, Ross H, Gosney JR, Donnelly RJ, Field JK. Allelotype of non-small cell lung cancer. Int J Oncol 1996; 9:533–539.
28. Neville EM, Stewart M, Myskow M, Donnelly RJ, Field JK. Loss of heterozygosity at 9p23 defines a novel locus in non-small cell lung cancer. Oncogene 1995; 11:581–585.
29. Field JK, Neville EM, Stewart MP, Swift A, Liloglou T, Risk JM, Ross H, Gosney JR, Donnelly RJ. Fractional allele loss data indicate distinct genetic populations in the development of non-small-cell lung cancer. Br J Cancer 1996; 74:1968–1974.
30. Loeb L. Mutator phenotype may be required for multistage carcinogenesis. Cancer Res 1991; 51:3075–3079.
31. Perucho M. Microsatellite instability: the mutator that mutates the other mutator. Nature Med 1996; 2(6):630–631.
32. Steiner G, Schoenberg MP, Linn JF, Mao L, Sidransky D. Detection of bladder cancer recurrence by microsatellite analysis of urine. Nature Med 1997; 3:621–624.
33. Chen XQ, Stroun M, Magnenat JL, Nicod LP, Kurt AM, Lyautey J, Lederrey C, Anker P. Microsatellite alterations in plasma DNA of small cell lung cancer patients. Nat Med 1996; 2:1033–1035.
34. Merlo A, Mabry M, Gabrielson E, Vollmer R, Baylin SB, Sidransky D. Frequent microsatellite instability in primary small cell lung cancer. Cancer Res 1994; 54:2098–2101.
35. Miozzo M, Sozzi G, Musso K, Pilotti S, Incarbone M, Pastorino U, Pierotti MA. Microsatellite alterations in bronchial and sputum specimens of lung cancer patients. Cancer Res 1996; 56:2285–2288.
36. Hollstein M, Sidransky D, Vogelstein B, Harris CC. p53 mutations in human cancers. Science 1991; 253:49–53.
37. Greenblatt MS, Bennett WP, Hollstein M, Harris CC. Mutations in the p53 tumor suppressor gene: clues to cancer etiology and molecular pathogenesis. Cancer Res 1994; 54:4855–4878.
38. Sidransky D, Hollstein M. Clinical implications of the p53 gene. Ann Rev Med 1996; 47:285–301.
39. Chiba I, Takahashi T, Nau MM, D'Amico D, Curiel DT, Mitsudomi T, Buchhagen DL, Carbone D, Piantadosi S, Koga H, Reissman PT, Slamon DJ, Holmes EC, Minna JD. Mutations

in the p53 gene are frequent in primary, resected non-small cell lung cancer. Oncogene 1990; 5:1603–1610.

40. Lehman TA, Bennett WP, Metcalf RA, Welsh JA, Ecker J, Modali RV, Ullrich S, Romano JW, Appella E, Testa JR, Gerwin BI, Harris CC. p53 mutations, ras mutations, and p53-heat shock 70 protein complexes in human lung carcinoma cell lines. Cancer Res 1991; 51:4090–4096.

41. Sameshima Y, Matsuno Y, Hirohashi S, Shimosato Y, Mizoguchi H, Sugimura T, Terada M, Yokota J. Alterations of the p53 gene are common and critical events for the maintenance of malignant phenotypes in small-cell lung carcinoma. Oncogene 1992; 7:451–457.

42. Suzuki H, Takahashi T, Kuroishi T, Suyama M, Ariyoshi Y, Takahashi T, Ueda R. p53 mutations in non-small cell lung cancer in Japan: association between mutations and smoking. Cancer Res 1992; 52:734–736.

43. Westra ES, Offerhaus GJA, Goodman SN, Slebos RJC, Polak M, Baas IO, Rodenhuis S, Hruban RH. Overexpression of the p53-tumor suppressor gene-product in primary lung adenocarcinomas is associated with cigarette smoking. Am J Surg Pathol 1993; 17:213–220.

44. Zheng J, Shu QP, Li ZH, Tsao JL, Weiss LM, Shibata D. Patterns of p53 mutations in squamous-cell carcinoma of the lung—acquisition at a relatively early age. Am J Pathol 1994; 145:1444–1449.

45. Carbone DP, Mitsudomi T, Chiba I, Piantadosi S, Rusch V, Nowak JA, McIntire D, Slamon D, Gazdar A, Minna J. p53 immunostaining positivity is associated with reduced survival and is imperfectly correlated with gene mutations in resected non-small cell lung cancer. A preliminary report of LCSG 871. Chest 1994; 106(6 suppl):377S–381S.

46. Mitsudomi T, Steinberg SM, Nau MM, Carbone D, Damico D, Bodner S, Oie HK, Linnoila RI, Mulshine JL, Minna JD, Gazdar AF. p53 gene-mutations in non-small-cell lung cancer cell-lines and their correlation with the presence of ras mutations and clinical features. Oncogene 1992; 7:171–180.

47. Takeshima Y, Seyama T, Bennett WP, Akiyama M, Tokuoka S, Inai K, Mabuchi K, Land CE, Harris CC. p53 mutations in lung cancers from nonsmoking atomic bomb survivors. Lancet 1993; 342:1520–1521.

48. Mitsudomi T, Oyama T, Kusano T, Osaki T, Nakanishi R, Shirakusa T. Mutations of the p53 gene as a predictor of poor prognosis in patients with non small cell lung cancer. J Natl Cancer Inst 1993; 85:2018–2023.

49. Ramet M, Castren K, Jarvinsen K, Pekkala K, Turpeenniemi-Hujanen T, Soini Y, Paakko P, Vahakangas K. p53 protein expression correlated with benzoapyrene-DNA adducts in carcinoma cell lines. Carcinogen 1995; 16:2117–2124.

50. Husgafvel-Pursiainen K, Ridanpaa M, Anttila S, Vainio H. p53 and ras gene mutations in lung cancer: implications for smoking and occupational exposures. J Occup Environ Med 1995; 37:69–76.

51. Liloglou T, Ross H, Prime W, Donnelly RJ, Spandidos DA, Gosney JR, Field JK. p53 gene aberrations in non-small cell lung carcinomas from a smoking population. Br J Cancer 1997; 75:1119–1124.

52. Lee LN, Shew JY, Sheu JC, Lee YC, Lee WC, Fang MT, Chang HF, Yu CJ, Yang PC, Luh KT. Exon-8 mutation of p53 gene associated with nodal metastasis in non-small cell lung cancer. Am J Respir Crit Care Med 1994; 150:1667–1671.

53. Wynder EL, Hoffmann D. Smoking and lung cancer: scientific challenges and opportunities. Cancer Res 1994; 54:5284–5295.

54. DeMarini DM, Shelton ML, Levine LG. Mutation spectrum of cigarette smoke condensate in Salmonella: comparison to mutations in smoking-associated tumours. Carcinogen 1995; 16:2535–2542.

55. Liloglou T, Scholes AGM, Spandidos DA, Vaughan ED, Jones AS, Field JK. p53 gene mutations in squamous cell carcinoma of the head and neck predominate in a subgroup of former and present smokers with a low frequency of genetic instability. Cancer Res 1997; 57: 4070–4074.

56. Zhou J, Mulshine JL, Unsworth EJ, Scott FR, Avis IM, Vos MD, Treston AM. Purification and characterization of a protein the permits early detection of lung cancer—identification of heterogeneous nuclear ribonucleoprotein A2/B1 as the antigen for monoclonal antibody 703D4. J Biol Chem 1996; 271:10760–10766.

57. Burd CG, Dreyfuss G. RNA specificity of hnRNP A1 significance high-affinity binding sites in pre-messenger RNA splicing. EMBO J 1994; 13:1197–1204.

58. Tockman MS, Prabodh KG, Myers JD, Frost JK, Baylin SB, Gold EB, Chase AM, Wilkinson PH, Mulshine JL. Sensitive and specific monoclonal antibody recognition of human lung cancer antigen on preserved sputum cells: a new approach to early lung cancer detection. J Clin Oncol 1988; 6:1685–1693.

59. Tockman MS. Development of labels of early lung cancer at the John K frost Center for Imaging of cells and Molecular markers. Lung Cancer Res Q 1991; 1:4–6.

60. Tockman MS, Gupta PK, Pressman PK, Mulshine JL. Cytometric validation of immunocytochemical observations in developing lung cancer. Diagn Cytopathol 1993; 9:615–622.

61. Tockman MS. Monoclonal antibody detection of premalignant lesions of the lung. In: Fortner JG, Sharp PA, eds. Accomplishments in Cancer Research–1995 Prize Year, General Motors Cancer Research Foundation. Philadelphia: Lippincott–Raven, 1996: 169–177.

62. Gonzalez FJ, Gelboin H. Role of human cytochrome P450s in risk assessment and susceptibility to environmentally based disease. J Toxicol Environ Health 1993; 40:289–308.

63. Ayesh SK, Ferne M, Flechner I, Babior BM, Matzner Y. Partial characterization of a C5A-inhibitor in peritoneal fluid. J Immunol 1990; 144:3066–3070.

64. Wolf CR, Smith CAD, Forman D. Metabolic polymorphisms in carcinogen metabolising enzymes and cancer susceptibility. Br Med Bull 1994; 50:718–731.

65. Brockmoller J, Reinhold K, Drakoulis N, Staffeldt B, Roots I. GSTM1 and its variants A and B as host factors of bladder cancer susceptibility: a case control study. Cancer Res 1994; 54:4103–4111.

66. Seidegard J, Voracheck WR, Perow RW, Pearson WR. Hereditary deficiencies in the expression of the human GST on trans-stilbene oxide are due to a gene deletion. Proc Natl Acad Sci USA 1988; 85:7293–7297.

67. Kihara M, Kihara M, Noda K. Lung cancer risk of GSTM1 null genotype is dependent on the extent of tobacco smoke exposure. Carcinogenesis 1994; 15:415–418.

68. Hayashi S, Watanabe J, Kawajiri K. High susceptibility to lung cancer in terms of combined genotypes of P4501A1 and Mu class GST genes. Jpn J Can Res 1992; 83:866–870.

69. Braun MM, Caporaso NE, Page WF, Hoover RN. Genetic component of lung cancer: cohort study of twins. Lancet 1994; 344:440–443.

19

Retinoids for Lung Cancer Intervention

UGO PASTORINO

European Institute of Oncology
Milan, Italy

I. Introduction

Cancer prevention has gained a more prominent role in experimental and clinical research by providing a new insight and better comprehension of the mechanisms of human carcinogenesis and improving the selectivity and efficacy of intervention. Lung cancer prevention covers different areas: primary prevention, aimed at eliminating the exposure to tobacco smoking and other known environmental carcinogens; secondary prevention, focused on early diagnosis and treatment of preneoplastic or preinvasive lesions; and pharmacological prevention or chemoprevention, aimed at suppressing or reverting the process of carcinogenesis and preventing the occurrence of invasive cancer by the administration of drugs or other natural substances, present in human physiology or normal diet. There is no doubt that widespread control of tobacco consumption represents the main target of lung cancer prevention. Pharmacological prevention could, however, offer a useful support to primary prevention. In fact, with the success of tobacco-control policies, an expanding cohort of ex-smokers will remain at high risk of lung cancer for 15–20 years, and there is an objective need for strategies aimed at reducing cancer mortality in individuals who have stopped smoking. Experimental data have consistently proved that chemoprevention of upper aerodigestive tract cancer is feasible, but the evidence of a beneficial effect in humans is still limited and controversial. Better selection of high-risk individuals and identification of more effective preventive agents remain crucial requirements for chemoprevention to become a reality (1). Despite all the difficulties encountered so far, research on prevention has a indisputable priority in a disease that is so common and poorly curable.

II. Dietary Factors in Lung Cancer

Guided by the observation of geographic and time trends in lung cancer incidence not attributable to tobacco consumption, epidemiological studies have correlated the risk of cancer with other lifestyle factors. Among these, dietary deficiency of vitamins, micronutrients, or specific foods has emerged as a potential modifier of lung cancer risk. A relative protection against lung cancer has been hypothesized for β-carotene and other substances belonging to the group of antioxidants, such as selenium or vitamin E (α-tocopherol). Individuals with a lower dietary consumption or serum levels of these nutrients consistently showed a higher risk of lung cancer in case-control studies.

Unfortunately, dietary questionnaires are neither accurate nor specific with respect to the individual substance with biological activity, and fruits and vegetables which are rich in β-carotene and other carotenoids also contain other substances with potential anticancer properties. Overall, the epidemiological data supported the hypothesis that a different lifelong intake of common dietary components could modulate the risk of lung cancer, but only prospective trials will clarify whether any change in dietary habits likely to occur later in life may have an effect on cancer risks (2).

III. Latency and Field Effect

Human epidemiology and experimental data on multistep carcinogenesis indicate that the development of invasive lung cancer requires a complex sequence of critical events. In fact, most epidemiological studies on time trends and human cohorts, as well as analytic case-control studies, consistently demonstrated that the interval between the beginning of the exposure to known carcinogens and the occurrence of lung cancer ranges from 10 to 30 years. Such a long phase of latency suggests a large potential space for intervention. Theoretically, it is possible to hypothesize a combination of selective chemopreventive agents aimed at the various phases of carcinogenesis: from the inhibition of early induction (metabolic activation, formation of DNA adducts, DNA repair) to the antagonism of tumor promotion and the reversal of progression to invasive cancer. The damage induced by inhaled carcinogens affects diffusely the respiratory and upper digestive epithelium, thereby inducing multiple areas of premalignant changes and in some individuals the occurrence of multiple primary cancers. Biological and clinical research related to chemoprevention is now trying to identify the preclinical steps of lung carcinogenesis and the genetic basis of individual susceptibility to tobacco exposure, with ultimate benefits in the collateral fields of screening of precancerous lesions and early diagnosis of invasive cancer. This prospect is of particular interest for those individuals who have stopped smoking after a long period of carcinogenic exposure.

IV. Experimental Activity of Retinoids

Experimental data have demonstrated that lung cancer can be pharmacologically prevented and progression to end-stage disease inhibited. Substances with potential chemopreventive properties, such as retinoids and antioxidants, have been investigated using nearly all the available systems for testing anticarcinogenic activity, in vitro and in vivo (3). Retinoids exert a strong regulatory effect upon the physiological mechanisms of cell proliferation and differentiation, being able to inhibit malignant transformation and suppress tumor promotion, particularly in the presence of indirect carcinogens such as benzopyrene or methylcholanthrene (4). The postinitiation effect of retinoids against tumor promotion and progression is of great interest in lung cancer for the possibility of interfering with the late stages of tumor development. Under specific conditions, retinoids have shown a direct antineoplastic effect (5,6), as well as growth factor inhibition (7,8). Recently, retinoids have been shown to suppress malignant cell growth and induce apoptosis in lymphoid and myeloid malignant cell lines (HL-60R and NB306) (9). Another potential mechanism of action is represented by the enhancement of immune response to cancer, both cell- and antibody-mediated (10–12). A synergistic effect between retinoids and other substances (selenium, α-tocopherol, β-carotene) has also been demonstrated in N-nitrosodiethylamine–induced adenosquamous lung carcinoma in Syrian golden hamsters (13,14). The new compound N-(4hydroxyphenyl) retinamide (4HPR) has demonstrated a strong capacity to induce apoptosis in several neoplastic systems such as small-cell lung cancer and head and neck squamous cell carcinoma (15,16). These features are of particular interest for chemoprevention as the mechanism of elimination of genetically altered cells through apoptosis may be more effective than differentiation or growth suppression and lead to permanent eradication of potentially clonogenic foci in the bronchial mucosa.

The experimental data on β-carotene are far less convincing, and a specific chemopreventive activity of carotenoids was demonstrated only for UV-induced skin tumors in mice (17).

V. Nuclear Receptors

The discovery of specific nuclear retinoic acid receptors (RARs) has dramatically increased our knowledge on the mechanisms of action of retinoids (18–20). RARs belong to the superfamily of ligand-activated nuclear receptors for steroid and thyroid hormones. They are DNA-binding, transcription-modulating proteins, whose expression may be induced by retinoic acid administration (21–24). Unlike other members of this family, retinoid receptors recognize two classes: RARs and RXRs, each containing α, β, and γ subtypes. RAR-α gene is located on chromosome 17q21, RAR-β on chromosome 3p24, and RAR-γ on chromosome 12q13 (25). Upregulation or downregulation of RARs may explain how retinoids can interfere with epithelial cell growth, differentiation, and apoptosis, or inhibit progression of premalignant cells to cancer, and offers a rational basis for selection of receptor-specific retinoids in chemoprevention (26,27). Different retinoids bind to the different receptor classes and subclasses with different affinities. Retinoid receptors are active only as dimers, in the forms of RAR/RXR heterodimers or RXR/RXR homodimers, which bind to specific DNA sequences causing induction or suppression of gene transcription (20). Specific ligand-binding patterns have been identified for the various retinoids: RARs bind ATRA and 9cRA, while RXRs only bind 9cRA. Quite interestingly, 13cRA is unable to bind nuclear receptors but needs to be transformed into ATRA. It appears that nuclear receptors subclasses are not evenly distributed in the various tissues: while RAR-γ is mainly expressed in the skin, RAR-β expression is of key relevance for the respiratory and upper digestive epithelia. Their concentration in target tissues also varies in pathological conditions, thus making them a suitable marker of carcinogenic damage.

VI. Clinical Development of Retinoids

Natural retinol, or vitamin A, has been available for experimental testing and clinical practice for over 60 years. The interest for retinol as a modulator of cell growth was generated by its physiologic properties, extending from the early phases of fetal development through adult life. In higher animals, vitamin A is essential for vision, reproduction, and maintenance of differentiated epithelia and mucus secretion (28,29). *Trans*-retinoic acid shares only some of these functions, and is unable to support vision and reproduction; therefore, animals maintained on retinoic acid as only source of vitamin A are both blind and sterile (30,31). Retinol, as well as other retinoids, has shown a definite clinical anticancer activity in different epithelial tumors, and particularly in skin cancer. Many studies have demonstrated that these substances, either topically or orally administered, could achieve a complete remission in a high proportion of patients with basal cell and advanced squamous cell carcinoma; the effect was, however, reversible and tumor growth have been reported after interruption of treatment (32–34). Starting in the late 1960s, industrial laboratories have made an enormous effort to produce synthetic analogs with higher, or more selective, activity and lower toxicity than natural vitamin A. In this research process, more than 1500 new retinoids have been produced and tested (35), using two biological assays: the in vitro reversal of tracheal keratinization on hamsters raised on vitamin A–deficient diet, and in vivo ability to reverse skin papillomas in mice (36). Of the hundreds of compounds examined, only a few ultimately entered thorough clinical investigation: retinyl esters (palmitate, acetate), all-*trans* retinoic acid (ATRA), 13-*cis*-retinoic acid (13-CRA), etretinate, and fenretinide (4-HPR).

Randomized placebo-controlled trials have proved that 13-*cis*-retinoic acid is an effective drug, but the toxicological profile in humans was less favorable than the one anticipated from the animal data (37–39). A great level of interest and expectation for chemoprevention of premalignant lesions in the upper aerodigestive tract has been generated by studies in oral leukoplakia. The first study demonstrated that 13-*cis*-retinoic acid (1–2 mg/kg daily for 3 months) could achieve major regression of leukoplakia in 67% of patients (vs. 10% for placebo) (40). Unfortunately, the majority of patients did not tolerate the treatment for more than 6 months, and relapse occurred in most cases after the interruption of treatment. A further study of isotretinoin, designed to overcome the problems of toxicity and relapse, included a 3-month induction treatment with high-dose isotretinoin (1.5 mg/kg/day) followed by randomization to a 9-month maintenance therapy with either low-dose isotretinoin (0.5 mg/k/day) or β-carotene (30 mg/day). This study showed that low-dose isotretinoin was more effective than β-carotene in maintaining clinical/histological remission (relapse rate of 6% vs. 58%), thus demonstrating that low-dose isotretinoin was an effective and well-tolerated maintenance therapy for oral premalignancy (41).

VII. Pharmacology and Toxicology

Natural retinol is stored in the liver in large amounts (>90% of one-year physiologic requirement) and is then released in the plasma and transported bound to a specific retinol-binding protein (RBP). The process of mobilization is controlled by the liver, although recycling from peripheral tissues and extravascular spaces may also play a role (42). Consequently, retinol plasma levels are maintained stable except in extreme conditions (e.g., chronic dietary deficiency, high dose supplementation). Due to such a tight homeostatic mechanism, the administration of moderate doses of vitamin A failed to show any significant change of retinol plasma levels in a number of studies (43–45). In a prospective randomized trial, a daily dose of 300,000 IU was associated with a 30% increase of the average plasma retinol and 60% increase of retinol-binding protein after 12 months of treatment (46). Intestinal absorption rate in humans is commonly estimated as 50–60% of total dietary retinol. In pharmacological supplementation, the level of absorption depends on the chemical structure (alcohol, esters) or the type of preparation (oily solution, emulsion), being as high as 80% for emulsified retinol, compared to 20% for oily solutions (47). Chemical and physical properties may also be implicated in the pattern of liver toxicity and bioavailability in extrahepatic tissues as natural retinol is almost entirely vehiculated by chylomicrons through the lymphatic system, while retinoic acid is directly transported to the liver through the portal system (48). One aspect that has generated in the past substantial confusion is the side effects and toxicity of vitamin A. The long-lasting concern for retinol toxicity, so common among the medical community, was not substantiated by controlled clinical studies. In nearly 50 years of clinical application in opthalmology and dermatology, there were only a few cases of serious intoxication and no deaths attributable to the so-called hypervitaminosis A syndrome

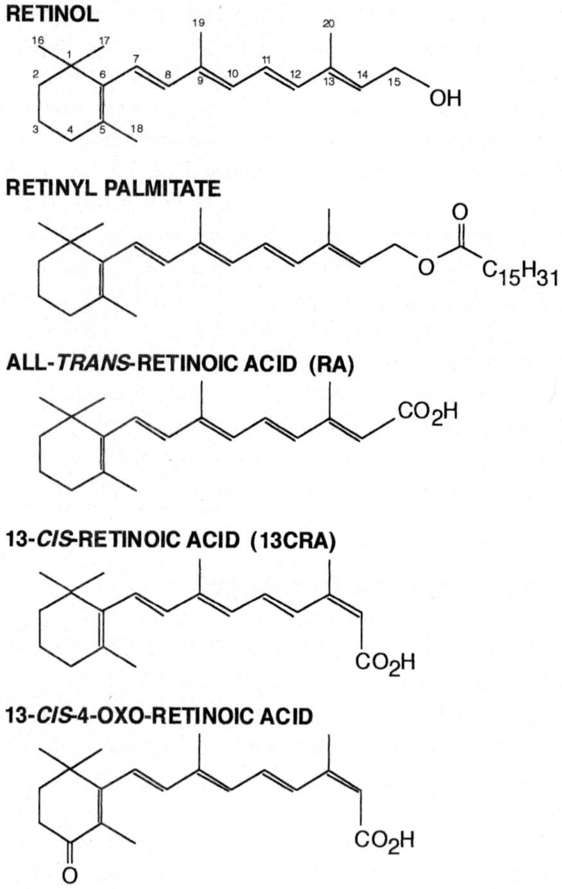

Figure 1   Chemical structure of different retinoids.

(49,50). Most of the typical side effects, such as mucocutaneous dryness, desquamation, or cheilitis, are a common feature of any retinoid treatment at proper pharmacological doses. Liver enlargement and rise of serum triglycerides are frequently observed, but invariably transient.

   With natural retinol, a daily dose of 25,000 I.U. has been considered adequate for large-scale intervention trials on healthy individuals, where side effects must be absent or negligible. For adjuvant trials in cancer patients, a much higher dose can be selected, based on efficacy data derived from other diseases (51–54). In a prospective randomized trial using emulsified retinyl palmitate at high dose (300,000 I.U./day) for a long period of time, we could not demonstrate a significant effect on liver function or objective liver toxicity measurable with repeated blood tests (55).

ETRETINATE

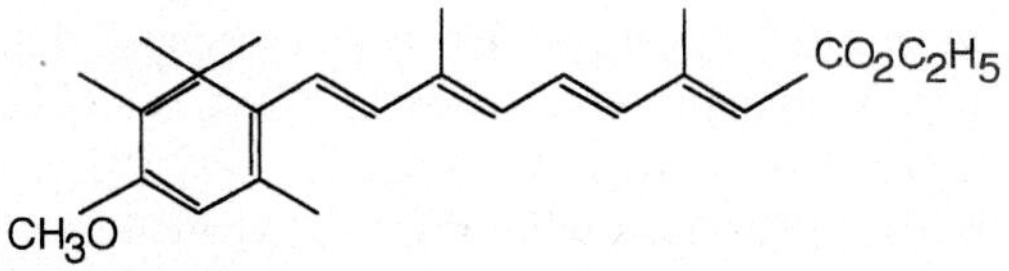

CH_3O

ACITRETIN

CH_3O

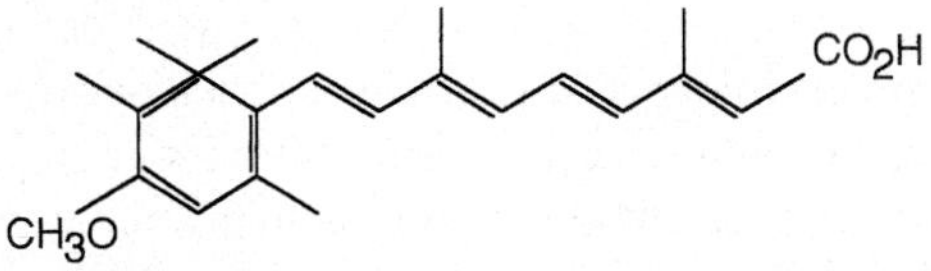

FENRETINIDE (4HPR)

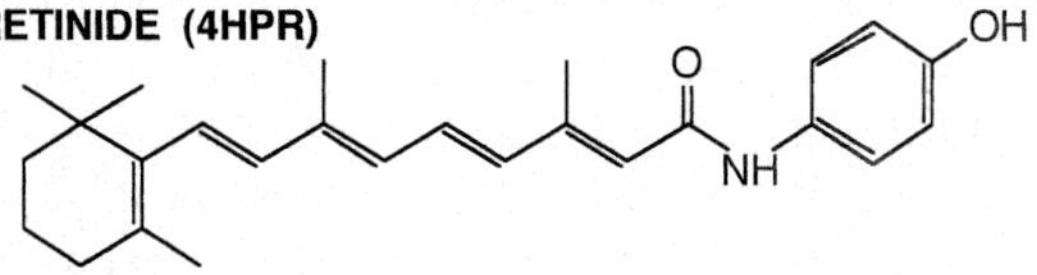

TEMAROTENE

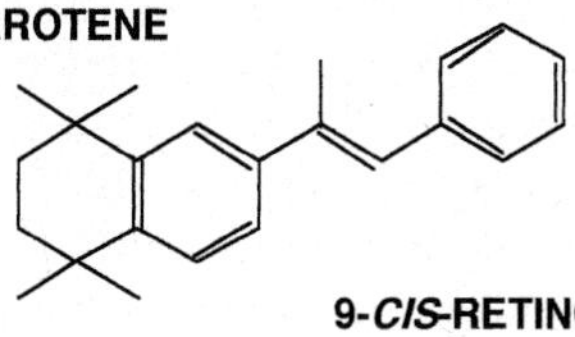

9-*CIS*-RETINOIC ACID

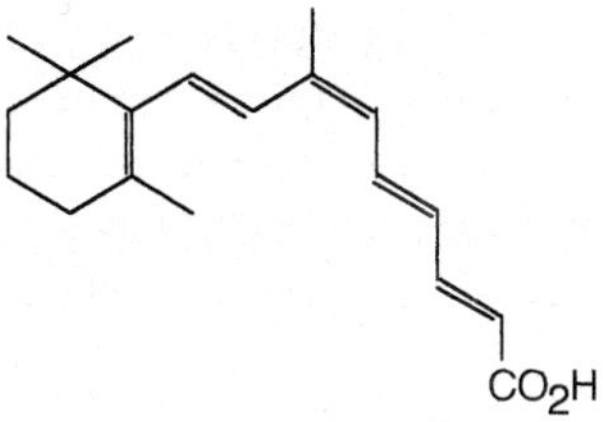

The group of synthetic retinoids includes a highly heterogeneous group of substances, with peculiar properties in terms of resorption, metabolism, pharmacokinetics, bioavailability, and toxicity. As an example, the plasma elimination half-life ranged from less than 1 hour for ATRA to 10 hours for 13CRA, and was greater than 120 days for etretinate. Overall, the available data suggested that plasma levels of 13CRA (the most widely tested retinoid) were relatively stable after multiple doses, and that long-term pharmacokinetic profile could be predicted from single dose data. Although recent animal data have demonstrated that oral administration of many retinoids, including 13CRA, causes significant and dose-proportional reduction of plasma retinol levels (56), clinical data on 13CRA are not conclusive (57,58).

Dry skin, itching, flaking, nasal stuffiness, xerostomia, and cheilitis are observed frequently with the use of 13-*cis*-retinoic acid. These reactions can usually be managed with topical lubricants and moisturizing agents; however, some patients may require a decrease in the drug dose. Bone pain may occur in patients receiving 13-*cis*-retinoic acid, and long-term treatment has been associated with formation of hyperostosis (bone spurs), particularly on the vertebral bodies and in the calcaneus (59,60). Hypercalcemia has also been reported occasionally (61,62). Hypertriglyceridemia has been observed with most retinoids, but hypercholesterolemia is less striking. Even in the case of 13-*cis*-retinoic acid, cardiovascular consequences related to hyperlipidemia have not been described; however, such complications may become evident after a more prolonged use in cancer chemoprevention. Hepatic toxicity may be manifested by a transient increase in serum transaminases, alkaline phosphatase, or bilirubin during the initial period of administration. Although these effects may persist for a few weeks after the drugs have been discontinued, they are usually readily reversible. Overall, the degree of toxicity observed in patients receiving 13-*cis*-retinoic acid at full dosage (1 mg/kg daily) was significant in chemoprevention studies, and most patients did not tolerate the treatment for more than 6 months (40). Overall, it is fair to say that the toxicological profile of synthetic retinoids has been less favorable than expected, and the degree of toxicity is still a limiting factor for chemoprevention studies. A possible exception may be represented by 4-HPR, the new synthetic derivative initially tested in breast cancer chemoprevention (63,64). Prospective clinical trials on patients with resected breast cancer have shown an excellent tolerability of 4-HPR, given orally at the daily dose of 200 mg. The only concern was related to lowered retinol serum levels and impaired dark adaptation in a significant proportion of treated patients (65,66). Although clinical data on direct efficacy of 4-HPR against cancer or premalignant diseases are scanty, a concurrent study conducted on patients surgically treated for oral leukoplakia has shown a significant reduction in the incidence of new leukoplakia lesions (67), thus making 4-HPR a good candidate for lung cancer intervention.

VIII. Selection of High-Risk Individuals and Optimal Endpoints

Primary chemoprevention trials have been designed for individuals at high risk of developing a lung cancer because of previous heavy exposure to smoking, asbestos, or other carcinogens, or volunteers with a high level of cultural motivation such as physicians or nurses. These studies tried to counteract a hypothetical deficiency of putative protective agents, such as β-carotene, retinol (vitamin A), or α-tocopherol (vitamin E). Many thousands of people had to be recruited, with a long period of observation (5–10 years), to reach an adequate number of events. The doses selected for preventive agents were relatively low, in order to avoid any side effects, obtain high recruitment and compliance rates. A second level of intervention involved subjects affected by precancerous or preinvasive lesions such as oral leukoplakia, bronchial metaplasia, or dysplasia. Aim of the intervention was to induce regression of preneoplastic disease and thereby prevent progression to invasive cancer. The third level of intervention was focused on prevention of new primary tumors, arising as a consequence of widespread exposure of the entire epithelial surface to carcinogenic insults (68–70) in patients cured for a prior cancer (71–75). In general, patients cured for a prior cancer show a high motivation to accept the intervention plan as part of their long-term follow-up, and side effects are better tolerated with a view to potential protective effect against relapse. Only tumors occurring in the target field of chemoprevention should be considered as relevant endpoints: upper aerodigestive tract tumors, all tobacco-related cancers (oral cavity, pharynx, larynx, lung, esophagus, and bladder) (76,77).

IX. Primary Chemoprevention Trials in Healthy Individuals

The comprehensive program of randomized trials on high-risk individuals funded by the National Cancer Institute has been discussed elsewhere in this book (1,78–80). In summary, the data suggest a possible unfavorable interaction between current smoking and β-carotene treatment. While a definitive judgment on the carcinogenic effect of β-carotene will require further investigation, it is clear that vitamin supplementation cannot replace primary prevention (81). Therefore, it appears reasonable to concentrate future chemoprevention programs on former smokers as part of tobacco-control programs in the same population.

X. Treatment of Precancerous Lesions

The potential efficacy of retinoids in bronchial premalignancy was suggested by a French pilot study where chronic smokers with squamous metaplasia of the bronchial epithelium, detected by bronchoscopy, were treated with etretinate, 25 mg/d, for 6 months (82). This trial showed a reduction of squamous metaplasia in patients treated with etretinate. Two randomized trials were subsequently conducted on heavy-smoker volunteers with the aim of reverting bronchial metaplasia and dysplasia with retinoids and both studies were negative. The first study tested the efficacy of etretinate on sputum cytology of heavy smokers: after 6 months of treatment, the degree of atypia measured in the sputum of etretinate-treated subjects was similar to that observed in the placebo group (83). The second trial tested the effect of 13-*cis*-retinoic acid versus placebo on 87 chronic smokers with bronchial dysplasia and/or metaplasia index greater than 15%, as assessed by multiple bronchoscopic biopsies. A new bronchoscopy, performed after 6 months of treatment, showed a significant decrease in the frequency of squamous metaplasia in those patients who had stopped smoking, but no difference between the two treatment arms (55 vs. 59%) (84). Although negative, these experiences have provided a methodological set-up for prospective investigation of bronchial premalignancy with intermediate biomarkers, and new research prospects are now being generated by innovative endoscopic instruments using spontaneous fluorescence to detect dysplastic areas and carcinoma in situ on the macroscopically normal bronchial mucosa.

XI. Trials on Chemoprevention of Second Primary Tumors

The potential benefit of retinoids as adjuvant treatment to reduce the occurrence of secondary primary tumors has been demonstrated by two independent randomized trials. The first study was conducted on 103 patients with previously treated head and neck cancer, randomized to receive either isotretinoin or placebo for 12 months (85). The incidence of second primary tumors was significantly lower in the treatment arm after a median follow-up of 32 months (4% vs. 24%) and persisted at a later analysis with 54 months median follow-up (14% vs. 31%).

The second trial was conducted on 307 patients with early-stage lung cancer, randomized after complete surgical resection to receive high-dose retinol palmitate for 12–24 months or no further treatment. The rationale for such a treatment schedule was discussed extensively in the first report of the trial (34). The dose of 300,000 I.U./day for a minimum of 12 months was then selected on the basis of two elements: the highest therapeutic effect achieved in the treatment of dermatological diseases (ichthyosis, psoriasis, and oral leukoplakia) and maximum tolerance in toxicological studies (4,000 I.U./kg/day). The emulsified preparation of retinol palmitate was chosen in consideration of its absorption properties and higher bioavailability. In this trial, after a median follow-up of 46 months, we observed a significant difference in the frequency of second primaries (12% vs. 21%) and total cancer failures (37% vs. 48%) in favor of the treatment arm (86) (Table 1). Despite our initial concerns and a very intense monitoring of side effects in the pilot phase of the study, the toxicity and tolerability profile of high-dose retinol palmitate was excellent. A high proportion of patients presented typical side effects such as skin desquamation or dryness of mucosae, but only in very few patients did the treatment

Table 1 Results of the First Randomized Trial on Lung Cancer Chemoprevention in Stage I NSCLC

	Retinol P (300,000 IU/day)	Control
All cancer failures	56 (37)	75 (48)
Recurrence	38 (25)	46 (29)
Locoregional	15 (10)	11 (7)
Distant	23 (15)	35 (22)
New primary	18 (12)	29 (18)
Deaths	55 (37)	64 (41)
Recurrence	37 (25)	39 (25)
New primary	7 (5)	14 (9)
Other cause	11 (7)	11 (7)

Source: Modified from Ref. 86.

need to be discontinued because of toxicity (55). The high frequency of easily detectable side effects convinced us to avoid a double-blind placebo-controlled design. In our opinion, the use of placebo would have been feasible and convenient only with a much lower dose, below the threshold of clinical side effects.

Based on this favorable pilot experiences, a series of trials have been designed with the purpose of preventing new primary malignancies after curative resection. The EUROSCAN cooperative study was set up in 1988 as a joint venture of the E.O.R.T.C. Lung Cancer and Head and Neck Cancer Cooperative Groups (87) to test the efficacy of retinol palmitate and NAC, given for 2 years with a 2 × 2 factorial design to patients with previous cancer of the larynx, oral cavity, and lung (NSCLC). The accrual was closed in 1994, with 2595 patients entered, and the first analysis was planned for 1997. A reassuring aspect of the EUROSCAN trial is the fact that only a minority (11%) of randomized patients with prior lung cancer continued or resumed smoking throughout the intervention period. The early analysis of smoking habits provided evidence that, regardless of the intervention program, smoking after treatment of the initial cancer was associated with a significant worsening of long-term survival. Another chemoprevention trial on resected stage I NSCLC was started by the U.S. Intergroup in 1992. This study is expected to enter over 600 patients per arm, to be treated with oral 13-*cis*-retinoic acid at the dose of 30 mg/day.

XII. Limits of Early Clinical Trials

In the early 1980s a worldwide program of clinical research has been launched by the NCI Chemoprevention Branch. Substantial resources were invested to identify and test specific dietary components and drugs for chemoprevention purposes, through a comprehensive program covering preclinical screening of new agents, assessment of efficacy and safety, and conduct of clinical trials in humans (88). The results of such a large effort may not be fully established before the next decade. Fifteen years later, the clinical evidence of a beneficial effect of chemoprevention in human lung cancer is still limited and controversial. In fact, this "first generation" of clinical trials has served as a test of reality for various experimental and epidemiological hypotheses. The failure of most prospective randomized trials, as well as the recent evidence of a possible detrimental effect of β-carotene in current heavy smokers, can only emphasize the limits of initial experiences in human chemoprevention and represent a challenge for future research and developments.

Many problems remain open: simplistic interpretation of epidemiological data on diet and cancer, low predictivity of animal models, unfavorable efficacy/toxicity profile of retinoids, reversibility of biological effect, lack of intermediate biological endpoints, difficulty to design proper phase II trials, low risk of cancer requiring prolonged intervention and huge number of subjects, and persisting exposure to known carcinogens such as tobacco smoking.

XIII. New Prospects of Retinoid Intervention

Ideally, a new generation of clinical trials should be based on innovative preclinical studies providing fresh data on the efficacy of new substances, alone and in combination with old agents, against bronchial premalignancy, as defined by new biomarkers. In particular, the lack of proper animal models for experimental development of lung cancer and preinvasive bronchial lesions represents an objective limitation in the design and planning of future chemoprevention trials. In the real world, more human-orientated experimental models are still beyond our reach, and the difficulty of inducing lung carcinomas in animals by tobacco smoking appears an unsurmountable paradox.

Several new agents are on pipeline and a few of them have gone through the steps of clinical toxicology. Natural dietary components such as genistein or curcumin appear very attractive on the safety ground, but new retinoids such as 4-HPR or 9-cisRA are also promising.

Topical application of retinoids is a logical way to circumvent systemic toxicity and increase pharmacological levels in target tissues. This is particularly sound for substances like vitamin A and retinoids with a view to their well-established capacity to induce complete regression of skin cancer (and other dermatological diseases) by topical application. Pilot studies on inhalation of aerosolized retinoids are ongoing in the United States with ATRA (89), and we have recently activated in the UK a research program using 13-*cis*-retinoic acid via aerosol.

After the experience of ATBC and CARET trials, overwhelming scientific and ethical problems strongly recommend to focus chemoprevention programs on former smokers or other individuals who are at high risk because of previous cancer or genetic susceptibility.

XIV. Biologic Markers and Intermediate Endpoints

To increase the cost/benefit ratio of intervention plans, specific subpopulations of very high-risk individuals must be identified on the basis of constitutive or acquired abnormalities detectable in the target tissues. Intermediate biomarkers are the hypothetical instrument to select high-risk populations on basis of tissue-specific genetic damage rather than of nonspecific carcinogenic exposure. In addition, biologic intermediate endpoints could fulfill the crucial need to monitor the efficacy of preventive strategies on premalignant lesions, well before the actual occurrence of invasive cancer (90–93). A number of genetic abnormalities have been consistently observed in lung cancer, premalignant lesions, and normal bronchial mucosa, and represent potential biomarkers for chemoprevention. Some of the new biomarkers, such as RAR-β or FHIT gene, display some very promising features: a high specificity for lung cancer, early occurrence in bronchial metaplasia or even microscopically normal mucosa, and detectability through routine sputum samples (94,95).

In practical terms, it is now conceivable to use a panel of specific markers (3p deletion, P53, EGFR, KRAS, MSI, FHIT) to select candidates for chemoprevention. In fact, with the present developments in research technology, such as immunocytochemistry, in situ hybridization (FISH), and PCR, even small samples collected through bronchoscopic biopsies, brushing, or sputum cytology will become suitable for systematic screening of high-risk individuals (93).

A large effort will be required in the coming years to test and validate such a large group of biomarkers through purpose designed, small-scale, controlled studies. In order to justify their systematic use, intermediate endpoints will have to prove specific for the process of carcinogenesis under study, correlate quantitatively or qualitatively with the degree of tumor progression, show a low rate of spontaneous regression, and be modulated by the selected preventive agent. Such biomarkers should also be easily measurable on small specimens, and the process of sampling tolerable at repeated intervals with minimal side effects.

XV. Conclusion

Despite all the difficulties encountered so far, research on cancer chemoprevention has provided a new insight and better comprehension of the mechanisms of human carcinogenesis and represents a indisputable priority, particularly in those diseases such as lung cancer that are common and poorly curable. The use of retinoids for cancer chemoprevention still must be considered experimental, and these substances should be administered with this purpose only in the framework of controlled clinical trials. There is an urgent need for greater investments in cancer chemoprevention programs exploiting the new resources available in the experimental and clinical fields.

References

1. Greenwald P, Stern HR. Role of biology and prevention in aerodigestive tract cancers. J Natl Cancer Inst Monogr 1992; 13:3–14.
2. Greenwald P, Sondik E, Lynch BS. Diet and chemoprevention in NCI's research strategy to achieve national cancer control objectives. Ann Rev Public Health 1986; 7:267–291.
3. Sporn MB, Newton DL. Chemoprevention of cancer with retinoids. Fed Proc 1979; 38:2528–2534.
4. Lotan R. Effects of vitamin A and its analogs (retinoids) on normal and neoplastic cells. Biochim Biophys Acta 1980; 605:33–91.
5. Trown PW, Buck MJ, Hansen R. Inhibition of growth and regression of a transplantable rat chrondrosarcoma by three retinoids. Cancer Treat Rep 1976; 60:1647–1653.
6. Lotan R. Different susceptibilities of human melanoma and breast carcinoma cell lines to retinoic acid-induced growth inhibition. Cancer Res 1979; 39:1014–1019.
7. Todaro GJ, DeLarco JE, Sporn MB. Retinoid blocks phenotypic cell transformation produced by sarcoma growth factor. Nature 1978; 276:272–278.
8. Gensler HL, Matrisian LM, Bowden GT. Effect of retinoic acid on the late-stage promotion of transformation in JB6 mouse epidermal cells in culture. Cancer Res 1985; 45:1922–1925.

9. Delia D, Aiello A, Lombardi L, Pelicci PG, Grignani F, Grignani F, Formelli F, Menard S, Costa A, Veronesi U, et al. N-(4-hydroxyphenyl)retinamide induces apoptosis of malignant hemopoietic cell lines including those unresponsive to retinoic acid. Cancer Res 1993; 53:6036–41.

10. Floersheim GL, Bollag W. Accelerated rejection of skin homografts by vitamin A acid. Transplantation 1972; 14:564–567.

11. Tachibana K, Sone S, Tsubura E, Kishino Y. Stimulatory effect of vitamin A on tumoricidal activity of rat alveolar macrophages. Br J Cancer 1984; 49:343–348.

12. Dennert G. Immunostimulation by retinoic acid. In: Retinoids, Differentiation and Disease. London: Ciba Foundation Symposium 113. Pitman, 1985:117–131.

13. Moon RC, Rao KV, Detrisac CJ, Kelloff GJ. Animal models for chemoprevention of respiratory cancer. Monogr Natl Cancer Inst 1992; 13:45–49.

14. Moon RC, Mehta RG, Rao KV. Retinoids and cancer in experimental animals. In: Sporn MB, Roberts AB, Goodman DS, eds. The Retinoids. 2d ed. New York: Raven, 1994:573.

15. Kalemkerian GP, Slusher R, Ramalingam S, Gadgeel S, Mabry M. Growth inhibition and induction of apoptosis by fenretinide in small-cell lung cancer cell lines. J Natl Cancer Inst 1995; 87:1674.

16. Oridate N, Lotan D, Xu X-C, et al. Differential induction of apoptosis by all-trans-retinoic acid and N-(4-hydroxyphenyl-retinamide in human head and neck squamous cell carcinoma cell lines. Clin Cancer Res 1996; 2:855.

17. Mathews-Roth MM. Antitumor activity of beta-carotene, cathaxanthin and phytoene. Oncology 1982; 39:33–37.

18. Evans RM. The steroid and thyroid hormone receptor superfamily. Science 1988; 240: 889–895.

19. Lotan R, Clifford JL. Nuclear receptors for retinoids: mediators of retinoid effects on normal and malignant cells. Biomed Pharmacother 1990; 45:145–156.

20. Chambon P. The retinoid signalling pathway: molecular and genetic analyses. Sem Cell Biol 1994; 5:115.

21. de The H, Marchio A, Tiollais P, Dejean A. Differential expression and ligand regulation of the retinoic acid receptor a and b genes. EMBO J 1989; 8:429–433.

22. Hu L, Gudas LJ. Cyclic AMP analogs and retinoic acid influence the expression of retinoic acid receptor a, b, and g mRNAs in F9 teratocarcinoma cells. Mol Cell Biol 1990; 10: 391–396.

23. Clifford J, Petkovich M, Chambon P, Lotan R. Modulation by retinoids of mRNA levels for nuclear retinoic acid receptors in murine melanoma cells. Molec Endocrinol 1990; 4:1546–1555.

24. Leid M, Kastner P, Chambon P. Multiplicity generates diversity in the retinoic acid signalling pathways. Trends Biochem Sci 1992; 17:427–433.

25. Mattei MG, Riviere M, Krust A, Ingvarsson S, Vennstrom B, Islam MQ, Levan G, Kautner P, Zelent A, Chambon P, Szpirer J, Szpirer C. Chromosomal assignment of retinoic acid receptor (RAR) genes in the human, mouse, and rat genomes. Genomics 1991; 10:1061–1069.

26. de The H, Vivanco-Ruiz MdM, Tiollais P, Stunnenberg H, Dejean A. Identification of a retinoic acid responsive element in the retinoic acid receptor b gene. Nature 1990; 343:177–180.

27. Lehman JM, Dawson MI, Hobbs PD, Husmann M, Pfahl M. Identification of retinoids with nuclear receptor subtype-selective activities. Cancer Res 1991; 51:4804–4809.

28. Wolbach SB, Howe PR. Tissue changes following deprivation of fat soluble A vitamin. J Exp Med 1925; 42:753–777.

29. Moon RC, McCormic DL, Mehta RG: Inhibition of carcinogenesis by retinoids. Cancer Res 1983; 43:2469–2475.

30. Dowling JE, Wald J. The biological function of vitamin A acid. Proc Natl Acad Sci USA 1960; 46:587–608.

31. Thompson JN, Howell JM, Pitt GAJ. Vitamin A and reproduction in rats. Proc R Soc Lond 1964; 159:510–535.

32. Bollag W. Therapy of chemically induced skin tumour of mice with vitamin A palmitate and vitamin A acid. Experientia 1971; 27:90–92.
33. Lippman SM, Kessler JF, Meyskens FL. Retinoids as preventive and therapeutic anticancer agents (part II). Cancer Tr Rep 1987; 71:493–515.
34. Pastorino U, Soresi E, Clerici M, Chiesa G, Belloni PA, Ongari M, Valente M, Ravasi G. Lung cancer chemoprevention with retinol palmitate. Acta Oncol 1988; 27:773–782.
35. Bollag W. Vitamin A and retinoid: from nutrition to pharmacotherapy in dermatology and oncology. Lancet 1983; 1:860–863.
36. Sporn MB, Dunlop NM, Newton DL, Henderson WR. Relationship between structure and activity of retinoids. Nature 1976; 263:110–113.
37. Peck GL, Olsen TG, Butkus D, Pandya M, Arnaud-Battandier J, Yoder F, Levis WR. Treatment of basal cell carcinomas with 13-cis retinoic acid. Proc Am Assoc Cancer Res 1979; 20:56.
38. Kamm JJ, Ashenfelter KO, Ehmann CW: Preclinical and clinical toxicology of selected retinoids. In: Sporn MB et al., eds. The Retinoids. Orlando: Academic Press, 1984: 287–326.
39. Pennes DR, Ellis CN, Madison KC, Voorhees JJ, Martel W. Early skeletal hyperostosis secondary to 13-cis-retinoic acid. Am J Radiol 1984; 141:979–983.
40. Hong WK, Endicott J, Itri L, et al. 13-cis-Retinoic acid in the treatment of oral leukoplakia. N Engl J Med 1986; 315:1501–1505.
41. Lippman SM, Batsakis JG, Toth BB, Weber RS, Lee JJ, Martin JW, Hays GL, Goepfert H, Hong WK. Comparison of low-dose isotretinoin with beta carotene to prevent oral carcinogenesis. N Engl J Med 1993; 328:15–20.
42. Blomhoff R, Green MH, Green JB, Berg T, Norum KR. Vitamin A metabolism: new perspectives on absorption, transport and storage. Physiol Rev 1991; 71:951–990.
43. Goodman GE, Alberts DS, Peng YM, Beaudry J, Leigh SA, Moon T. Plasma kinetics of oral retinol in cancer patients. Cancer Treat Rep 1984; 68:1125–1133.
44. Wald NJ, Cuckle HS, Barlow RD, Thompson P, Nanchahal K, Blow RJ, Brown I, Harling CC, McCulloch WJ, Morgan J, Reid AR. The effect of vitamin A supplementation on serum retinol and retinol-binding protein levels. Cancer Lett 1985; 29:203–213.
45. Plezia PM, Alberts DS, Peng YM, Xu MJ, Sayers S, Davis BT, Surwit EA, Meyskens F: The role of serum and tissue pharmacology studies in the design and interpretation of chemoprevention trials. Prev Med 1989; 18:680–687.
46. Infante M, Pastorino U, Chiesa G, Bera E, Pisani P, Valente M, Ravasi G. Laboratory evaluation during high-dose vitamin A administration: a randomised study on lung cancer patients after surgical resection. J Cancer Res Clin Oncol 1991; 117:156–162.
47. Korner WF, Vollm J. New aspects of the tolerance of retinol in humans. Int J Vit Nutr Res 1975; 45:363–372.
48. Fidge NH, Shiratori T, Ganguly J, Goodman DS. Pathways of absorption of retinal and retinoic acid in the rat. J Lipid Res 1968; 9:103–109.
49. Bauernfeind JC. The Safe Use of Vitamin A: A Report of the International Vitamin A Consultative Group (IVAG). Washington, DC: The Nutrition Foundation, 1980.
50. Bendich, Langseth L. Safety of vitamin A. Am J Clin Nutr 1989; 49:358–371.
51. Rapaport HG, Herman H, Lehman E: Treatment of ichtyosis with vitamin A. J Pediatr 1942; 21:733–746.
52. Frey JR, Schoch MA. Therapeutische Versuche bei Psoriasis mit Vitamin A, zugleich ein Beitrag zur A-Hypervitaminose. Dermatologicala 1952; 104:80–86.
53. Silverman S, Renstrup G, Pindborg J. Studies in oral leukoplakias: III. Effects of vitamin A comparing clinical, histopathological, cytologic, and hematologic responses. Acta Odont Scand 1963; 21:271–292.
54. Schimpf A, Jansen KH. Hochdosierte Vitamin-A-Therapie bei Psoriasis und Mycosis fungoides. Fortschr Ther 1972; 90:635–639.
55. Pastorino U, Chiesa G, Infante M, Soresi E, Clerici M, Valente M, Belloni PA, Ravasi G. Safety of high-dose vitamin A. Randomized trial on lung cancer chemoprevention. Oncology 1991; 48:131–137.

56. Berni R, Clerici M, Malpeli G, Cleris L, Formelli F. Retinoids: in vitro interaction with retinol-binding protein and influence on plasma retinol. FASEB J 1993; 7:1179–1184.

57. Kerr IG, Lippman ME, Jenkins J, Myers C. Pharmacology of 13-cis-retinoic acid in humans. Cancer Res 1982; 42:2069–2073.

58. Goodman GE, Alberts DS, Peng YM, Beaudry J, Einspahr J, Leigh S, Miles NJ, Davis TP, Meyskens FL. Pharmacokinetics and phase I trial of retinol and 13-cis-retinoic acid. In: Modulation and Mediation of Cancer by Vitamins. Basel: Karger, 983:311–316.

59. DiGiovanna J, Helfgott R, Gerber L, et al. Extraspinal tendon and ligament calcification associated with long-term therapy with etretinate. N Engl J Med 1986; 315:1177–1182.

60. Kilcoyne R. Effects of retinoids on bone. J Am Acad Dermatol 1988; 19:212–216.

61. Akiyama H, Nakamura N, Nagasaka S, Sakamaki H, Onozawa Y. Hypercalcaemia due to all-trans retinoic acid. Lancet 1992; 339:308–309.

62. Niesvizky R, Siegel D, Straus D, et al. Hypercalcemia and increased serum interleukin-6 (IL-6) levels induced by all-trans retinoic acid (ATRA) in patients with multiple myeloma. Proc Am Soc Clin Oncol 1993; 12:407.

63. Moon RC, Thompson HJ, Becci PL, et al. N-(4-Hydroxyphenyl)retinamide, a new retinoid for prevention of breast cancer. Cancer Res 1979; 39:1339–1346.

64. Paulson JD, Oldham JW, Preston RF, et al. Lack of genotoxicity of the cancer chemopreventive agent N-(4-hydroxyphenyl)retinamide. Fundam Appl Toxicol 1985; 5:144–150.

65. Formelli F, Carsana R, Costa A, Buranelli F, Campa T, Dossena G, Magni A, Pizzichetta M. Plasma retinol level reduction by the synthetic retinoid fenretinide: a one year follow-up study of breast cancer patients. Cancer Res 1989; 48:6149–6152.

66a. Veronesi U, De Palo G, Costa A, et al. Chemoprevention of breast cancer with retinoids. INCI Monogr 1992; 12:93–97.

66b. Berni R, Formelli F. In vitro interaction of fenretinide with plasma retinol binding protein and its functional consequences. FEBS Lett 1992; 308:43–45.

67. Chiesa F, Tradati N, Marazza M, Rossi N, Boracchi P, Mariani L, Clerici M, Formelli F, Barzan L, Carrassi A, Pastorini A, Camerini T, Giardini R, Zurrida S, Minn FL, Costa A, DePalo G, Veronesi U. Prevention of local relapses and new localisations of oral leukoplachias with the synthetic retinoid fenretinide (4-HPR). Preliminary results. Oral Oncol Eur J Cancer 1992; 28B:97–102.

68. Hong WK, Bromer RH, Amato DA. Patterns of relapse in locally advanced head and neck cancer patients who achieved complete remission after combined modality therapy. Cancer 1985; 56:1242–1245.

69. de Vries N. The magnitude of the problem. In: de Vries N, Glukman JL, eds. Multiple primary tumors in the head and neck. Stuttgart: Thieme, 1990:1–29.

70. Slaughter DP, Southwick HW, Smejkal W. "Field cancerization" in oral stratified squamous epithelium: clinical implications of multicentric origin. Cancer 1953; 6:963–968.

71. de Vries N, van der Waal I, Snow GB, Multiple primary tumors in oral cancer. Int J Maxillofac Surg 1986; 15:85–87.

72. McDonald S, Haie C, Rubin P, Nelson D, Divers LD. Second malignant tumors in patients with laryngeal carcinoma: diagnosis, treatment and prevention. Int J Radiat Oncol Biol Phys 1989; 17:457–465.

73. Auerbach O, Stout AP, Hammond EC, et al. Multiple primary bronchial carcinomas. Cancer 1967; 20:699.

74. Fontana RS. Early diagnosis of lung cancer. Am Rev Respir Dis 1977; 116:399–402.

75. Femeck BK, Flehinger BJ, Martini N. A retrospective analysis of 10-year survivors from carcinoma of the lung. Cancer 1984; 53(6):1405–1408.

76. Chung KY, Mukhopadhyay T, Kim J, Casson A, Ro JY, Goepfert H, Hong WK, Roth JA. Discordant p53 gene mutations in primary head and neck cancers and corresponding second primary cancers of the upper aerodigestive tract. Cancer Res 1993; 53:1676–1683.

77. Sozzi G, Miozzo M, Pastorino U, et al. Genetic evidence for an independent origin of multiple preneoplastic and neoplastic lung lesions. Cancer Res 1995; 55:135–140.

78. The alpha-tocopherol, beta-carotene cancer prevention study group. The effect of vitamin E and beta-carotene on the incidence of lung cancer and other cancers in male smokers. N Engl J Med 1994; 330:1029–1035.

79. Omenn GS, Goodman GE, Thornquist MD, Balmes J, Cullen MR, Glass A, et al. Effects of a combination of beta-carotene and vitamin A on lung cancer and cardiovascular disease. N Engl J Med 1996; 334:1150–1155.

80. Hennekens CH, Buring JE, Manson JE, Stampfer M, Rosner B, Cook NR, et al. Lack of effect of long-term supplementation with beta-carotene on the incidence of malignant neoplasms and cardiovascular disease. N Engl J Med 1996; 334:1145–1149.

81. Pastorino U. Re: B-carotene and the risk of lung cancer [letter]. J Natl Cancer Inst 1997; 89(6):456–457.

82. Misset JL, Mathe G, Santelli G, et al. Regression of bronchial epidermoid metaplasia in heavy smokers with etretinate treatment. Cancer Detect Prev 1986; 9:167.

83. Arnold AM, Browman GP, Levine MN, D'Souza T, Johnstone B, Skingsley P, Turner-Smith L, Cayco R, Booker L, Newhouse M, Hryniuk WM. The effect of the synthetic retinoid etretinate on sputum cytology: results from a randomised trial. Br J Cancer 1992; 65: 737–743.

84. Lee JS, Benner SE, Lippman SM, Lee JJ, Ro JY, Lukeman JM, Morice RC, Peters EJ, Pang AC, Hittelman HM, Hong WK. A randomised placebo-controlled chemoprevention trial of 13-cis-retinoic acid (cRA) in bronchial squamous metaplasia. Proc ASCO 1993; 13:1117.

85. Hong WK, Lippman JM, Itri L, et al. Prevention of second primary tumors with isotretinoin in squamous cell carcinoma of the head and neck. N Engl J Med 1990; 323:795–801.

86. Pastorino U, Infante I, Maioli, M, Chiesa G, Buyse M, Firket P, Rosmentz N, Clerici M, Soresi E, Valente M, Belloni PA, Ravasi G. Adjuvant treatment of stage I lung cancer with high dose vitamin A. J Clin Oncol 1993; 11:1216–1222.

87. De Vries N, Van Zandwijk N, Pastorino U. The EUROSCAN Study. Br J Cancer 1991; 64:985–989.

88. Kelloff GJ, Boone CW, Crowell JA, et al. Chemopreventive drug development: perspectives and progress. Cancer Epidemiol Biomarkers Prev 1994; 3:85–98.

89. Brooks AD, Benedetti F, Tong WP, Miller VA, Burt M, Kris MG, Warrel RP. Chemoprevention of respiratory tract cancers. Proc Am Assoc Cancer Res (ASCO) 1997; 38:86.

90. Sundaresan V, Ganly P, Hasleton P, Rudd R, Sinha G, Bleehen NM, Rabbitts P. p53 and chromosome 3 abnormalities, characteristic of malignant lung tumours, are detectable in preinvasive lesions of the bronchus. Oncogene 1992; 7:1989–1997.

91. Sozzi G, Miozzo M, Tagliabue E, Calderone C, Lombardi L, Pilotti S, Pastorino U, Pierotti MA, Della Porta G. Cytogenetic abnormalities and overexpression of receptors for growth factors in normal bronchial epithelium and tumor samples of lung cancer patients. Cancer Res 1991; 51:400–404.

92. Lee JS, Lippman SM, Hong WK, Ro JY, Kim SY, Lotan R, Hittelman WN. Determination of biomarkers for intermediate end points in chemoprevention trials. Cancer Res 1992; 52(9 suppl):2707s–2710s.

93. Miozzo M, Sozzi G, Musso K, Pilotti S, Incarbone M, Pastorino U, Pierotti MA. Microsatellite alterations in bronchial and sputum specimens of lung cancer patients. Cancer Res 1996; 56:2285–2288.

94. Sozzi G, Veronese ML, Negrini M, Baffa R, Cotticelli MG, Inoue H, Tornielli S, Pilotti S, De Gregorio L, Pastorino U, Pierotti MA, Ohta M, Huebner K, Croce CM. The FHIT gene at 3p14.2 is abnormal in lung cancer. Cell 1996; 85:117–126.

95. Xu CS, Sozzi G, Lee JS, Pastorino U, Pilotti S, Kurie JM, Hong WK, Lotan R. Suppression of retinoic acid receptor b in non-small cell lung cancer in vivo: implications for lung cancer development. J Natl Cancer Inst 1997;

20

Antioxidants and the Chemoprevention of Lung Cancer

NICO VAN ZANDWIJK and L. VAN 't VEER

Netherlands Cancer Institute
Amsterdam, The Netherlands

I. Introduction

The term *chemoprevention* has been used for almost two decades and has, together with the advances in molecular biology and their application to cancer, become more and more popular in recent years. Chemoprevention is defined as the prevention of cancer in individuals at risk through the administration of compounds that inhibit the process of carcinogenesis. It should be distinguished from the broader term *chemoprophylaxis*, which also includes the elimination of malignant cell lines by any nonsurgical means. It should also be distinguished from the ingestion of certain food components as a part of the normal diet. Simply stated, chemoprevention is the utilization of noncytotoxic natural or synthetic agents to reverse, suppress, or prevent carcinogenesis and its progression toward invasive cancer. This approach to cancer prevention recognizes that cancer is not caused by one single threshold event, but is an evolving multistep molecular and cellular process characterized by a latent period of many years between the initiation of carcinogenesis and the onset of invasive and metastatic cancer.

Cancer of the lung, the most frequent cancer-related cause of death in the western world, is ±90% the result of smoking. For most individuals there is at least a 30-year interval between the commencement of smoking and the onset of a clinically demonstrable tumor (1,2). Continuous exposure to cigarette smoke must therefore be a prerequisite, since stopping of smoking is followed by a steady diminution in the risk of lung cancer. A series of smoking-induced events is required before the appearance of clinical cancer. Oxidants and other reactive chemicals, which are abundantly present in cigarette smoke, have been connected to several of these steps. For any individual it is obvious that the most important preventive "medicine" is smoking cessation, but additional strategies such as chemoprevention with antioxidants might be helpful.

II. Carcinogenesis

Epithelial carcinogenesis proceeds through multiple distinct stages, each characterized by specific molecular and cellular alterations. These stages have been identified as (1) initiation, the rapid irreversible damage to a cell through mutation of genetic material following exposure to carcinogens; (2) promotion, the lengthy process of (reversible) selective growth stimulation and clonal expansion; and (3) progression, when the irreversible steps leading to invasive cancer occur. This classical view of carcinogenesis, although very important for our understanding, is rather simplistic. In reality there may be many more independent events involving genetic and epigenetic changes (3).

In recent years a great deal of research has focused on the identification of cancer-causing genes, and gradually the precise molecular events involving tumor suppressor genes and dominant oncogenes are becoming unraveled. Exposure to cigarette smoke in lung and head and neck cancer has been shown to be correlated to specific mutations of certain oncogenes (K-*ras* and *p53*) found in lung and head and neck cancer (4–6). Interestingly, B(a)P adducts were found on those spots where *p53* mutation is encountered (7). Experimental studies have also shown that mutations resulting from DNA damage elicited by reactive oxygen species frequently involve C-T transitions (8).

III. Oxidative Stress

There is accumulating evidence that one of the major (pro)mutagenic threats faced by many human cells, including especially those of the respiratory tract, which are by virtue of their function already exposed to high oxygen concentrations, is that of (chronic) oxidative stress. Oxidative stress refers to a disturbance in the prooxidant/antioxidant balance in favor of the prooxidants, leading to potential damage (9). Reactive oxygen species arise in most cells as a result of normal metabolic processes such as respiration, but they may also have exogenous sources. These highly reactive chemical molecules include superoxide anion radicals, hydroxyl radicals alkoxyl, and peroxyl radicals. Each has its own distinct chemistry and cellular distribution, and all of them have the potential to alter nucleotide residues. Upon reaction with DNA, oxygen radicals produce a large number of different adducts (10), protein and lipid addition products, and inter- and intrastrand cross-links. Thus, there are potentially hundreds of different types of chemical changes in the DNA resulting from oxygen free radicals that could be mutagenic and contribute to carcinogenesis.

A. Mechanisms to Overcome Oxidative Stress

To protect cellular components, the body has evolved a number of systems to counterbalance oxidative stress. These systems are involved in preventing initial generation of oxidants, trapping oxidants once they have been formed, or repairing the oxidant-induced damage. Table 1 shows a list of common reactive oxygen species and the major free radical–scavenging enzymes, and Figure 1 depicts sites where these enzymes are active. There are two superoxide dismutase (SOD) enzymes, one of which is cytosolic and dependent on copper and zinc. The other is localized in the mitochondria and is manganese dependent. The hydrogen peroxide that results from SOD catalyzation is removed by the enzymes catalase and glutathione (GSH) peroxidase. The highest concentration of catalase is found in the peroxisomes, while GSH peroxidase is predominantly found in the cytoplasm. There are two forms of GSH peroxidase, one requiring selenium as a cofactor and hydrogen peroxide as a substrate. The other form, which is selenium independent, catalyzes the degradation of organic peroxides. The reduction of these peroxides is coupled to the oxidation of reduced GSH. The supply of GSH is replenished by the action of the NADPH-dependent enzyme glutathione reductase. GSH maintains the pool of reduced ascor-

Table 1 Reactive Oxygen Species and the Major (Free) Radical Scavenging Enzymes

Reactive oxygen species[a]	Nonradicals
Superoxide, $O_2^{\cdot-}$	Hydrogen peroxide, H_2O_2
Hydroxyl, $OH^{\cdot}$	Hypochlorous acid, $HOCl$
Peroxyl, $RO_2^{\cdot}$	Ozone, O_3
Alkoyl, $RO^{\cdot}$	Singlet oxygen, $^1\Delta g$
Hydroperoxyl, $HO_2^{\cdot}$	

Free radical–scavenging enzymes	Reaction
Superoxide dismutase	$2O_2^{\cdot-} + 2H^+ \rightarrow H_2O_2 + O_2$
Catalase	$2H_2O_2 \rightarrow 2H_2 + O_2$
Glutathione peroxidase	$ROOH^b + 2\ GSH \rightarrow ROH + H_2O + GSSG$

[a]A collective term that includes both oxygen radicals[c] and certain nonradicals that are oxidizing agents and/or are easily converted into radicals ($HOCl$, O_3, $ONOO-$, $^1O_2$, H_2O_2).
[b]Lipid hydroperoxide.
[c]A radical is defined as an atom or molecule with an unpaired electron.
Source: Adapted from Ref. 12.

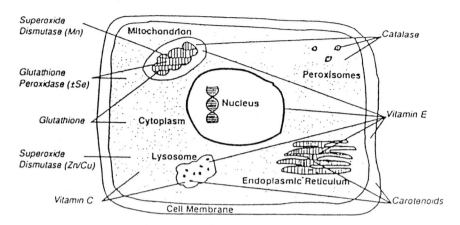

Figure 1 Antioxidants and their cellular location.

bic acid, which in turn is available to quench free radicals and contributes to the ability of GSH peroxidase to remove peroxides. Peroxides may also be eliminated by the conjugating action of glutathione-S-transferase. GSH conjugates have lost metabolic activity and are excreted. GSH has been regarded as one of the most important elements in antioxidant protection as hydroxyl radicals may only be neutralized by nonenzymatic quenching by GSH. In the lung GSH plays a prominent role as very high concentrations of GSH are found in the epithelial lining fluid (ELF). GSH levels are far higher than that found in the circulating blood, and it is thought that these levels are maintained by active release from intracellular stores of pulmonary epithelial cells. Interestingly GSH levels in the ELF have been found to increase (after an initial decrease) after exposure to cigarette smoke and chronic hyperoxia (11-13) (Fig. 1, Table 1).

B. Reactive Oxygen Species

Oxygen exists in several states depending on the number of electrons and how they are paired (12). The superoxide radical is formed in aerobic cells by the transfer of electrons to oxygen as a by-product of electron transport. During phagocytosis the superoxide radical, produced by NADPH oxidase, helps to kill bacteria. The superoxide dismutase enzymes limit the effects of superoxide radicals by inducing a transformation to H_2O_2. The toxicity of H_2O_2, which can easily cross membranes, is limited by H_2O_2-removing enzymes such as catalase. The most serious cellular damage will occur when superoxide radicals and H_2O_2 are converted to more reactive species, such as the hydroxyl radical. The hydroxyl radical is formed by metal (iron)-dependent decomposition of H_2O_2 (Fenton and Haber-Weiss reactions). The hydroxyl radical is so reactive that it will cause damage at, or very close to, the site where it is formed.

C. Metals and Trace Elements

As mentioned above, trace elements and metals are important components of free radical–scavenging metalloenzymes. They may, however, also catalyze oxidation of biomolecules. The metals most important in oxidant/antioxidant balance include iron, copper, zinc, manganese and selenium. The proteins that bind these metals have been considered as primary antioxidants because they prevent the metals from participating in free radical formation (14). Two thirds of the body's iron occurs in hemoglobin or is bound by proteins such as transferrin, lactoferrin, myoglobin, and ferritin. These proteins that chelate or complex iron help to regulate the iron-dependent formation of the hydroxyl radical. Radical reactions seem to be catalytically stimulated by tissue injury or other processes that enable the release of iron. For example, cytostatic drugs increase the amount of free iron in the circulation. The released iron could then participate in Fenton and Haber-Weiss type reactions to cause further acceleration of tissue damage. Copper is bound to the plasma protein ceruloplasmin and is incorporated into other copper-dependent proteins, such as superoxide dismutase and cytochrome oxidase. Albumin binds up to 5% of plasma copper. Although oxygen free radical damage may occur locally to albumin, albumin is actually protecting other important molecules, such as DNA, against oxidative damage (14).

IV. Cigarette Smoke and Air Pollution

The most important sources of oxidative stress for the epithelial cells in the lung and the upper aerodigestive tract include cigarette smoke and air pollution. Cigarette smoke is a complex mixture of over 4000 chemical compounds, including high concentrations of free radicals in both the gas and tar phases and other oxidants (15). Gas-phase radicals are both inorganic and organic, including reactive oxygen species and various other free radicals. Cigarette tar contains high concentrations of stable radicals, and at least four different species have been identified with electron paramagnetic resonance (EPR) (16,17). The most interesting is a semiquinone in equilibrium with quinones and hydroquinones in a low molecular weight tar matrix (18). Hydroquinones and semiquinones can react with molecular oxygen to produce superoxide, and superoxide can dismutate to form hydrogen peroxide. Hydrogen peroxide can directly oxidize and inactivate the protein α_1-proteinase inhibitor by nonradical mechanisms, but it can also be reduced to the hydroxyl radical. As previously mentioned, the superoxide and hydroxyl radicals are unstable and may elicit DNA damage. Thus, apart from the well-known (pro)carcinogens like benzo(*a*)pyrene and tobacco-specific nitrosamine (NNKs) radicals present in cigarette tar appear to be an additional source for mutagenicity and carcinogenicity (9). Smoke also induces an influx of neutrophils and macrophages into the lung with the potential to release oxidants (19). It is therefore not surprising that lung cancer is much more frequent among individuals suffering from oxidant-induced pulmonary disease such as chronic obstructive pulmonary disease (COPD) (20,21).

It is far more difficult to prove the relationship between air pollution and lung cancer. Some ecological studies, however, have shown a higher incidence of lung cancer in urban areas when compared with rural areas (22,23). Air pollution, although not very well defined, is at least characterized by increased levels of a number of oxidants.

V. Carcinogen Metabolism

Many of the known carcinogens are environmental chemicals that enter the body as procarcinogens requiring metabolic activation in order to start the initiation process. The critical importance of this activation became clear from studies in the 1970s demonstrating that ultimate carcinogens, like reactive oxygen species, are electrophilic and may enter into damaging reactions with the DNA (adduct formation), thus exerting promutagenic effects (24). Metabolic activation generally involves one or more of the family of inducible cytochromes P-450 (designated phase I enzymes) that mainly carry out oxidation and reduction reactions. Although some of the cytochromes are involved in the conversion of promutagens, such as benzopyrene, to the highly carcinogenic diolepoxides, most of the reactions catalyzed by P-450 do not lead to metabolic activation, but to the formation of more water-soluble, non-electrophilic detoxification products.

Protection of cells against the (reactive) electrophilic metabolites and other xenobiotic products may be provided by high intracellular levels of GSH (acting as a noncritical electrophile scavenger) and phase II enzymes that inactivate electrophiles by conjugation with glutathione (glutathione S-transferase GST) or glucuronic acid, or by hydrolysis. Another important detoxification enzyme is reduced nicotinamide adenine dinucleotide phosphate (NADPH), or quinone oxidoreductase (NQ01), which catalyzes quinones and thereby shields cells against the damaging electrophilicity of quinones and their ability to generate oxidative stress (25). The balance between activation and detoxification of a carcinogen is clearly important, and there is an increasing number of reports suggesting that heritable differences in

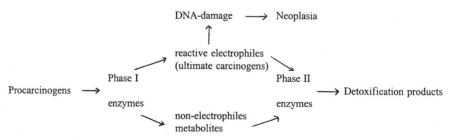

Figure 2 A simplified scheme for the role of phase I and phase II enzymes in carcinogen metabolism.

the genes coding for certain enzymes (GST, NQ01) are responsible for the interindividual differences in the predisposition to and familial clustering of lung cancer (26–28) (Fig. 2).

VI. Diet

Diet can affect lung cancer risk. A large body of epidemiological evidence, together with data from animal and in vitro studies, strongly supports the relationships between dietary constituents and the risk of specific cancers. In a review of 32 published epidemiological studies it was apparent that the quarter of the population with low dietary intake of fruits and vegetables had double the cancer rate of those with high intake for the most common types of cancer, including cancer of the lung (29). This preventive effect of fruits and vegetables has been attributed to (the antioxidant) β-carotene (30). Dietary intake of carotenoids is reflected in serum carotene levels, and low serum levels of β-carotene have clearly correlated with an excess risk of lung cancer (31,32).

In recent years, other micronutrients have also been identified as having the potential to decrease human cancer risk, including vitamin E, folic acid, vitamin C, and the trace element selenium. It is important to emphasize that there is a lack of consistency in some of the correlations found, with some epidemiological studies reporting an effect on cancer incidence but others being unable to demonstrate this (33,34). It is apparent that the human diet is varied and complex and cannot be easily assessed. The accuracy of information collected by dietary interview is not only limited by the human capacity for recall, but also by the complex methodology of dietary questionnaires. Diet records are laborious to maintain and can only be collected on a limited number of individuals over a brief period of time. Estimations of levels of micronutrients in biological samples provide objective measurements. However, their relevance to eating habits is not always clear. Moreover, samples have generally been obtained at one point in time. For many nutrients, few or no data are available regarding the relationship of a single biological measurement of one micronutrient level to long-term nutrient status or to the carcinogenic process. It may also be theorized that the outcome of the measurement of a potential dietary preventive agent in cancer patients may rather be a reflection of the disease on the serum level of that agent (35). Thus, abnormal levels should be interpreted with caution, and the definite tests of dietary preventive agents should be conducted under controlled conditions, where the agents serve as the only variable between the treated and control groups.

Thus far, large clinical trials have provided disappointing results (see below), and, despite many retrospective suggestive epidemiological studies addressing the issue of smoking-related cancer and nutrition, there is no conclusive evidence for a preventive effect of the antioxidant vitamins β-carotene and α-tocopherol. On the other hand, it is gradually becoming clear that oxidative stress by cigarette smoke is not simply leading to decreased levels of one or two antioxidants but that it may involve a complex sequence of events with natural antioxidants such as β-carotene, α-tocopherol, and vitamin C. These substances may also have prooxidant effects with a consequent stimulus of oxidative stress. Recent studies have shown that inverse relations between ascorbate and α-tocopherol may exist in vitamin E–supplemented subjects (36,37), that α-tocopherol may also have prooxidant function, and that tocopherol radicals can be reduced by ascorbate (38). Moreover, it has been suggested that administration of high amounts of an antioxidant like α-tocopherol might influence the tissue delivery of other antioxidants (39).

Isolating the effects of certain food constituents has been shown to be difficult. On the other hand, many preclinical studies confirm that certain chemicals from fruits and vegetables are able to inhibit experimental tumors. Many of these substances do have antioxidative properties or are able to induce detoxification, and in some cases synthetic analogs have also proven to be preventive in preclinical studies. Examples of this last category are N-acetylcysteine, an antioxidant sulfur compound and GSH agonist widely used in Europe for the (preventive) treatment of COPD and an effective rescue agent for paracetamol intoxication (40), and Oltipraz, a dithiolethione with detoxifying properties (41). A list of potential chemopreventive agents, many of which are phytochemicals, is given in Table 2. Interestingly, most of them share stimulating effects on phase II enzymes or inhibiting action on phase I inducers.

VII. Chemoprevention Studies

Large-scale, randomized, controlled chemoprevention trials using the antioxidants β-carotene and α-tocopherol include the physicians health study (PHS), the β-carotene and retinol efficacy trial (CARET), and the α-tocopherol, β-carotene cancer prevention study (ATBC).

The PHS study (double-blind, placebo-controlled) evaluated the prevention of cancer and cardiovascular disease by β-carotene (50 mg on alternate days) and aspirin supplementation in 22,071 U.S. physicians. After an average of 12 years of intervention with β-carotene (the aspirin part was terminated in 1987, as a clear preventive effect on the first heart attack was noted), no significant evidence of benefit or harm from this intervention could be found. There were no significant differences in the number of deaths from lung cancer among current or former smokers (42). It has to be emphasized, however, that this study was conducted in a population of well-educated, well-nourished, healthy (89% were nonsmokers) men.

CARET and ATBC were both conducted in a population at high risk for lung cancer. CARET (double-blind, placebo-controlled) tested the efficacy of a combination of β-carotene and retinyl palmitate in male and female (heavy) smokers, former smokers, and workers exposed to asbestos (total of 18,314 individuals). CARET was stopped earlier than planned after an average of 4 years of supplementation as a 28% higher incidence of lung cancer was observed in participants receiving the

Table 2 Antioxidants (Phytochemicals) and Chemopreventive Action

Category	Source	Agent	Chemopreventive action	Experimental evidence	Clinical experience
Carotenoids	Fruit Vegetables	Lutein Lycopene	High antioxidant capacity (oxidated metabolites in vivo)	—	Epidemiologic evidence
Dithiolethiones	Cruciferous vegetables	1.2-Dithiole-3 thiones[a]	Stimulation of detoxification (phase II enzymes incl. GST)	Preventive in several exp. models, incl. inhibition of exp. lung tumors (BaP and NNK induced)	
		Oltipraz			Phase II (ongoing)[53]
Isothiocyanates		Benzyl isothiocyanate (BITC) Phenethyl isothiocyante (PEITC)	Selective inhibition of (cytochrome p450) phase I and stimulation of phase II enzymes (GST)		
Flavonoids/ Polyperols	Fruits (berries) Nuts Tea Turmeric Vegetables	Quercitin Myricetin Curcumin Catechin Gallic acid			
Sulfur compounds	Garlic Onion	Diallyl sulfide			
		N-acetylcysteine[a]	High antioxidant capacity induction and replenishment of GSH stores Enhancement of detoxification	Several animal models inhibition exp. lung tumors and DNA adducts	Phase III (Euroscan, ongoing)
Terpenes	Citrus fruits	Limonene	Induction of phase I and phase II enzymes	Prevention of rat mammary carcinomas	Phase I (ongoing)

[a]Synthetic.
Source: Ref. 52.

β-carotene/retinyl palmitate combination (43). ATBC, a trial in a population of 29,133 male smokers from Finland, investigated the efficacy of vitamin E (α-tocopherol) alone, β-carotene alone, or the combination of the two compounds in preventing lung cancer (44). ATBC (double-blind, placebo-controlled) also showed a 16% higher incidence of lung cancer in the β-carotene–supplemented population. This increased risk translated into a 8% higher risk of death, primarily due to deaths from lung cancer and ischemic heart disease. No evidence of an interaction between β-carotene and α-tocopherol with respect to the incidence of lung cancer was found. Interestingly in this study α-tocopherol conferred some protection against prostate cancer. In contrast with the CARET and ATBC studies, a large number (29,548) of individuals involving the general population of Linxian (China) with antioxidants (β-carotene, α-tocopherol, and selenium) demonstrated a 13% reduction of cancer (45). This reduction of cancer in a rural population with subclinical deficiencies of several nutrients and high incidence of esophageal and gastric cancer was mainly due to a lower gastric cancer rate.

The different outcomes of these large studies have elicited a lot of reactions, some pointing to the confounding effect of smoking (Table 2) (46), others to the relatively short duration of intervention in comparison with life-long smoking (47). The contrast between the long latency period of lung cancer and the relative short follow-up period (6 years) in the ATBC study has also been noted. Some of the lung cancers found during follow-up might have already been present at the time of randomization.

Notwithstanding these arguments, the increased risk of lung cancer in those individuals who continued to smoke in the CARET and ATBC studies points to the fact that we still lack insight in the complex area of oxidative stress by smoking and antioxidative preventive mechanisms. Prooxidative effects of antioxidants like β-carotene, α-tocopherol, and vitamin C as well as their interactions must be further investigated. It may be argued that the cancer-protective effect observed for vegetables and fruits is dependent on interactions of a number of constituents in these foods and that we must focus on other groups of antioxidants present in fruits and vegetables (Table 3).

One of the major problems with large-scale intervention studies with cancer as an endpoint is that it is so many years before a conclusion can be reached. In recent years, smaller studies with intermediate markers of carcinogenesis as surrogate endpoints have been advocated. Another approach might be found in the identification of individuals with a significant increased risk for specific cancers. For example, this approach has been used in studies on patients who received curative treatment for primary cancer of the head and neck (48) or lung (49) when there is an increased risk for a second cancer in the same field (50). One of these studies, the Euroscan study, is already almost 10 years underway studying the preventive effects of *N*-acetylcysteine and retinyl palmitate in a population of patients curatively treated for lung and head and neck cancer at risk for second primary tumor (51).

Table 3 Lung Cancer Incidence and Overall Mortality (per 10,000 person-years) and Proportion of Smokers at Entry

Trial and reference	β-Carotene[a]	Control	Smokers at entry (%) Current	Former
PHS				
Lung cancer incidence	6	6	11	39
Total mortality	74	73		
ATBC				
Lung cancer incidence	56	47	100	0
Total mortality	218	201		
CARET				
Lung cancer incidence	59	46	60	39
Total mortality	144	119		

[a]Combined with retinol in CARET.
PHS = Physicians Health Study; ATBC = Alpha-Tocopherol, Beta-Carotene Cancer Prevention Study; CARET = Beta-Carotene and Retinol Efficacy Trial.
Source: Adapted from Ref. 47.

VIII. Conclusion

The process of continuous damage to the respiratory epithelium by cigarette smoke leading to lung cancer is gradually being illucidated. It is apparent that metabolic processes, including the activation of xenobiotics to electrophilic reactants and scavenging of reactive oxygen species, are important in the multistep process of pulmonary carcinogenesis. Diet and genetic metabolic factors seem to influence these processes, which may explain why only about 18% of lifetime smokers will become victims of lung cancer. Although our understanding of pulmonary carcinogenesis has increased, recent chemoprevention studies have shown that the prescription of one or two antioxidants during a relatively limited period are insufficient to counterbalance the detrimental effects of smoking and may even augment the risk of lung cancer. It is therefore likely that future research will focus on early intervention for nonsmoking individuals who still have an increased risk for lung cancer. There are many phytochemicals with antioxidative properties in addition to synthetic analogs, which have already gone through extensive preclinical testing to be incorporated in clinical studies.

References

1. Sporn MB. Approaches to prevention of epithelial cancer during the preneoplastic period. Cancer Res 1976; 36:2699–2702.
2. Pierce JP, Thurmond L, Rosbrook B. Projecting international lung cancer mortality rates: first approximations with tobacco-consumption data. Monogr J Natl Cancer Inst 1992; 12:45–49.

3. Loeb LA, Eruster VL, Warner KE, Abbotts J, Laszio J. Smoking and lung cancer: an overview. Cancer Res 1984; 44:5940–5958.
4. Greenblatt MS, Reddel RR, Harris CC. Carcinogenesis and cellular and molecular biology of lung cancer. In: Roth JA, Ruckdeschel JC, Weisenburger TH, eds. Thoracic Oncology. 2d ed. Philadelphia: W.B. Saunders, 1995:5–25.
5. Brennan J, Boyle JO, Koch WM, Goodman SN, Hruban RH, Eby YJ, Couch MJ, Forastiere AA, Sidransky D. Association between cigarette smoking and mutation of the p53 gene in squamous-cell carcinoma of the head and neck. N Engl J Med 1995; 332:712–717.
6. Slebos R, Hruban RH, Dalesio O, Mooi WJ, Otterhaus GJA, Rodenhuis S. Relationship between k-ras oncogene activation and smoking in adenocarcinoma of the lung. J Natl Cancer Inst 1991; 83:1024–1027.
7. Westra WH, Offerhaus GJ, Goodman SN, Slebos RJ, Polak M, Baas IO, Rodenhuis S, Hruban RH. Overexpression of the p53 tumor suppressor gene product in primary lung adenocarcinomas is associated with cigarette smoking. Am J Surg Pathol 1993; 17:213–220.
8. Denissenko MF. Preferential formation of benzo(a)pyrene adducts at lung cancer hotspots in p53. Science 1996; 374:430–432.
9. Feig DI, Reid TM, Loeb LA. Reactive oxygen species in tumorigenesis. Cancer Res 1994; 54(suppl):1890S–1894S.
10. Sies H. Oxidative stress: introduction. In: Sies H, ed. Oxidative Stress: Oxidants and Antioxidants. San Diego: Academic Press, 1991:15–22.
11. Halliwell B, Aruoma O. DNA damage by oxygen-derived species. FEBS Lett 1991; 281: 9–19.
12. Chow CK, Cigarette smoking and oxidative damage in the lung. Ann NY Acad Sci 1993; 686:289–298.
13. Rahman I, MacNee W. Role of oxidants/antioxidants in smoking-induced lung diseases. Free Radical Biol Med 1996; 21:669–681.
14. Halliwell B. Antioxidants: the basics. In: Sies H, ed. Antioxidants in Disease Mechanisms and Therapy. Advances in Pharmacology. Vol. 38. San Diego: Academic Press, 1997:3–20.
15. Mulholland CW, Strain JJ. Serum total free radical trapping ability in acute myocardial infarction. Clin Biochem 1991; 24:437–441.
16. U.S. Department of Health and Human Services (DHHS). The health consequences of smoking: 25 years of progress. Washington DC: DHSS. Public Health Service Center for Disease Control and Prevention, Office on Smoking and Health DHHS Publication No. (CDC) 89–8411, 1989.
17. Pryor WA. Cigarette smoke and the involvement of free radicals reactions in chemical carcinogenesis. Br J Cancer 1987; 8(suppl):19–23.
18. Pryor WA, Prier DG, Church DF. Electron-spin resonance study of mainstream and sidestream cigarette smoke: nature of free radicals in gas-phase smoke and cigarette tar. Environ Health Perspect 1983; 47:345–355.
19. Stone K, Pryor WA. The effects of cigarette smoke free radicals. In: Pass HI, Mitchell JB, Johnson DH, Turrisi AT, eds. Lung Cancer. Principles and Practice. Lippincott-Raven 1996:323–328.
20. MacNee W, Wiggs B, Berzberg AS, Hogg JC. The effects of cigarette smoking on neutrophil kinetics in human lungs. N Engl J Med 1989; 321:924–928.
21. Tockman MS, Anthonisen NR, Wright EC, Donithan MG. Airways obstruction and the risk for lung cancer. Ann Intern Med 1987; 106:512–518.
22. Nomura A, Stemmermann GN, Chyou PH, Marcus EB, Buist AB. Prospective study of pulmonary function and lung cancer. Am Rev Respir Dis 1991; 144:307–311.
23. Vena JE. Air pollution as a risk factor in lung cancer. Am J Epidemiol 1982; 116:42–56.
24. Friis S, Storm HH. Urban-rural variation in cancer incidence in Denmark 1943–1987. Eur J Cancer 1993; 29A:538–544.
25. Miller EC. Some current perspectives on chemical carcinogenesis in humans and experimental animals: presidential address. Cancer Res 1978; 38:1479–1496.
26. Prochaska HJ, Talalay P. Role of NAD(P)H: quinone reductase in protection against the toxicities of quinones and related agents. In: Sies H, ed. Oxidative stress, Oxidants and Antioxidants. London: Academic Press, 1991:195.

27. Law MR. Genetic predisposition to lung cancer. Br J Cancer 1990; 61:195–206.
28. McWilliams JE, Sanderson BJ, Harris EL, Richert-Boe KE, Henner WD. Glutathione S-transferase M_1 ($GSTM_1$) deficiency and lung cancer risk. Cancer Epidemiol Biomarkers Prev 1995; 4:589–594.
29. Wiencke JK, Spitz MR, McWilliams A, Kelsey KT. Lung cancer in Mexican-Americans and African-Americans is associated with the mild-type genotype of the NAD(P)H quinone oxido reductase polymorphism. Cancer Epidemiol Biomarkers Prev 1997; 6:87–92.
30. Block G, Patterson B, Subar A. Fruit, vegetables, and cancer prevention: a review of the epidemiological evidence. Nutr Cancer 1992; 18:1–29.
31. Peto R, Doll R, Buckley JD, Sporn MB. Can dietary beta-carotene materially reduce human cancer rates? Nature 1981; 290:201–208.
32. Menkes MS, Comstock GW, Vuilleumier JP, Helsing KJ, Rider AA, Brookmeyer R. Serum beta-carotene, vitamin A and E, selenium, and the risk of lung cancer. N Engl J Med 1986; 315:1250–1254.
33. Wald NJ, Thompson SG, Densem JW, Boreham J, Bailey A. Serum beta-carotene and subsequent risk of cancer: results from the BUPA study. Br J Cancer 1988; 57:428–433.
34. Greenwald P, Nixon DW, Malone WF, Kelloff GJ, Stern HR, Witkin KM. Concepts in cancer chemoprevention research. Cancer 1990; 65:1483–1490.
35. Hunter DJ, Willett WC. Human epidemiological evidence on the nutritional prevention of cancer. In: Moon TE, Micozzi MS, eds. Nutrition and Cancer Prevention: Investigating the Role of Micronutrients. New York: Marcel Dekker, 1989:83–100.
36. Robinson MF, Godfrey PJ, Thomson CD. Blood selenium and glutathion peroxidase activity in normal subjects and in surgical patients with and without cancer in New Zealand. Am J Clin Nutr 1979; 32:1477–1485.
37. Brown KM, Morrice PC, Duthie GG. Erythrocyte vitamin E and plasma ascorbate concentrations in relation to erythrocyte peroxidation in smokers and non-smokers: dose response to vitamin E supplementation. Am J Clin Nutr 1997; 65:496–502.
38. Waldeck AR, Stocker R. Radical-initiated lipid peroxidation in low density lipoproteins: insights obtained from kinetic modeling. Chem Res Toxicol 1996; 9:954–964.
39. Handelman GJ, Macklin LJ, Fitch K, Weiter JJ, Dratz EA. Oral α-tocopherol supplements decrease plasma g-tocopherol levels in humans. J Nutr 1985; 115:807–813.
40. Cross GE, Traber MG. Cigarette smoking and antioxidant vitamins: the smoke screen continues to clear but has a way to go. Am J Clin Nutr 1997; 65:562–563.
41. Van Zandwijk N. N-Acetylcysteine for lung cancer prevention. Chest 1995; 107:1437–1441.
42. Kensler TW, Helzloner KJ. Oltipraz: clinical opportunities for cancer prevention. J Cell Biochem 1995; suppl 22:101–107.
43. Hennekens CH, Buring JE, Manson JE, Stampfer M, Rosner B, Cook NR, Belanger C, LaMotte F, Gaziano JM, Ridker PM, Willett W, Peto R. Lack of effect of long-term supplementation with beta carotene on the incidence of malignant neoplasms and cardiovascular disease. N Engl J Med 1996; 334:1145–1149.
44. Omenn GS, Goodman GE, Thornquist MD, Balmes J, Cullen MR, Glass A, Keogh JP, Meyskens FL, Valanis B, Williams JH, Barnhart S, Hammar S. Effects of combination of beta carotene and vitamin A on lung cancer and cardiovascular disease. N Engl J Med 1996; 334:1150–1155.
45. The alpha-tocopherol, beta-carotene cancer prevention study group. The effect of vitamin E and beta carotene on the incidence of lung cancer and other cancers in male smokers. N Engl J Med 1994; 330:1029–1035.
46. Blot WJ, Li JY, Taylor PR, Guo W, Dawsey S, Wang GQ, Yang CS, Zheng SF, Gail M, Li GY et al. Nutrition intervention trials in Linxian: supplementation with specific vitamin/mineral combinations, cancer incidence and disease-specific mortality in the general population. J Natl Cancer Inst 1993; 85:1483–1492.
47. Pastorino U. Beta-carotene and the risk of lung cancer. J Natl Cancer Inst 1995; 89:456–457.
48. Pryor WA. Letter to the editor. N Engl J Med 1994; 331:621.
49. Hong WK, Lippmann SM, Itri LM, Karp DD, Lee JS, Beyers RM, Schantz SP, Kramer AM, Lotan R, Peters LJ et al. Prevention of second primary tumors with isoretinoin in squamous cell carcinoma of the head and neck. N Engl J Med 1990; 323:795–801.

50. Pastorino U, Infante M, Maioli M, Chiesa G, Buyse M, Firket P, Rosmentz N, et al. Adjuvant treatment of stage I lung cancer with high-dose vitamin B. J Clin Oncol 1993; 11:1216–1222.
51. Lippman SM, Benner SE, Hong WK. Cancer chemoprevention. J Clin Oncol 1994; 12: 851–873.
52. Van Zandwijk N, Pastorino U, De Vries N, Dalesio O. Euroscan. The European organization for research and treatment of cancer. Chemoprevention study in lung cancer. Lung Cancer 1993; 9:351–356.
53. Cancer chemopreventive agents: drug development status and future prospects. Kellof GJ, Boone CW (guest eds.). J Cell Biochem 1995; supplement 22.
54. Jacobson LP, Zhang B, Zhu W, Wang J, Wu Y, Zhang Q, Yu L, et al. Oltipraz chemoprevention trial in Qidong, People's Republic of China: study design and clinical outcomes. Cancer Epidemiol Biomarkers Prev 1997; 6:257–265.

21

Integrated Approach to the Management of Early Lung Cancer

**JAMES L. MULSHINE, ANTHONY M.
TRESTON, and FRANK CUTTITTA**

National Cancer Institute
National Institutes of Health
Bethesda, Maryland

MELVYN S. TOCKMAN

University of South Florida
Tampa, Florida

I. Introduction

Lung cancer is the most commonly fatal cancer worldwide. The current mortality rate for this cancer approaches 90%, with the overwhelming majority of this disease caused by exposure to tobacco combustion products (1). While improved measures to successfully reduce youth smoking are essential to limit the extent of this problem, unfortunately the current burden of tobacco consumption in the world today and the long incubation time of lung cancer mean that the high death rate from this disease will not change for decades despite any level of success of primary smoking prevention measures. Significantly more effective lung cancer clinical management approaches are required. In some instances, there is a perception that fostering early detection and intervention research will compromise the allocation of sufficient resources to allow successful primary prevention. The research needs of lung cancer prevention are twofold, with a complementary focus on both reducing tobacco consumption as well as measures to improve the outcome of individuals afflicted with this cancer. In the United States at a number of major lung cancer centers, the frequency of newly diagnosed cases of lung cancer in former smokers exceeds the number of new lung cancer cases in current smokers (2). If this trend continues without the ability to better manage these new lung cancer cases, then the incentive for current smokers to stop smoking will be reduced. In reality, effective reduction of lung cancer mortality, especially in the near-term, will require more than primary prevention measures. Improved early lung cancer detection capability assumes central importance in moving from the current problem of routinely diagnosing new cases of lung cancer only after metastatic disease has already occurred.

The current clinical management dilemma with lung cancer patients who have already developed regional or distant metastatic cancer at the time of initial detection is due to the existing diagnostic technology. This systemic phase of lung cancer is usually treated with combination chemotherapy. Despite some improvement in outcome with newer agents, especially with better control of the drug side effects, chemotherapy for metastatic lung cancer is rarely curative. The persistent high mortality of lung cancer is therefore due to the inability of existing diagnostic imaging technology to routinely detect premetastatic lung cancer. This reflects the evolution of lung cancer in the tracheobronchial tree, where it is obscured by the complex anatomy of the thoracic cavity. This is a problem that is not likely to be overcome by any of the existing imaging modalities. Efforts to improve the early detection of lung cancer have been ongoing for decades with a major aspect of this effort coming into focus with the National Cancer Institute–sponsored study conducted at Johns Hopkins, Mayo Clinic, and Memorial Sloan Kettering (3,4). In that landmark study, the benefit of adding cytological evaluation of sputum specimens to serial chest x-ray was evaluated to determine if the combined screening approach would allow at least a 50% reduction in lung cancer mortality. This trial resulted in an improvement of many clinical parameters except for the most important endpoint of cancer-related survival. In the wake of this negative trial, efforts to improve early lung cancer detection virtually evaporated (5). To this day, the vast majority of research energy for lung cancer has been channeled into the improvement of the treatment of advanced lung cancer. Unfortunately, the net result of this effort has been that the mortality of lung cancer has only marginally improved over the last 30 years. While acknowledging that even a 1% reduction in lung cancer mortality means 1500 additional lives saved, the improvement in 5-year survival over the last 30 years has been significant. Given the level of research effort, the expectation was that a considerably greater improvement in 5-year lung cancer survival rate should have been achieved.

II. Considerations in Improved Lung Cancer Outcomes

The concept of field carcinogenesis has surprisingly powerful implications in shaping the requirements of early detection research. In general, lung cancer arises in response to chronic exposure of the bronchial epithelium to tobacco combustion products. In the 1950s the head and neck cancer surgeon D. P. Slaughter noted that a resected surgical specimen contained multifocal areas of severe tissue injury in addition to the primary cancer (6). The suggestion was that the entire epithelium was injured by the exposure to the carcinogenic tobacco smoke, and the entire area of involvement was called field cancerization. This concept has been validated on a histological level, and the cytological correlate of this concept is the basis for the success of cytomorphologic detection of lung cancer as reported by Saccomanno et al. (7). Yet cytomorphological detection failed to change cancer-related lung cancer mortality in the previously mentioned large, three-institution early lung cancer detection trial (3,4). The failure, however, was due to the complex biology of lung cancer as reflected by the finding that only a fraction of lung cancer (all sputum cytology-detected cases were squamous cell cancer) could be detected with conventional sputum-based cytomorphological detection. No standard criteria have been developed for the cytomorphological characteristics of early small-cell, adenocarcinoma, or large-cell lung cancer, which explains why these cancer histologies were not detected with this assay. The basis for the failure of this trial to reduce lung cancer mortality is still not generally understood. Approaches to cytomorphologic lung cancer detection, even with computer-assisted image analysis, to this day are only successful with squamous cell lung cancer (8,9). With the frequency of squamous cell lung cancer decreasing relative to the other lung cancer histologies, other approaches that are effective in identifying all lung cancer histologies are required.

III. Where Does Early Lung Cancer Start?

The bronchial epithelium is the only site in the body that is thought to be involved in the early stages of lung cancer development. The implication of this is that the epithelium can provide evidence of involvement with carcinogenesis decades before the development of metastatic disease. This reality provides a potential "window of opportunity" for early lung cancer detection. Overwhelming clinical evidence shows that metastatic disease is lethal, so the identification of lung cancer prior to metastatic spread becomes a functional requirement for useful early lung cancer detection. Fortunately, the research literature is full of examples of new molecular tools that can be used to demonstrate extensive, multifaceted cellular injury. Several groups have shown extensive genetic injury (chromosomal duplications as well as deletions and mutations) in the airway cells of smokers as well as in individuals with lung cancer (10,11). An important research focus is in establishing the precise sequence of molecular events that leads to the development of a new lung cancer. The biology of the respiratory epithelium as it relates to carcinogenesis will be considered in this article relative to the opportunity to establish better approaches to early lung cancer detection. A number of additional developmental issues will come into play as we begin to translate specific scientific information into the basis of new lung cancer detection tools.

In the field of lung cancer biology, we are now aware of a bewildering array of biological changes that may occur in the airway cells of subjects chronically exposed to combusted tobacco products. We also know that the process of developing a lung cancer can take decades. Critical, initial steps of early carcinogenesis could be obscured by the accumulation of genetic injuries found at the time a primary tumor is large enough to be clinically detected. A thoughtful discussion on how to approach these complex issues has been provided through a series of workshops conducted by the International Association for the Study of Lung Cancer (12,13). The working assumption is that the biological mediators of early lung cancer would provide a series of rational targets to exploit for marker-based early cancer detection. Our own research has been driven by the hypothesis that the molecular events occurring on the bronchial epithelium should also be reflected by comparable molecular findings evident in the exfoliated cells recovered in the sputum from an individual with field cancerization (14).

A sputum specimen is a useful target for screening analysis since it can be obtained from an individual without an invasive diagnostic procedure. The technical challenge in using sputum as a screening assay target is inherent to any detection assay in that the earlier in the natural history one analyzes, the lower the percentage of positive cells contained in the specimen. Specifically a sputum will provide only a limited number of cells of demonstrable bronchial epithelial origin and only a limited proportion of those cells may betray the presence of field carcinogenesis. However, when a large numbers of subjects are to be screened, sputum acquisition is so much less expensive and less intrusive than performing either bronchoscopy or a computerized tomography that it becomes the assay of choice. The kind of in vitro assay analysis contemplated for definitive early lung cancer detection in a cost-effective fashion requires an instrumentation platform that can rapidly ascertain biomarker expression status for a restricted subset of informative bronchial epithelial cells contained in the complex cellular mixture routinely seen with sputum specimens. A related type of image analysis technology has been recently approved in certain settings with cervical cytology analysis, but the cellular environment in the cervix is somewhat simpler than the range of cell types encountered in the airway. To ensure economic viability, population-based cancer screening tools will require developmental refinement. Validation of every step from specimen acquisition through assay analysis is essential, since important management issues are involved. Careful attention to quality assurance measures may permit the general public to feel comfortable with this new management paradigm. While such a sophisticated analytical tool has not yet been perfected, the world of diagnostic technology is in the midst of an unprecedented period of progress.

Critical analysis of the processes required to be successful with early lung cancer detection have received relatively minor attention considering the proportional contribution of this cancer to overall cancer mortality. In the field of early lung cancer detection research, the principal effort to date has been a focus on finding the appropriate marker to identify incipient lung cancer. This issue, while of enormous importance, is interwoven with other critical research and development issues that are fundamental to the success of early detection efforts. When the proposed clinical application involves such vast numbers at risk for the disease, the economic aspects of the diagnostic technology must be considered. In addition, a new therapeutic management approach would be required to manage the early cancer cases detected with new diagnostic technology. In attempting to understand what research direction for reduction of lung cancer mortality is most promising, a careful consideration of these issues is warranted. Indeed there is a certain irony in the current situation as perceived by the commercial development community. Improved intervention measures only have value if the diagnostic techniques improve, but the incentives to improve the diagnostic technology are inhibited by the current lack of appropriate clinical intervention approaches.

IV. Placing Early Lung Cancer Detection in a Clinical Context

Positive developments in the world of diagnostic technology may present new opportunities to move from the current situation. Newer and more efficient diagnostic platforms may supersede the discussion regarding the most appropriate target to identify early lung cancer (15–17). As the cost of molecular diagnostics has already fallen dramatically, this trend could well accelerate as the ability to perform multiple analyses on a single specimen expands. Yet while this is exciting new technology, without other complementary treatment developments to successfully change the natural history of the detected early cancer, no clinical benefit will occur. This concern is similar to the preliminary experience with the development of sputum-based immunocytologic approach to early lung cancer detection. In three independent clinical populations, we have found that the immunodetection of a ribonuclear protein called heterogeneous nuclear, ribonucleoprotein A2/B1 results in the correct classification of cancer status in at least two thirds of the subjects (14,18,19). Until some clinical intervention is actually shown to improve the outcome of those detected lung cancer, the interest in the diagnostic assay is modest.

An understanding of the conceptual foundation for the success of this assay is emerging in conjunction with our growing understanding of the biological basis for early lung cancer. Table 1 lists a series of statements summarizing what is known about the process of lung cancer early detection (20–22). The long disease incubation period, which often lasts for more than a decade and occurs on a vast epithelial surface area, imposes an enormous challenge for identifying reliable diagnostic reagents. In this regard, the selection process used to identify our informative ribonucleoprotein marker may be of general interest. The validating procedure used to establish the early detection utility of this marker involved the use of a sputum archive. This resource was prospectively acquired with annual sputum sampling from a clinical trial population accrued based on their statistically high risk of developing lung cancer (14). At the time we performed the validation analysis, 8 years of clinical follow-up permitted the true cancer outcome status of the reference population to be known. This permitted precise correlation of marker expression and eventual cancer outcome. There are several excellent reviews in general as well as throughout this book that will discuss the biological rationale for a large number of the potentially interesting lung cancer markers (23,24). For instance, the expression of the ribonucleoprotein in field carcinogenesis and in fetal lung development is consistent

Table 1 Concepts for Early Detection

The toxicity of tobacco combustion products leads to many types of cellular injury.

From inception in the airway to clinical detection lung cancer takes years to decades.

Cancer arises from the chronic exposure of the bronchial epithelial cells to inhaled carcinogens when critical genotoxic injury occurs.

Area at risk includes all cells washed by the carcinogen stream or "the field of cancer."

This "field cancerization" model provides a range of biological targets for early cancer detection.

Many molecular changes in the epithelium precede morphologic change.

The presence of an oncogene, loss of a chromosome does not mean cancer.

Discrimination of informative markers of carcinogenesis can only be validated clinically.

Through successive marker validation clinical trials, a molecular signature of cancer may emerge.

Technology of efficient tissue analysis progressing rapidly.

New diagnostic technology can facilitate marker validation trials.

Large numbers of individuals could be found to have the "molecular signature" of cancer.

with this family of ribonucleoproteins playing an important but previously unappreciated role in carcinogenesis (19,25). Using a tissue archive serially acquired in advance of clinical cancer when the long-term cancer status of the monitored individuals will eventually be known is a definitive way to establish which markers have clinical utility in the detection of early lung cancer. The appropriate conclusion about this approach is not only the potential utility of this ribonucleoprotein but also the process of validation. Given the complexity of cancer especially in regard to finding early cancer markers, carefully characterized material containing evolving stages of carcinogenesis is the gold standard for marker validation where eventual clinical correlation regarding ultimate cancer status establishes the linkage to true field carcinogenesis.

The developments of diagnostic technology may accelerate using this validation approach with clinical/pathological archives, as a large number of markers that may have some utility in early lung cancer detection will be identified. The availability of an economical, efficient diagnostic platform will allow easy evaluation of marker panels devised by adding individuals markers that convey independent information about the process of carcinogenesis (15–17). The accuracy of this multiple marker analysis may also be essential in allowing population-based screening, since only highly multiplexed early detection assays may be informative enough to allow high levels of user confidence with this approach.

Given the dynamic state of the developing early lung cancer detection approaches, consideration of how this technology might be integrated clinically is essential. From the cumulative impact of the diagnostic research developments discussed above, the ability to routinely identify the complex, multidimensional picture of progressive carcinogenesis should emerge. As the vast numbers of individuals that should be evaluated with a successful early detection test come into evaluation, it may become evident that the process of carcinogenesis can be obscured by a range of genetic and epigenetic factors such as intercurrent infection. These considerations have tempered our view regarding the suitability of all early detection assay. Many aspects of these are generic concerns which represent general challenges for population-based studies for any early detection of any epithelial cancer. We also recognize the preliminary nature of this work, but there has been only limited discussion of research strategies in this fledgling field. To the extent that this area is currently enjoying much broader attention from serious investigators, the prospects for accelerating the rate of progress in this field improve.

V. Integrating Chemoprevention Approaches to Manage Preinvasive Lung Cancer

Pioneering work by the research groups from M.D. Anderson and Milan have suggested that the administration of vitamin A or its analogs may be of benefit in reducing the development of lung cancers (26–28). While not all of the trials with retinoids have been positive, there is growing interest in this chemoprevention approach. Large prospective validation trials are ongoing, but irrespective of the outcome, certain aspects of management have to improve. In particular, the doses of 13-*cis*-retinoic acid used in the M.D. Anderson trials are consistently associated with a range of nonlethal but noxious side effects. The side effects range from headaches and severe itching to hyperlipidemia. A follow-up study of 13-*cis*-retinoic acid chemoprevention suggests that chronic retinoid administration beyond a year is going to be required, highlighting the problem posed by the side effect profile of 13-*cis*-retinoic acid (29). For chemoprevention application, the occurrence of frequent debilitating side effects compromises utility, as asymptomatic individuals will not tolerate side effects like individuals with advanced cancer. As with chemotherapy research, finding a potent drug to arrest cancer biology without causing serious side effects is an enormous challenge.

Based on some of our research on the impact on retinoid-albumin interactions on bioavailability, we have speculated that the optimal route of administration for retinoid administration may be to avoid delivery through the systemic circulation. Aerosolizing the drug could allow direct delivery of high drug concentrations to the injured bronchial tissue while resulting in minimal systemic side effects (30,31). In a recent article, we reviewed the theoretical basis for considering epithelial-directed chemoprevention delivery as an appropriate option when attempting to achieve high local concentrations of chemoprevention agent while minimizing the likelihood of systemic side effects. The technology to accomplish aerosolized delivery was recently reviewed (32). An important consideration is to ensure that adequate delivery of the active agent occurs throughout the entire air column, especially in the area of peak cigarette smoke exposure. The value of any early detection approach will be greatly enhanced if an effective chemoprevention agent is defined. By delivery of chemoprevention agents via the airway that is the same route of administration for the tobacco combustion products, a consistent pharmacologic advantage over systemic drug deliveries may be realized. A range of drugs may ultimately be directly administered to the bronchial epithelium as aerosolized chemoprevention agents so that the clinician can arrest lung cancer before lethal metastatic progression occurs. As shown in Figure 1, research progress for both biomarker and intervention technology is required prior to reductions in lung cancer mortality.

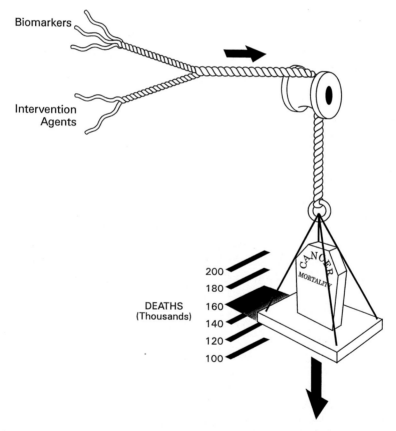

Figure 1 The interaction of diagnostic technology with intervention technology is represented schematically. The ability to control the progression of early cancer is thought to be essential to reducing the high mortality related to the consequences of metastatic disease.

The ability to determine if airway-directed chemoprevention approaches work will require another application of multiple-marker screening technology. Monitoring for changes in the pattern of mutational injury or differentiation status of the airway epithelium through analysis of shed bronchial epithelial cells may use the same diagnostic technology as was discussed for early lung cancer detection. If multiple molecular targets can be analyzed from a single, small clinical specimen to reliably establish response to chemoprevention agent, it would be an important breakthrough in early lung cancer clinical management. To the extent that biomarker panels are validated as reflecting the biological status of the entire airway epithelium, this greatly facilitates the process of conducting clinical trial to identify useful agents capable of arresting early lung cancer progression.

The positive developments in the area of high-density, probe-based molecular diagnostics have exciting possibilities for early lung cancer care (15,22). This technology could allow a major shift in lung cancer management if the preinvasive phase of cancer can be routinely identified. While we await these promising developments, continued efforts at improving both tobacco control and treatment of advanced disease should be maintained. As it is predicted that with current trends, one in five adults alive today will die of premature tobacco-related mortality, the public health dimension of this research is transcendent (33). Increased efforts to elucidate the mechanisms driving the earliest phases of lung cancer are critical, as this information could potentially accelerate progress in preventative strategies for lung cancer and ultimately reduce the burden of lung cancer mortality.

References

1. Parker SL, Tong T, Bolden S, Wingo PA. Cancer statistics, 1997. CA Cancer J Clin 1997; 47:5–25.
2. Strauss G, DeCamp M, Dibiccaro E, Richards W, Harpole D, Healey E, Sugarbaker D. Lung cancer diagnosis is being made with increasing frequency in former cigarette smokers. Proc Am Soc Clin Oncol 1995; 14:362.
3. Bailar JC. Early lung cancer cooperative study group: early lung cancer detection. Summary and conclusion. Am Rev Respir Dis 1984; 130:565.
4. Bailar JC. Screening for lung cancer—where are we now? Am Rev Respir Dis 1984; 130:541.
5. Mulshine Jl, Tockman MS, Smart CR. Consideration in the development of lung cancer screening tools. J Natl Cancer Inst 1989; 81:900.
6. Slaughter DP, Southwick HW, Smejkal W. "Field cancerization" in oral stratified squamous epithelium. Cancer 1953; 6:963–968.
7. Saccomanno G, Saunders RP, Ellis H. Concentration of carcinoma or atypical cells in sputum. Acta Cytol 1963; 7:305–310.
8. Payne PW, Sebo TJ, Doudkine A, Garner D, MacAulay C, Llam S, LeRiche JC, Palcic B. Sputum screening by quantitative microscopy: a reexamination of the National Cancer Institute Cooperative Early Lung Cancer Study. Mayo Clin Proc 1997; 72:697–704.
9. Tockman MS, Mulshine JL. Sputum screening by quantitative microscopy: a new dawn for detection of lung cancer. Mayo Clin Proc 1997; 72:788–790.
10. Mao L, Lee JS, Kurie J, Lee JJ, Ro JY, Broxson A, Yu R, Morice RC, Kemp BL, Khuri FR, Walsh GL, Hittelman WN, Hong WK. Clonal genetics alterations in the lungs of current and former smokers. J Natl Cancer Inst 1997; 89:857–862.

11. Wistuba II, Gazdar AF. Molecular abnormalities in the sequential development of lung carcinoma. In: Martinet Y, Martinet N, Vignaud JM, Hirsch F, Mulshine JL, eds. Clinical and Biological Basis of Lung Cancer Prevention. Basel: Birkhauser Verlag AG, 1997:

12. Battey J, Brown PH, Gritz E, Hong WK, Johnson BE, Karp D, Mulshine JL, Shaw GL, Shopland D, Sunday M, Szabo E. Primary and secondary prevention of lung cancer: an International Association for the Study of Lung Cancer workshop. Lung Cancer 1995; 12:91–103.

13. Hirsch FR, Brambilla E, Gray N, Gritz E, Kelloff GJ, RI Linnoila, Pastorino U, Mulshine JL. Prevention and early detection of lung cancer-clinical aspects. Lung Cancer 1997; 17: 163–174.

14. Tockman MS, Gupta PK, Myers JD, Frost JK, Baylin SB, Gold EB, Chase AM, Wilkinson PH, Mulshine J. Sensitive and specific monoclonal antibody recognition of human lung cancer antigen on preserved sputum cells: a new approach to early lung cancer detection. J Clin Oncol 1988; 6:1685–1693.

15. Eggers M, Hogan M, Reich RK, et al. A microchip for quantitative detection of molecules utilizing luminescent and radioisotope reporter groups. BioTechniques 1994; 17:516.

16. Schena M, Shalon D, Heller R, Chai A, Brown PO, Davis RW. Parallel human genome analysis: microarray-based expression monitoring of 1000 genes. Proc Natl Acad Sci USA 1996; 93:10614–10619.

17. Yershov G, Barsky V, Belgovskiy A, et al. DNA analysis and diagnostics on oligonucleotide microchips. Proc Natl Acad Sci 1996; 93:4913.

18. Tockman MS, Mulshine JL, Piantadosi S, Erozan YS, Gupta P, Ruckdeschel J, Taylor P, Zhukov T, Zhou W, Qiao Y, Yao SX, LCEWDG and YTC Investigators. Prospective detection of preclinical lung cancer: preliminary results from two studies of hnRNP overexpression. Clin Cancer Res 1997;

19. Zhou J, Mulshine JL, Unsworth EJ, Avis I, Cuttitta F, Treston A. Identification of a heterogeneous nuclear ribonucleoprotein (hnRNP) as an early lung cancer detection marker. J Biol Chem 1996; 271:10760–10766.

20. Tockman MS, Gupta PK, Pressman NJ, Mulshine JL. Considerations in bringing a cancer biomarker to clinical application. Cancer Res 1992; 52(suppl):2711s–2718s.

21. Tockman MS, Gupta PK, Pressman NJ, Mulshine JL. Cytometric validation of immunocytochemical observations in developing lung cancer. Diagn Cytopathol 1993; 9(6):615–622.

22. Mulshine JL, Zhou J, Treston AM, Szabo E, Tockman MS, Cuttitta F. New approaches to the integrated management of early lung cancer. Med Clin North Am 1997; 11:235–252.

23. Brambilla E. Molecular markers of early lung cancer. In: Martinet Y, Martinet N, Vignaud JM, Hirsch F, Mulshine JL, eds. Biological Basis of Lung Cancer Prevention. Basel: Birkhauser Verlag AG, 1997.

24. Papadimitrakopoulou VA, Hong WK. Biomarkers as intermediate endpoints in chemoprevention trials. In: Martinet Y, Martinet N, Vignaud JM, Hirsch F, Mulshine JL, eds. Biological Basis of Lung Cancer Prevention. Basel: Birkhauser Verlag AG, 1997.

25. Zhou J, Jensen SM, Steinberg SM, Mulshine JL, Linnoila RI. Expression of early lung cancer detection marker p31 in neoplastic and non-neoplastic respiratory epithelium. Lung Cancer 1996; 14:85–97.

26. Hong WK, Lippman SM, Itri LM, Karp DD, Lee JS, Byers RM, Schantz SP, Kramer AM, Lotan R, Peters LJ. Prevention of second primary tumors with isotretinoin in squamous-cell carcinoma of the head and neck. N Engl J Med 1990; 323:795–801.

27. Pastorino U, Infante M, Maioli M, Chiesa G, Buyse M, Firket P, Rosmentz N, Clerici M, Soresi E, Valente M, Belloni PA, Ravasi G. Adjuvant treatment of stage I lung cancer with high-dose vitamin A. J Clin Oncol 1993; 11:1216–1222.

28. Lippman S, Benner S, Hong W. Cancer chemoprevention. J Clin Oncol 1994; 12:851.

29. Benner SE, Pajak TF, Lippman SM, Earley C, Hong WK. Prevention of second primary tumors with isotretinoin in patients with squamous cell carcinoma of the head and neck: long-term follow-up. J Natl Cancer Inst 1994; 86:140–141.

30. Avis I, Mathias A, Unsworth E, Miller MJ, Cuttitta F, Mulshine J, Jakowlew S. Analysis of small cell lung cancer cell growth inhibition by 13-cis retinoic acid: importance of bioavailability. Cell Growth Diff 1995; 6:485–492.

31. Mulshine JL, De Luca LM, Dedrick RL. Regional delivery of retinoids: a new approach to early lung cancer intervention. In: Martinet Y, Martinet N, Vignaud JM, Hirsch F, Mulshine JL, eds. Clinical and Biological Basis of Lung Cancer Prevention. Basel: Birkhauser Verlag AG, 1997:
32. Service RE. Drug delivery takes a deep breath. Science 1997; 277:1199–1200.
33. Peto R, Lopez AD, Boreham J, Thun M, Heath C Jr. Mortality from Smoking in Developed Countries 1950–2000. Indirect Estimates from National Vital Statistics. Oxford: Oxford University Press, 1994.

22

Role of Growth Factors in the Stromal Reaction in Non–Small-Cell Lung Carcinoma

JEAN-MICHEL VIGNAUD, YVES MARTINET, AND NADINE MARTINET

Laboratoire d'Anatomie Pathologique and INSERM U14
Université Henri-Poincaré
Vandoeuvre les Nancy, France

I. Introduction

Neoplastic cells require an appropriate pericellular environment, called stroma, in order to constitute a solid tumor. The stroma is a specialized connective tissue, consisting of an extracellular matrix (ECM) and of a cellular compartment made of inflammatory, mesenchymal, and endothelial cells. It is now currently accepted that stroma acts for tumor cells as a physical support, a feeding support and pathway for metabolic waste products, an actor in the control of tumor cell differentiation, proliferation, adhesion, and migration, and ultimately as a promotor of the tumor invasive phenotype and the metastatic process, although a number of histochemical studies have demonstrated the presence of infiltrating immune cells within carcinomas. The stroma is qualitatively distinct from the connective tissue developing in inflammatory conditions: in particular, stromal inflammatory and mesenchymal cells have distinct phenotypic characteristics, and specific spliced variants of ECM components have been reported. Stroma processing is the result of a spacially and temporally changing imbalance between agonist and antagonist mechanisms that also control the tumor progression. In this process, growth factors (GF) and cytokines play a key role by connecting carcinoma cells with stromal cells and ECM components via a complex network of extracellular signals. Although the in vivo functions of many GF/cytokines are not fully understood, their net effect is to enhance the establishment of the stromal compartment by stimulating both the deposition of ECM and the development of a blood supply through the angiogenesis process. These GF are synthesized by carcinoma cells and stromal cells that collaborate for stroma production. GF release by tumor cells has been extensively reviewed (1,2) and will be considered shortly, as well as the angiogenesis process further developed in this book. In this chapter we focus on the role of the interactions occurring between ECM components and mesenchymal cells, and more specifically inflammatory cells, in the development of stroma.

II. Growth Factors Functional Status in Carcinoma: A Multistep Regulated Process

GF have been loosely defined as molecules that influence the division, differentiation, and survival of cells. They are closely related to cytokines, but can be distinguished from cytokines insofar as their production is mainly constitutive and their preferential targets are not hematopoietic cells in origin. These molecules have a wide spectrum of activities on cultured cell types, but the in vivo functions of only a few GF are known with certainty. Indeed, once released in the extracellular environment, a GF/cytokine can interact with a rich network of molecules susceptible to critically influence its activity (3). In this regard a substantial pool of GF is maintained outside the cells in an inactive form, as complexed to binding proteins, or as linked to ECM components, and GF activity regulation cannot be limited to the control of these GF and their specific plasma membrane receptor expression. Indeed, ECM components, specifically proteoglycans, are an important reservoir of bound GF maintained in an inactive form, and many GF can be complexed with binding proteins, such as insulin-like growth factors (IGF) with IGF-binding proteins (IGF-BPs), or as part of a propeptide for transforming growth factor-β (TGF-β). Soluble receptors interfering with GF activities, by competing with cell surface receptors, have also been described for different GF including epidermal growth factor (EGF), tumor necrosis factor (TNF), and basic-fibroblast growth factor (b-FGF). Furthermore, GF such as platelet-derived growth factor (PDGF) (4) and TNF-α (5) can be complexed with α_2-macroglobulin plasma protein.

These interactions of GF with ECM and diverse binding molecules can strongly modulate GF functions by controlling their diffusion, increasing their stability, protecting them from proteolytic degradation, and allowing a slow release. For instance, in vitro, heparin protects acid-FGF (a-FGF) and b-FGF from heat or acid inactivation (6) and proteases and allows a 100-fold increase of the half-life of a-FGF (7). Independent of these mechanisms, interfering with the disponibility in active form of GF, the cell response also depends upon the combination with other GF with distinct functions, the level of expression of cell surface receptors, and the receptor transduction pathways. Considering more specifically the last point, synergistic effects between polypeptidic GF, neuropeptides, and cytokines have been documented in a variety of cultured cell types. This is in agreement with the fact that cell proliferation can be stimulated through multiple independent signal transduction pathways acting in a synergistic and combinatorial fashion. Thus, the numerous levels of regulation of GF function explain the difficulties encountered in reliably attributing an in vivo observed biological event to a specific GF.

III. The Extracellular Matrix: A Reservoir of Bound Growth Factors

A wide range of stromal ECM patterns has been described, each of them broadly related to an histologic type: for instance, while abundant in non–small-cell lung cancer (NSCLC) the stroma is slender in bronchioloalveolar carcinomas and in neuroendocrine carcinomas, especially SCLC. These distinct patterns are mainly supported by qualitative and quantitative differencies within the four major classes of ECM components (collagens, elastin, proteoglycans and hyaluronic acid, and glycoproteins), contributing to the constitution of a very complex network of molecules. The presence of homologous sequences repeated in different proteins of the ECM has reduced the great diversity of ECM proteins to a relatively small number of distinct modules such as EGF, fibronectin (FN) type III, and proteoglycan tandem repeat. These modules can play both a structural and functional role. For instance, ECM proteins (such as laminin) containing EGF precursor repeats have been implicated in cell division (8).

Carcinoma cell–ECM interactions are mediated by cell surface receptors: integrins, nonintegrins, and cell surface proteoglycans. Integrins play an important role in both tumor cell–ECM and carcinoma cell–stromal cell interactions, especially with endothelial cells and leukocytes. It is now well established that survival of many cell types requires integrin-mediated adhesion to ECM. In the absence of appropriate ECM contacts, most cells undergo apoptosis (9). But it is likely that tumor cells escape this mechanism of control as suggested by the extensive changes that integrins undergo during malignant transformation and tumor progression. Several studies have shown that GF receptor signaling and integrins can interfere. For instance, cell adhesion can downregulate EGF-receptor (EGF-R) signals (10), and the signals due to some integrins may require a priming from GF (11).

Proteoglycans (PGs), *the reservoir of bound growth factors,* are macromolecules consisting of a core protein covalently linked to one or several glycosaminoglycan (GAG) side chains that are, sulfated or nonsulfated, repeating disaccharide units. GAG have a strongly negative charge that makes them able to bind growth factors, but also proteins specific to a GAG (for instance, hyaluronic acid is the ligand for CD 44). Many PGs are constituents of the ECM, such as aggrecan, decorin, fibromodulin, and perlecan. They modulate GF activities (12,13): decorin, associated with type I collagen, binds TGF-β in an inactive form through its core protein as does biglycan (14). PDGF-B and the PDGF-A$_L$ isoform may also interact with heparan sulfate PGs in the ECM (15). The binding of TGF-β and PDGF-A and -B is reversible; as a consequence, PGs may form a reservoir for these GF that are clearly involved in stroma processing. In the same way, perlecan, a basement membrane PG, interacts with b-FGF, a-FGF (16), and granulocyte-macrophage colony-stimulating factor (GM-CSF) (17). Hepatocyte growth factor/scatter factor (HGF/SF), a potent mitogenic and motogenic factor for different cell types, is secreted as an inactive precursor that binds the ECM. Vascular endothelial growth factor (VEGF), the main angiogenic factor for NSCLC, is a heparin-binding glycoprotein with diverse isoforms resulting from an alternative splicing. $VEGF_{189}$ and $VEGF_{260}$ are completely sequestered in the ECM (18); $VEGF_{165}$, the main isoform, binds to heparin with a lower affinity. These three isoforms are released in a soluble form by heparinase, and the long forms may also be released by plasmin (19). The ability of ECM to function as a slow release reservoir for GF may explain how molecules released over a short period of time can stimulate processes, such as angiogenesis, that take days. GF interactions with matrix molecules may also be required for the binding of the GF to its receptor. In this regard, perlecan, by promoting the binding of b-FGF to its receptor, is a potent inducer of angiogenesis (20). In addition, some PGs can generate their own signal, such as versican, that has EGF-like domains possibly involved in cell division (21). It has also been suggested that the hyaluronic acid accumulation in tumors, providing a well-hydrated matrix, may favor carcinoma cell growth and migration (22) by creating a loose hydrated extracellular pathway conducive to cell migration (23). NSCLC are highly enriched in hyaluronan (24), and it seems that tumor cells stimulate stromal mesenchymal cells to synthesize PGs rather than to produce PGs themselves. Finally, GF such as PDGF, TGF-β, EGF, and IGF stimulate the production of hyaluronan (25).

Thus, an increased stromal PG content could, through the reservoir bound of growth factors, promote ECM production, the angiogenesis process, and tumor cell growth.

IV. ECM Production by Stromal Fibroblasts

Tumor-associated fibroblasts/myofibroblasts (TAF) represent an important subpopulation of stromal cells in NSCLC, synthesizing collagen, elastic fibers, GAG, and glycoproteins. TAF are phenotypically distinct from their counterparts in healthy tissues. In particular, they exhibit an extended in vitro life span (26) and express fetal-specific cell surface antigens (27). They synthesize tumor-specific isoforms of ECM components (e.g., EDB fibronectin) and can produce proteases [particularly stromelysin-3, gelatinase-A and -B (28,29)] that participate in ECM degradation, as well as GF/cytokines such as interleukin (IL)-6 and -8, b-FGF, IGF, HGF/SF, and VEGF (30). However, these fetal-like TAF are not tumor-specific and represent a phenotypically heterogeneous population in respect to their distribution inside the tumor (39). It is likely that the factors that allow TAF to express such phenotypic characteristics involve the complex interactions of cytokines and matrix molecules.

In this regard, TAF can respond to different effectors, including chemokines [such as growth-related oncogene-α (GRO-α)], and to several GF clearly involved in ECM synthesis (PDGF-A and -B, b-FGF, and TGF-β). For instance in NSCLC, tumor-associated macrophages (TAM), and to a lower extent tumor cells, strongly express PDGF-A and -B proteins, and TAF constantly express PDGF receptor α and β subunits. In addition, the sites where PDGF-producing TAM are present in high concentration are the sites where TAF are replicating. These observations strongly suggest the role of PDGF in TAF growth (32). Other growth factors, such as TGF-β (33), increase collagen and fibronectin synthesis and secretion by several fibroblast cell lines (34,35) and very likely do so in vivo. It has been reported that TGF-β stimulates FN synthesis and, especially for the EDB+, EDA+ containing isoforms and the III C-S variant 2, encoding for FNs that initiate the fibrillogenesis of the ECM (36). The TAF capacity to synthesize ECM components is counterbalanced by their ability to produce proteases. In this regard, in NSCLC, TAF express matrix metalloproteinase (MMP)-2, -9, stromelysin-1, -3, and matrilysin (37). This protease production could be induced by tumor cell–derived factors, such as the tumor cell–derived collagenase-stimulating factor. Thus TAF, by interacting with extracellular and plasma membrane signals provided by inflammatory cells and carcinoma cells, direct ECM production, and remodeling, favor the angiogenic process and consequently tumor progression.

V. Stromal Inflammatory Cells in Stroma Processing

Tumor-infiltrating lymphocytes (TIL) and TAM are the main inflammatory cell populations infiltrating lung carcinoma. Potent producers of GF/cytokines they are strongly involved in stroma production, without underestimating the role of other cell populations such as Langerhans cells, polymorphonuclear leukocytes, and mastocytes.

A. Tumor Infiltrating Lymphocytes

TIL are a heterogeneous population, consisting mainly of CD3+ T lymphocytes (T-Ly), a minority of B lymphocytes, and a few natural killer (NK) cells, respectively representing, in NSCLC, an average of 80%, 20%, and 1% of TIL population. TIL are mainly CD8+, with a low (15–30%) CD4/CD8 ratio (personal data). CD8+ TIL may potentially kill carcinoma cells that express peptides derived from mutated genes and presented in association with class I major histocompatibility complex (MHC) molecules. The lytic capacity of CD56+ NK cells, MHC-unrestricted, is increased by interferon-γ (IFN-γ), TNF-α, IL-2, and IL-12. Therefore, their cytotoxic potential may depend upon the simultaneous activation of CD4+ T-Ly, tumor cells, and TAM producing these cytokines. CD4+ T-Ly are necessary for a successful antitumor immune response mediated via the cytokines secreted by Th1 (IL-2, IFN-γ, TNF-β) and Th2 subsets (IL-4, -5, -10, -13) (38), regulating the induction of immune cells. Both subsets can produce IL-3, TNF-α, and GM-CSF. TNF-α and IFN-γ can increase tumor cell class I MHC expression and sensitivity to lysis by CD8+ TIL. However,

1. Class I MHC molecule in vivo expression is strongly downregulated on epidermoid and lung adenocarcinoma cells (personal data), as well as in SCLC (39), so that efficient complexes of processed tumor antigen peptides and MHC molecules required for CD8+ T-Ly recognition cannot be formed.
2. Using RT-PCR a decreased mRNA expression has been shown for IL-2, -4, -6, GM-CSF, and IFN-γ in TIL freshly isolated from lung adenocarcinoma versus peripheral blood lymphocytes (40).
3. Moreover, using iododeoxuridine technique to appreciate TIL in vivo kinetics, we observed a low replication rate of these cells (32).
4. Finally, it has been shown, in vitro, that pulmonary macrophages could suppress TIL proliferation and cytotoxicity (41).

These observations suggest that TIL are partially functionally deficient in their capacity to mediate a strong antitumor cytotoxicity, to release cytokines, and to proliferate, although it has also been shown that NSCLC carcinoma cells express a type 2 lymphocyte-like cytokine pattern (42) that can facilitate the immune response.

In addition to their immune functions, CD4+ T-Ly, through the complex network of cytokines they produce, interfere with the mechanisms regulating ECM production and the functions of tumor cells and other inflammatory cells. For instance, IL-1β, -1α, and -6 (43,44) have been shown to induce VEGF expression in several cell lines including smooth muscle cells (SMC) (43). IL-1 via PDGF stimulates TAF and SMC proliferation, but on the contrary inhibits endothelial cell replication. IL-8 is also mitogenic for SMC and chemotactic for both SMC and TAF, while IL-4 is an inhibitor of TAF proliferation. IL-12 strongly inhibits neovascularization. This inhibition is mediated by IFN-γ (45), which is also a potent stimulator of TAM activities and may therefore determine several GF release by macrophages. TNF-α, in in vivo models, interferes with the angiogenesis process (46) and the proteolytic mechanisms of ECM degradation (47). Thus, the interactions between TIL and other stromal cells and cancer cells are far from fully understood, but clinical trials of adoptive immunotherapy have nevertheless already been conducted.

B. Tumor-Associated Macrophages in Stroma Production

TAM, representing an average of 30% of stromal inflammatory cells in NSCLC, play many, sometimes contradictory functions (48). These pleiotropic cells have the capacity to modulate ECM production and remodeling, to exert cytotoxic activity but also to promote carcinoma cell growth, and to favor the angiogenesis process. Currently some evidence suggests that the protumor effects of TAM dominate their cytotoxic functions.

1. *Macrophage tumor infiltration is mainly relevant to a superfamily of cytokines called chemokines* produced by tumor cells as well as stromal cells including mononuclear phagocytes. Indeed, TAM are weakly replicating in NSCLC (32), but are mainly recruited at tumor site (49). Monocyte chemotactic protein-1 (MCP-1), a chemoattractant for monocytes, but inactive on lymphocytes, is a representative of the α and β chemokine families, including other members such as MCP-2, -3, macrophage inflammatory protein-1α and -β, and GRO-α. The local inoculation of MCP-1 induced monocyte infiltration in rats (50), and MCP-1 gene transfer into murine tumor cells resulted in an increased infiltration by blood monocytes in nude mice (51). Factors other than chemokines, such as M-CSF and GM-CSF, are also involved in TAM recruitment, as demonstrated by gene transfer experiments in mouse (52). TIL and tumor cells produce GM-CSF in NSCLC (53) and participate in monocyte recruitment, but anti-inflammatory cytokines such as TGF-β and IL-10 could counterbalance the action of these chemokines.

2. *The activation of macrophages is a prerequisite for cellular cytotoxicity.* Many factors produced by carcinoma cells and T-Ly are potent activators of TAM, such as IFN-γ, TNF-α and -β, and GM-CSF (54). Appropriately activated macrophages can overcome cancer cells via different mediators, including cytokines (IL-12, TNF-α, IL-6) and reactive oxygen or nitrogen intermediates. The cytolytic process is dependent upon cell-cell contact, mediated by specific cell-surface receptors present on macrophages. Adhesion molecules, particularly of the β-integrin family, are clearly involved in several forms of TAM–tumor cell interactions, including antibody-independent as well as dependent forms. Sixty-four percent of TAM from NSCLC express low affinity Fc receptor III (CD16) (55), which makes them potent effectors for killing antibody-sensitized carcinoma cells. However, this cytolytic potential may be modulated by the fact that TAM, in lung cancer, are relatively poor producers of IL-12 and TNF-α (40). Furthermore, carcinoma cells produce IL-10 (56), which has varied immunosuppressive bioactivities, including alteration of monocyte cytotoxicity, downregulation of class II MHC molecule expression, and inhibition of proinflammatory cytokine production.

3. *TAM interactions with carcinoma cell growth and ECM production take place through GF synthesis and interplay within the intratumoral cytokine network.* TAM are capable of producing high amounts of GF, such as EGF, GM-CSF, IL-1, -6, -12, PDGF, TGF-α, TNF-α, b-FGF, and VEGF and can respond to effectors such as GM-CSF, INF-γ, IL-3, -4, -7, -10, MCP-1, PDGF, TGF-β, TNF-α, and VEGF. It is therefore not surprising that these cells, in association with cytokines produced by the other stromal cells and by the carcinoma cells themselves (57), can promote the in vitro growth of tumor cells, favor ECM production, and participate in the angiogenesis process. However, in this tightly meshed network, the key cytokines that control stroma development are not known. It can be hypothesized that GF directly involved in ECM production and the angiogenesis process play a central role. From this point of view, PDGF and TGF-β are serious candidates for the control of ECM

regulation, since NSCLC cell lines expressing these genes induce a significant tumor stroma when injected into nude mice (58).

PDGF

PDGF is a potent chemotactic and growth factor for mesenchymal cells and endothelial cells. PDGF is composed of two chains, A and B, the B chain being coded for by the *c-sis* proto-oncogene. PDGF interacts on target cells with a receptor composed of two subunits, α and β. Beside being involved, in a paracrine fashion, in different human fibrotic disorders, especially lung fibrosis (59,60), PDGF has been suggested to participate, in an autocrine and paracrine fashion, in both the production of ECM and the replication of endothelial cells and cancer cells in NSCLC (32). In this process, TAM may play a central role. In 92% of lung cancer, TAM express PDGF-A and -B chain genes (Fig. 1A(c)) and produce PDGF proteins (Fig. 1A(a)). These PDGF-producing TAM are mainly found in the peripheral part of the tumor, in close connection with the normal surrounding lung tissue. In this area, 10–25% of PDGF-positive TAM are observed. TAM also express both PDGF receptor α and β subunits. Furthermore, stromal mesenchymal cells, as well as endothelial cells, strongly express PDGF receptors (Fig. 1A(e) and (f)). In addition, 30% of NSCLC express PDGF genes and proteins at carcinoma cell level (Fig. 1A(d) and (b)) with frequent co-expression of receptors. Thus, a sequence of events participating in stroma formation is proposed (Fig. 1B) (32): (1) recruitment of TAM from blood monocytes by the release by tumor cells of chemotactic factors such as MCP-1, followed by (2) recruitment and local proliferation of mesenchymal and endothelial cells due to the release of PDGF by TAM and, to a lesser extent, by tumor cells. This concept is further supported by the fact that the higher levels of PDGF-producing TAM and of replicating endothelial and mesenchymal cells are observed in the same areas.

TGF-β

TGF-β1, both a stimulator and inhibitor of cell replication, may control the production of many components of the ECM, as well as modulate cell differentiation, angiogenesis, and cellular migration (61,62). In NSCLC, the major sources of TGF-β1 are tumor cells, ECM components, and to a lesser extent TAM. TGF-β1, the most abundant isoform of TGF-β, is a multifunctional cytokine, acting in both autocrine and paracrine ways, producing a wide range of frequently opposing effects on different cells and human tissues. TGF-β1, secreted as a latent complex (LTGF-β1), is activated when cleaved from the LTGF-β1 complex by acidification or proteolysis. The active form of TGF-β1 binds to TGF-β receptors (I, II, and III) virtually present on all cells.

TGF-β interfere with stromal cells and carcinoma cell proliferation. Most of the knowledge comes from investigations carried out in cell cultures and has clearly demonstrated the growth inhibitory effect of TGF-β for cells of ectodermal origin and, on the contrary, its ability to stimulate the growth of most cells of mesodermal origin such as fibroblastic cell lines. Its growth stimulatory action is thought to be

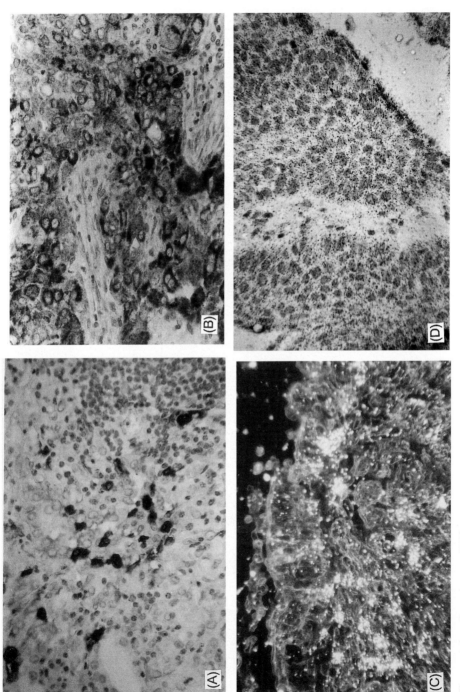

Figure 1 (continued on p. 356).

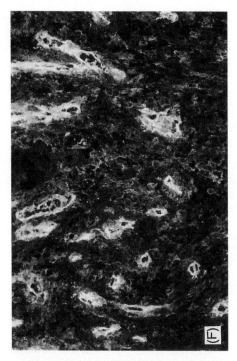

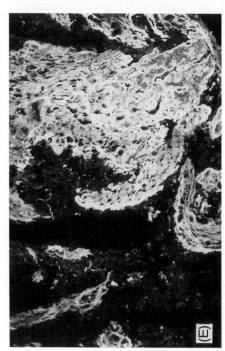

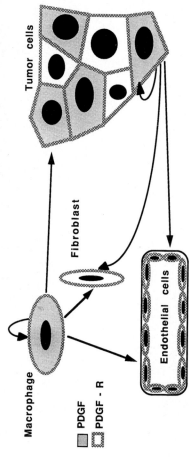

due to the induction of PDGF synthesis (63). Thus PDGF, in addition to its ability to induce carcinoma cell proliferation, may counterbalance the inhibitory effect of TGF-β1 on carcinoma cells. This hypothesis correlates with the fact that in vivo, in NSCLC (especially in adenocarcinomas), both TGF-β1 (64,65) and PDGF-A and -B chains (32) are strongly expressed by tumor cells and TAM. In NSCLC cell lines, a variety of TGF-β1 effects has been shown including growth inhibition (66), increased in vitro invasion, and cell attachment (67).

TGF-β1 stimulates the expression of a wide range of ECM proteins, including FN, laminin, elastin, thrombospondin, and various collagens (68). It modulates the expression of these proteins at transcriptional or posttranscriptional levels. ECM synthesis and deposition, in turn, regulate TGF-β1 expression leading to a negative feedback mechanism (69). It has been shown that central fibrosis appearance in lung adenocarcinoma is significantly related to positive staining for TGF-β1, suggesting that TGF-β1 plays some role in central fibrosis formation (70). In addition to the induction of ECM proteins, TGF-β1 also increases the amount of ECM by inhibiting ECM degradation especially by inducing the release of protease inhibitors (71). Furthermore, TGF-β1 stimulates the adhesiveness of both normal and malignant cells, in part by modulating the integrin-mediated adhesion.

TGF-β stimulates angiogenesis (72), although TGF-β1 exerts on endothelial cells a pronounced in vitro antiproliferative effect by increasing production of thrombospondin, an ECM associated antiangiogenic protein (73). Several studies have confirmed the in vivo angiogenic effect of TGF-β. TGF-β1–transfected rodent cells inoculated into nude mice were found to induce a marked angiogenesis, which was completely abolished by TGF-β1–neutralizing antibodies (74). The ability of TGF-β to induce macrophage urokinase-type plasminogen activator expression and the plasmin-dependent release of matrix-bound b-FGF may provide one mechanism by which TGF-β stimulates angiogenesis (75).

Other GF

In addition to PDGF and TGF-β, several other GF produced by TAM can also contribute to stroma development, such as GM-CSF, b-FGF, and also VEGF. GM-CSF

Figure 1 The role of platelet-derived growth factor production by tumor-associated macrophages and carcinoma cells in tumor stroma formation in lung cancer. A: Strong staining of (a) TAM and (b) carcinoma cells with an anti-PDGF-B chain antibody. In situ hybridization with a PDGF-B chain antisense probe: mRNA expression in (c) TAM (dark field examination) and (d) tumor cells. Immunofluorescence study with an anti-PDGF receptor β-subunit antibody: strong staining of (e) mesenchymal cells and (f) endothelial cells. B: One representative example obtained from a patient with squamous cell lung carcinoma shows expression of PDGF-A and -B chains by TAM and carcinoma cells, as well as PDGF receptor α and β subunits by carcinoma cells and stromal mesenchymal cells, which provide a paracrine mechanism for stroma development and an autocrine loop for carcinoma cell proliferation.

produced by carcinoma cells and some mononuclear phagocytes in NSCLC (76) has also been suggested to contribute to the formation of tumor stroma. This function is related to the local macrophage accumulation induced by GM-CSF. The local application of GM-CSF in rat subcutaneous tissue induces the formation of a typical granulation tissue; in addition, it has been shown that the growth of primary tumor of transplanted Lewis lung carcinoma is impaired in *op/op* mice, which have no endogenous GM-CSF, most likely because of a reduced stroma response (77). VEGF, the major angiogenic factor for NSCLC, produced both by TAM and carcinoma cells, with a potent mitogenic function restricted to endothelial cells, plays another major role in allowing the induction of plasma protein leakage (30). TAM, via the expression of clotting factors (factors II, V, VII, X, and XII) (78), promote the fibrin formation and deposition from the extravased fibrinogen, and thus directly contribute to stroma formation.

VI. Contribution of GF Released by Tumor Cells to Stroma Development

There are many more quantitative than qualitative differences between the range of GF that carcinoma cells and stromal cells produce, although great variations can be observed from one tumor to another. The implication of GF in the autocrine growth of cancer cells has been extensively studied in NSCLC (1,2). But their effective role in stroma development, clearly demonstrated for PDGF and TGF-β, as previously related, is still questionable for many of them. In particular, the in vivo expression on stromal cells of the corresponding GF receptors is not always clearly established or has to be confirmed by more extensive studies. b-FGF, beside being involved in the fibrotic process, is one of the most important angiogenic factors. Several immunohistochemical studies have shown that b-FGF and its high-affinity type I receptor (FGFR-1) are coexpressed in 50% of lung adenocarcinomas (79). Stromal TAF were also shown to be stained for b-FGF and FGFR-1, suggesting for this growth factor a role in ECM production, in addition to its angiogenic properties. EGF and TGF-α are strongly expressed as is their common receptor (EGF-R) by carcinoma cells. But we, like others (80), failed to localize EGF-R protein and mRNA in stromal cells. However, EGF and TGF-α, in some models, have been shown to promote angiogenesis through the induction of VEGF secretion (81) or of tissue-type plasminogen activator production (82). IGFs are autocrine growth factors for NSCLC (83) with a frequent coexpression of IGF-I and -II and IGF-I and -II receptors on carcinoma cells, although soluble and membrane-associated IGF-BP-2 compete with IGF receptors. If IGF-I is a major fibroblast mitogen in vitro, there is no consistent in vivo result definitively demonstrating the expression of IGF receptors on stromal cell. A strong overexpression and activation of HGF/SF and the corresponding c-*Met* oncogene–encoded receptor has also been reported in carcinoma cells compartment of NSCLC (84). This potent mitogenic and motogenic factor could also ˙ a role in stroma development if further studies demonstrate c-*Met* expression ˙mal cells.

Many other GFs such as nerve growth factor, neuropeptides, and other angiogenic factors produced by some NSCLC have not yet been investigated for their participation in stroma formation in vivo.

VII. Growth Factor Participation in ECM Degradation by Proteases

The stroma is characterized by both simultaneous active degradation and synthesis of ECM components. Matrix degradation is controlled by proteases and protease inhibitors, provided by cancer cells, inflammatory cells, and TAF. Proteases are grouped in four main classes: serin-proteases, cystein-proteases, aspartyl-proteases, and MMPs. The latter are a family of zinc atom–dependent endopeptidases, mainly produced by peritumoral fibroblasts, with specific and selective activities against many components of the ECM (85,86). They favor the progression of cancer cells through the ECM, but also the release of ECM-bound GF, in particular TGF-β, b-FGF, and VEGF, and of GF/cytokine domains from ECM components. The functions of MMPs in ECM can be regulated at many stages, from gene activation to pro-enzyme activation and inactivation, by a group of inhibitors. Gelatinase-A excepted, MMP production is induced by IL-1 β, TNF-α, PDGF, VEGF, TGF-α, EGF, and b-FGF. However, most of these reagents stimulate only one or two MMPS, and many are repressed by TGF-β (85). For instance, VEGF induces metalloprotease interstitial collagenase in endothelial cells that facilitate their migration and sprouting (87).

VIII. Conclusion

By connecting stromal cells with carcinoma cells, the intratumoral network of GF/cytokines produced by both types of cells tightly regulates tumor cell proliferation and migration, angiogenesis, as well as ECM deposition and remodeling. Although rapid progress has been made in the understanding of how GF act in a complex environment, caution must be exerted in interpreting data, especially from in vitro experiments, since the overall GF/cytokine balance is likely to strongly vary within and between different tumor types. However, we can expect that a more advanced deciphering of this network will facilitate, in the near future, the design of new anticancer treatments.

Acknowledgments

This work was supported in part by grants from the Programme Hospitalier de Recherche Cinique 95 from Ministère des Affaires Sociales, de la Santé et de la Ville, France, and from the Ligue Nationale contre le Cancer (Comités de Moselle et Meuse).

References

1. Kelly K, Lane MA, Bunn PA Jr. Growth factors in lung cancer: possible etiologic role and clinical target. Med Ped Oncol 1991; 19:449–458.
2. Sethi T, Woll PJ. Growth factors and lung cancer. In: Hansen HH, ed. Lung Cancer. Amsterdam: Kluwer Academic Publishers. 1994:111–130.
3. Schubert D. Collaborative interactions between growth factors and the extracellular matrix. Trends Cell Biol 1992; 2:63–66.
4. Huang JS, Huang SS, Deuel T. Specific covalent binding of platelet-derived growth factor to plasma alpha$_2$-macroglobulin. Proc Natl Acad Sci USA 1984; 81:342–346.
5. Wollenberg GK, LaMarre J, Rosendale S, Gonias SL, Hayes MA. Binding of tumor necrosis factor to activated forms of human plasma alpha$_2$-macroglobulin. Am J Pathol 1991; 138:265–272.
6. Gospodarowicz D, Cheng J. Heparin protects basic and acidic FGF from inactivation. J Cell Physiol 1986; 128:475–484.
7. Damon DH, Lobb RR, D'Amore PA, Wagner JA. Heparin potentiates the action of acidic fibroblast growth factor by prolonging its biological half life. J Cell Physiol 1989; 138:221–226.
8. Panayotou G, End P, Aumailley M, Timpl R, Engel J. Domains of laminin with growth-factor activity. Cell 1989; 56:93–101.
9. Meredith JE, Schwartz MA. Integrins, adhesion and apoptosis. Trends Cell Biol 1997; 7:146–150.
10. Cybulsky AV, McTavish AJ, Cyr MD. ECM modulates epidermal growth factor receptor activation in rat glomerular epithelial cells. J Clin Invest 1994; 94:68–78.
11. Hotchin NA, Hall A. The assembly of integrin adhesion complexes requires both extracellular matrix and intracellular rho/rac GTPases. J Cell Biol 1995; 131:1857–1865.
12. Ruoslahti E, Yamagucchi Y. Proteoglycans as modulators of growth factor activities. Cell 1991; 64:867–869.
13. Ruoslahti E, Yamaguchi Y, Hildebrand A, Border WA. Extracellular Matrix/Growth Factor Interactions. Cold Spring Harbor Symposia on Quantitative Biology; Volume LVII. Cold Spring Harbor, NY: Cold Spring Harbor Laboratory Press, 1992.
14. Yamaguchi Y, Mann DM, Ruoslahti K. Negative regulation of transforming growth factor-β by the proteoglycan decorin. Nature 1990; 346:281–284.
15. Raines EW, Ross R. Compartmentalization of PDGF on extracellular binding sites dependent on exon-6-encoded sequences. J Cell Biol 1992; 116:533–543.
16. Burgess WH, Maciag T. The heparin-binding (fibroblast) growth factor family of proteins. Annu Rev Biochem 1989; 58:575–606.
17. Roberts R, Gallagher J, Spooncer E, Allen TD, Bloomfield F, Dexter TM. Heparan sulphate bound growth factor: a mechanism for stromal cell mediated haemopoiesis. Nature 1988; 332:376–378.
18. Park JE, Keller GA, Ferrara N. The vascular endothelial growth factor (VEGF) isoforms: differential deposition into the subepithelial extracellular matrix and bioactivity of ECM-bound VEGF. Mol Biol Cell 1993; 4:1317–1326.
19. Houck KA, Leung DW, Rowland AM, Winer J, Ferrara N. Dual regulation of vascular endothelial growth factor bioavailability by genetic and proteolytic mechanisms. J Biol Chem 1992; 267:26031–26037.
20. Aviezer D, Hecht D, Safran M, Eisinger M, David G, Yayon A. Perlecan, basal lamina proteoglycan, promotes basic fibroblast growth factor-receptor binding, mitogenesis, and angiogenesis. Cell 1994; 79:1005–1013.
21. Krusius T, Gehlsen KR, Ruoslahti E. A fibroblast chondroitin sulfate proteoglycan core protein contains lectin-like and growth factor-like sequences. J Biol Chem 1987; 262:13120–13125.
    Turley EA, Tretiak M. Glycosaminoglycan production by murine melanoma variants *in vivo* and *in vitro*. Cancer Res 1985; 45:5098–5105.

23. Underhill CB. CD44: the hyaluronan receptor. J Cell Sci 1992; 103:293–298.

24. Knudson W, Knudson CB. Overproduction of hyaluronan in the tumor stroma. In: Adany R, ed. Tumor Matrix Biology. New York: CRC Press, 1995:55–79.

25. Teder P, Bergh J, Heldin P. Functional hyaluronan receptors are expressed on a squamous cell lung carcinoma cell line but not on other lung carcinoma cell lines. Cancer Res 1995; 55:3908–3914.

26. Wynford-Thomas D, Smith P, Williams ED. Prolongation of fibroblast lifespan associated with epithelial rat tumor development. Cancer Res 1986; 46:3125–3127.

27. Bartal AH, Lichtig C, Cardo CC, Feit C, Robinson E, Hirshaut Y. Monoclonal antibody defining fibroblasts appearing in fetal and neoplastic tissue. J Natl Cancer Inst 1986; 76: 415–419.

28. Basset P, Bellocq JP, Wolf C. A novel metalloproteinase gene specifically expressed in stromal cells of breast carcinoma. Nature 1990; 348:699–704.

29. Urbanski SJ, Edwards DR, Maitland A, Leco KJ, Watson A, Kossakowska AE. Expression of metalloproteinases and their inhibitors in primary pulmonary carcinomas. Br J Cancer 1992; 66:1188–1194.

30. Ferrara N, Davis-Smyth T. The biology of vascular endothelial growth factor. Endoc Rev 1997; 18:4–25.

31. Schor SL. Fibroblast subpopulations as accelerators of tumor progression: the role of migration stimulating factor. In: Goldberg ID, Rosen EM, eds. Epithelial Mesenchymal Interactions in Cancer. Basel: Birkhauser Verlag, 1995:273–296.

32. Vignaud JM, Marie B, Klein N, Plénat F, Pech M, Borrelly J, Martinet N, Duprez A, Martinet Y. The role of platelet-derived growth factor production by tumor-associated macrophages in tumor stroma formation in lung cancer. Cancer Res 1994; 54:5455–5463.

33. Norgaard P, Hougaard S, Poulsen HS, Spang-Thomsen M. Transforming growth factor-β and cancer. Cancer Treat Rev 1995; 21:367–403.

34. Ignotz RA, Massagué J. Transforming growth factor-beta stimulates the expression of fibronectin and collagen and their incorporation in the extracellular matrix. J Biol Chem 1986; 261:4337–4345.

35. Ignotz RA, Endo T, Massagué J. Regulation of fibronectin and type I collagen mRNA levels by transforming growth factor-β. J Biol Chem 1987; 262:6443–6446.

36. Magnuson VL, Young M, Schattenberg DG, Mancini MA, Chen D, Steffensen B, Klebe RJ. The alternative splicing of fibronectin pre-mRNA is altered during aging and in response to growth factors. J Biol Chem 1991; 266:14654–14662.

37. Bolon I, Devouassoux M, Robert C, Moro D, Brambilla C, Brambilla E. Expression of urokinase-type plasminogen activator, stromelysin 1, stromelysin 3, and matrilysin genes in lung carcinomas. Am J Pathol 1997; 150:1619–1629.

38. Yoong KF, Adams DH. Tumour infiltrating lymphocytes: insights into tumour immunology and potential therapeutic implications. J Clin Pathol Mol Pathol 1996; 49:M256–267.

39. Doyle A, Martin WJ, Funa K, Gazdar A, Carney D, Martin SE, Linnoila I, Cuttitta F, Mulshine J, Bunn P, Minna J. Markedly decreased expression of class I histocompatibility antigens, protein, and mRNA in human small-cell lung cancer. J Exp Med 1985; 161:1135–1151.

40. Gingras MC, Roussel E, Roth JA. Little expression of cytokine mRNA by fresh tumour-infiltrating mononuclear leucocytes from glioma and lung adenocarcinoma. Cytokine 1995; 7:580–588.

41. Swhiher SG, Kiertscher SM, Golub SH, Carmack Holmes E, Roth MD. Pulmonary macrophages suppress the proliferation and cytotoxicity of tumor-infiltrating lymphocytes. Am J Respir Cell Mol Biol 1993; 8:486–492.

42. Huang M, Wang J, Lee P, Sharma S, Mao JT, Meissner H, Uyemura K, Modlin R, Wollman J, Dubinett SM. Human non-small cell lung cancer cells express a type 2 cytokine pattern. Cancer Res 1995; 55:3847–3853.

43. Li J, Perrella MA, Tsai JC, Yet SF, Hsieh CM, Yoshizumi M, Patterson C, Endego WO, Zhou F, Lee M. Induction of vascular endothelial growth factor gene expression by interleukin-1 beta in rat aortic smooth muscle cells. J Biol Chem 1995; 270:308–312.

44. Cohen T, Nahari D, Cerem LW, Neufeld G, Levi BZ. Interleukin 6 induces the expression of vascular endothelial growth factor. J Biol Chem 1996; 271:736–741.

45. Voest EE, Kenyon BM, O'Reilly MS, Truitt G, D'Amato RJ, Folkman J. Inhibition of angiogenesis *in vivo* by interleukin 12. J Natl Cancer Inst 1995; 87:581–586.

46. Fajardo LF, Kwan HH, Kowalski J, Prionas SD, Allison AC. Dual role of tumor necrosis factor-alpha in angiogenesis. Am J Pathol 1992; 140:539–544.

47. Niedbala MJ, Stein M. Tumor necrosis factor induction of urokinase-type plasminogen activator in human endothelial cells. Biomed Biochim Acta 1991; 50:427–436.

48. Mantovani A. Tumor-associated macrophages in neoplastic progression: a paradigm for the in vivo function of chemokines. Lab Invest 1994; 71:5–16.

49. Martinet N, Beck G, Bernard V, Plénat F, Vaillant P, Schooneman F, Vignaud JM, Martinet Y. Mechanism for the recruitment of macrophages to cancer site: *in vivo* concentration gradient of monocyte chemotactic activity. Cancer 1992; 70:854–860.

50. Zachariae CO, Anderson AO, Thompson HL, Appella E, Mantovani A, Oppenheim JJ, Matsushima K. Properties of monocyte chemotactic and activating factor (MCAF) purified from a human fibrosarcoma cell line. J Exp Med 1990; 171:2177–2182.

51. Bottazzi B, Walter S, Govoni D, Colotta F, Mantovani A. Monocyte chemotactic cytokine gene transfer modulates macrophage infiltration, growth, and susceptibility to IL-2 therapy of a murine melanoma. J Immunol 1992; 148:1280–1285.

52. Dorsch M, Hock H, Kunzendorf U, Diamantstein T, Blankenstein T. Macrophage colony-stimulating factor gene transfer into tumor cells induces macrophage infiltration but not tumor suppression. Eur J Immunol 1993; 23:186–190.

53. Tazi A, Bouchonnet F, Grandsaigne M, Boumsell L, Lance AJ, Soler P. Evidence that granulocyte macrophage-colony-stimulating factor regulates the distribution and differentiated state of dendritic cells/langerhans cells in human lung and lung cancers. J Clin Invest 1993; 91:566–76.

54. Adams DO, Hamilton TA. Macrophages as destructive cells in host defense. In: Gallin JI, Goldstein IM, Snyderman R, eds. Inflammation: Basic Principles and Clinical Correlates. New York: Raven Press, 1992:637–661.

55. Van Ravenswaay Claasen HH, Kluin PM, Fleuren GT. Tumor infiltrating cells in human cancer. On the possible role of CD16+ macrophages in antitumor cytotoxicity. Lab Invest 1992; 67:166–174.

56. Smith DR, Kunkel SL, Burdick MD, Wilke CA, Orringer MB, Whyte RI, Strieter RM. Production of interleukin-10 by human bronchogenic carcinoma. Am J Pathol 1994; 145: 18–25.

57. Betsholtz C, Berg J, Bywater M, Petterson M, Johnsson A, Heldin CH, Ohlsson R, Knott TJ, Scott J, Bell GI, Westermark B. Expression of multiple growth factors in a human lung cancer cell line. Int J Cancer 1987; 39:502–507.

58. Berg J. The expression of the platelet-derived and transforming growth factor genes in human non-small lung cancer lines is related to tumor stroma formation in nude mice tumors. Am J Pathol 1988; 133:434–439.

59. Martinet Y, Rom W, Grotendorst GR, Martin GR, Crystal RG. Exaggerated spontaneous release of plateled-derived growth factor by alveolar macrophages of patients with idiopathic pulmonary fibrosis. N Engl J Med 1987; 317:202–209.

60. Vignaud JM, Allam M, Martinet N, Pech M, Plénat F, Martinet Y. Presence of platelet-derived growth factor in normal and fibrotic lung is specifically associated with interstitial macrophages while both interstitial macrophages and alveolar epithelial cells express the *c-sis* proto-oncogene. Am J Respir Cell Mol Biol 1991; 5:531–538.

61. Mooradian DL, McCarthy JB, Komandduri KV, Furcht LT. Effects of transforming growth factor-beta 1 on human pulmonary adenocarcinoma cell adhesion, motility, and invasion in vitro. J Natl Cancer Inst 1992; 84:523–527.

62. Pertovaara L, Kaipainen A, Mustonen T, Orpana A, Ferrara N, Saksela O, Alitalo K. Vascular endothelial growth factor is induced in response to transforming growth factor-beta in fibroblastic and epithelial cells. J Biol Chem 1994; 269:6271–6274.

63. Moses HL, Yang EY, Pientenpol JA. TGF-β stimulation and inhibition of cell proliferation: new mechanistic insights. Cell 1990; 63:245–247.

64. Takanami I, Imamura T, Hashizume T, Kikuchi K, Yamamoto Y, Kodaira S. Transforming growth factor-beta 1 as a prognostic factor in pulmonary adenocarcinoma. J Clin Pathol 1994; 47:1098–1100.

65. Inoue T, Ishida T, Takenoyama M, Sugio K, Sugimachi K. The relationship between the immunodetection of transforming growth factor-beta in lung adenocarcinoma and longer survival rates. Surg Oncol 1995; 4:51–57.

66. Newman MJ. Inhibition of carcinoma and melanoma cell growth by type 1 transforming growth factor-β is dependent on the presence of polyunsaturated fatty acids. Proc Natl Acad Sci USA, 1993; 87:5543–5547.

67. Mooradian DL, McCarthy JB, Komanduri KV, Furcht LT. Effects of transforming growth factor-β1 on human pulmonary adenocarcinoma cell adhesion motility and invasion *in vitro*. J Natl Cancer Inst 1992; 84:523–527.

68. Roberts AB, McCune BK, Sporn MB. TGF-β: regulation of extracellular matrix. Kidney Int 1992; 41:557–559.

69. Streuli CH, Schmidhauser C, Kobrin M, Bissell MJ, Derynck R. Extracellular matrix regulates expression of the TGF-β1 gene. J Cell Biol 1993; 120:253–260.

70. Asakura S, Kato H, Fujino S, Konishi T, Asada Y, Tezuka N, Mori A. Immunohistochemical study of transforming growth factor-beta and central fibrosis in T1 adenocarcinoma of the lung. Nippon Kyo Geka Gak Zas 1995; 43:1924–1928.

71. Roberts AB, Sporn MB. Peptide Growth Factors and Their Receptors. Handbook of Experimental Pharmacology. 95th ed. Heidelberg: Springer-Verlag, 1990:419–472.

72. Yang EY, Moses HL. Transforming growth factor-β1-induced changes in cell migration, proliferation, and angiogenesis in the chicken chorioallantoic membrane. J Cell Biol 1990; 111:731–741.

73. Ray Chaudhury A, Frazier WA, D'Amore PA. Comparison of normal and tumorigenetic endothelial cells: differences in thrombospondin production and responses to transforming growth factor-beta. J Cell Sci 1994; 107:39–46.

74. Ueki N, Nakazato M, Okhawa T, Ikeda T, Amuro Y, Hada T, Higashino K. Excessive production of transforming growth-factor β1 can play an important role in the development of tumorigenesis by its action for angiogenesis: validity of neutralizing antibodies to block tumor growth. Biochem Biophys Acta 1992; 1137:189–196.

75. Falcone DJ, McCaffrey TA, Haimovitz-Freidman A, Garcia M. Transforming growth factor-β1 stimulates macrophages urokinase expression and release of matrix-bound basic fibroblast growth factor. J Cell Physiol 1993; 155:595–605.

76. Tazi A, Bouchonnet F, Grandsaigne M, Boumsell L, Hance AJ, Soler P. Evidence that granulocyte macrophage-colony-stimulating factor regulates the distribution and differentiated state of dendritic cells/Langerhans cells in human lung and lung cancers. J Clin Invest 1993; 91:566–576.

77. Nowicki A, Szenajch J, Ostrowska G, Wojtowicz A, Wojtowicz K, Kruszewski AA, Maruszynski M, Aukerman SL, WIktor-Jedrezejczak W. Impaired tumor growth in colony-stimulating factor 1 (CSF-1)-deficient, macrophage-deficient *op/op* mouse: evidence for a role of CSF-1-dependent macrophages in formation of tumor stroma. Int J Cancer 1996; 62:112–119.

78. Adany R, Kappelmayer J, Berényi E, Szegedi A, Fabian E, Muszbek L. Factors of the extrinsic pathway of blood coagulation in tumour associated macrophages. Thromb Haemost 1989; 62:850–855.

79. Takanami I, Tanaka F, Hashizume T, Kijuchi K, Yamamoto Y, Yamamoto T, Kodaira S. The basic fibroblast growth factor and its receptor in pulmonary adenocarcinomas: an investigation of their expression as prognostic markers. Eur J Cancer 1996; 32A:1504–1509.

80. Rusch V, Baselga J, Cordon-Cardo C, Orazem J, Zaman M, Hoda S, McIntosh J, Kurie J, Dmitrovsky E. Differential expression of the epidermal growth factor receptor and its ligands

in primary non-small cell lung cancers and adjacent benign lung. Cancer Res 1993; 53:2379–2385.

81. Goldman CK, Kim J, Wong WL, King V, Brock T, Gillespie GY. Epidermal growth factor stimulates vascular endothelial growth factor production by human malignant glioma cells: a model of glioblastoma multiforme pathophysiology. Mol Biol Cell 1993; 4:121–133.

82. Sato Y, Okamura K, Morimoto A, Hamanaka R, Hamaguchi K, Shimada T, Ono M, Kohno K, Sakata T, Kuwano M. Indispensable role of tissue-type plasminogen activator in growth factor-dependent tube formation of human microvascular endothelial cells *in vitro*. Exp Cell Res 1993; 204:223–229.

83. Reeve JG, Morgan J, Schwander J, Bleehen NM. Role for membrane and secreted insulin-like growth factor-binding protein-2 in the regulation of insulin-like growth factor action in lung tumors. Cancer Res 1993; 53:4680–4685.

84. Olivero M, Rizzo M, Madeddu R, Casadio C, Pennacchietti S, Nicotra MR, Prat M, Maggi G, Arena N, Natali PG, Comoglio PM, Di Renzo MF. Overexpression and activation of hepatocyte growth factor/scatter factor in human non-small-cell lung carcinomas. Br J Cancer 1996; 74:1862–1868.

85. Birkedal-Hansen H, Moore WGI, Bodden MK. Matrix metalloproteinases: a review. Crit Rev Oral Biol Med 1993; 4:197–250.

86. Ray JM, Stetler-Stevenson WG. The role of matrix metalloproteases and their inhibitors in tumour invasion, metastasis and angiogenesis. Eur Respir J 1994; 7:2062–2072.

87. Unemori EN, Ferrara N, Bauer EA, Amento EP. Vascular endothelial growth factor induces interstitial collagenase expression in human endothelial cell. J Cell Physiol 1992; 153:557–562.

23

Tumor Angiogenesis

FABRICE SONCIN and BERNARD VANDENBUNDER

Institut de Biologie de Lille
Lille, France

The formation of new blood vessels, or angiogenesis, is essential for the transport of oxygen, nutrients, and metabolites wherever organogenesis occurs. The need for nutrients and elimination of metabolites is such that the heart and the vascular system are among the first functional organs to be formed in the embryo. A similar situation exists in solid tumors: the development of a tumor beyond a size of approximately one to two cubic millimeters is dependent on the formation of new blood vessels. These vessels directly connect the growing tumor to the circulation and allow the exchange of elements essential for its growth. In addition, the tumor uses these vessels as a way to spread by metastasis; the blood circulation subsequently transports the pioneer cancer cells to their target organs (1). Angiogenesis is therefore a necessary step for tumor development.

I. Morphogenesis of the Vascular Tree

In the embryo, the vascular tree is formed by two different mechanisms, angiogenesis and vasculogenesis (2,3). Vasculogenesis describes the differentiation of mesoderm-derived endothelial precursors in situ and their association to form the first blood vessels. It occurs during the initial stages of embryonic development and during the vascularization of organs that derive from the mesoderm and endoderm, such as the lungs, pancreas, and intestine. Angiogenesis is the process by which endothelial cells form new capillaries by sprouting from existing blood vessels. During embryonic development, it is responsible for the extension of the vascular tree, in particular within the kidney, the limb buds, and the brain (4). The formation of the vascular tree involves not only the budding of new capillaries but also intussusception, i.e., the splitting of existing vessels by transcapillary pillars, and the trimming of superfluous microvascular sprouts (4–7). Endothelial cell precursors, or angioblasts that participate in new capillaries where they originally differentiated, are also able to migrate great distances in the embryo (8). A recent report suggests the existence of endothelial cell precursors in the adult peripheral blood, which would be able to differentiate as endothelial cells in vitro and to participate to angiogenesis in vivo (9). These cells, isolated using CD34- or Flk-1–coated magnetic beads, are able to aggregate and to form capillary-like structures on a fibronectin or collagen substrate. They can also take part in the formation of collateral blood vessels that develop after severe ischemia induced in the rabbit or mouse limb. Potentially, these endothelial cell precursors could be used as angiogenesis-targeting therapeutic vectors. The formation of new blood vessels is therefore a complex process involving not only differentiated endothelial cells from established vessels but also potential precursors, which may originate far from the angiogenic stimulus and participate in the formation of new capillaries.

Angiogenesis is not restricted to embryonic development. In the adult, it occurs normally during would healing, cyclic repair of the endometrium, corpus luteum formation (6), as well as in several pathologies like retinopathies or tumor formation (10). Tumor microvessels in rapidly growing tumors show a series of severe structural abnormalities: a lack of organization, with incomplete endothelial lining, tortuous vessels, blind ends, and arterio-venous shunts (11). Interstitial fluid pressure is high, due to the high vascular permeability and to the absence of a lymphatic network to drain the excess of fluid. This higher pressure is a barrier to the penetration of anticancer drugs and is also an advantage for the exportation of tumor components (12), including metastatic cells. Inadequate oxygenation is also a characteristic of solid tumors and is an angiogenic stimulus per se.

II. From the Budding of a Capillary to the Irrigation of a Tumor

The histological observation of angiogenic models reveals the existence of several distinct phases; first there is an increase in vascular permeability resulting in the extravasation of plasma proteins and a degradation of the surrounding extracellular matrix. Second, the endothelial cells that line the luminal side of the established ~ssels begin to migrate from the parent blood vessel toward the angiogenic stimu-
Endothelial cells located behind this front of migration proliferate, whereas cells
ᵗ at the most proximal part of the new capillary begin to differentiate into a
The newly formed tube will eventually open to the blood stream (13).

Whereas some capillaries extend progressively, others receiving a lower flow retract and disappear (13). Aside from the repair processes mentioned earlier, the endothelium is a very quiescent lineage in the adult: a proliferation index below 0.01% and 0.14% has been measured in capillaries irrigating the retina and the myocardial muscle, respectively, in the rat (14). However, in pathological processes such as the vasoproliferative or diabetic retinopathy, rheumatoid arthritis or tumor development, the proliferation index of the endothelium reaches 9–20% (10).

The effect of new perfusion on tumor growth has been evidenced in the ear chamber and in cornea models (for review, see Ref. 1): a few days after its implantation in the avascular area of the cornea, a tumor fragment induces the growth of new capillaries from the limbus (15). When the newly formed small arteries reach the tumor, connect with small veins, and support a functional perfusion (Fig. 1), the volume of the tumor begins to increase exponentially. ^{3}H-thymidine incorporation studies have shown that the mitotic index of cancer cells within a tumor implanted in the mouse is higher in cells located around the blood vessels and that the growth rate of endothelial cells is approximately 2000-fold higher in tumors than in normal blood vessels of corresponding tissues (16).

It has been shown that micrometastases developing in the lung after subcutaneous injection of Lewis lung carcinoma cells in mice remain quiescent because the rate of apoptosis is high. In that model, angiogenesis induces micrometastasis outgrowth by providing survival factors that drastically reduce the rate of apoptosis (17). A correlation between the presence of a dense vasculature and a bad prognosis in melanomas, lung, prostate, head and neck, and especially breast cancers has been demonstrated, and some authors have suggested the use of vessel density calculation in the prognosis of cancer. However, these data are controversial: indeed, some benign tumors like adrenal adenocarcinoma are also highly vascularized. The associa-

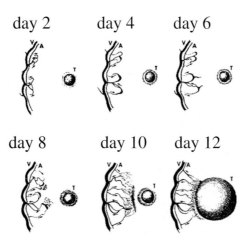

Figure 1 Chronology of the irrigation of a tumor fragment implanted into the cornea. From Muthukkaruppan K, Auerbach R. Science 1979; *205*:1416–1418.

tion between tumor angiogenesis and the risk of metastasis or tumor recurrence must therefore be evaluated for each type of cancer.

III. Angiogenic Factors

Since implanted solid tumors are able to attract new blood vessels (1), it has been postulated that a solid tumor secretes soluble angiogenic factors, which diffuse and induce the proliferation and migration of endothelial cells toward it. Indeed, a number of angiogenic factors have been initially isolated from tumor extracts or tumor cell conditioned media, based on their capacity to induce endothelial cell proliferation in vitro (18). Most of these factors when assayed in experimental conditions in vivo have angiogenic properties on the chick chorio-allantoid membrane (19) or in the rabbit cornea (20). More than a dozen such factors are known today (Table 1). FGF-2 was the first identified and isolated on its capacity to induce the growth of endothelial cells and to be angiogenic in vivo (21,22). Its effect, however, is not restricted to endothelial cell proliferation, since it stimulates the growth of a wide variety of other cells. The vascular endothelial cell growth factor/vascular permeability factor (VEGF/VPF) has all the expected hallmarks of an angiogenic factor. It was identified by its ability to induce vascular permeability (23,24) and to support endothelial cell proliferation (25,26). VEGF/VPF is present as four glycosylated dimer proteins with molecular weights ranging from 35 to 45 kDa, produced by a variety of normal and tumor cells (26–29). It was initially shown that VEGF/VPF is mitogenic for most endothelial cells but not for corneal endothelial cells, smooth muscle

Table 1 Angiogenic Factors

	Proliferation	Migration
FGF-1	+	+
Angiogenin	0/+	0
FGF-2	+	+
HGF/SF	+	+
Interleukin-8	+	+
Placental growth factor	+	+
PDGF	+	+
PD-ECGF/TP	0	+
TGF-α	+	+
TGF-β	−	−
TNF-α	−	+
VPF/VEGF	−	+
	+	+
VCAM		+
selectin		+
nt SPARC	−	+

cells, granulosa cells, fibroblasts, keratinocytes, or epithelial cells (25). However, it does have a mitogenic effect on cells from the pigmented epithelium of the retina and it is an autocrine factor for hair dermal papilla cells (30). VEGF/VPF is angiogenic in the chick chorio-allantoid membrane (26,31) and it induces the formation of capillaries by endothelial cells in vitro (32). Two types of receptors for VEGF/VPF, Flt-1 (VEGFR-1) and Flk-1/KDR (VEGFR-2), expressed by endothelial cells in vitro and during embryonic development have been isolated, and several lines of evidence suggest that Flk-1/KDR is responsible for the proliferative response of endothelial cells to VEGF/VPF (for review, see Ref. 33).

Angiogenic factors are not always endothelial cell growth factors. Transforming growth factor-β (TGF-β) inhibits their growth (34), while angiogenin or platelet-derived endothelial cell growth factor/thymidine phosphorylase (PD-ECGF/TP) have, respectively, a weak or no effect on the proliferation of these cells (35,36), although all of these factors proved to be angiogenic in various in vivo assays. A probable explanation for this apparent paradox is that these molecules induce by a paracrine effect the expression of factors, which in turn induce endothelial cell growth (18). On the other hand, endothelial cell proliferation is not strictly necessary for the formation of new blood vessels in vivo (37).

A number of molecules related to the extracellular matrix are also involved in the regulation of angiogenesis. In vitro, fibronectin, laminin, and collagens stimulate the migration of endothelial cells (38) and laminin supports the formation of capillaries by endothelial cells (39). Heparan sulfates are constituents of the endothelial-produced extracellular matrix, which takes part in the regulation of the binding of FGFs and VEGF/VPF to their high-affinity receptors. Also, most angiogenic proteins isolated so far bind to the glycosaminoglycan heparin, and heparin itself can be angiogenic (40) or can prevent angiogenesis (41), depending on the conditions. Thus, in normal and tumor angiogenesis, the extracellular matrix acts both as an adhesion and migration substrate and as a reservoir for angiogenic factors (for review, see Ref. 42).

IV. The Role of the Angiogenic Factors In Vivo

In vitro, most angiogenic factors are able to stimulate not only endothelial cells but other cell lineages as well. Over the past few years, however, several studies have shown that VEGF/VPF is probably one of the most specific angiogenic factors in vivo (33). In situ hybridization and immunolocalization studies have shown that the expression of VEGF/VPF, and not of FGF-1 or 2, correlates with the formation of new blood vessels in the embryo. In addition, the expression of VEGF/VPF receptors Flt-1 (VEGFR-1) and Flk-1/KDR (VEGFR-2) is observed in endothelial cells at the beginning of embryogenesis (43). Finally, the inactivation of the gene encoding VEGF/VPF gene or its receptors showed a crucial role for this factor in angiogenesis. Embryos die in utero between E8.5 and E9.5 (44); when the VEGFR-2 gene is inactivated, the formation of hemangioblasts, the common precursors to both hematopoietic and endothelial cell lineage, is blocked (45), whereas the formation of blood vessels is disrupted when VEGFR-1 gene is knocked out (46).

The role for VEGF/VPF in tumor angiogenesis has also been extensively documented. Thus, in various brain tumors, VEGF/VPF expression is upregulated (47–49) and transfection of MCF-7 breast cancer cells with a VEGF/VPF gene results in a stronger angiogenic phenotype and a better growth of the tumors formed after subcutaneous injection in nude mice (50). Indeed, besides VEGF/VPF, a variety of other angiogenic factors are also specifically expressed in human tumors, suggesting that angiogenesis involves a coordinate regulation of several vascular growth factors (51).

The family of receptors Tie (Tie-1) and Tek (Tie-2) is another group of molecules specifically expressed in the endothelium (52,53). In contrast to the inactivation of VEGFR-2, which results in the blockage of endothelial precursor formation, the inactivation of Tie-1 or -2 receptor genes affects blood vessel integrity. Tie-1 or Tie-2 $-/-$ embryos die from hemorrhage around E13.5 and E10, respectively (54,55). Recently a ligand for Tie-2 has been identified (56). This factor, named angiopoietin, does not induce endothelial cell growth or capillary formation in vitro, but the inactivation of its gene shows that it plays a role in the interactions between endothelial cells and extracellular matrix during development (57).

V.   The Induction of Angiogenesis by Hypoxia

The excessive rate of aerobic glycolysis results in a high oxygen consumption in tumor tissues (12). Several lines of evidence suggest that a low oxygen tension (hypoxia) induces VEGF/VPF expression. VEGF/VPF mRNA level is dramatically increased within a few hours following exposure of various cell cultures to hypoxia. In glioblastomas, the expression of VEGF/VPF is detected in the periphery of necrotic areas, in tumor cells that presumably experience the most severe hypoxia, whereas the expression of VEGFR-1 and -2 is localized in the blood vessels (47,48). The induction of VEGF/VPF mRNA accumulation by hypoxia results from an increase of both mRNA transcription and stability. The promoter/enhancer of the VEGF/VPF gene (58) as well as of other hypoxia-responsive genes such as the erythropoietin gene (59) contain functional binding sites for the hypoxia-inducible factor-1 (HIF-1α) (60). HIF-1α forms heterodimers with the arylhydrocarbon-receptor nuclear translocator (ARNT) (61) for the control of the VEGF/VPF gene transcription. In ARNT $-/-$ embryonic stem cells, VEGF/VPF gene is no longer induced by hypoxia. ARNT $-/-$ embryos die around E9 and show defects in yolk sac angiogenesis and brachial arcs, a phenotype close to the angiogenic abnormali-
~ observed in VEGF/VPF $-/-$ or tissue factor (TF) $-/-$ mice. In addition, the
~ssion of VEGF/VPF in the yolk sac and other tissues of ARNT $-/-$ embryos
~(62). Natural development of the retinal vasculature is also considered to be
~y oxygen. Physiological levels of hypoxia are thought to be detected by
~ls that secrete VEGF/VPF, and during the formation of the retina in the

newborn rat, the reduction in VEGF/VPF expression induced by artificial hyperoxia is responsible for vascular regression (63).

VI. Angiogenesis in Lung Cancer

Angiogenic factors may play a role in the development of lung cancer by supporting both the proliferation of stroma and of cancer cells as well as by promoting angiogenesis. A high vessel density correlates with the stage of non–small-cell lung cancer progression (64), metastasis (65), and survival (66). However, the direct correlation between vessel density and bad prognosis remains a subject of controversy. Regarding angiogenic factors, the expression of VEGF/VPF is detected in approximately 60% of non–small-cell cancer, including in the tumor stroma (67), and approximately 60% of epidermoid lung carcinoma (68). Also, PD-ECGF/TP expression correlates with blood vessel density in non–small-cell lung cancer (69). In addition, the expression pattern of the platelet-derived growth factor (PDGF) suggests that it plays an autocrine or paracrine role in the development of this type of cancer. Normal lung epithelial cells do not express PDGF receptors (70); in contrast, half of the non–small-cell lung cancer analyzed show the expression of PDGF receptors (71) and the transfer of the PDGF receptor gene to normal cells leads to transformation into fibrosarcoma (72). It seems likely that in this type of cancer, PDGF expression by stroma cells like macrophages, but also by cancer cells in certain cases, may support the growth of lung tumors.

VII. The Inhibitors of Angiogenesis

Analysis of tumor development in transgenic mouse models of multistage carcinogenesis showed that tumor formation is preceded by a phase of intense vascularization (73). The visualization of the vasculature in preneoplastic stages of human breast and cervix cancer also suggests the existence of an angiogenic switch that becomes activated during tumor progression (74). It has been proposed that this switch is dependent on the balance between angiogenic factors and inhibitors (75) (Fig. 2). Heparin and its fragments and protamine were among the first tumor-induced angiogenesis inhibitors to be isolated (Table 2) (41,76). Angiogenic inhibitors have been sought in avascular tissues such as the cartilage; chondrocytes in culture produce a potent inhibitor of neovascularization, TIMP-1, which also inhibits collagenase I (77).

Certain angiogenic inhibitors are expressed by normal cells and are underexpressed when these cells adopt a cancerous phenotype (78,79). Other inhibitors of angiogenesis are fragments of larger molecules, which have no effect themselves on angiogenesis. For example, a fragment of thrombospondin, an extracellular matrix glycoprotein, has been shown to inhibit angiogenesis (78). This category also includes a 16 kDa fragment of prolactin (80), a 29 kDa fragment of fibronectin (74), as well as angiostatin, a fragment of plasminogen (17) and endostatin, a fragment of collagen XVIII (81). Platelet factor-4, itself a weak angiogenic inhibitor, contains a

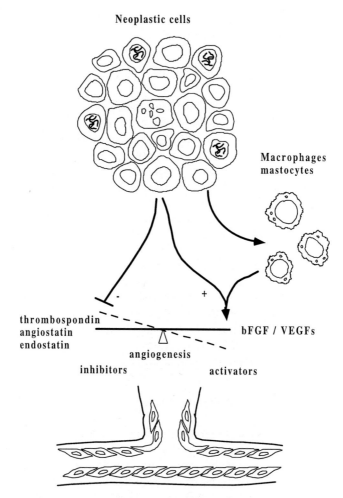

Figure 2   Balance between activators and inhibitors of angiogenesis.

fragment that is 50-fold more potent at inhibiting angiogenesis (reviewed in Ref. 74). These molecules can be considered as cryptic inhibitors, which might be released rapidly by proteolysis when angiogenesis needs to be regulated.

VIII.   The Response of Endothelial Cells to Angiogenic Stimuli

As already mentioned above, in the adult, endothelial cells are mostly quiescent. It is the imbalance between angiogenic activators and inhibitors that is responsible for the activation of endothelial cells. At the gene level, little is known about the tran-

Table 2   Inhibitors of Angiogenesis

IFN-α/β
Platelet factor-4

Angiostatin
Endostatin
16 kDa prolactin fragment
Thrombospondin fragment

Cartilage-derived inhibitor
TIMP-1 & -2
Glioma-derived angiogenesis inhibitor

Heparin, protamine,
steroids, 2-methoxyestradiol
AGM 1470, fumagillin analog
thalidomide, genistein, taxol

scriptional regulation that takes place in endothelial cells during angiogenesis. The Ets 1 transcription factor is expressed in endothelial cells during embryonic development and tumor growth (82,83) and is able to activate the VEGFR-1 gene promoter (84). The expression of the NFkB/IkB system was also detected in the vasculature and its activation shown to correlate with endothelial regeneration after wounding (85).

During the initial phases of angiogenesis, the permeability and motility of endothelial cells increase. Angiogenic factors induce a change in cell-cell and cell-matrix interactions, as well as the degradation and remodeling of this extracellular matrix. All of these steps are essential to the initial migration of endothelial cells toward the angiogenic stimulus. Molecules that mediate endothelial cell adhesion have been identified. Among those, VE-cadherin and PECAM reside at interendothelial cell junctions (86). A number of integrins that are extracellular matrix molecule receptors, primarily β1 and β3 subunits, have been involved in angiogenesis. The integrin αv-β3, a receptor for fibrinogen, vitronectin, fibronectin, thrombospondin, and laminin, is a marker of new blood vessel formation in the embryo and during wound-healing (42).

The histological observation of the establishment of new capillaries suggests that degradation and remodeling of the ECM are essential to the initial steps of angiogenesis. This degradation was initially thought to be mediated by the urokinase type plasminogen activator (u-PA) and collagenase I (MMP1) since their expression as well as the expression of their inhibitors is stimulated by angiogenic factors such as FGF-2 and TGF-β in cultured endothelial cells (87,88). However, neither gene is specifically expressed in endothelial cells during embryonic development or during most tumor formation (89,90). In the tumor stroma, these proteases are essentially expressed by fibroblasts as inactive proenzymes. Upon binding to its receptor at the surface of endothelial cells stimulated by angiogenic factors, pro u-PA is activated. Indeed, several proteases cooperate in the regulation of angiogenesis: the 72 kDa gelatinase A (MMP2) binds to the αv-β3 integrin and is subsequently activated on the surface of endothelial cells (91).

At the onset of angiogenesis, plasma proteins extravasate in the surrounding tissues, due to a greater permeability of the endothelium and a modification of the extracellular matrix (42,92). These blood components take part in vessel development by interacting with proteins induced by angiogenic factors in endothelial cells. For example, TF, a major blood-coagulation factor receptor secreted by endothelial cells after VEGF/VPF stimulation, is found in vessels irrigating malignant tumors, but not benign ones (93). In the embryo, the knock-out of the TF (or of factor V) gene is lethal at E9.5, probably due to a defect in yolk sac vascularization (94). Together with extravasated coagulation factors, TF activates thrombin, which converts fibrinogen into fibrin, thus modifying the composition of the extracellular matrix (95). Plasma vitronectin and fibronectin bind to αv-β3 integrin on the surface of endothelial cells and modulate the adherence and proliferation properties of these cells. u-PA bound to its receptor promotes the activation of extravasated plasminogen at the periphery of endothelial cells. Subsequently, plasmin takes part in the activation of MMP zymogens expressed locally, triggers the digestion of the underlying extracellular matrix, and opens the way to the migration of endothelial cells and the release ECM-trapped growth factors.

Angiogenesis involves the interaction between endothelial cells and factors secreted by neighboring cells, released from the underlying extracellular matrix and from the circulation. The description of this network of interactions in the various environments where angiogenesis takes place represents a formidable challenge.

IX. Antiangiogenesis as a Potential Therapeutic Strategy

At the beginning of the 1970s, Judah Folkman suggested that the growth of tumors depended on the formation of new blood vessels. According to this hypothesis, it should be possible to block tumor growth by shutting off these vessels. The studies on the various aspects of angiogenesis that followed have brought a growing base of knowledge on its molecular mechanism and allowed the elaboration of precisely targeted drugs. Various experimental approaches intended to prevent angiogenesis in vivo have been used successfully to inhibit tumor development in mouse tumorigenesis models. Each step in the formation of a capillary is a potential target for this approach (Fig. 3). Indeed, blocking antibodies specific for angiogenic factors like FGF-2 (96), VEGF/VPF or angiogenin (97), as well as soluble or mutated forms of VEGF/VPF receptors (98,99) have been used to inhibit tumor-induced angiogenesis or tumor growth. This list also includes various angiogenic inhibitors like angiosta-

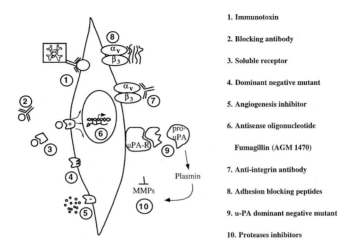

1. Immunotoxin

2. Blocking antibody

3. Soluble receptor

4. Dominant negative mutant

5. Angiogenesis inhibitor

6. Antisense oligonucleotide

   Fumagillin (AGM 1470)

7. Anti-integrin antibody

8. Adhesion blocking peptides

9. u-PA dominant negative mutant

10. Proteases inhibitors

Figure 3 Potential targets of antiangiogenesis therapy.

tin (100) and endostatin (81), interferon-alpha and the fumagillin analog AGM 1470 (101), antisense oligonucleotides, antibodies blocking the function of αv-β3 integrins (102), u-PA antagonists (103), or protease inhibitors such as Marimastat.

Whether results that look so promising in mice will be obtained in human remains a major question. Most studies in mouse models were done with rapidly growing tumors; indeed the hastily formed microvessels in these tumors and the vessels irrigating tumors that have been growing for years in humans have a different structure, and presumably a different response towards antiangiogenic agents. In most studies, the antiangiogenic agents were subcutaneously injected together with cancer cells; it may be difficult to initiate an antiangiogenic treatment at the time of tumor outgrowth in humans. However, with several treatments the regression of preexisting tumors has been obtained. Thus, when cancer cells are engineered to induce in nearby endothelial cells the expression of class II antigen, a protein that they do not make normally, immunotoxin coupled to antibodies against this antigen causes complete occlusion of the tumor vasculature and a dramatic regression in large solid tumors (104). However, tumor collapse was followed by a regrowth 7–10 days later. Primary tumors 100–400 mm^3 in size also regressed to dormant microscopic lesions upon treatment with angiostatin (100) or endostatin (81). After discontinuation of angiostatin or endostatin therapy, a tumor recurred at the primary site within 1–2 weeks.

These results suggest that long-term antiangiogenic treatments would be necessary to keep micrometastases dormant after the surgical resection of a primary tumor, if metastasis is suspected. One may worry that a long-term systemic injection of antiangiogenic factors will induce severe side effects on wound healing, on the female reproductive pathway (105), and on the regeneration of the arterial wall at the branching points where the turbulence of flow is the highest.

Tumor regrowth after cessation of anti-angiogenic treatment may be the result of the selection of more aggressive cancer cells, such as p53 mutant cells, which are resistant to killing by hypoxia (106) and become predominant. These difficulties, as well as the complications due to long-term antiangiogenic treatments, could be avoided by combining therapies targeting blood vessels and cancer cells. Indeed, one report illustrates the potentiation of a cytotoxic drug by several antiangiogenic agents (107); when tumor-specific and tumor endothelium–specific immunotoxins are used in combination, five out of eight treated animals clear their tumors and remain disease-free (104). Again, these results cannot be extrapolated without caution. A successful attack against endothelial and cancer cells requires a reconciliation between two antagonistic desires: increasing the blood flow to improve oxygen delivery for radiotherapy or drug delivery for chemotherapy, and shutting down the blood flow to achieve anoxia and tumor necrosis (108). In order to combine efficiently these two strategies in humans, clinical investigations dealing with the microcirculatory parameters, the oxygen and nutrient supply, and the interstitial fluid pressure within the different tumors will be necessary (12).

Several inhibitors of angiogenesis are currently studied in phase 1 or 2 clinical trials. During the past few years, our understanding of the molecular mechanisms of angiogenesis has steadily increased. One may foresee that new inhibitors specific for the various steps of the angiogenic process will become available. The approach of targeting endothelial cells and more generally the tumor stroma will require the understanding of the tumor as a system, which will come from both molecular and physiological studies.

Acknowledgments

We would like to thank Eric Maire for the figures and all the laboratory members for our discussions. Our work is supported by the Centre National de la Recherche Scientifique, l'Institut Pasteur de Lille, l'Institut National de la Santé et de la Recherche Médicale, la Ligue contre le Cancer, l'Association pour la Recherche sur le Cancer, le GEFLUC and l'AICR.

References

1. Blood CH, Zetter BR. Tumor interactions with the vasculature: angiogenesis and tumor metastasis. Biochem Biophys Acta 1990; 1032:89–118.
2. Coffin JD, Poole TJ. Embryonic vascular development: immunohistochemical identification of the origin and subsequent morphogenesis of the major vessels primordia in quail embryos. Development 1988; 102:735–748.
3. Pardanaud L, Altmann C, Kitos P, Dieterlen-Lièvre F, Buck CA. Vasculogenesis in the early quail blastodisc as studied with a monoclonal antibody recognizing endothelial cells. Development 1987; 100:339–349.
4. Pardanaud L, Yassine F, Dieterlen-Lièvre F. Relationship between vasculogenesis, angiogenesis and haemopoiesis during avian ontogeny. Development 1989; 105:473–485.

5. Ausprunk DH, Falterman KJF. The sequence of events in the regression of corneal capillaries. Lab Invest 1978; 38:284–294.
6. Risau W, Flamme I. Vasculogenesis. Annu Rev Cell Dev Biol 1995; 11:73–91.
7. Risau W. Mechanisms of angiogenesis. Nature 1997; 386:671–674.
8. Noden DM. Embryonic origins and assembly of blood vessels. Am Rev Respir Dis 1989; 140:1097–1103.
9. Asahara T, Murohara T, Sullivan A, et al. Isolation of putative progenitor endothelial cells for angiogenesis. Science 1997; 275:964–967.
10. D'Amore PA, Thompson RW. Mechanisms of angiogenesis. Ann Rev Physiol 1987; 49:453–464.
11. Less J, Skalak T, Sevick EM, Jain R. Microvascular architecture in a mammary carcinoma: branching patterns and vascular dimensions. Cancer Res 1991; 51:265–273.
12. Vaupel P, Schlenger K, Höckel M. Blood flow and tissue oxygenation of human tumors: an update. Adv Exp Med Biol 1992; 317:139–151.
13. Folkman J. Angiogenesis. Biology of endothelial cells. Jaffe E. A., 1984:412–428.
14. Engerman RL, Pfaffenbach D, Davis MD. Cell turnover of capillaries. Lab Invest 1967; 17:738–743.
15. Gimbrone MAJ, Leapman SB, Cotran RS, Folkman J. Tumor angiogenesis: iris neovascularization at a distance from experimental intraocular tumors. J Natl Cancer Inst 1973; 50:219–228.
16. Tannock IF. Population kinetics of carcinoma cells, capillary endothelial cells, and fibroblasts in a transplanted mouse mammary tumor. Cancer Res 1970; 30:2470–2476.
17. O'Reilly MS, Holmgren L, Shing Y, et al. Angiostatin: A novel angiogenesis inhibitor that mediates the suppression of metastases by a Lewis lung carcinoma. Cell 1994; 79:315–328.
18. Folkman J, Klagsbrun M. Angiogenic factors. Science 1987; 235:442–447.
19. Ausprunk DH, Knighton DR, Folkman J. Vascularization of normal and neoplastic tissues grafted to the chick chorioallantois. Role of host and preexisting graft blood vessels. Am J Pathol 1975; 79:597–618.
20. Gimbrone MA, Cotran RS, Leapman SB, Folkman J. Tumor growth and neovascularization: an experimental model using the rabbit cornea. J Natl Cancer Inst 1974; 52:413–427.
21. Shing Y, Folkman J, Sullivan R, Butterfield C, Murray J, Klagsbrun M. Heparin affinity: purification of a tumor-derived capillary endothelial cell growth factor. Science 1984; 223:1296–1299.
22. Shing Y, Folkman J, Haudenschild C, Lund D, Crum R, Klagsbrun M. Angiogenesis is stimulated by a tumor-derived endothelial cell growth factor. J Cell Biochem 1985; 29: 275–287.
23. Senger DR, Galli SJ, Perruzz CA, Harvey VS, Dvorak HF. Tumor cells secrete a vascular permeability factor that promotes accumulation of ascites fluid. Science 1983; 219: 983–985.
24. Keck PJ, Hauser SD, Krivi G, et al. Vascular permeability factor, an endothelial cell mitogen related to PDGF. Science 1989; 246:1309–1312.
25. Ferrara N, Henzel WJ. Pituitary follicular cells secrete a novel heparin-binding growth factor specific for vascular endothelial cells. Biochem Biophys Res Commun 1989; 161:851–858.
26. Leung DW, Cachianes G, Kuang WJ, Goeddel DV, Ferrara N. Vascular endothelial growth factor is a secreted angiogenic mitogen. Science 1989; 246:1306–1309.
27. Senger DR, Perruzzi CA, Feder J, Dvorak HF. A highly conserved vascular permeability factor secreted by a variety of human and rodent tumor cell lines. Cancer Res 1986; 46:5629–5632.
28. Gospodarowicz D, Abraham JA, Schilling J. Isolation and characterization of a vascular endothelial cell mitogen produces by pituitary-derived folliculo stellate cells. Proc Natl Acad Sci USA 1989; 86:7311–7315.
29. Conn G, Soderman DD, Schaeffer M-T, Wile M, Hatcher VB, Thomas KA. Purification of a glycoprotein vascular endothelial cell mitogen from a rat glioma-derived cell line. Proc Natl Acad Sci USA 1990; 87:1323–1327.
30. Guerrin M, H. M, Chollet P, et al. Vasculotropin/vascular endothelial growth factor is an au-

tocrine growth factor for human retinal pigment epithelial cells cultured in vitro. J Cell Physiol 1995; 164:385–394.

31. Plouët J, Schilling J, Gospodarowicz D. Isolation and characterization of a newly identified endothelial cell mitogen produced by AtT-20 cells. EMBO J 1989; 8:3801–3806.

32. Pepper MS, Ferrara N, Orci L, Montesano R. Potent synergism between vascular endothelial growth factor and basic fibroblast growth factor in the induction of angiogenesis in vitro. Biochem Biophys Res Commun 1992; 189:824–831.

33. Thomas KA. Vascular endothelial growth factor, a potent and selective angiogenic agent. J Biol Chem 1996; 271:603–606.

34. Baird A, Durkin T. Inhibition of endothelial cell proliferation by type β-transforming growth factor: interactions with acidic and basic fibroblast growth factors. Biochem Biophys Res Commun 1986; 138:476–482.

35. Hu GF, Riordan JF, Vallee BL. A putative angiogenin receptor in angiogenin-responsive human endothelial cells. Proc Natl Acad Sci USA 1997; 94:2204–2209.

36. Moghaddam A, Bicknell R. Expression of platelet-derived endothelial cell growth factor in Escherichia coli and confirmation of its thymidine phosphorylase activity. Biochemistry 1992; 31:12141–12146.

37. Sholley MM, Ferguson GP, Seibel HR, Montour JL, Wilson JD. Mechanisms of neovascularization. Vascular sprouting can occur without proliferation of endothelial cells. Lab Invest 1984; 51:624–634.

38. Terranova VP, DiFlorio R, Lyall RM, Hic S, Friesel R, Maciag T. Human endothelial cells are chemotactic to endothelial cell growth factor and heparin. J Cell Biol 1985; 101:2330–2334.

39. Grant DS, Tashiro K-I, Segui-Real B, Yamada Y, Martin GR, Kleinman HK. Two different laminin domains mediate the differentiation of human endothelial cells into capillary-like structures in vitro. Cell 1989; 58:933–943.

40. Raju KS, Alessandri G, Ziche M, Gullino PM. Ceruloplasmin, copper ions, and angiogenesis. J Natl Cancer Inst 1982; 69:1183–1188.

41. Folkman J, Langer R, Linhardt RJ, Haudenschild C, Taylor S. Angiogenesis inhibition and tumor regression caused by heparin or a heparin fragment in the presence of cortisone. Science 1983; 221:719–725.

42. Polverini PJ. Cellular adhesion molecules; newly identified mediators of angiogenesis. Am J Pathol 1996; 148:1023–1029.

43. Mustonen T, Alitalo K. Endothelial receptor tyrosine kinases involved in angiogenesis. J Cell Biol 1995; 129:895–898.

44. Ferrara N, Carver-Moore K, Chen H, et al. Heterozygous embryonic lethality induced by targeted inactivation of the VEGF gene. Nature 1996; 380:439–442.

45. Shalaby F, Rossant J, Yamaguchi TP, et al. Failure of blood-island formation and vasculogenesis in Flk-1-deficient mice. Nature 1995; 376:62–66.

46. Fong G-H, Rossant J, Gertsenstein M, Breitman ML. Role of the Flt-1 receptor tyrosine kinase in regulating the assembly of vascular endothelium. Nature 1995; 376:66–70.

47. Shweiki D, Itin A, Soffer D, Keshet E. Vascular endothelial growth factor induced by hypoxia may mediate hypoxia-initiated angiogenesis. Nature 1992; 359:843–845.

48. Plate KH, Breier G, Weich HA, Risau W. Vascular endothelial growth factor is a potential tumour angiogenesis factor in human gliomas in vivo. Nature 1992; 359:845–848.

49. Berkman RA, Merrill MJ, Reinhold WC, et al. Expression of the vascular permeability factor/vascular endothelial growth factor gene in central nervous system neoplasms. J Clin Invest 1993; 91:153–159.

50. Zhang H-T, Craft P, Scott PAE, et al. Enhancement of tumor growth and vascular density by transfection of vascular endothelial cell growth factor into MCF-7 human breast carcinoma cells. J Natl Cancer Inst 1995; 87:213–219.

51. Relf M, Lejeune S, Scott PAE, et al. Expression of angiogenic factors vascular endothelial cell growth factor, acidic and basic fibroblast growth factor, tumor growth factor β-1, platelet-derived endothelial cell growth factor, placenta growth factor, and pleiotrophin in

human primary breast cancer and its relation to angiogenesis. Cancer Res 1997; 57: 963–969.

52. Partanen J, Armstrong E, Mäkelä TP, et al. A novel endothelial cell surface receptor tyrosine kinase with extracellular epidermal growth factor homology domains. Mol Cell Biol 1992; 12:1698–1707.

53. Schnürch H, Risau W. Expression of tie-2, a member of a novel family of receptor tyrosine kinases, in the endothelial cell lineage. Development 1993; 119:957–968.

54. Puri MC, Rossant J, Alitalo K, Bernstein A, Partanen J. The receptor tyrosine kinase TIE is required for integrity and survival of vascular endothelial cells. EMBO J 1995; 14:5884–5891.

55. Sato TN, Tozawa Y, Deutsch U, et al. Distinct roles of the receptor tyrosine kinases Tie-1 and Tie-2 in blood vessel formation. Nature 1995; 376:70–74.

56. Davis S, Aldrich TH, Jones PF, et al. Isolation of angiopoietin-1, a ligand for the Tie2 receptor by secretion-trap expression cloning. Cell 1996; 87:1161–1169.

57. Suri C, Jones PF, Patan S, et al. Requisite role of Angiopoietin-1, a ligand for the Tie2 receptor, during embryonic angiogenesis. Cell 1996; 87:1171–1180.

58. Forsythe JA, Jiang BH, Iyer NV, et al. Activation of vascular endothelial growth factor gene transcription by hypoxia-inducible factor 1. Mol Cell Biol 1996; 16:4604–4613.

59. Wang GL, Semenza GL. Purification and characterization of hypoxia-inducible factor 1. J Biol Chem 1995; 270:1230–1237.

60. Ema M, Taya S, Yokotani N, Sogawa K, Matsuda Y, Fujii-Kuriyama Y. A novel bHLH-PAS factor with close sequence similarity to hypoxia-inducible factor 1 alpha regulates the VEGF expression and is potentially involved in lung and vascular development. Proc Natl Acad Sci USA 1997; 94:4273–4278.

61. Wang GL, Jiang BH, Rue EA, Semenza GL. Hypoxia-inducible factor 1 is a basic-helix-loop-helix-PAS heterodimer regulated by cellular O_2 tension. Proc Natl Acad Sci USA 1995; 92:5510–5514.

62. Maltepe E, Schmidt JV, Baunoch D, Bradfield CA, Simon MC. Abnormal angiogenesis and responses to glucose and oxygen deprivation in mice lacking the protein ARNT. Nature 1997; 386:403–407.

63. Alon T, Hemo I, Itin A, Pe'er A, Stone J, Keshet E. Vascular endothelial growth factor acts as a survival factor for newly formed retinal vessels and has applications for retinopathy of prematurity. Nature Med 1995; 1:1024–1028.

64. Yuan A, Yang P-C, Yu C-J, et al. Tumor angiogenesis correlates with histologic type and metastasis in non-small cell lung cancer. Am J Crit Care Med 1995; 152:2157–2162.

65. Macchiarini P, Fontanini G, Hardin MJ, Squartini F, Angeletti CA. Relation of neovascularisation to metastasis of non-small-cell lung cancer. Lancet 1992; 340:145–146.

66. Fontanini G, Bigini D, Vignati S, et al. Microvessel count predicts metastatic disease and survival in non-small cell lung cancer. J Pathol 1995; 177:57–63.

67. Mattern J, Koomägi R, Volm M. Vascular endothelial growth factor expression and angiogenesis in non-small cell lung cancer. Int J Oncol 1995; 6:1059–1062.

68. Mattern J, Koomägi R, Volm M. Association of vascular endothelial cell growth factor expression with intratumoral microvessel density and tumour cell proliferation in human epidermoid lung carcinoma. Br J Cancer 1996; 73:931–934.

69. Koukourakis MI, Giatromanolaki A, O'Byrne KJ, et al. Platelet-derived endothelial cell growth factor expression correlates with tumour angiogenesis and prognosis in non-small-cell lung cancer. Br J Cancer 1997; 75:477–481.

70. Vignaud JM, Allam M, Martinet M, Pech M, Plénat F, Martinet Y. Presence of platelet-derived growth factor in normal and fibrotic lung is specifically associated with interstitial macrophages while both interstitial macrophages and alveolar epithelial cells express the c-sis proto-oncogene. Am J Respir Cell Mol Biol 1991; 5:531–538.

71. Vignaud J-M, Marie B, Klein N, et al. The role of platelet-derived growth factor production by tumor-associated macrophages in tumor stroma formation in lung cancer. Cancer Res 1994; 54:5455–5463.

72. Pech M, Gazit A, Aaronson SA. Generation of fibrosarcomas in vivo by a retrovirus that expresses the normal B chain of platelet-derived growth factor and mimics the alternative splice pattern of the v-sis oncogene. Proc Natl Acad Sci USA 1989; 86:2693–2697.

73. Folkman J, Watson K, Ingber D, Hanahan D. Induction of angiogenesis during the transition from hyperplasia to neoplasia. Nature 1989; 339:58–61.

74. Hanahan D, Folkman J. Patterns and emerging mechanisms of the angiogenic switch during tumorigenesis. Cell 1996; 86:353–364.

75. Folkman J, Shing Y. Angiogenesis. J Biol Chem 1992; 267:10931–10934.

76. Taylor S, Folkman J. Protamine is an inhibitor of angiogenesis. Nature 1982; 297:307–312.

77. Moses MA, Sudhalter J, Langer R. Identification of an inhibitor of neovascularization from cartilage. Science 1990; 248:1408–1410.

78. Good DJ, Polverini PJ, Rastinejad F, et al. A tumor suppressor-dependent inhibitor of angiogenesis is immunologically and functionally indistinguishable from a fragment of thrombospondin. Proc Natl Acad Sci USA 1990; 87:6624–6628.

79. Van Meir EG, Polverini PJ, Chazin VR, H.-J. SH, de Tribolet N, Cavence WK. Release of an inhibitor of angiogenesis upon induction of wild type p53 expression in glioblastoma cells. Nature Gen 1994; 8:171–176.

80. Clapp C, Martial JA, Guzman RC, Rentier-Delrue F, Weiner RI. The 16-kilodalton N-terminal fragment of human prolactin is a potent inhibitor of angiogenesis. Endocrinology 1993; 133:1292–1298.

81. O'Reilly MS, Boehm T, Shing Y, et al. Endostatin: an endogenous inhibitor of angiogenesis and tumor growth. Cell 1997; 88:277–285.

82. Vandenbunder B, Pardanaud L, Jaffredo T, Mirabel MA, Stehelin D. Complementary patterns of expression of c-ets1, c-myb and c-myc in the blood-forming system of the chick embryo. Development 1989; 107:265–274.

83. Wernert N, Raes MB, Lassalle P, et al. The c-ets 1 proto-oncogene is a transcription factor expressed in endothelial cells during tumor vascularisation and other forms of angiogenesis in man. Am J Pathol 1992; 140:119–127.

84. Wakiya K, Stehelin D, Begue A, Shibuya M. A cyclic AMP response element and an ETS motif are involved in the transcriptional regulation of flt-1 tyrosine kinase (VEGF receptor 1) gene. J Biol Chem 1996; 271:30823–30828.

85. Lindner V, Collins T. Expression of NF-kB and IkB-alpha by aortic endothelium in an arterial injury model. Am J Pathol 1996; 148:427–438.

86. Breier G, Breviario F, Caveda L, et al. Molecular cloning and expression of murine vascular endothelial-cadherin in early stage development of cardiovascular system. Blood 1996; 87:630–641.

87. Moscatelli D, Presta M, Rifkin DB. Purification of a factor from human placenta that stimulates capillary endothelial cell protease production, DNA synthesis, and migration. Proc Natl Acad Sci USA 1986; 83:2091–2095.

88. Saksela O, Moscatelli D, Rifkin DB. The opposing effects of basic fibroblast growth factor and transforming growth factor beta on the regulation of plasminogen activator activity in capillary endothelial cells. J Cell Biol 1987; 105:957–963.

89. Mattot V, Raes M, Henriet P, et al. Expression of interstitial collagenase is restricted to skeletal tissue during mouse embryogenesis. J Cell Sci 1995; 108:529–535.

90. Sappino AP, Huarte J, Vassalli JD, Belin D. Sites of synthesis of urokinase and tissue-type plasminogen activators in the murine kidney. J Clin Invest 1991; 87:962–970.

91. Brooks PC, Strömblad S, Sanders L, et al. Localization of matrix metalloproteinase MMP-2 to the surface of invasive cells by interaction with integrin $\alpha v\beta 3$. Cell 1996; 85:683–693.

92. Dvorak HF. Tumors: wounds that do not heal. N Engl J Med 1986; 315:1650–1659.

93. Contrino J, Hair G, Kreutzer D, Rickles FR. *In situ* detection of expression of tissue factor in vascular endothelial cells: correlation with the malignant phenotype of human breast tissue. Nature Med 1996; 2:209–215.

94. Carmeliet P, Mackman N, Moons L, et al. Role of tissue factor in embryonic blood vessel development. Nature 1996; 383:73–75.

95. Senger DR. Molecular framework for angiogenesis. Am J Pathol 1996; 149:1–7.

96. Hori A, Sasada R, Matsutani E, et al. Suppression of solid tumor growth by immunoneutralizing monoclonal antibody against human basic fibroblast growth factor. Cancer Res 1991; 51:6180–6184.

97. Olson KA, Fett JW, French TC, Key ME, Vallee BL. Angiogenin antagonists prevent tumor growth in vivo. Proc Natl Acad Sci USA 1995; 92:442–446.

98. Aiello LP, Pierce EA, Foley ED, et al. Suppression of retinal neovascularization *in vivo* by inhibition of vascular endothelial growth factor (VEGF) using soluble VEGF-receptor chimeric proteins. Proc Natl Acad Sci USA 1995; 92:10457–10461.

99. Millauer B, Shawver LK, Plate KH, Risau W, Ullrich A. Glioblastoma growth inhibited *in vivo* by a dominant-negative Flk1 mutant. Nature 1994; 367:576–579.

100. O'Reilly MS, Holmgren L, Chen C, Folkman J. Angiostatin induces and sustains dormancy of human primary tumors in mice. Nature Med. 1996; 2:689–692.

101. Ingber D, Fujita T, Kishimoto S, et al. Synthetic analogues of fumagillin that inhibit angiogenesis and suppress tumour growth. Nature 1990; 348:555–557.

102. Brooks PC, Montgomery AMP, Rosenfeld M, et al. Integrin $\alpha v \beta 3$ antagonists promote tumor regression by inducing apoptosis of angiogenic blood vessels. Cell 1994; 79:1157–1164.

103. Min HY, Doyle LV, Vitt CR, et al. Urokinase receptor antagonists inhibit angiogenesis and primary tumor growth in syngeneic mice. Cancer Res 1996; 56:2428–2433.

104. Burrows FJ, Thorpe PE. Eradication of large solid tumors in mice with an immunotoxin directed against tumor vasculature. Proc Natl Acad Sci USA 1993; 90:8996–9000.

105. Klauber N, Rohan RM, Flynn E, D'Amato RJ. Critical components of the female reproductive pathway are suppressed by the angiogenesis inhibitor AGM-1470. Nature Med 1997; 3:443–446.

106. Graeber TG, Osmanian C, Jacks T, et al. Hypoxia-mediated selection of cells with diminished apoptotic potential in solid tumours. Nature 1996; 379:88–91.

107. Teicher BA, Holden SA, Ara G, Sotomayor EA, Dong HZ. Potentiation of cytotoxic cancer therapies by TNP-470 alone and with other antiangiogenic agents. Int J Cancer 1994; 57:1–6.

108. Jain RK. Delivery of molecular medicine to solid tumors. Science 1996; 271:1079–1080.

24

Angiogenesis in Lung Cancer

FRANCESCO PEZZELLA

University College London
London, England

KEVIN C. GATTER

Oxford University
Oxford, England

UGO PASTORINO

European Institute of Oncology
Milan, Italy

I. Introduction

A. Angiogenesis and Tumors

In 1971 Folkman formulated the hypothesis that tumor growth is dependent on angiogenesis (1). Subsequently he demonstrated that tumors can initially grow without inducing neovascularization (avascular phase), but they do not become larger than 1 or 2 mm: any further increase in size must be supported by the production of new vessels (2). In more recent years, the essential role played by angiogenesis in neoplastic growth has become increasingly evident (3,4).

Since than, other evidence that tumors are angiogenesis dependent has been collected (3,5). It has become clear that angiogenesis is under the control of a number of positive and negative regulators (3). The normal cells are nonangiogenic and a switch from nonangiogenic to angiogenic status must occur, either in the preneoplastic phase or after neoplastic transformation, for the tumor to grow.

Growth of new vessels is not an isolated phenomenon. It is part of a complex process that involves destruction of the existing normal parenchyma by enzymes such as metalloproteinases and remodeling of extracellular matrix surrounding the vessels from which new vascular buds emerge. Production of newly formed extracellular matrix, the so-called tumor-associated stroma, must occur to support both the new vessels and the neoplastic cells (6–8). To trigger this series of events, the tumor cells must be able to produce a variety of enzymes, growth factors, and angiogenic factors as well as inhibiting the synthesis of other molecules that possess antiangiogenic activity (7).

The study of angiogenesis in tumors has not remained confined to basic biology but has now entered into clinical applications: the evaluation of intratumor vessel density as a prognostic marker and the development of therapeutic strategies using antiangiogenic drugs.

The finding, in a variety of different malignancies, that the higher the microvessel density (MVD), the poorer the clinical outcome (7,10–12) has highlighted the clinical relevance of intratumor MVD. All these studies have considered tumor vascularization to be synonymous with neo-angiogenesis. This assumption is based on the fact that the normal tissue has been replaced by the neoplasm and that new vessels have developed supplying the malignancy, leading to the conclusion that, in order to grow, a tumor needs to induce production of new vessels and that the richer its vascularization, the more successful the growth.

B. Microvessel Density: What Is It and How Is It Scored?

When we talk about evaluation of angiogenesis in tumors, we refer to the quantification of the intratumor microvessels, which it is assumed reflect the intensity of neo-angiogenesis. Microvessel count in tumors is performed according to different systems, but they all share the search for the areas with the highest amount of endothelial cells after immunostaining with an antibody against endothelial cells (so-called hot spots) (13–15).

II. Microvessel Density in Lung Tumors

As in other types of tumor, several studies have been carried out in non–small-cell lung carcinoma (NSCLC) looking at the relationship between microvessel density, prognosis, and stage of the disease (Table 1). These investigations are rather heterogeneous but can be divided into two groups: series including patients at different pathological stages and series including only patients with the same stage of disease. This difference is important because stage is the best predictor of outcome in NSCLC (16).

A. Studies Including NSCLC Patients at Different Stages of Disease

One group of studies deals with mixed series in which patients at different stages are present. The number of cases studied in each report is highly variable (from 48 to 407 cases).

Fontanini et al. (17) reported data concerning a large series of 407 patients with stage I–III disease looking at the relationship between microvessel density with both disease-free and overall survival at 2 years. In univariate analysis microvessel

Table 1 Survival and Microvessel Density in Non–Small-Cell Lung Carcinoma

Authors (Ref.)	No. of cases	Stage	FU (months)	MVD and nodes involvement at presentation		Univariate analysis		Multivariate analysis		MVD and relapse
				Univariate	Multivariate	RFS	OS	RFS	OS	
Fontanini et al. (17)	407	I–III	29(15–60)				$p < 0.00001$		$p = 0.00001$	
Fontanini et al. (18)	253	I–IIIB	16 (2–41)	$p < 0.000001$	$p = 0.000003$		$p = 0.00067$	$p = 0.03$		
follow up	94		>=24							$p = 0.003$
Giatromanalaki et al. (19)	107	I–II	45 (2–96)	$p = 0.0001$			$p = 0.0004$		$p = 0.19$	
Yan et al. (20)	55	I–IIIB		$p = 0.001$						$p < 0.001$
Yamazako et al. (21)	42	I–IV	71(39–107)	$p = 0.97$						$p = 0.027$
Pastorino et al. (22)	488	I	64(1–239)			$p = 0.77$	$p = 0.47$			
Harpole et al. (23)	275	I	>=68				$p = 0.006$		$p = 0.021$	
Angeletti et al. (25)	96	IIIA	24(3–50)				$p = 0.00076$		$p = 0.024$	
Macchiarini et al. (24)	87	I								$p < 0.0001$
Giatromanalaki et al. (19)	75	I					$p = 0.07$			
Giatromanalaki et al. (19)	38	II					$p = 0.33$			
Macchiarini et al. (26)	28	IIIB	42 (8–145)			$p = 0.0011$	$p = 0.0005$	$p = 0.008$	n.s.	

RFS = Relapse-free survival; OS = overall survival.

density was associated with overall survival alongside tumor size (T), node status, and stage. Multivariate analysis shows that tumor size, node involvement, and microvessel density retain independent values as a prognostic factors.

In a previous study (18) on a smaller group of 253 patients in stages I to IIIB, the same authors correlate MVD with the presence of node metastasis at the presentation of the disease. A high MVD in the primary tumor was associated with a high incidence of metastasis in hilar and mediastinal nodes at presentation. Other parameters were associated with lymph node metastasis (sex, histotype, tumor size, and vascular invasion), but MVD was the strongest independent marker for nodal involvement at presentation. For 94 patients longer follow-up was available (at least 24 months) to investigate the correlation between microvessel density and development of distant metastases. MVD was associated with both shorter overall survival and disease-free survival, but again it was dependent on the nodal status.

Another study (19) of a series of 107 patients with stage I and II confirmed the results reported by Fontanini and coworkers: MVD was correlated with node involvement and was dependent on the nodal status as a prognostic marker. The authors also looked independently at squamous cell carcinoma and adenocarcinoma. No evidence of a correlation between MVD and prognosis was found in the latter, although only 38 cases of adenocarcinoma were studied.

Yuan et al. (20) have investigated the relationship between MVD, tumor stage, lymph node involvement, and disease-free survival in 55 NSCLC at various stages of disease. Once again, high MVD correlated with advanced stage, nodal status, and early relapse. Furthermore, the authors reported higher MVD in adenocarcinoma, suggesting that it could be responsible for their more aggressive behavior with respect to squamous cell carcinoma. The last of these studies (21) focused on 42 cases of adenocarcinoma (stage I to IV) without detecting any association between MVD, survival, and node metastasis: MVD was only related to the occurrence of distant metastases.

B. Studies Stratifying Patients According to Disease Stage

Another group of papers has investigated patients with the same stage of disease: four studies looked at stage I patients and three others reported data on series with more advanced disease.

In a recent study (22) we investigated NSCLC from 515 patients with stage I with a median clinical follow-up of 102 months. Tumors were analyzed for a variety of biomarkers. Microvessel density count was successful in 488 cases but failed to show any correlation between MVD in the hot spots and either overall survival or disease-free survival. Tumor size (T1 vs. T2) was the strongest independent prognostic predictor.

Harpole et al. (23) investigated 275 cases with follow-up of at least 68 months for surviving patients. In univariate analysis tumor size (T) and vascular infiltration are the strongest predictors of overall survival ($p = 0.0001$). Microvessel density shows a better overall survival for patients with a lower MVD, ($p =$ 0.001). However, two different multivariate analyses were carried out: one included so-called histologic factors (including T but not microvessel density) and the other included microvessel density and other so-called biologic markers (p53, erb-2, and Ki67) but did not include T and vascular invasion: in this multivariate analysis microvessel density had a weak ($p = 0.021$) significance.

Studies on stage I tumors include a report from Macchiarini et al. (24) in which 87 stage I patients (T1 N0 M0) were investigated. The median follow-up was for relapsing patients 29 months and for patients free of disease 95 months. The authors showed that the risk of relapse was directly proportional to the MVD in the primary tumor. On multivariate analysis MVD was the only independent factor predicting metastasis. Tumor size had no predictive value for relapse. No survival curves or logrank tests were done. In contrast, Giatromanolaki et al. (19) did not find any correlation between MVD and survival in 75 patients with stage I disease.

Three studies were concerned with patients with more advanced disease. The largest included 96 patients with stage IIIA (T1-T3 N2 M0) NSCLC treated by radical surgery and adjuvant therapy with a median follow-up of 24 months. Microvessel density was reported as the only independent prognostic factor (25). In a series of 28 patients, all with NSCLC invading the thoracic inlet, the relationship between MVD and survival and disease-free interval was investigated. For both these parameters univariate and multivariate analyses showed that MVD was the only prognostic factor (26). Finally Giatromanolaki et al. (19) analyzed 32 patients with stage II (T1, T2 N1 M0) disease and found no correlation between MVD and overall survival.

While a broad agreement emerges from all the studies on patients at different stages that microvessel density is directly associated with a more advanced stage of disease at presentation and therefore with prognosis, there is a confusing picture as far as the value of microvessel density is concerned in patients with the same stage of disease. Most of the studies looking at homogeneous series are small: two have fewer than 50 patients, two others have fewer than 100, and only two have larger series (275 and 488 patients). Furthermore, the follow-up time varied greatly (Table 1). Therefore, the main reason for the observed discrepancies is likely to be due to problems connected with study design and statistical analysis. A meta-analysis of the published papers could be helpful.

Another statistical problem common to all the studies examined is the use of multivariate analysis: different studies include different parameters, making the results not comparable. Some authors (14) have questioned the way MVD is evaluated in order to explain the differences observed between different studies. We believe that differences in the use of statistics and the small number of cases investigated in some of the studies, in addition to making them poorly comparable, are likely to represent a more important reason for the discrepancies observed than differences in vessel-counting techniques.

III. The Switch to Angiogenic Phenotype in Hyperplastic and Dysplastic Lesions

The induction of angiogenesis during the progression from hyperplasia to neoplasia was first demonstrated in a mouse model (27,28). In the first of these two studies (27), the model employed was a transgenic mouse expressing an oncogene in the pancreatic β-cells. As a result these mice developed first hyperplasia and then a neoplasia of these cells. Neoangiogenesis appeared first in some of the hyperplastic islets, while it was present in all the malignant tumors developing later. In another study (28) on a transgenic mouse developing mild fibromatosis, then an aggressive fibromatosis of the skin, a similar observation was made. Normal skin and mild fibromatosis showed a comparable localization and density of microvessels, while an increased number of irregularly distributed capillaries appeared in aggressive fibromatosis and fibrosarcoma. Such an increase in vascularization is due, in this tumor model, to the release from inside the cells of an angiogenic molecule, the basic fibroblast growth factor (bFGF).

It has been postulated that a switch to angiogenic phenotype occurs during tumor progression. Such a switch is not synonymous with malignancy since benign tumors can be highly vascularized, nor is it essential to full neoplastic transformation, but it is believed to be essential for a tumor to grow sufficiently to be clinically detectable (3).

This experimental evidence prompted a number of clinico-pathological studies. In the cervix (29) a higher number of vessels is present in the basal membrane underlying CINIII compared to CINI. In breast (30,31) a trend of correlation between a higher number of vessels around in situ carcinoma and a higher risk of subsequently developing invasive tumors has been found.

In two recent papers (32,33) microvessel density in the lamina propria of the bronchial tree has been investigated in relationship to the status of the bronchial epithelium. Normal bronchial epithelium, hyperplastic mucosa, squamous metaplasia, dysplasia, and in situ carcinoma have investigated. Although the series are not large (68 and 86 patients), both studies show a trend of increasing microvessel density in the lamina propria from normal epithelium to in situ carcinoma throughout hyperplasia, metaplasia, and dysplasia.

IV. Angiogenic and Nonangiogenic Primary Tumors of the Lung

In the previous paragraphs we have summarized the evidence in the literature that neoplastic transformation is not dependent on angiogenesis but successful further growth is. Furthermore, it has been shown that the switch to angiogenic phenotypes can occur both before and after full neoplastic transformation. Once the switch has occurred, the release of angiogenic factors causes new capillaries to sprout from nearby vessels and infiltrate the tumor, allowing its growth.

Another hypothesis is that if a tumor can obtain an efficient blood supply from a suitable vascular bed that already exists, it could grow without the immediate need for switching to the angiogenic phenotype. The switch could be delayed to a later stage of tumor progression, perhaps after its clinical presentation. It could even not occur at the primary site but be delayed as late as the time of occurrence of distant metastases. Some data have already supported this possibility. The association between high MVD and poor prognosis has not been demonstrated in all tumors. In squamous cell carcinoma of the tongue (34) no association has been found with overall survival and node metastases. The hypothesis above could explain these contradictory findings. If in highly vascularized organs, like the tongue, the preexisting vessels were able to provide the blood supply essential for tumor progression, they, rather than the intratumor newly formed vessels, could dictate the clinical course of the tumor (10).

Another interesting clue comes from Miliaris et al. (35). Comparing microvessel density in the primary tumor with vascular density in synchronous node metastases, they have found that the microvessel density in the metastases is not higher but lower than in the primary tumor. This demonstrates that in lymph nodes a poorly angiogenic clone can easily produce metastases. Reactive lymph nodes are well vascularized organs, and a possible explanation could be that in some cases the neoplastic cell metastasizing in the node grows by exploiting the local vessels.

Further supporting evidence has been published by O'Reilly et al. (36). In a mouse model in which the Lewis lung cancer cell line was grown, it was shown that resection of the primary tumor leads to a faster growth of metastatic lesions. This is because of the production by the primary tumor of a new angiogenic inhibiting factor called angiostatin. How does the primary tumor escape the angiostatin inhibition? An explanation put forward by the authors is that the primary tumor has a production of VEGF which can overrun, locally but not in distant sites, angiostatin. This would explain local growth but distant inhibition. Another hypothesis is that the primary tumor, which has not switched to an angiogenic phenotype, could be growing, exploiting, at least in part, local vessels.

We have reported (22,37,38) that immunostaining of endothelial cells in non–small-cell lung carcinomas highlights four distinct patterns of vascularization. Three patterns (basal, papillary, and diffuse) have in common the destruction of the normal lung parenchyma and the production of newly formed vessels and stroma. The fourth pattern, called alveolar or nonangiogenic, was characterized by a lack of parenchymal destruction, tumor-associated stroma, or new intratumoral vessels. The only vessels we observed were in the alveolar septi, and their staining highlighted throughout the whole lesion the alveolar network of the lung parenchyma "frozen" by the neoplastic cells (Fig. 1).

We will now discuss this group of putative nonangiogenic tumors in relation to the three types of angiogenic tumors. Finally, we will summarize the preliminary data concerning the clinical and biological characteristics associated with these four patterns of tumor.

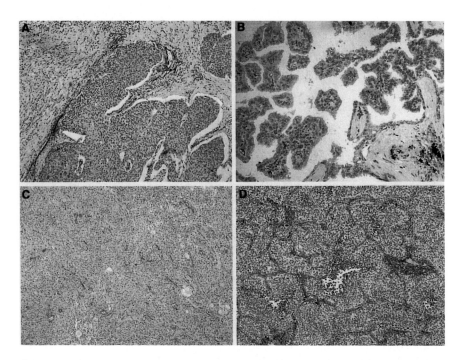

Figure 1 Immunostaining for CD31 (antibody JC70) immunoperoxidase/AEC method. (A) Basal pattern, nests of neoplastic epithelial cells are surrounded by stroma in which vessels are present, beneath the neoplastic epithelium. (B) Papillary pattern: the tumor is made up by a fibrous stalk lined by neoplastic cells. Immunostaining for CD31 shows vessels in the stalk. (C) Diffuse pattern: a diffuse neoplastic proliferation, without any identifiable architecture is seen, vessels and stroma are randomly scattered throughout the tumor, mixed with neoplastic epithelial cells. (D) Alveolar pattern, nonangiogenic: staining for CD31 shows the alveolar vessels highlighting the normal lung architecture. This pattern is present throughout the whole lesion. The alveolar spaces are now filled by neoplastic epithelial cells.

A. Nonangiogenic Tumors (Alveolar Pattern)

In this group of NSCLC the only vessels evident after immunostaining for CD31, an endothelial marker, arise from the alveolar septa and highlight the alveolar network of the lung entrapped by neoplastic cells which grow filling the alveolar spaces. Their identification as alveolar vessels is made possible not only by the recognition of the normal lung architecture, but also by the anthracite pigment present within them. The tumor grows in a solid fashion, filling the alveolar spaces. Neither endothelial cells nor tumor-associated stroma are present alongside the neoplastic cells. An alveolar pattern of spread at the periphery of lung tumors is common and has been reported previously (39,40). We have classified as alveolar (nonangiogenic) cases only those presenting this pattern throughout the whole tumor and not just on the edge.

B. Angiogenic Tumors and Their Topographical Organization

In the other cases the classical signs associated with neoangiogenesis were present: the tumor grows, destroying the host organ, there is production of tumor-associated stroma and formation of a network of newly formed vessels. Immunostaining of the vessels shows three patterns of vascular organization reflecting three different architectural arrangement of the tumors:

1. Basal. The basic structure of a mucosa is reproduced. Neoplastic cells are arranged in epithelial nests surrounded by connective tissue. Most of the vessels are in the connective tissue beneath the neoplastic epithelium.
2. Papillary. In this pattern the vessels are in a stromal stalk, which is covered by neoplastic cells, mostly as a monolayer. The normal lung alveolar pattern is usually recognizable in some areas of the tumor but remodeling of the alveolar structure with disruption of normal lung and papillary growth invariably occurs.
3. Diffuse. The normal lung architecture is diffusely replaced. New vessels and stroma are produced intimately admixed with neoplastic cells but without any recognizable architectural structure.

C. The Edge of the Tumors

As mentioned above, it is common in lung tumors with an otherwise angiogenic pattern to find at the edge a pattern of growth represented by filling of alveoli, while deeper in the tumor the destruction of lung parenchyma with remodeling and neoangiogenesis occurs. This pattern of growth suggests that exploiting the local vasculature in lung is a common event but in most cases switches to the angiogenic phenotype as the neoplastic cells are trapped inside the tumor. Hypoxia is the factor most likely to trigger this angiogenesis, which occurs in the majority of lung cancer cases. At the moment this explanation of angiogenic and nonangiogenic histological findings remains a hypothesis and will need further investigation.

D. Comparison of the Characteristics of the Four Patterns

Clinical Correlations

In a recent study (22) we evaluated a series of biologic and pathological factors as prognostic markers in stage I lung NSCLC. Pathological stage (i.e., T1 vs. T2) was the only independent predictor of overall and disease-free survival. Bcl-2 expression is associated with longer disease-free survival in univariate analysis (RR 0.59, $p = 0.03$) but dropped out the multivariate analysis. The only other notable biologic marker is the division into angiogenic and nonangiogenic tumors. Patients with nonangiogenic patterns appear to have a higher incidence of metastases and a shorter disease-free survival, although the former shows only weak significance ($p < 0.025$) and the second does not (RR 1.44, $p = 0.06$). In patients with earlier stages of cancer (i.e., T1) in the univariate analysis the nonangiogenic tumors have a shorter disease-free ($p = 0.02$) and overall survival ($p = 0.02$). Other significant markers appears to be bcl-2, p53, and EGFr. On multivariate analysis only the division into nonangiogenic and angiogenic maintains its value on both overall (RR1.91, $p = 0.04$) and disease-free (RR3.18, $p = 0.007$) survival.

Other Clinical and Biological Correlations

We have also reported some characteristics of these tumors according to their vascular patterns (38). No differences were found when comparing patients with angiogenic versus nonangiogenic tumours for sex, age, mean of daily cigarettes, and smoking status. Incidence of nonsmokers was lower in patients with the basal pattern and higher than expected in patients with a papillary pattern. The average microvessel density in angiogenic and nonangiogenic tumors is the same, although it should be kept in mind that the vessels counted in the nonangiogenic tumors are the normal lung vessels trapped by the tumor. No differences were found in relation to the stages of the tumor.

A significant association is found between vascular patterns and histological tumor type (Table 2). The basal pattern was associated with squamous cell carcinomas and the papillary with adenocarcinomas while the diffuse and the alveolar patterns were equally represented in both. Among the more rare histotype, as shown in Table 2, almost all cases diagnosed as bronchioalveolar have a papillary pattern, while the majority of the other types have a diffuse pattern but never a papillary. Yuan et al. (20) reported an analogous finding. They noticed that in squamous cell carcinomas the microvessels were located mainly at the margin of the tumor nests while in adenocarcinoma the microvessels were present around the gland-like structures or in the stroma of neoplastic papillary proliferations. Also, the grading was significantly associated with pattern: papillary was associated with well-

Table 2 Histological Type of Tumor According to Vascular Pattern

| Histotype (total) | Basal | Angiogenic patterns | | Nonangiogenic alveolar | p value |
		Papillary	Diffuse		
Adenocarcinoma (210)	35	59	77	39	<0.0005[a]
Squamous cell carcinoma (245)	152	5	54	34	
Others (45)	11	7	20	7	
Bronchioalveolar (11)	—	7	1	3	
Large cell (15)	2	—	10	3	
Adeno squamous (3)	2	—	1	—	
Muco epidermoid (16)	7	—	8	1	
Total (500)	198	71	151	80	

[a]p value calculated by the rxc frequency table.
Source: Modified from Ref. 38.

differentiated while diffuse and alveolar were present mainly in poorly differentiated carcinomas.

The relationship between vascular patterns and selected biological markers has been looked at as well. An association has been found between all four markers investigated and vascular patterns. The basal pattern has a higher incidence of bcl-2 and laminin receptor expression. The papillary pattern shows lower bcl-2, p53, and EGFr expression. Lower bcl-2 and lower laminin receptor expression characterizes the diffuse pattern, while the alveolar has a higher incidence of bcl-2–positive cases. In this series of non–small-cell carcinomas we have also examined (unpublished data) but failed to find any association between bcl-2 and/or p53 expression and microvessel density as has recently been suggested (41–44).

V. Angiogenic Factors in Lung Cancers

All studies summarized to date are concerned with the description and quantifications of vessels in tumors. A recent small group of studies has started to look at the expression of some of the most important angiogenic factors. Three vascular growth factors have been investigated so far in NSCLC: platelet-derived growth factor, vascular endothelial growth factor, and hepatocyte growth factor. Presence of VEGF has been documented by immunohistochemistry in a series of 152 NSCLC: low expression of VEGF is reported in 102 of 154 cases and high expression in 52 of 154 (45). More recent results from the same group are reported in a study of 91 squamous cell carcinomas of the lung. Expression of VEGF, mostly cytoplasmic, was detected in 59% of the cases. Microvessel count in these VEGF-positive tumors was found to be higher than in VEGF-negative cases (46). This finding has been recently confirmed by Fontanini et al. (44). VEGF mRNA has also been reported in a few cases from a smaller series (47).

Expression of PD-ECGF has been investigated in 116 non–small-cell lung carcinomas and 22 small-cell lung carcinomas (48). All of the small-cell carcinomas were negative, while 32% of the squamous cell carcinomas and 42% of the adenocarcinomas were positive. Areas of squamous metaplasia were also positive. The staining was cytoplasmic, but occasional nuclear positivity was found. In normal lung tissue occasional staining was found in bronchiolar epithelium on basal and columnar cells. The alveolar epithelium is negative, while alveolar macrophages are positive. Comparison of PD-ECGF expression and microvessel density showed a clear correlation (49).

The third growth factor investigated is the hepatocyte growth factor/scatter factor, which stimulates the invasive growth of epithelial cells throughout the c-MET oncogene–encoded receptor (50). Expression of HGF/SF in its activated form and of its receptor, met, was found in 23 out 42 cases. In three more cases only the expression of the receptor was found.

These results must be considered preliminary. A main problem with the interpretation of this data is that histochemical localization of anti-angiogenic factors is not yet possible. A second point is that the final angiogenic status of one tumor is likely to be due to the balanced effect of angiogenic and antiangiogenic factors. It is likely that the quantification of both these factors by biochemical means will be necessary, together with functional essays, to evaluate the angiogenic ability of the neoplastic cells.

VI. Metastatic Disease

The lung is not only home to one of the most common primary malignancies but is also one of the most frequent places for secondary localization of other tumors. No longer seen as an inevitably incurable disease (51), the clinical and biological investigation of lung metastases could hopefully result in progress in their treatment. In a preliminary study (37) we have started to investigate lung metastases from carcinomas arising in other organs. The data we collected require cautious interpretation because we have not yet been able to study both primary and metastatic lesions in each patient.

Our first observation is that microvessel density in lung metastases is higher than in lung primary tumors. This is in agreement with the prediction that distant metastases are made up of more angiogenic clones, while primary tumors are usually a mixture of highly and poorly vascularized areas. The second result is that there are exceptions to this "rule." A group of lung metastases from both breast and colon carcinoma are actually indistinguishable as far as vascularization is concerned from the nonangiogenic primary non–small-cell carcinomas of the lung. Therefore they are likely to be made up by cells in which the angiogenic phenotype is switched off. If this is the case, it means that poorly angiogenic clones can still produce distant metastases and are likely to be resistant to antiangiogenic treatment.

References

1. Folkman J. Tumour angiogenesis: therapeutic implication. N Engl J Med 1971; 285:1182–1186.
2. Knighton D, Ausoprunk D, Tapper D, Folkman J. Avascular and vascular phase of tumour growth in the chick embryo. Br J Cancer 1977; 35:347–356.
3. Folkman J. Tumour angiogenesis. In: Mendelshon J, Howley PM, Israel MA, Liotta LA, eds. The Molecular Basis of Cancer. Philadelphia: W.B. Saunders, 1995:206–232.
4. Folkman J. Angiogenesis in cancer, vascular, rheumatoid and other disease. Nature Med 1995; 1:27–31.
5. Folkman J. What is the evidence that tumours are angiogenesis dependent? J Natl Cancer Inst 1990; 82:4–6.
6. Blood CH, Zetter BR. Tumor interactions with the vasculature: angiogenesis and tumour metastasis. Biochem Biophys Acta 1990; 1032:89–118.
7. Hart IR, Saini A. Biology of tumour metastasis. Lancet 1992; 339:1453–1457.
8. Ellis LM and Fidler IJ. Angiogenesis and metastasis. Eur J Cancer 1996; 32A:2451–2460.

9. Weidner N. Tumour angiogenesis; review of current applications in tumour prognostication. Sem Diag Path 1993; 10:302–313.
10. Weidner N. Intratumor microvessel density as a prognostic factor in cancer. Am J Pathol 1995; 147:9–19.
11. Gasparini G, Harris AL. Clinical importance of the determination of tumor angiogenesis in breast carcinoma: much more than a new diagnostic tool. J Clin Oncol 1995; 13:765–782.
12. Craft PS, Harris AL. Clinical prognostic significance of tumour angiogenesis. Ann Oncol 1994; 5:305–311.
13. Fox SB, Leek RD, Weekes MP, Whitehouse RM, Gatter KC, Harris AL. Quantitation and prognostic value of breast cancer angiogenesis: comparison of microvessel density, Chalkly count and computer image analysis. J Pathol 1995; 177:275–283.
14. Fox SB. Tumour angiogenesis and prognosis. Histopathology 1997; 30:294–301.
15. Vermeulen PB, Gasparini G, Fox SB, Toi M, Martin L, McCulloch P, Pezzella F, Viale G, Weidner N, Harris AL, Dirix LY. Quantification of angiogenesis in solid human tumours; an international consensus on the methodology and criteria of evaluation. Eur J Cancer 1996; 32A:2474–2484.
16. Naruke T, Goya T, Tsuchiya R, Guemasu K. Prognosis and survival in resected lung carcinoma based on the new international staging system. J Thorac Cardiovasc Surg 1988; 96:440–447.
17. Fontanini G, Licchi M, Vignati S, Mussi A, Ciardiello F, De Laurentiis M, De Placido S, Basolo F, Angeletti CA, Bevilacqua G. Angiogenesis as a prognostic indicator of survival in non-small cell lung carcinoma: a prospective study. J Natl Cancer Inst 1997; 89: 881–886.
18. Fontanini G, Bigini D, Vignati S, Basolo F, Mussi A, Lucchi M, Chine S, Angeletti CA, Harris AL, Bevilacqua G. Microvessel count predicts metastatic disease and survival in non-small cell lung cancer. J Pathol 1995; 177:57–63.
19. Giatromanolaki A, Koukourakis M, O'Byrne K, Fox S, Whitehouse R, Talbot D, Harris AL, Gatter KC. Angiogenesis is a significant prognostic marker in operable non small cell lung cancer. J Pathol 1995; 179:80–88.
20. Yuan A, Yng PC, Yu CJ, Lee YC, Yao YT, Chen CL, Lee LN, Kuo SH, Luh KT. Tumour angiogenesis correlates with histologic type and metastasis in non-small cell lung cancer. Am J Respir Crit Care Med 1995; 152(6 Pt 1):2157–2162.
21. Yamazaki K, Abe S, Takekawa H, Sukoh N, Watanabe N, Ogura S, Nakajima I, Isobe H, Inoue K, Kawakami Y. Tumor angiogenesis in human lung adenocarcinoma. Cancer 1994; 74:2245–2250.
22. Pastorino U, Andreola S, Tagliabue E, Pezzella F, Incarbone M, Sozzi G, Buyse M, Menard S, Pierotti M, Rilke F. Immunocytochemical markers in stage I lung cancer (NSCLC): relevance to prognosis. J Clin Oncol. 1997; 15:2858–2865.
23. Harpole DH, Richards WG, Hernedon JE, Sugarbaker DJ. Angiogenesis and molecular biologic substaging in patients with stage I non-small cell lung cancer. Ann Thorac Surg 1996; 61:1470–1476.
24. Macchiarini P, Fontanini G, Hardin MJ, Squartini F, Angeletti CA. Relation of neovascularisation to metastasis of non small cell lung cancer. Lancet 1992; 340:145–146.
25. Angeletti CA, Lucchi M, Fontanini G, Mussi A, Chella A, Ribechini A, Vignati S, Bevilacqua G. Prognostic significance of tumoral angiogenesis in completely resected late stage lung carcinoma (stage IIIA-N2). Cancer 1996; 78:409–415.
26. Macchiarini P, Fontanini G, Dulmet E, de Montpreville V, Chapelier AR, Cerrina J, Ladurie FL, Dartvelle PG. Angiogenesis: an indicator of metastasis in non-small cell lung cancer invading the thoracic inlet. Ann Thor Surg 1994; 57:1534–1539.
27. Folkman J, Watson K, Ingber D, Hanahan. Induction of angiogenesis during the transition from hyperplasia to neoplasia. Nature 1989; 339:58–61.
28. Kandel J, Bossy-Wetzel E, Radvanyi F, Klagsbrun M, Folkman J, Hanahan D. Neovascularization is associated with a switch to the export of bFGF in the multistep development of fibrosarcoma. Cell 1991; 66:1095–1104.

29. Smith-McCune K, Weidner N. Demonstration and characterization of the angiogenic property of cervical dysplasia. Cancer Res 1994; 54:800–804.

30. Guidi AJ, Fischer L, Harris JA, Schnitt SJ. Microvessel density and distribution in ductal carcinoma in situ of the breast. J Natl Cancer Inst 1994; 86:614–619.

31. Engels K, Fox SB, Whitehouse RM, Gatter KC, Harris AL. Distinct angiogenic patterns are associated with high-grade in situ ductal carcinomas of the breast. J Path 1997; 181:207–212.

32. Fisseler-Eckhoff A, Rothstein D, Muller K-M. Neovascularization in hyperplastic, metaplastic and potentially preneoplastic lesions of the bronchial mucosa. Virchows Arch 1996; 429:95–100.

33. Fontanini G, Vignati S, Bigini D, Lucchi M, Mussi A, Basolo F, Angeletti CA, Bevilacqua G. Neoangiogenesis: a putative marker of malignancy in non-small-cell lung cancer (NSCLC) development. Int J Cancer 1996; 67:615–619.

34. Leedy DA, Trune DR, Kronz JD, Weidner N, Cohen JI. Tumor angiogenesis, the p53 antigen and cervical metastasis in squamous carcinoma. Otolaryngol Head Neck Surg 1994; 111: 417–422.

35. Miliaris D, Kamas A, Kalekou H. Angiogenesis in invasive breast carcinoma: is it associated with parameters of prognostic significance? Histopathology 1995; 26:165–169.

36. O'Reilly MS, Holmgren L, Shing Y, Chen C, Rosenthal RA, Moses M, Lane WS, Cao Y, Sage EH, Folkman J. Angiostatin: a novel angiogenesis inhibitor that mediates the suppression of metastases by a Lewis lung carcinoma. Cell 1994; 79:315–328.

37. Pezzella F, Di Bacco A, Andreola S, Nicholson AG, Pastorino U, Harris AL. Angiogenesis in primary lung cancer and lung secondaries. Eur J Cancer 1996; 32A:2494–2500.

38. Pezzella F, Pastorino U, Tagliabue E, Andreola S, Sozzi G, Gasparini G, Menard S, Gatter KC, Harris AL, Fox S, Buyse M, Pilotti S, Pierotti M, Rilke F. Non-small cell lung carcinoma tumour-growth without morphological evidence of neo angiogenesis. Am J Pathol 1997; 151:1417–1423.

39. Colby TV, Koss MN, Travis WD. Tumours of the lower respiratory tract. Atlas of Tumor Pathology. Washington, DC: Armed Forces Institute of Pathology, 1994.

40. Paakko P, Risteli J, Risteli L, Autio-Harmainen H. Immunohistochemical evidences that lung carcinomas grow on alveolar basement membranes. Am J Surg Pathol 1990; 14:464–473.

41. Dameron KM, Volpert OV, Tainsky MA, Bouck N. Control of angiogenesis in fibroblasts by p53 regulation of thrombospondin-1. Science 1994; 265:1582–1584.

42. Kieser A, Weich HA, Brandner G, Marme' D, Kolch W. Mutant p53 potentiates protein kinases C induction of vascular endothelial growth factor expression. Oncogene 1994; 9: 963–969.

43. O'Byrne KJ, Koukourakis MI, Giatromanalaki A, Whitehouse R, Talbot DC, Gatter KC, Harris AL. Correlation of bcl-2 expression with tumour angiogenesis in non-small cell lung cancer. (abst) Proc ASCO 1996; 15:383.

44. Fontanini G, Vignati S, Lucchi M, Mussi A, Calcinai A, Boldrini L, Chine' S, Silvestri V, Angeletti CA, Basolo F, Bevilacqua G. Neoangiogenesis and p53 protein in lung cancer: their prognostic role and their relation with vascular endothelial growth factor (VEGF) expression. Br J Cancer 1997; 75:1295–1301.

45. Volm M, Koomagi R, Mattern J. Interrelationship between microvessel density, expression of VEGF and resistance to doxorubicin of non-small lung cell carcinoma. Anticancer Res 1996; 16:213–217.

46. Mattern J, Koomagi R, Volm M. Association of vascular endothelial growth factor expression with intratumoral microvessel density and tumour cell proliferation in human epidermoid lung carcinoma. Br J Cancer 1996; 73:931–934.

47. Berger DP, Hersbritt L, Dengler WA, Marme D, Mertelsmann R, Fiegig HH. Vascular endothelial growth factor (VEGF)mRNA expression in human tumour models of different histologies. Ann Oncol 1995; 6:817–825.

48. Giatromanalaki A, Koukourakis MI, Comley M, Kaklamanis L, Turley H, O'Byrne K, Harris AL, Gatter KC. Platelet-derived endothelial growth factor (thymidine phosphorylase) expression in lung cancer. J Pathol 1997; 181:196–199.

49. Koukourakis MI, Giatromanalaki A, O'Byrne K, Comley M, Whitehouse RM, Talbot DC,

Gatter KC, Harris AL. Platelet-derived endothelial cell growth factor expression correlates with tumour angiogenesis and prognosis in non-small-cell lung cancer. Br J Cancer 1997; 75:477–481.

50. Olivero M, Rizzo M, Madeddu R, Casadio C, Pennacchietti S, Nicotra MR, Prat M, Maggi G, Arena N, Natali PG, Comoglio PM, Di Renzo MF. Overexpression of hepatocyte growth factor/scatter factor in human non-small-cell lung carcinomas. Br J Cancer 1996; 74:1862–1868.

51. The International Registry of Lung metastases. Long term results of lung metastasectomy: prognostic analyses based on 5206 cases. J Thorac Cardiovasc Surg 1997; 113:37–49.

25

Matrix Proteases and Transcription Factors in the Process of Dissemination

ISABELLE BOLON and CATHERINE ROBERT

CJF INSERM 97-01, Institut Albert Bonniot
La Tronche, France

I. Introduction

The genetic alterations involved in lung cancer development including *c-myc* gene family activation and tumor suppressor gene inactivation (1–4) lead to the uncontrolled proliferation necessary for both primary tumor and metastasis expansion. However, unrestrained growth does not, by itself, cause invasion and metastasis. Progression from a bronchial in situ carcinoma (a preinvasive step) to an invasive and metastatic lung carcinoma involves extensive interaction between tumor and host, including breakdown of the basement membrane, invasion of surrounding tissue, intravasation into a lymph or blood vessel, extravasation out of the vessel, and invasion of a secondary tissue (Fig. 1). Because each of these processes involves extracellular matrix (ECM) proteolysis, tissue remodeling, or tissue invasion, matrix proteases (MPs) have been examined for their potential role in tumor progression. New capillary blood vessels are needed if a tumor is to expand in three dimensions beyond 2 mm (5). This angiogenesis, in addition to cell migration, may play an important role in determining chance of metastasis. In lung carcinomas the degree of angiogenesis, as assessed by counting microvessels of the primary tumor, has proved to be predictive for metastatic disease (6–9).

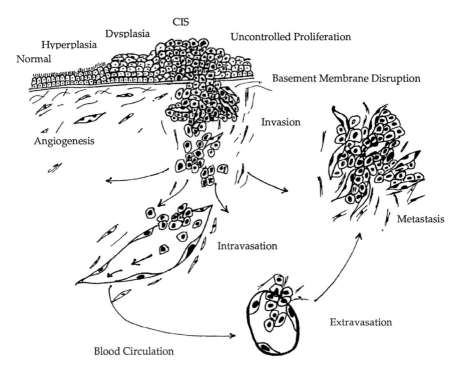

Figure 1   Hyperplasia, metaplasia, dysplasia, and CIS are benign proliferative disorders of the bronchus. They are all characterized by a continuous basement membrane separating the epithelium from the chorion. In contrast, cancer invasion and metastasis involve angiogenesis of the primary tumor, neoplastic cells intravasation, systemic dissemination via the blood circulation, and extravasation into the target organ. During intravasation and extravasation, the tumor cells must penetrate the subendothelial basement membrane. Thus, the enzymatic degradation of ECM is a prerequisite for cancer cell dissemination.

The transcription factor c-Ets-1, the founder of the Ets family, appears to be expressed during angiogenesis and invasive processes in normal and pathological development (for review, see Ref. 10). Since several in vitro studies showed that c-Ets-1 and c-Ets-2 activate MP promoters (11–13), it was of interest to analyze in vivo the link between these transcription factors and MP expression during lung tumor invasion.

In the study of the dissemination process, lung carcinomas are of considerable interest. They are subdivided in a wide diversity of histological types (14) with varying degree of aggressiveness. Tumors exhibiting a neuroendocrine (NE) differentiation extend from the rather benign carcinoids to the highly aggressive large-cell neuroendocrine carcinomas (LCNECs) and small-cell lung carcinomas (SCLCs). Non-NE lung carcinomas include on the one hand squamous carcinomas, adenocarcinomas, and large-cell carcinomas, which have an unpredictable metastatic behavior, and on the other hand basaloid carcinomas, which have been distinguished from a population of poorly differentiated squamous carcinomas because of their poor prognosis (15,16). In addition, preinvasive steps for squamous lung carcinoma, the most frequent histological type, have been well defined starting from metaplasia to dysplasia and carcinoma in situ (CIS) (17,18). These intraepithelial lesions are valuable materials to study the molecular mechanisms involved in the transition of preinvasion to invasion.

The focus of this chapter has been placed on matrix-degrading proteases and their promoter-related Ets-1 and Ets-2 transcription factors elaborated by human lung cancer and their precursor bronchial lesions in relation to recent studies investigating the importance of cellular sources of enzymes.

II. Matrix Proteases Produced by Lung Carcinomas

Human lung carcinomas produce the same matrix-degrading enzymes as those that have been implicated in normal invasive processes, such as embryonic development, tissue repair, and inflammation and in the biology of other malignant tumors. These proteolytic enzymes are classified according to the nature of their active sites as serine proteases, metalloproteases (MMPs), and cysteine proteases. For each subclass we analyzed the link between MP secretion and histological class or phenotype of lung cancer and the influence of MP secretion on local progression and metastasis.

A. Plasminogen Activators

The two known plasminogen activators, urokinase-type (u-PA) and tissue-type (tPA) plasminogen activator, are serine proteases that cleave the ubiquitous zymogen plasminogen and generate plasmin. Plasmin is a broad-acting serine protease that can degrade fibrin and the matrix glycoproteins fibronectin and laminin (19) and is also able to contribute to matrix degradation by activating some latent MMPs (20,21). The plasminogen activator/plasmin system is tightly controlled by specific inhibitors including the plasminogen activator inhibitors (PAI-1, PAI-2). Pericellular plasminogen activation is enhanced on the cell surface and is regulated by cell surface receptors, as has been most clearly demonstrated for the u-PA receptor (u-PAR) (22).

The role of plasminogen activator system components in the malignant behavior of carcinoma has been the subject of a large number of recent studies. It has been shown that u-PA and PAI-1 levels in tissue of breast (23), ovarian (24), and gastric (25) cancer are independent and significant prognostic markers, and high levels of each of these parameters are associated with poor prognosis.

In non-NE lung cancer extracts, u-PA gene expression was found to be overexpressed when compared with non-neoplastic counterparts (26–28). Sappino et al. showed a significant correlation between elevated u-PA mRNA content and the presence of regional lymph node metastases (27). However, there is no consensus when u-PA protein content of whole extracts is compared with clinicopathological param-

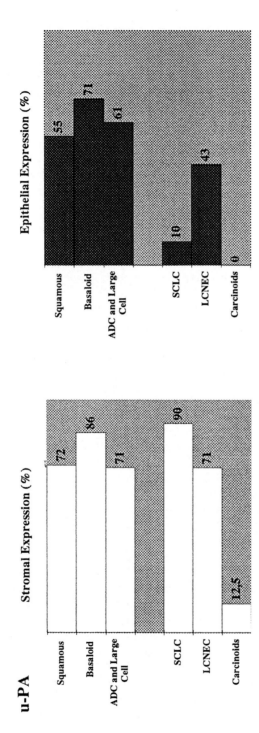

Figure 2 Pattern of u-PA mRNA expression in the different histological types of lung carcinoma including non-NE and NE tumors. Each bar represents the percentage of cases where a stromal (on the left and in white) or an epithelial (on the right and in dark) expression of u-PA gene was observed. (1) u-PA expression is frequent and predominated in stromal cells in all histological types. (2) u-PA stromal expression is more frequent in SCLCs and LCNECs than in carcinoids, therefore is inversely correlated with NE tumor aggressivity. (3) u-PA epithelial expression is significantly more frequent in non-NE than NE tumors ($p = 0.0002$).

eters (26,28–30). Although u-PA protein has been localized in lung cancer cells (28,31–33), using in situ hybridization and immunohistochemistry we have reported that cancer and stromal cells (fibroblasts, inflammatory cells) could synthesize u-PA (Figs. 2,3). Stromal expression predominated in all the histological types, whereas epithelial expression of u-PA was mainly restricted to non-NE cancer cells (Fig. 2) (34,35). Interestingly in NE and non-NE lung tumors, high levels of u-PA mRNA expression in stromal cells, but not in neoplastic cells, were significantly correlated with the presence of lymph node metastases. The greater localization of u-PA in stromal rather than cancer cells in patients with cervical cancer of the uterus (36) or breast carcinoma (37) is also a predictor of early relapse and poor prognosis. These observations emphasize the active stromal cell participation in the degradative process of cancer metastasis.

The disruption of the balance between u-PA and the two main u-PA inhibitors, PAI-1 and PAI-2, may influence the progression of lung cancer. Using enzyme-linked immunosorbent assays, Pedersen et al. reported in vivo increase of PAI-1 gene expression in adenocarcinomas, squamous, and large-cell carcinomas (29,30). There was a significant correlation between high PAI-1 levels and short-duration overall survival in the subgroup of adenocarcinomas (30). In a small series of lung cancer, PAI-1 and PAI-2 proteins have been localized in cancer cells (28,33). Recently, we analyzed PAI-1 and PAI-2 expression using immunohistochemistry in a large series of lung carcinomas. These proteins were overexpressed more frequently

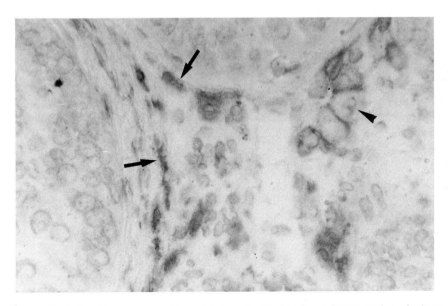

Figure 3 Indirect immunoperoxidase staining of u-PA protein on frozen section of a lung adenocarcinoma (×300): cytoplasmic u-PA staining of fibroblasts surrounding tumor lobules (arrow) and cell-surface staining of macrophages (arrowhead).

in non-NE than in NE tumors (unpublished results). PAI-1 protein was detected in cancer cells, fibroblasts, and in the ECM, whereas PAI-2 was exclusively expressed in stromal cells (fibroblasts and endothelial cells). In agreement with Pedersen et al. (30), the presence of PAI-1 was a poor prognosis factor since it was significantly correlated to a high tumor size, lymph node metastasis, and late stages. Interestingly in cancer cells, PAI-1 and u-PA expression were strongly associated ($p = 0.003$). This suggests that PAI-1 might play a role in cancer invasion by protecting the cancer tissue itself against the destructive effect of u-PA. Moreover, lung cancers that co-expressed PAI-1 and u-PA were more frequently seen in patients with lymph node metastasis than in those expressing only u-PA or PAI-1 ($p = 0.04$). These results emphasize a synergistic effect of u-PA and PAI-1 proteins on lung cancer invasion. At present it is unknown how PAI-1 promotes migration. One possible explanation is that formation of a complex between PAI-1 and u-PA may result in loss of PAI-1 affinity for vitronectin and thus may restore integrin-dependent cell migration, as has been demonstrated in vitro (38).

On the opposite to PAI-1, PAI-2 expression was inversely correlated to lymph node (data not shown). Moreover, lung cancers that co-expressed PAI-2 and u-PA were more frequently seen in patients without lymph node metastasis than in those expressing only u-PA ($p = 0.009$), supporting the effective role of PAI-2 in inhibiting u-PA–mediated cancer cell migration.

Receptor binding of u-PA leads to a strong enhancement of plasmin generation (22). It is through this same receptor that u-PA can act like a growth factor and stimulate cellular proliferation and migration. The expression of u-PAR has been reported in tissue extracts of squamous and large-cell lung carcinoma (29,39), however, the cellular source of this receptor in lung carcinoma is currently unknown. High u-PAR levels in patients with squamous cell lung cancer were significantly associated with short overall survival (29). Moreover, the combination of high u-PAR and high PAI-1 levels in squamous cancer has a particular significant association with short overall survival (29). Both u-PAR and PAI-1 are able to bind to vitronectin. Interestingly, in vitro PAI-1 was found to block binding of u-PAR-bearing cells to vitronectin and thus to promote cellular detachment (40). So, excess PAI-1 in vivo may facilitate metastasis ·by reducing cell adhesion to the ECM. Supporting this view, PAI-1 protein was frequently found deposited in the ECM in our series of lung cancer (unpublished results).

In conclusion, u-PA–mediated cell migration require tightly controlled interactions between u-PA, PAI-1, PAI-2, u-PAR, and ECM molecules. In addition "stromal" u-PA might catalyze the activation of the abundant zymogen plasminogen into plasmin. Since plasmin can initiate in a proteolytic cascade the activation of proMMPs (20,21) it was of interest to analyze also the localization of these proenzymes in lung cancer.

B. Matrix Metalloproteinases

The MMPs constitute a family of 17 or more extracellular zinc-dependent matrix-degrading enzymes, all of which are secreted or localized at the cell surface (41).

Based on substrate specificity, they are subdivided into four subclasses: (1) the collagenases (interstitial (MMP-1), neutrophil (MMP-8) and type 3 (MMP-13) collagenases) are the only members able to cleave fibrillar collagens in gelatin; (2) type IV collagenases/gelatinases (gelatinase A (MMP-2) and gelatinase B (MMP-9)) have specificity for type IV basement membrane collagen but also for denatured collagens (gelatins); (3) stromelysins, including stromelysin 1 (ST1)(MMP-3), stromelysin 2 (ST2)(MMP-10), and matrilysin (MMP-7), have a broad specificity and degrade most of the ECM components (proteoglycans, glycoproteins, fibronectin, laminin). [The only physiological substrates of stromelysin 3 (ST3)(MMP-11) are serine protease inhibitors: α_1-protease inhibitor and α_2-antiplasmin (42). However, Noel et al. (43) showed that a truncated form of ST3 exhibits a proteolytic activity against casein, laminin, and type IV collagen.] (4) Sato et al. (44) discovered a cell surface MMP (MT-MMP1)(membrane-type MMP) which specifically cleaves and activates progelatinase A (45) and procollagenase 3 (46).

With the exception of ST3, whose activation is achieved by an intracellular furin-dependent mechanism (47,48), MMPs are secreted in a proenzyme form and cooperate for their mutual activation (41). The activity of secreted MMPs is inhibited by tissue inhibitors of metalloproteinases (TIMP), a family of glycoproteins with two well-characterized members: TIMP-1 and TIMP-2 (49).

We analyzed for the first time the expression of several MMP family members in NE lung carcinomas (34,35). Transcripts for collagenase 1, ST1, and matrilysin were seldom or never detected in these cancers, whereas ST3 gene was frequently expressed in the stroma of all NE histological types including carcinoids (Fig. 4). However, the levels of ST3 mRNAs expression were not correlated with clinicopathological parameters (35). In contrast, non-NE lung carcinomas were reported to produce almost all MMPs. In tissue extracts of non-NE lung cancer, elevated levels of mRNAs for gelatinase A and B (50), for collagenase 1, ST1, ST2, ST3, and matrilysin (50–52), and for MT-MMP1 (53) were detected. Excepted for matrilysin, these enzymes are mainly synthesized by stromal cells, i.e., fibroblasts or inflammatory cells (gelatinase B) (34,35,54,55) (Fig. 4). Of particular interest was the characteristic pattern of expression of ST3 in fibroblasts. The highest levels of ST3 gene expression were not found at the invasive front of tumors but in thin stromal trabeculae inside the tumoral mass (Fig. 5A) and in close contact with cancer cells (Fig. 5) (35,52). This suggests a role for ST3 in the remodeling processes involved in the building of the stromal architecture which indirectly contribute to the tumor expansion. Among invasive carcinomas, the ST3 gene is usually strongly expressed in tumors exhibiting high local invasiveness such as skin basal cell carcinoma (56) and head and neck squamous cell carcinomas (57), or in tumors known to have a poor prognosis. Indeed, in breast cancer, high levels of expression of ST3 mRNA or protein have been associated with patient fatality due to metastatic disease (58,59). In non-NE lung carcinoma, whereas the levels of expression of ST1, collagenase 1, and matrilysin were not correlated with clinical variables, high levels of fibroblastic expression of ST3 mRNAs were correlated with tumor size and lymph node metastasis (35). Thus, in the same manner as u-PA, it is the fibroblastic expression

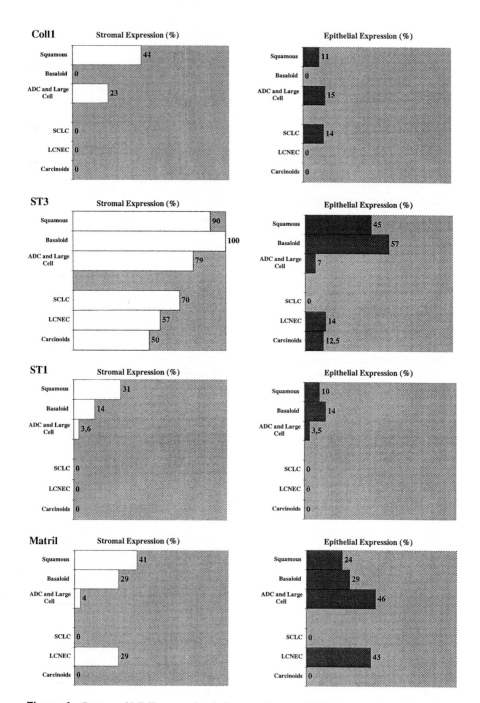

Figure 4 Pattern of MMP expression in lung carcinomas. Each bar represents the percentage of cases where a stromal (on the left and in white) or an epithelial (on the right and in dark) expression of collagenase 1 (coll1), stromelysin 3 (ST3), stromelysin 1 (ST1), and matrilysin (Matril). (1) Stromal expressions are predominant. (2) In NE tumors, epithelial expression of MMP is either absent (ST1) or significantly less frequent than in non-NE tumors.

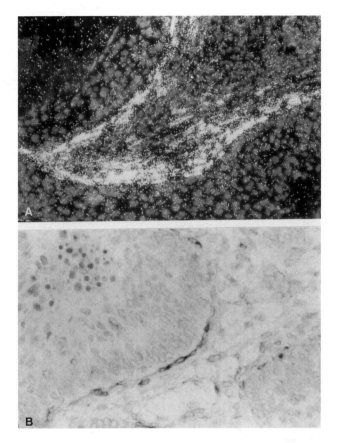

Figure 5 Pattern of ST3 expression in lung cancer. (A) Well-differentiated squamous carcinoma showing ST3 mRNAs in a stromal band infiltrating a lobule. The highest levels of ST3 expression are found in fibroblasts underlying cancer cells. Dark field photomicrograph of section counterstained with Hoechst 33258 after in situ hybridization with 35S-labeled antisense RNA probe (×150). (B) Adenocarcinoma: ST3 protein expression is restricted to the row of fibroblasts immediately adjacent to the cancer cells. Bright-field view (×300).

of ST3 rather than its epithelial expression that may allow the local metastatic dissemination.

Epithelial expression of MMPs, mainly observed in non-NE cancer cells, was linked to cell phenotype (Fig. 4). For example, ST1, ST3, gelatinase B, and MT-MMP1 epithelial expression was characteristic of squamous and squamous-related (basaloid) carcinomas, whereas matrilysin epithelial expression was predominant in adenocarcinomas (35,53,55). These specific patterns of expression may reflect the physiological expression of MMPs in non-neoplastic lung. ST3 is expressed in bronchial epithelial cells repairing a wound (60). Matrilysin is normally expressed in various human glandular epithelium including peribronchial glands (61).

TIMP-1 and TIMP-2 were found to be highly expressed in extracts of lung cancer and at a lower level in non-neoplastic lung tissue; their transcripts were localized to host stroma (50). Since this work was carried out in a small series of cases, the prognostic impact of MMP inhibitor in lung cancer progression has not been reported. In a preliminary immunohistochemical study we detected TIMP-1 and TIMP-2 proteins in endothelial cells, fibroblasts, and ECM of NE and non-NE lung carcinomas. Interestingly, TIMP-1 and TIMP-2 were strongly co-expressed ($p < 0.0001$) and co-localized on tissue sections. Surprisingly, although several in vitro and in vivo experimental models suggested a role for TIMPs in preventing tumor cell invasion (49), we found a positive correlation between TIMP-1 and TIMP-2 expression and lymph node metastasis ($p = 0.036$ and 0.032, respectively). However, TIMP expression has also been associated with poor prognosis in human breast, bladder, and colon cancer (62–64). This positive relationship between TIMP expression and cancer is paradoxical. But recent studies have shown that TIMP-2 plays a role in the activation of progelatinase A by MT-MMP-1 (45). Alternatively, TIMP-1 and TIMP-2 were shown to possess in vitro mitogenic activity for several cells, including transformed fibroblasts (49). Further investigations are needed to analyze the prognostic value of the balance between the levels of stromal MMPs and TIMPs during the course of lung tumor invasion.

Several studies showed that u-PA and MMPs cooperate for their mutual activation (20,21,65). Since u-PA and MMPs, including the membrane receptor (MT-MMP1), are predominantly associated with stromal cells, they may interact in a proteolytic cascade. We reported that lung cancers that co-expressed u-PA, ST1, ST3, and matrilysin mRNAs were more frequently seen in patients with lymph node metastasis than in those expressing no or less than four proteases ($p = 0,05$) (35). In vitro, MT-MMP1 mediates activation of progelatinase A on the cell surface (45), and indirect evidence suggests that this activation might occur in vivo in lung carcinoma. Northern blot analysis showed a parallel expression of MT-MMP1 and gelatinase A transcripts in lung cancer (53). The progelatinase A mRNA has been demonstrated in tumor stroma, while the protein has been immunolocalized to the surface of lung cancer cells themselves (54).

The specific pattern of expression of some MPs such as ST3 in the depth of the tumor mass suggests a role of stromal enzymes not only in the disruption of the ECM but also in the formation of tumor stroma. Matrix degradation may result in the release and/or activation of stored growth, angiogenesis, or motility factors. Indeed proteoglycans provide local tissue-bound reservoir of numerous growth factors: heparan sulfate is a ligand for bFGF and EGF, decorin for TGFβ, β-glycan for bFGF and TFG-β, or syndecan for aFGF, bFGF, and GMCSF (66). u-PA–mediated proteolysis is involved in the release of biologically active bFGF from the matrix (67). u-PA is required for the maturation to the active form of the inactive hepatocyte growth factor/scatter factor (68). Thus, extracellular proteinases produced by stromal cells in lung carcinomas may act like growth signals necessary for primary tumor expansion.

C. Other Matrix-Degrading Enzymes

Cathepsin B, L, and H are lysosomal cysteine proteinases that are active at acidic pH. Tumor cells frequently release cathepsins, which can act as ectopeptidases on various proteins in the ECM. Cathepsin B activity has been positively correlated with the metastatic ability of tumor cell lines and with tumor progression (69). Expression and activity of cathepsin B and L were detected in vitro in non-NE lung cancer cell lines (70). In vivo, cathepsin B activity is enhanced in non-NE lung cancer, when compared to normal lung parenchyma (71–73). Increased cathepsin B activity was related to shorter survival rates of the patients (71,73). Using immunohistochemistry, cathepsin B was detected in cancer cells in lung adenocarcinoma, and this overexpression was significantly associated with lymph node metastasis (74) and with distant metastasis (75).

III. Matrix Proteases in Lung Preneoplasia

MPs are frequently overexpressed in lung carcinoma. However, the temporal sequence of their expression during the morphological transformation process remained indefined. Squamous lung carcinomas are thought to arise from the progressive malignant transformation of the bronchial mucosa, which steps are hyperplasia, metaplasia, considered as reactive changes, and dysplasia and CIS of risk for malignant progression (16–18). In these intraepithelial lesions, the cell populations on either side of the basement membrane do not intermix. Only during the transition from in situ to invasive carcinoma do tumor cells penetrate epithelial basement membrane and enter the underlying interstitial stroma to interact with the stromal cells (76).

Recently, we reported that MPs were early expressed during the development of squamous lung carcinoma (77). Using in situ hybridization and immunohistochemistry, collagenase 1, ST1, ST3, matrilysin, and u-PA expression could be detected in intraepithelial bronchial lesions, whereas no obvious disruption of the basal lamina was seen with laminin immunostaining. Of particular interest was the restricted expression of mRNAs encoding ST3 and u-PA in dysplasia and CIS. Thus expression of these two enzymes seems to be highly predictive of an evolution toward invasion. In contrast, ST1 expression, which was seen in histologically normal bronchial epithelium as well as in all types of intraepithelial lesions, may reflect a nonspecific response to cellular injury.

Curiously, MPs were predominantly expressed in epithelial cells in the preinvasive lesions (Figs. 6,7), whereas this expression was relayed by a fibroblastic expression in the corresponding squamous lung carcinomas (Fig. 8). This early epithelial expression of MPs during squamous lung tumor development could be a direct or indirect result of the activation of oncogenes and the loss of tumor suppressor genes responsible for tumor initiation. Indeed, several reports mentioned the frequent alterations of p53 gene in dysplasia and CIS (78–80). Chromosome 3p deletion (81) and overexpression of c-ErbB1 (80) were also observed in bronchial precancerous lesions. Cellular transformation induced by oncogenes (v-src, ras) or

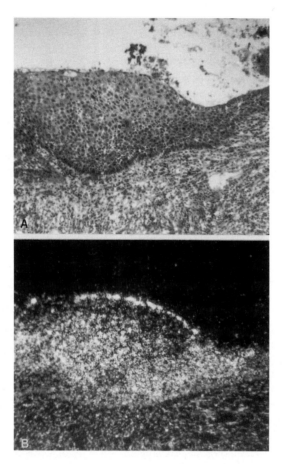

Figure 6   (A) Hematoxylin-eosin-safran staining of a bronchial CIS (×70). (B) On a serial section, the expression of u-PA mRNAs is detected in the upper layer cells of the CIS and in the desquamated cells in the bronchial luminae. Dark field epifluorescent view after in situ hybridization (×70).

tumor promoters (phorbol esters) in vitro leads to an expression of several MPs (82,83). In the same way, wild-type p53 may repress u-PA transcription (84) in normal tissues. However, we could not find a relationship between p53 mutation and u-PA expression in the preinvasive lesions (data not shown).

The epithelial expression of MPs in dysplasia and CIS that remains underlined by an intact basal lamina is striking. It has been shown that ST3 expression in breast malignant cells promotes the tumor take of these cancer cells in nude mice, and it was suggested that ST3 contributes to cell survival and implantation in host tissues (85). Therefore, in the epithelium of preinvasive bronchial lesions, ST3 might have effects on squamous lung tumor establishment.

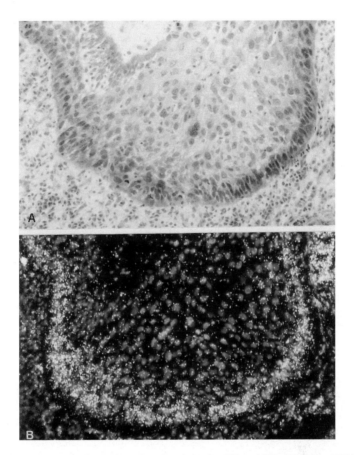

Figure 7 (A) Hematoxylin-eosin-safran staining of a CIS (×150). (B) ST3 mRNAs are localized in the basal and suprabasal epithelial cells. Dark field epifluorescent view after in situ hybridization (×150).

MP genes were subsequently expressed in fibroblasts in microinvasive and invasive bronchial lesions. ST3 gene expression in submucosal fibroblasts, early detected in bronchial CIS (Fig. 9), seems to be particularly related to the invasive process since it was also observed in two thirds of comedo-type breast CIS (a more agressive lesion) and uncommonly observed in less invasive lobular CIS (86). Several mechanisms could be involved in the inductive events for fibroblastic expression in preinvasive and invasive bronchial lesions: (1) the influence on fibroblasts of mechanical force as a result of the increasing thickness of the precancerous lesion, (2) secretion of soluble, paracrine factors from the epithelial cells or from infiltrating inflammatory cells: indeed, most MP genes are inducible by growth factors such as PDGF or EGF synthesized by bronchial neoplastic cells or by inflammatory cy-

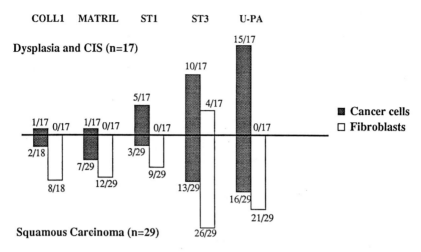

COLL1   MATRIL   ST1   ST3   U-PA

Dysplasia and CIS (n=17)

■ Cancer cells
□ Fibroblasts

Squamous Carcinoma (n=29)

Figure 8   Comparison of the frequency of MP expression in epithelial cells and/or in fibroblasts in preinvasive bronchial lesions (i.e., dysplasia and CIS) and in the corresponding squamous lung carcinomas. MPs are mainly expressed in epithelial cells in the preinvasion. This epithelial expression is relayed by a fibroblastic expression in the invasive lesions.

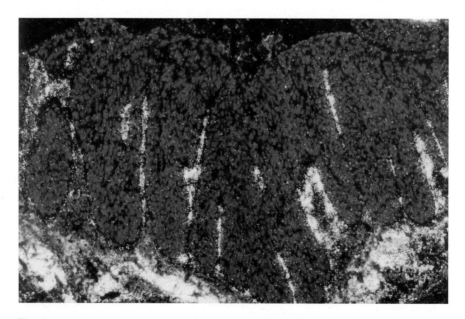

Figure 9   ST3 mRNAs expression in thin stromal trabeculae inside a CIS. In this case epithelial cells are negative for ST3 expression. Dark field epifluorescent view after in situ hybridization (×70).

tokines such as IL-1 and TNF-α (82,83), (3) cell-cell contact between invading cancer cells and surrounding stromal fibroblasts, once the basement membrane has been disrupted, could induce the expression of some MPs like it has been reported in vitro (87,88).

Although intraepithelial preneoplastic bronchial lesions may lead to the development of a squamous cancer, they have also been described in patients with SCLC (89) and adenocarcinoma (90). In our series, intraepithelial preneoplastic bronchial lesions were either adjacent to a squamous lung carcinoma or distant from invasive tumors of another histological type. We reported that high levels of u-PA and ST3 expression in the epithelial cells of preinvasive bronchial lesions might be predictive of an invasion in the vicinity of the preneoplastic lesion, implying the presence of a signaling molecule in preneoplastic cells that is absent in carcinoma cells.

The proteinases that appear to be necessary for invasion can be expressed in preinvasive steps, indicating their potential applications as markers of irreversibility of these lesions and as targets for therapeutic intervention.

IV. Expression of ETS Transcription Factors

MPs are known to be transcriptionally regulated by oncogenes, and it was widely assumed that MP expression in tumor tissue is the direct result of transforming events (41). Thus, it is somewhat surprising that MP expression in the malignant epithelium of lung cancers is limited to matrilysin expression and to sporadic and/or cell phenotype-specific expression of u-PA, ST1, collagenase 1, gelatinase B, and ST3. It is expected that elements that control tissue-specific expression will be identified in MMP promoters. From the data presented in this study, the expression of most MPs is rather consistent with regulation via a stromally derived host response to the presence of neoplastic cells.

The Ets gene family encodes transcription factors and includes over 30 members. c-Ets-1 and c-Ets-2 are closely related proteins that contain the highly conserved Ets DNA-binding domain (91). c-ets-1 gene expression has been linked to invasive processes and angiogenesis (10). This transcription factor is expressed in fibroblasts when mesenchymal-epithelial interactions occur such as during tumor invasion (92,93). It is also expressed in proliferating endothelial cells during the formation of new blood vessels in human embryos (92) and when angiogenesis resumes in adult tissues, i.e., in granulation tissue and vascularization of tumors (92,93). c-ets-2 has been involved in cell cycle control (94,95). It is ubiquitously expressed in embryos in most proliferating tissue including epithelia but not in endothelial cells (96). c-ets-2 products are abundant in young proliferating tissues and are greatly reduced in terminally differentiated tissues (97). The distinct expression pattern for each of these genes suggests a specific role.

Juxtaposed binding sites for Ets and AP1 proteins have been described in gene promoters of collagenase 1 (11), ST1 (12), matrilysin (98), and u-PA enhancer (99). The c-Ets-1 and c-Ets-2 proteins, in cooperation with other transcription factors such as AP-1, are known to be able to upregulate in transient transfection assays the activity of collagenase 1 and ST1 promoters (11–13). Interestingly, adjacent binding sites for AP-1 and Ets are also involved in the regulation of protease inhibitor genes such as murine TIMP-1 gene promoter (100) and the novel serpin called maspin (101). Thus, expression of proteases and protease inhibitors might be regulated by the same mechanisms.

Using in situ hybridization, we have analyzed the mRNA expression of c-ets-1 (34,77) and c-ets-2 (unpublished results) in lung carcinomas and in their precursors. Expression of c-ets-1 gene was particularly related to the invasive process since it was frequent in lung cancer and seldom in precancerous bronchial lesions. In agree-

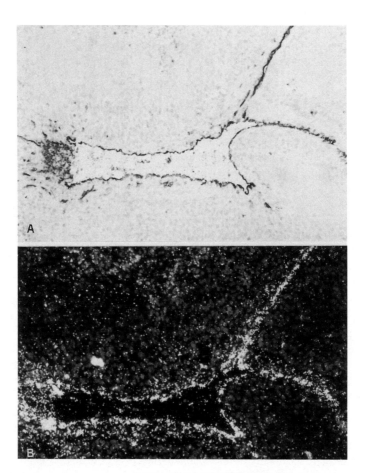

Figure 10   Section of a stromal vessel in a squamous cell lung carcinoma (×70). (A) Endothelial cells stained with an anti-CD31 antibody (B) exhibit a strong hybridization signal with c-ets-1 probe. (A) Bright field view. (B) Dark field epifluorescent view after in situ hybridization.

ment with previous results (92,93), c-ets-1 transcripts were mainly observed in stromal cells (fibroblasts and endothelial cells) (Fig. 10) in all the histological types (Fig. 11). Epithelial expression of this gene was characteristic of NE lung cancer (Fig. 11). It is the first report on c-ets-2 expression in tumor. The c-ets-2 gene was expressed in 59% of lung carcinomas. In contrast to c-ets-1 mRNAs, c-ets-2 transcripts predominated in neoplastic cells (NE and non-NE) (Fig. 11) and were not detected in endothelial cells. Interestingly, the frequency of c-ets-1 and c-ets-2 gene epithelial expression were significantly higher in advanced clinical stages (stages III and IV and metastasis) as compared with stages I and II ($p = 0.0065$ and 0.0054, respectively). Thus, c-ets-1 and c-ets-2 expression might favor cancer cells invasion, but the exact mechanism is currently unknown. The c-ets-1 gene expression has been reported in normal and neoplastic mammary epithelial cells and this epithelial expression was also associated with cell invasion (102). In the same way, transfection of MCF7 cells with another member of the Ets family, E1AF, induced the expression of gelatinase B and the scattering of these cells in vitro and in vivo

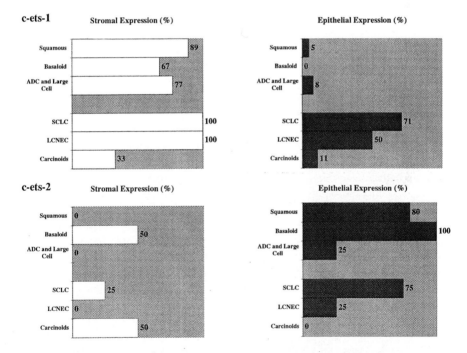

Figure 11 Pattern of c-ets-1 and c-ets-2 mRNA expression in the different histological types of lung carcinoma including non-NE and NE tumors. Each bar represents the percentage of cases where a stromal (on the left and in white) or an epithelial (on the right and in dark) expression of c-ets-1 and c-ets-2 gene was observed. (1) c-ets-1 mRNAs are more often seen in stromal cells whereas c-ets-2 mRNAs predominated in cancer cells. (2) Epithelial expression of c-ets-1 is significantly more frequent in NE than in non-NE tumors ($p = 0.0059$).

(103). Since c-ets-1 and c-ets-2 are potential markers of lung tumor aggressivity, we compared their expression with expression of molecules involved in cancer progression. No correlation was found between epithelial expression of c-ets-1 or c-ets-2 and altered expression of p53 and Rb, overexpression of apoptotic genes (Bc12, Bax and the ratio Bc12/Bax), and expression of cellular proliferation markers (Ki67) (unpublished data).

The tissue-specific expression patterns of c-Ets-1 and c-Ets-2 suggest that these two proteins play distinct biological roles and consequently transactivate different downstream cellular genes. We compared the pattern of expression of these two genes with two of their target genes, collagenase 1 and u-PA. In fibroblasts, the good concordance between c-ets-1 and collagenase 1 transcript localization confirms in vivo the possibility that c-Ets-1 might transactivate collagenase 1 gene. In neoplastic cells, no co-localization of MP transcripts and c-ets-1 or c-ets-2 mRNAs was noted.

In agreement with previous results, the predominant expression of c-ets-2 in lung neoplastic cells confirms the potential role of c-ets-2 in cell proliferation. One possibility is the involvement of c-ets-2 in the transactivation of promoters of genes encoding for cyclin D1 (98) or cdc2 kinase (97) as has been reported in vitro.

All these descriptive and correlative studies on tissue section need further experimental studies to confirm the determinant role of these transcription factors in the progression of carcinomas.

V. Future Directions

It was previously thought that MPs were produced by malignant cells in order to dissolve the occluding matrix, thus enabling the cancer cells to migrate into the interstitial matrix of the mesenchyme at the site of a primary tumor and to cross the basement membrane of blood vessels in the process of intra- and extravasation. However, this review of recent studies emphasized that extracellular proteinases implicated in the progression of human lung carcinoma are predominantly expressed by stromal and not by cancer cells. Since MPs can cleave some molecules implicated in the control of growth factor activities, the role of these enzymes during cancer progression may not be limited to faciliting malignant cell migration but may also participate in epithelial cell proliferation and stroma formation and maintenance. Thus, influence of the stromal environment on the growth, angiogenesis, and invasive capacity of tumor cells may play a significant role in lung cancer progression.

For many years, all efforts to treat lung cancer have concentrated on the inhibition or destruction of tumor cells. Strategies both to treat the tumor cells (chemotherapy and immunotherapy) and to modulate the host microenvironment (tumor vasculature and secretion of degradative enzymes) could provide an additional approach for cancer treatment. Therapeutic potential of MP inhibitors in controlling MP-dependent pathological processes may be quite considerable. The targeting of stromal proteinases will make possible more efficient drug delivery and may lead to a "soil" suppression. Synthetic inhibitors of MMPs have proven remarkably effective in blocking malignant tumor growth in animals (104). One of them, the marimastat, is currently tested in phase III clinical studies for human pancreatic (105) and gastric cancer and for SCLC.

Acknowledgments

This work was supported by French Health Ministery, Paris, Ligue contre le cancer, Isère, Association pour la Recherche sur le Cancer, Paris. I. Bolon was a recipient of a grant from Société de Pneumologie de Langue Française, Paris.

References

1. Gazzeri S, Brambilla E, Jacrot M, Chauvin C, Benabid AL, Brambilla C. Activation of myc gene family in human lung carcinomas and during heterotransplantation into nude mice. Cancer Res 1991; 51:2566–2571.
2. Gazzeri S, Brambilla E, Caron De Fromentel C, Gouyer V, Jacrot M, Brambilla C. Abnormalities of p53 gene and expression in human lung carcinomas. Int J Cancer 1994; 58:24–32.
3. Brambilla E, Gazzeri S, Moro D, Caron De Fromentel C, Gouyer V, Jacrot M, Brambilla C. Immunohistochemical study of p53 in human lung carcinomas. Am J Pathol 1993; 143:199–210.
4. Gouyer V, Gazzeri S, Brambilla E, Bolon I, Moro D, Perron P, Benabid AL, Brambilla C. Loss of heterozygozity at the Rb locus correlates with loss of Rb protein in primary malignant neuroendocrine lung carcinomas. Int J Cancer 1994; 58:818–824.
5. Folkman J. The role of angiogenesis in tumor growth. Semin Cancer Biol 1992; 3:65–71.
6. Macchiarini P, Fontanini G, Hardin MJ, Squartini F, Angeletti CA. Relation of neovascularization to metastasis of non-small-cell lung cancer. Lancet 1992; 340:145–146.
7. Yamazaki K, Abe S, Takekawa H, Sukoh N, Watanabe N, Ogura S, Nakajima I, Isobe H, Inoue K, Kawakami Y. Tumor angiogenesis in human lung adenocarcinoma. Cancer 1994; 74:2245–2250.
8. Fontanini G, Bigini D, Vignati S, Basolo F, Mussi A, Lucchi M, Chine S, Angeletti CA, Harris AL, Bevilacqua G. Microvessel count predicts metastatic disease and survival in non-small cell lung cancer. J Pathol 1995; 177:57–63.
9. Yuan A, Yang PC, Yu CJ, Lee YC, Yao YT, Chen CL, Lee LN, Kuo SH, Luh KT. Tumor angiogenesis correlates with histologic type and metastasis in non-small-cell lung cancer. Am J Respir Crit Care Med 1995; 152:2157–2162.
10. Vandenbunder B, Queva C, Desbiens X, Wernert N, Stehelin D. Expression of the transcription factor c-ets-1 correlates with the occurence of invasive processes during normal and pathological development. Invasion Metastasis 1995; 14:198–209.
11. Gutman A, Wasylyk B. The collagenase gene promoter contains a TPA and oncogene-responsive unit encompassing the PEA3 and AP-1 binding sites. EMBO J 1990; 9:2241–2246.
12. Wasylyk C, Gutman A, Nicholson R, Wasylyk B. The c-ets oncoprotein activates the stromelysin promoter through the same elements as several non-nuclear oncoproteins. EMBO J 1991; 10:1127–1134.
13. Butticé G, Kurkinen M. Oncogenes control stromelysin and collagenase gene expression. Contrib Nephrol 1994; 107:101–107.

14. Sobin LH, Yesner R. Histological Typing of Lung Tumors. International Histological Classification of Tumors. Geneva: World Health Organization, 1981.
15. Brambilla E, Moro D, Veale D, Brichon PY, Stoebner P, Paramelle B, Brambilla C. Basaloid carcinomas of lung a new phenotypic entity with prognosis significance. Human Pathol 1992; 23:993–1003.
16. Moro D, Brichon PY, Brambilla E, Veale D, Labat F, Brambilla C. Basaloid bronchial carcinoma. A histologic group with a poor prognosis. Cancer 1994; 73:2734–2739.
17. Auerbach O, Hammond EC, and Garfinkel L. Changes in bronchial epithelium in relation to cigarette smoking, 1955–1960 vs 1930–1977. N Engl J Med 1979; 300:381–385.
18. Trump BF, McDowell EM, Glaxin F, Barret LA, Becci PJ, Schürch W, Kaiser HE, Harris CC. The respiratory epithelium III. Histogenesis of epidermoid metaplasia and carcinoma in situ in the human. J Natl Cancer Inst 1978; 61:563–575.
19. Mackay AR, Corbitt RH, Hartzler JL, Thorgeirsson UP. Basement membrane type IV collagen degradation: evidence for the involvement of a proteolytic cascade independent of metalloproteinases. Cancer Res 1990; 50:5997–6001.
20. Mignatti P, Robbins E, Rifkin DB. Tumor invasion through the human amniotic membrane: requirement for a proteinase cascade. Cell 1986; 47:487–498.
21. Reich R, Thompson EW, Iwamoto Y, Martin GR, Deason JR, Fuller JC, Miskin R. Effects of inhibitors of plasminogen activators, serine proteinases, and collagenase IV on the invasion of basement membrane by metastatic cells. Cancer Res 1988; 48:3307–3312.
22. Blasi F. Urokinase and urokinase receptor: a paracrine/autocrine system regulating cell migration and invasiveness. Bioessays 1993; 15:105–111.
23. Jänicke F, Schmitt M Pache L, Ulm K, Harbeck N, Höfler H, Graeff H. Urokinase (u-PA) and its inhibitor PAI-1 are strong and independent prognostic factors in node-negative breast cancer. Breast Cancer Treat 1993; 24:195–208.
24. Pujade-Lauraine E, Lu H, Mirshahi S, Soria J, Soria C, Bernadou A, Kruithoff EKO, Lijnen HR, Burtin P. The plasminogen-activation system in ovarian tumors. Int J Cancer 1993; 55:27–31.
25. Nekarda H, Schmitt M, Ulm K, Wenninger A, Vogelsang H, Becker K, Roder JD, Fink U, Siewert JR. Prognostic impact of urokinase-type plasminogen activator and its inhibitor PAI-1 in completely resected gastric cancer. Cancer Res 1994; 54:2900–2907.
26. Markus G, Takita H, Camiolo S, Corasanti J, Evers J, Hobika GH. Content and characterization of plasminogen activators in human lung tumors and normal lung tissue. Cancer Res 1980; 40:841–848.
27. Sappino AP, Busso N, Belin D, Vassalli JD. Increase of urokinase-type plasminogen activator gene expression in human lung and breast carcinomas. Cancer Res 1987; 47:4043–4046.
28. Nagayama M, Sato A, Hayakawa H, Urano T, Takada Y, Takada A. Plasminogen activators and their inhibitors in non-small cell lung cancer. Cancer 1994; 73:1398–1405.
29. Pedersen H, Brunner N, Francis D, Osterlind K, Ronne E, Hansen HH, Dano K, Grondahl-Hansen J. Prognostic impact of urokinase, urokinase receptor, and type 1 plasminogen activator inhibitor in squamous and large cell lung cancer tissue. Cancer Res 1994; 54:4671–4675.
30. Pedersen H, Grondahl-Hansen J, Francis D, Osterlind K, Hansen HH, Dano K, Brünner N. Urokinase and plasminogen activator inhibitor type I in pulmonary adenocarcinoma. Cancer Res 1994; 54:120–123.
31. Ornstein DL, Zacharski LR, Memoli VA, Kisiel W, Kudryk BJ, Hunt J, Rousseau SM, Stump DC. Coexisting macrophage-associated fibrin formation and tumor cell urokinase in squamous cell and adenocarcinoma of the lung tissues. Cancer 1991; 68:1061–1067.
32. Oka T, Ishida T, Nishino T, Sugimachi K. Immunohistochemical evidence of urokinase-type plasminogen activator in primary and metastatic tumors of pulmonary adenocarcinoma. Cancer Res 1991; 51:3522–3525.
33. Gris JC, Scved JF, Marty-Double C, Mauboussin JM, Balmes P. Immunohistochemical study of tumor cell-associated plasminogen activators and plasminogen activator inhibitors in lung carcinomas. Chest 1993; 104:8–13.

34. Bolon I, Gouyer V, Devouassoux M, Vandenbunder B, Wernert N, Moro D, Brambilla C, Brambilla E. Expression of c-ets-1, collagenase 1, and urokinase-type plasminogen activator genes in lung carcinomas. Am J Pathol 1995; 147:1298–1310.

35. Bolon I, Devouassoux M, Robert C, Moro D, Brambilla C, Brambilla E. Expression of urokinase-type plasminogen activator, stromelysin 1, stromelysin 3, and matrilysin genes in lung carcinomas. Am J Pathol 1997; 150:1619–1629.

36. Kobayashi H, Fujishiro S, Terao T. Impact of urokinase-type plasminogen activator and its inhibitor type 1 on prognosis in cervical cancer of the uterus. Cancer Res 1994; 54:6539–6548.

37. Visscher DW, Sarkar F, LoRusso P, Sakr W, Ottosen S, Wykes S, Crissman JD. Immunohistologic evaluation of invasion-associated proteases in breast carcinoma. Mod Pathol 1993; 6:302–306.

38. Stefansson S, Lawrence DA. The serpin PAI-1 inhibits cell migration by blocking integrin a5b3 binding to vitronectin. Nature 1996; 383:441–443.

39. Veale D, Needham G, Harris A. Urokinase receptors in lung cancer and normal lung. Anticancer Res 1990; 10:417–422.

40. Waltz DA, Natkin LR, Fujita RM, Wei Y, Chapman HA. Plasmin and plasminogen activator inhibitor type 1 promote cellular motility by regulating the interaction between the urokinase receptor and vitronectin. J Clin Invest 1997; 100:58–67.

41. Matrisian LM. The matrix-degrading metalloproteinases. Bioessays 1992; 14:455–462.

42. Pei D, Majmudar G, Weiss SJ. Hydrolytic inactivation of a breast carcinoma cell-derived serpin by human stromelysin-3. J Biol Chem 1994; 269:25849–25855.

43. Noël A, Santavicca M, Stoll I, L'Hoir C, Staub A, Murphy G, Rio MC, Basset P. Identification of structural determinant controlling human and mouse stromelysin-3 proteolytic activities. J Biol Chem 1995; 270:22866–22872.

44. Sato H, Takino T, Okada Y, Cao J, Shinagawa A, Yamamoto E, Seiki M. A matrix metalloproteinase expressed on the surface of invasive tumour cells. Nature 1994; 370:61–65.

45. Strongin AY, Collier I, Bannikov G, Marmer BL, Grant GA, Goldberg GI. Mechanism of cell surface activation of 72 kDa type collagenase: isolation of the activated form of the membrane metalloprotease. J Biol Chem 1995; 270:5331–5338.

46. Knäuper V, Will H, Lopez-Otin C, Smith B, Atkinson SJ, Stanton H, Hembry RM, Murphy G. Cellular mechanisms for human procollagenase-3 (MMP-13) activation. J Biol Chem 1996; 271:17124–17131.

47. Pei D, Weiss SJ. Furin-dependent intracellular activation of the human stromelysin-3 zymogen. Nature 1995; 375:244–247.

48. Santavicca M, Noel A, Angliker H, Stoll I, Segain JP, Anglard P, Chretien M, Seidah N, Basset P. Characterization of structural determinants and molecular mechanisms involved in prostromelysin-3 activation by 4-aminophenylmercuric acetate and furin-type convertases. Biochem J 1996; 315:953–958.

49. DeClerck YA, Imren S. Protease inhibitors: role and potential therapeutic use in human cancer. Eur J Cancer 1994; 30A:2170–2180.

50. Urbanski SJ, Edwards DR, Maitland A, Leco KJ, Watson A, Kossakowska AE. Expression of metalloproteinases and their inhibitors in primary pulmonary carcinomas. Br J Cancer 1992; 66:1188–1194.

51. Muller D, Breathnach R, Engelmann A, Millon R, Bronner G, Flesch H, Dumont P, Eber M, Abecassis J. Expression of collagenase-related metalloproteinase genes in human lung or head and neck tumours. Int J Cancer 1991; 48:550–556.

52. Anderson IC, Sugarbaker DJ, Ganju RK, Tsarwhas DJ, Richards WG, Sunday M, Kobzik L, Shipp MA. Stromelysin-3 is overexpressed by stromal elements in primary non-small cell lung cancers and regulated by retinoic acid in pulmonary fibroblasts. Cancer Res 1995; 55:4120–4126.

53. Polette M, Nawrocki B, Gilles C, Sato H, Seiki M, Tournier JM, Birembaut P. MT-MMP expression and localisation in human lung and breast cancers. Virchows Arch 1996; 428:29–35.

54. Soini Y, Pääkkö P, Autio-Harmainen H. Genes of laminin B1 chain, a1(IV) chain of type IV collagen, and 72-kd type IV collagenase are mainly expressed by the stromal cells of lung carcinomas. Am J Pathol 1993; 142:1622–1630.

55. Canete-Soler R, Litzky L, Lubensky I, Muschel RJ. Localization of the 92 kd gelatinase mRNA in squamous cell and adenocarcinomas of the lung using in situ hybridization. Am J Pathol 1994; 164:518–527.

56. Wolf C, Chenard MP, De Grossouvre D, Bellocq JP, Chambon P, Basset P. Breast cancer-associated stromelysin 3 gene is expressed in basal cell carcinoma and during cutaneous wound healing. J Invest Dermatol 1992; 99:870–872.

57. Muller D, Wolf C, Abecassis J, Millon R, Engelmann A, Bronner G, Rouyer N, Rio MC, Eber M, Methling, Chambon P, Basset P. Increased stromelysin 3 gene expression is associated with increased local invasiveness in head and neck squamous cell carcinomas. Cancer Res 1993; 53:165–169.

58. Engel G, Heselmeyer K, Auer G, Bäckdahl M, Eriksson E, Linder S. Correlation between stromelysin-3 mRNA level and outcome of human breast cancer. Int J Cancer 1994; 58:830–835.

59. Chenard MP, O'Siorain L, Shering S, Rouyer N, Lutz Y, Wolf C, Basset P, Bellocq JP, Duffy J. High levels of stromelysin-3 correlate with poor prognosis in patients with breast carcinoma. Int J Cancer 1996; 69:448–451.

60. Buisson AC, Gilles C, Polette M, Zahm JM, Birembaut P, Tournier JM. Wound repair-induced expression of stromelysins is associated with the acquisition of a mesenchymal phenotype in human respiratory epithelial cells. Lab Invest 1996; 74:658–669.

61. Saarialhokere UK, Crouch EC, Parks WC. Matrix metalloproteinase matrilysin is constitutively expressed in adult human exocrine epithelium. J Invest Dermatol 1995; 105: 190–196.

62. Grignon DJ, Sakr W, Ravery V, Angulo J, Shamsa F, Pontes JE, Crissman JC, Fridman R. High levels of tissue inhibitor of metalloproteinase-2 (TIMP-2) expression are associated with poor outcome in invasive bladder cancer. Cancer Res 1996; 56:1654–1659.

63. Zeng ZS, Cohen AM, Zhang ZF, Stetler-Stevenson WG, Guillem JG. Elevated tissue inhibitor of metalloproteinase 1 RNA in colorectal cancer stroma correlates with lymph node and distant metastases. Clin Cancer Res 1995; 1:899–906.

64. Visscher DW, Hoyhtya M, Ottosen SK, Liang CM, Sarkar FH, Crissman JD, Fridman R. Enhanced expression of tissue inhibitor of metalloproteinase-2 (TIMP-2) in the stroma of breast carcinomas correlates with tumor recurrence. Int J Cancer 1994; 59:339–344.

65. Marcotte PA, Kozan IM, Dorwin SA, Ryan JM. The matrix metalloproteinase Pump-1 catalyses formation of low molecular weight (pro)urokinase in culture of normal human kidney cells. J Biol Chem 1992; 267:13803–13806.

66. Ruoslahti E, Yamaguchi Y. Proteoglycans as modulators of growth factor activities. Cell 1991; 64:867–869.

67. Rifkin DB, Moscatelli D, Bizik J, Quarto N, Blei F, Dennis P, Flaumenhaft R, Mignatti P. Growth factor control of extracellular proteolysis. Cell Diff Dev 1990; 32:313–318.

68. Naldini L, Tamagnone L, Vigna E, Sachs M, Hartmann G, Birchmeier W, Daikuhara Y, Tsubouchi H, Blasi F, Comoglio PM. Extracellular proteolytic cleavage by urokinase is required for activation of hepatocyte growth factor/scatter factor. EMBO J 1992; 11:4825–4833.

69. Sloane BF. Cathepsin B and cystatins: evidence for a role in cancer progression. Semin Cancer Biol 1990; 1:137–152.

70. Spiess E, Brüning A, Gack S, Ulbricht B, Spring H, Trefz G, Ebert W. Cathepsin B activity in human lung tumor cell lines: ultrastructural localization, pH sensitivity, and inhibitor status at the cellular level. J Histochem Cytochem 1994; 42:917–929.

71. Krepela E, Kasafirek E, Novak K, Viklicky J. Increased cathepsin G activity in human lung tumors. Neoplasma 1990; 37:61–70.

72. Sedo A, Krepela E, Kasafirek E. Dipeptidyl peptidase IV, propyl endopeptidase and cathepsin B activities in primary human lung tumours and lung parenchyma. J Cancer Res Clin Oncol 1991; 117:249–253.

73. Ebert W, Knoch H, Werle B, Trefz G, Muley T, Spiess E. Prognostic value of increased lung tumor tissues cathepsin B. Anticancer Res 1994; 14:895–899.
74. Sukoh S, Abe S, Nakajima I, Ogura S, Isobe H, Inoue K, Kawakami S. Immunohistochemical distributions of cathepsin B and basement membrane antigens in human lung adenocarcinoma: association with invasion and metastasis. Virchows Archiv 1994; 424:33–38.
75. Ozeki Y, Takishima K, Takagi K, Aida S, Tamai S, Mamiya G, Ogata T. Immunohistochemical analysis of cathepsin B expression in human lung adenocarcinoma: the role in cancer progression. Jpn J Cancer Res 1993; 84:972–975.
76. Barsky SH, Siegal GP, Janotta F, Liotta LA. Loss of basement membrane components by invasive tumors but not by their benign counterparts. Lab Invest 1983; 49:140–147.
77. Bolon I, Brambilla E, Vandenbunder B, Robert C, Lantuejoul S, Brambilla C. Changes in the expression of matrix proteases and of the transcription factor c-ets-1 during progression of precancerous bronchial lesions. Lab Invest 1996; 75:1–13.
78. Bennet WP, Colby TV, Travis WD, Borkowski A, Jones RT, Lane DP, Metcalf RA, Samet JM, Takeshima Y, Gu JR, Vähäkangas KH, Soini Y, Pääkkö P, Welsh JA, Trump BF, Harris CC. p53 accumulates frequently in early bronchial neoplasia. Cancer Res 1993; 53:4817–4822.
79. Walker C, Robertson LJ, Myskow MW, Pendleton N, Dixon GR. p53 expression in normal and dysplastic bronchial epithelium and in lung carcinomas. Br J Cancer 1994; 70:297–303.
80. Rush V, Klimstra D, Linkov I, Dmitrovsky E. Aberrant expression of p53 or the epidermal growth factor receptor is frequent in early bronchial neoplasia, and coexpression precedes squamous cell carcinoma development. Cancer Res 1995; 55:1365–1372.
81. Sundaresan V, Ganly P, Haselton P, Rudd R, Sinha G, Bleehen NM, Rabbits P. p53 and chromosome 3 abnormalities, characteristic of malignant lung tumours, are detectable in preinvasive lesions of the bronchus. Oncogene 1992; 7:1989–1997.
82. Laiho M, Keski-Oja J. Growth factors in the regulation of pericellular proteolysis: A review. Cancer Res 1989; 49:2533–2553.
83. Mauviel A. Cytokine regulation of metalloproteinase gene expression. J Cell Biochem 1993; 53:288–295.
84. Kunz C, Pebler S, Otte J, Von Der Ahe D. Differential regulation of plasminogen activator and inhibitor gene transcription by the tumor suppressor p53. Nucleic Acid Res 1995; 23:3710–3717.
85. Noël AC, Lefebvre O, Maquoi E, VanHoorde L, Chenard MP, Mareel M, Foidart JM, Basset P, Rio MC. Stromelysin-3 expression promotes tumor take in nude mice. J Clin Invest 1996; 97:1924–1930.
86. Wolf C, Rouyer N, Lutz Y, Adida C, Loriot M, Bellock JP, Chambon P, Basset P. Stromelysin 3 belongs to a subgroup of proteinases expressed in breast carcinoma fibroblastic cells and possibly implicated in tumor progression. Proc Natl Acad Sci USA 1993; 90:1843–1847.
87. Borchers AH, Powell MB, Fusenig NE, Tim Bowden G. Paracrine factor and cell-cell contact-mediated induction of protease and c-ets gene expression in malignant keratinocyte/dermal fibroblast cocultures. Exp Cell Res 1994; 213:143–147.
88. Ito A, Nakajima S, Sasaguri Y, Nagase H, Mori Y. Co-culture of human breast adenocarcinoma MCF-7 cells and human dermal fibroblasts enhances the production of matrix metalloproteinases 1, 2 and 3 in fibroblasts. Br J Cancer 1995; 71:1039–1045.
89. Yoneda K, Boucher LD. Bronchial epithelial changes associated with small cell lung carcinoma of the lung. Hum Pathol 1993; 24:1180–1183.
90. Solomon MD, Greenberg SD, Spjut HJ. Morphology of bronchial epithelium adjacent to adenocarcinoma of the lung. Mod Pathol 1990; 3:684–687.
91. Wasylyk B, Hahn SL, Giovane A. The Ets family of transcription factors. Eur J Biochem 1993; 211:7–18.
92. Wernert N, Raes MB, Lassalle PH, Dehouck MP, Gosselin B, Vandenbunder B, Stehelin D. c-ets-1 proto-oncogene is a transcription factor expressed in endothelial cells during tumor vascularization and other forms of angiogenesis in humans. Am J Pathol 1992; 140:119–127.

93. Wernert N, Gilles F, Fafeur V, Bouali F, Raes MB, Pyke C, Dupressoir T, Seitz G, Vanden-bunder B, Stéhelin D. Stromal expression of c-ets1 transcription factor correlates with tumor invasion. Cancer Res 1994; 54:5683–5688.

94. Wen SC, Ku DH, De Luca A, Claudio PP, Giordano A, Calabretta B. Ets-2 regulates cdc2 kinase activity in mammalian cells: coordinated expression of cdc2 and cyclinA. Exp Cell Res 1995; 217:8–14.

95. Albanez C, Johnson J, Watanabe G, Eklund N, Vu D, Pestell RG. Transforming p21 ras mutants and c-Ets-2 activate the cyclin D1 promoter through distinguishable regions. J Biol Chem 1995; 270:23589–23597.

96. Maroulakou IG, Papas TS, Green JE. Differential expression of ets-1 and ets-2 proto-oncogenes during murine embryogenesis. Oncogene 1994; 9:1551–1565.

97. Bhat NK, Fisher RJ, Fujiwara S, Ascione R, Papas TS. Temporal and tissue-specific expression of mouse ets genes. Proc Natl Acad Sci USA 1987; 84:3161–3165.

98. Gaire M, Zenaida M, McDonnell S, McNeil L, Lovett DH, Matrisian L.M. Structure and expression of the human gene for the matrix metalloproteinase matrilysin. J Biol Chem 1994; 269:2032–2040.

99. Nerlov C, Rorth P, Blasi F, Johnsen M. Essential AP-1 and PEA3 binding elements in the human urokinase enhancer display cell type-specific activity. Oncogene 1991; 6:1583–1592.

100. Edwards DR, Rocheleau H, Sharma RR, Wills AJ, Cowie A, Hassel JA, Heath JK. Involvement of AP1 and PEA3 binding sites in the regulation of murine tissue inhibitor of metalloproteinases-1 (TIMP-1) transcription. Biochim Biophys Acta 1992; 1171:41–55.

101. Zhang M, Maass Nicolai, Magit D, Sager R. Transactivation through Ets and Ap1 transcription sites determines the expression of the tumor-suppressing gene Maspin. Cell Growth Diff 1997; 8:179–186.

102. Delannoy-Courdent A, Fauquette W, Dong-Le Bourhis XF, Boilly B, Vandenbunder B, Desbiens X. Expression of c-ets-1 and u-PA genes is associated with mammary epithelial cell tubulogenesis or neoplastic scattering. Int J Dev Biol 1996; 40:1097–1108.

103. Kaya M, Yoshida K, Higashino F, Mitaka T, Ishii S, Fujinaga K. A single ets-related transcription factor, E1AF, confers invasive phenotype on human cancer cells. Oncogene 1996; 12:221–227.

104. Wang X, Fu X, Brown PD, Crimmin MJ, Hoffman RM. Matrix metalloproteinase inhibitor BB-94 (Batimastat) inhibits human colonic tumor growth and spread in a patient-like orthotopic model in nude mice. Cancer Res 1994; 54:4726–4728.

105. Bramhall SR. The matrix metalloproteinases and their inhibitors in pancreatic cancer. From molecular science to a clinical application. Int J Pancreatol 1997; 21:1–12.

26

Adhesion Molecules

JEAN-LOUIS PUJOL and PASCAL DEMOLY

Centre Hospitalier Universitaire
Montpellier, France

I. Introduction

In normal tissues, adhesion molecules are important effectors involved in cell-to-cell relationships but also in cell-to-extracellular matrix relationships. They act as regulators of tissue homeostasis. The progression of lung cancer, as in other human malignancies, depends on the ability of some cell subpopulations to migrate, colonize other tissues, and yield metastases. The microenvironment surrounding the malignant cells regulates their growth and, consequently, might represent a cornerstone of invasion and metastatic process. One of the fundamental properties of metastatic cells is their ability to transgress the extracellular matrix, which normally acts as a barrier against tumor progression (1). The detachment of malignant cells from the matrix depends on their ability to synthetize metalloproteinases which induce matrix lysis, but it also depends on the modification of the expressed adhesion molecules (1). These altered expressions yielding putative consequences for the cell-to-cell relationship and tumor progression may be roughly classified into three categories: overexpression (e.g., overexpression of the neural cell adhesion molecule [NCAM] by small cell lung cancer); heterotopic expression (e.g., NCAM expression by non-small cell lung cancer), or underexpression. Integrins and cadherins fall in the latter category. Structurally, there are four different adhesion molecule families: the integrin family, the cadherin family, the immunoglobulin superfamily, and the selectin family. In this chapter we will discuss current knowledge of adhesion molecule expression and their putative role in lung cancer development with particular focus on the NCAM which, in 1998, is the most widely studied adhesion molecule in lung cancer.

II. Integrins

Integrins are a family of transmembrane glycoproteins which normally act as regulators of interaction between cell and extracellular matrix. They act as receptors for a wide variety of extracellular matrix proteins including laminins (through $\alpha2,3,6$ integrin subunits) or fibronectin (through αv subunit) and for members of the immunoglobulin superfamily such as ICAM and VCAM molecules. They are involved in tissue homeostasis and cell differentiation, and they participate in the regulation of tissue growth fraction. There is a marked variability of integrin expression among the different lung carcinoma cell lines, which does not dramatically differ from what Mette et al. observed in clustered human bronchial epithelial cells (2). At cell surface, non–small-cell lung cancer cells express fewer integrins when compared with normal respiratory epithelial cells (3). The integrin subunits which serve as collagen-laminin receptors ($\alpha1$, $\alpha2$, $\alpha3$, $\alpha6$) and fibronectin-fibronogen receptors (αv) are predominantly expressed (2,3). In vitro, non–small-cell lung cancer cell lines, which do not express integrins, are also less adherent to the extracellular matrix proteins (2). From these experiments, it is suggested that integrins play a key role in the adhesion of tumor cells to the extracellular matrix, supporting the hypothesis that the lack of integrin expression may promote tumor progression. However, in vivo, there is no direct correlation between the metastatic potential of a xenograft and its panel of expressed integrins. It is thus likely that integrins are only one of the numerous adhesion molecules regulating cell–extracellular matrix relationships.

III. Cadherins

Cadherins are a family of Ca^{2+}-dependent cell-to-cell adhesion molecules involved in the segregation of cells into different tissues. This family includes, among others, E-cadherin, P-cadherin, A-CAM, and L-CAM (4). Besides their role in morphogenesis, altered expression of cadherins is recognized as a factor of invasion and metastasis.

Among them, E-cadherin has been widely investigated in both small-cell and non–small-cell carcinomas. In advanced lung adenocarcinomas, E-cadherin expression is reduced or altered (5), and both transcriptional and posttranslational events are involved. An E-cadherin–associated protein, α-catenin, is detectable in lung neoplasms with altered E-cadherin protein expression. A recent study found that the E-cadherin expression pattern is, in fact, more frequently altered in poorly differentiated squamous cell carcinomas and in small-cell carcinomas of the lung when compared with adenocarcinomas. In addition, a spotty pattern of expression was observed in metastastic tissues leading to a reduced or altered E-cadherin expression in tumors sharing the most aggressive clinical behavior (6). G protein–coupled receptors may regulate processes involving cadherin-mediated adhesion, such as embryonic development and cancer metastasis (7).

Finally, there might be a histology-specific cadherin alteration as P-cadherin has been found to be underexpressed in adenocarcinoma but not in small-cell lung cancer (8), and the reverse is true for N-cadherin (9).

IV. Carcinoembryonic Antigen

This 180 kDa transmembrane glycoprotein belongs to the immunoglobulin superfamily. Carcinoembryonic antigen (CEA) is a complex of CEA itself, nonspecific cross-reacting antigen (NCA), and biliary glycoprotein 1. All genes belonging to this family are localized to chromosome 19 (10). In vitro, cell lines raised from both small-cell and non–small-cell lung cancers expressed carcinoembryonic antigen, with a particularly high level of mRNA and protein in classic small-cell lung cancer cell lines (11). In this view, NCA constitutes the most prominent CEA immunoreactive molecule. In lung cancer cell lines, CEA is involved as a Ca^{2+}-independent adhesion molecule in homotypic and heterotypic cell-to-cell binding.

The CEA has been widely investigated as a serum tumor marker of many human malignancies, including lung cancer (12). Although its serum level is correlated with tumor stage in both small-cell and non–small-cell lung cancer, its ability to help the prognostication and management of lung cancer is controversial. In addition, iodine[131]-labeled anti-CEA immunoscintigraphy does not add information to the computerized tomography in assessing lung cancer staging, particularly for lymph node metastases (13).

V. Neural Cell Adhesion Molecules

Neural cell adhesion molecules (NCAM) are likely to be involved in the progression of lung cancer and, above all, in the phenotypic diversification of non–small-cell lung cancer. They are sialylated glycoproteins belonging to the immunoglobulin superfamily (Fig. 1) (14). Their physiological role has been widely investigated, and it is now well recognized that NCAM are important molecules in the homotypic cell-to-cell relationship during the embryonic development of the brain. NCAM are composed of an intracellular domain and a transmembrane and extracellular domain. A single gene localized on the 11q23 chromosome codes for all types of the NCAM family and alternative splicing of the large RNA segment result in different isoforms of NCAM, which differ by their molecular weight (between 115 and 180 kDa). Above all, posttranscriptional modification of the molecule results in different NCAM characterized by the length of an α2,8 polysialic acid (PSA) chain linked up

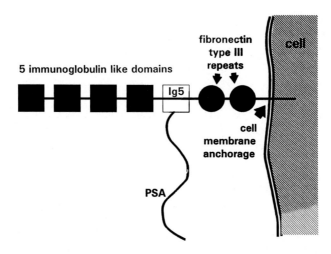

Figure 1 PSA NCAM is composed of five immunoglobulinlike domains and two fibronectin type III repeats near the membrane attachment. The fifth immunoglobulin domain contains two sites of polysialic acid anchorage.

to the extracellular domain of the molecule. This PSA branch is strikingly involved in the negative regulation of cell-to-cell adhesion.

A. Neural Cell Adhesion Molecule as a Marker of Neuroendocrine Differentiation of Lung Cancer

As NCAM are constantly expressed at the cell surface of almost all small-cell lung cancer cell lines, it was first suggested that they could be used as markers of neuroendocrine differentiation. Immunohistochemical studies of reactivity of NCAM antibodies in lung cancer tissue sections have clearly demonstrated that NCAM expression cannot be considered as a tool to distinguish small-cell from non–small-cell lung cancers, however. In fact, the latter group expresses the NCAM with a frequency of up to 20% of non–small-cell lung cancer specimens (Fig. 2) (15,16). Consequently, what first appeared as a convenient tool to segregate the two major groups of lung cancers (small-cell versus non–small-cell) not only failed to help the pathologist and the clinician but also resulted in new questions: Why does a subgroup of non–small-cell lung cancers express a so-called neuroendocrine differentiation antigen? Is there a particular behavior of the NCAM-positive non–small-cell lung cancer?

B. Phenotypic Heterogeneity of Lung Cancer

The heterotopic NCAM expression at the cell surface of non–small-cell lung cancers has added a new observation to the list of evidence that the lung cancer phenotype of some tumors transgresses the frontier conveniently introduced between small-cell

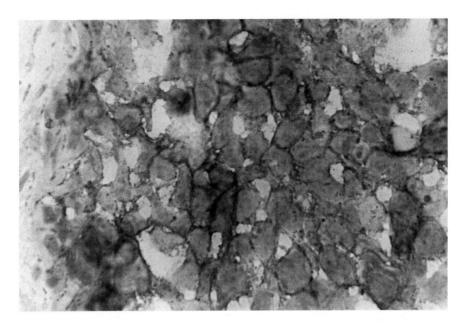

Figure 2 Indirect immunoperoxidase reaction of Mab MOC-1 (cluster 1 antibody) on a poorly differentiated SQC: All cells demonstrate strong membrane staining (magnification 400×).

and non–small-cell lung cancer. For instance, the classification of lung cancer recognizes the possible occurrence of foci of squamous cell lung cancer or adenocarcinoma in small-cell lung cancer. Such multidifferentiated tumors are called combined small-cell–non-small-cell lung cancer (17) and their frequency is probably underestimated. For instance, in autopsy studies of patients who died due to recurrent small-cell lung cancer, a large proportion of non–small-cell lung cancer foci have been observed in pathological tumor remainders (18). This suggests that the diversification of the lung cancer phenotype probably increases during tumor progression and is more evident when large specimens are analyzed rather than in small biopsies such as those obtained by fiberoptic bronchoscopy. Alternatively, treatment might be partly responsible for the phenotypic diversification (19).

Another related observation demonstrating the importance of phenotypic diversification has been added by a classical study, which demonstrated that up to 10% of so-called non–small-cell lung cancers contain, in fact, a small-cell lung cancer component observed when surgical specimens are exhaustively analyzed by conventional microscopy (20). In this regard, NCAM expression by non–small-cell lung cancer may appear as an additional tool to explore the phenotypic heterogeneity of lung cancer (15).

C. Mechanisms Sustaining the Heterotopic Expression Phenotypic of NCAM by Non–Small-Cell Lung Cancer

The "Y" hypothesis of lung cancer differentiation as proposed by Yesner suggests that all histological types of lung cancer arise from a common endodermal origin and that small-cell lung cancer, adenocarcinoma, and squamous cell carcinoma are all part of a single spectrum of differentiation allowing frequent overlaps between different ways (21). According to this hypothesis, large-cell carcinoma would be located at the central point of this "Y." Early studies using histology (21) or electronic microscopy (22) have demonstrated that mixed small-cell–non-small-cell lung cancer may be observed, although the frequency of combined histology is low. Patients suffering from this particular histology (combined small-cell–large-cell carcinoma) proved to have a shorter survival than those with pure histological small-cell lung cancer, suggesting that this heterogeneity has clinical relevance (23). The concept of phenotypic heterogeneity of lung cancer presumably hits a basic property of malignant cells: the genomic instability. Although all cancers derive from monoclonal origin, this genomic instability leads to the diversification of malignant cells. Whereas some subclones become rapidly extinct due to host immunological and nonimmunological defenses, others progress owing to their malignant properties, especially metastatic and resistant phenotypes (24). In a classic paper, Nicolson proposed a hypothesis linking the diversification of tumor phenotype and tumor progression (25): in malignant tumors with low invasive potential, the phenotype diversifies slowly, whereas in highly malignant tumors, this phenotypic diversification occurs early in the natural history of the tumor leading to the appearance of a metastatic phenotype. If chromosomal instability could be considered as a mover of the phenotypic diversification by allowing expression of genes unrelated to cell lineage, there might be a link between phenotypic heterogeneity and tumor progression (Fig. 3).

In one study, the phenotype diversification and ploidy of lung cancers were assessed in parallel (15). We prospectively analyzed the expression of neuroendocrine related antigens by immunohistochemistry and the cell DNA content in frozen specimens from patients who had undergone complete surgical resection of primary non–small-cell lung cancer in an attempt (1) to characterize the phenotypic heterogeneity and (2) to determine whether this heterogeneity is correlated with aneuploidy and clinical staging. Three cluster 1 antibodies were used in association to characterize adequately the expression of the intracellular domain of NCAM (S-L 11.14, MOC-1, and NE-25). Reactivity of these monoclonal antibodies (Mabs) in small-cell lung cancer and in lung carcinoid tissue sections was used as positive control. All small-cell lung cancers and almost all lung carcinoids tested were homogeneously positive with Mabs S-L 11.14, MOC-1, and NE-25. Thirty-two percent of the non–small-cell lung cancers were homogeneously positive and some additional specimens focally positive with Mabs S-L 11.14, MOC-1, and NE-25. The frequence of this abnormal phenotype was significantly higher in poorly differentiated squamous cell carcinomas when compared with well-differentiated ones. In addition, pathological stage III non–small-cell lung cancer and tumors involving me-

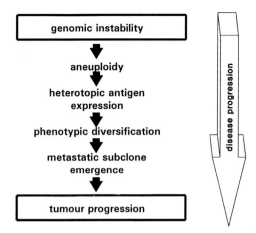

Figure 3 Link between genotypic instability, diversification, and progression to the metastatic phenotype. (Adapted from Ref. 25.)

diastinal lymph nodes proved to express NCAM more frequently when compared with the opposite conditions of each variable.

Taking the percentage of cells in the modal DNA of G0G1 phase as a criterium of ploidy, we observed that NCAM-positive non–small-cell lung cancers demonstrated more frequently an aneuploid pattern when compared with other tumors not expressing NCAM. We conclude that neuroendocrine differentiation in non–small-cell lung cancer is mainly observed in poorly differentiated tumors and in advanced clinical stages. This heterotopic phenotype is correlated with aneuploidy. The relatively high frequency of NCAM expression by non–small-cell lung cancers suggests a possible underestimation of phenotypic heterogeneity of malignant lung tumors when it is analyzed by conventional microscopy. However, its clinical significance cannot be definitively established by this study.

Several retrospective studies have been conducted in order to determine whether or not NCAM expression yields a more aggressive clinical behavior (26,27). They generally came to the conclusion that patients suffering from lung cancer expression NCAM possibly had a shorter survival. In our prospective study (28), the prognostic significance of the expression of NCAM in lung cancer was analyzed by the indirect immunoperoxidase method in 97 surgically treated patients. Reactivity of MOC-1 and S-L 11.14 was positive in 9 out of 9 small-cell lung cancers and in 16 out of 88 (18%) non–small-cell lung cancers. Again, for the latter group, this expression demonstrated a phenotypic heterogeneity, which was mainly observed in poorly differentiated squamous cell carcinomas and in N2 non–small-cell lung cancers. Patients with NCAM-positive non–small-cell lung cancer proved to have a shorter survival than those with a negative one (Fig. 4). Cox's model multivariate analysis revealed that nodal status and histology were the main independent determinants of prognosis, however.

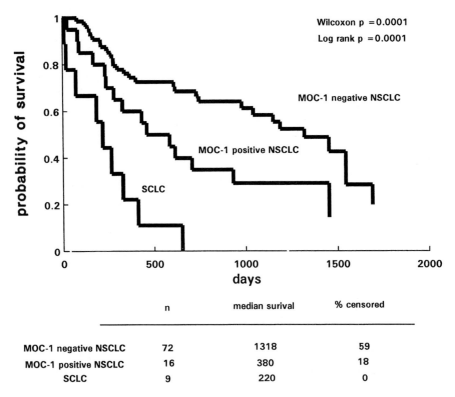

Figure 4 Effect of NCAM expression and histological grouping on survival of surgically resected lung cancer. (From Ref. 28.)

The poor survival of non–small-cell lung cancer patients with positive NCAM expression observed in this study is a clue in favor of the negative prognostic effect of the phenotypic instability of lung cancer. This is in accordance with the hypothesis that the diversification of lung cancer phenotype leads to tumor progression and brings a negative prognosis (25). However, the results of the multivariate analysis weakened the possible use of NCAM as an additional prognostic factor. Nodal status remains the most important prognostic variable, suggesting that NCAM expression is only one of many biological events that promote tumor progression.

An additional clue to the possible role of NCAM expression in the metastatic phenotype has been provided by in vitro experiments demonstrating that variant small-cell lung cancer cell lines, a transitional subgroup from small-cell lung cancer to non–small-cell lung cancer, lose the expression of NCAM (29,30). According to a study by Mabry, this NCAM expression loss can be reproduced by transfecting variant small-cell lung cancer cell lines with the v-Ha-*ras* oncogene (31).

D. Isoforms of NCAM

Cell surface glycoproteins such as NCAM undergo some transformations during the course of cell differentiation and development. Two different polysialyltransferase enzymes (PST and STX) produce polysialic acid (PSA) chain on NCAM (32). Of the different types of NCAM molecule, those that share a PSA chain play a key role inasmuch as PSA-NCAM negatively regulates the homotypic cell-to-cell adhesion by acting as a heavily hydrated negative charge (Fig. 5); (33). In addition, PSA inhibit cell-to-cell interaction induced by other adhesion molecules and receptors. The embryonic brain contains high amounts of PSA-NCAM, and this molecule allows the plasticity of neurogenesis. Polysialic acid is particularly crucial during synaptic rearrangement and neurite outgrowth. It is tempting to speculate that an analog role might be played by PSA-NCAM in lung cancer leading to the loss of cell-to-cell adhesion and facilitation of tumor cell detachment and progression. Such a mechanism might allow the migration of clonogenic tumor cells and promote the emergence of a metastatic phenotype (34). Small-cell lung cancer cell lines that express high amounts of PSA-NCAM proved to form many more colonies in vitro when compared with cell lines that express nonsialylated NCAM (32). In addition, xenografts of the former lines produce more metastases than the latter. As PSA-NCAM is detectable in the serum of lung cancer patients (35), the development of specific anti-

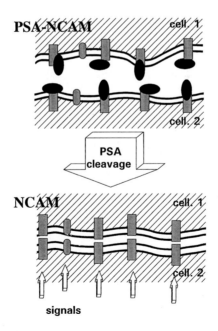

Figure 5 Regulation of cell-to-cell interactions by the degree of polysialylation of NCAM. (Modified from Ref. 33.)

PSA-NCAM antibodies deserves further study to determine whether or not PSA-NCAM expression is correlated with metastatic disease and poor prognosis.

VI. Perspectives

It is too early to expect any therapeutic applications specifically targeted to adhesion molecules or to the control of cell-to-cell and cell-to-matrix adhesion. Meanwhile, advances in comprehending host-tumor relationships will allow a better definition of lung cancer prognosis.

References

1. Cottam DW, Rees RC. Regulation of matrix metalloproteinases: their role in tumor invasion and metastasis (review). Int J Oncol 1993; 2:861–872.
2. Mette SA, Pilewski J, Buck CA, Albelda SM. Distribution of integrin cell adhesion receptors on normal bronchial epithelial cells and lung cancer cells in vitro and in vivo. Am J Respir Cell Mol Biol 1993; 8:562–572.
3. Damjanovich L, Albelda SM, Mette SA, Buck CA. Distribution of integrin cell adhesion receptors in normal and malignant lung tissue. Am J Respir Cell Mol Biol 1992; 6:197–206.
4. Broers JLV, Ramaekers FCS. Differentiation markers for lung-cancer sub-types. A comparative study of their expression in vivo and in vitro. Int J Cancer 1994; 8:134–137.
5. Bongiorno PF, Al-Kasspooles M, Lee SW, Rachwal WJ, Moore JH, Whyte RI, Orringer MB, Beer DG. E-cadherin expression in primary and metastatic thoracic neoplasms and Barret's oesophagus. Br J Cancer 1995; 71:166–172.
6. Bohm M, Totzeck B, Wieland I. Differences of E-cadherin expression levels and patterns in human lung cancer. Ann Hematol 1994; 68:81–3.
7. Williams CL, Hayes VY, Hummel AM, Tarara JE, Halsey TJ. Regulation of E-cadherin-mediated adhesion by muscarinic acetylcholine receptors in small cell lung carcinoma. J Cell Biol 1993; 121:643–54.
8. Shimoyama Y, Hirohashi S, Hirano S, Noguchi M, Shiosato Y, Takeichi M, Abe O. Cadherin cell-adhesion in human epithelial tissues and carcinomas. Cancer Res 1989; 49:2128–2133.
9. Rygaard K, Moller C, Bock E, Spang-Thomsen M. Expression of cadherin and NCAM in human small cell lung cancer lines and xenografts. Br J Cancer 1992; 65:573–577.
10. Zimmermann W, Weber B, Ortlied B, Rudert F, Schempp W, Fiebig HH, Shively JE, Von Kleist S, Thompson JA. Chromosomal localization of the carcinoembryonic antigen gene family and differential expression in various tumors. Cancer Res 1988; 48:2550–2554.
11. Kim J, Kaye FJ, Henslee JG, Sheverly JE, Park JG, Lai SL, Linnoila RI, Mulshine JL, Gazdar AF. Expression of carcinoembryonic antigen and related genes in lung and gastrointestinal cancers. Int J Cancer 1992; 52:718–725.
12. Buccheri G, Ferrigno D, Sartoris AM, Violante B, Vola F, Curcio A. Tumor markers in bronchogenic carcinoma. Superiority of tissue polypeptide antigen to carcinoembryonic antigen and carbohydrate antigenic determinant 19–9. Cancer 1987; 60:42–50.
13. Boilleau G, Pujol JL, Ychou M, Faurous P, Marty-Ane C, Michel FB, Godard P. Detection of lymph node metastasis in lung cancer: comparison of iodine131 labelled anti-CEA anti-CA 19–9 immunoscintigraphy versus computed tomography. Lung Cancer 1994; 11:209–219.
14. Michalides R, Kwa B, Springall D, Van Zandwijk N, Koopman J, Hilkens J, Mooi W. NCAM and lung cancer. Int J Cancer 1994; 8:34–37.
15. Pujol JL, Simony J, Laurent JC, Richer G, Bousquet J, Godard Ph, Mary H, Michel FB. Phenotypic heterogeneity studied by immunohistochemistry and aneuploidy in non-small cell lung cancers. Cancer Res 1989; 49:2797–802.

16. Broers JLV, Rot MK, Oostendorp T, Huysmans A, Wagenaar SS, Wiersma-van Tilburg AJM, Vooijs P, Ramaekers FCS. Immunohistochemical detection of human lung heterogeneity using antibodies to epithelial, neuronal and neuroendocrine antigens. Cancer Res 1987; 47:3225–3234.

17. Hirsch FR, Matthews MJ, Aisner S, Campobasso O, Elema JD, Gazdar AF, Mackay B, Naseill M, Shimosato Y, Steele RH, Yesner R, Zettergren L. Histopathologic classification of small cell lung cancer. Cancer 1988; 62:973–977.

18. Brereton, HD, Mathews MM, Costa J, Kent CH, Johnson RE. Mixed anaplastic small cell and squamous cell carcinoma of the lung. Ann Intern Med 1978; 88:805–806.

19. Brambilla E, Moro D, Gazzeri S, Brichon PY, Nagy-Mignotte H, Morel F, Jacrot M, C Brambilla. Cytotoxic chemotherapy induces cell differentiation in small cell lung carcinoma. J Clin Oncol 1991; 9:50[6]1.

20. Roggli VL, Vollmer RT, Greenberg SD, McGavran MH, Spjut HJ, Yesner R. Lung cancer heterogeneity: a blinded and randomized study of 100 consecutive cases. Human Pathol 1985; 16:569–579.

21. Yesner R, Carter D. Pathology of carcinoma of the lung. Changing patterns. Clin Chest Med 1982; 3:257–89.

22. Gould VE, Linnoila RI, Memoli VA, Warren WH. Biology of disease: neuroendocrine components of the bronchopulmonary tract: hyperplasias, dysplasias and neoplasms. Lab Invest 1983; 49:519–37.

23. Radice PA, Matthews MJ, Ihde DC, et al. The clinical behavior of "mixed' small cell/large cell bronchogenic carcinoma compared to "pure" small cell subtypes. Cancer 1982; 50: 2894–902.

24. Tubiana M. The growth and progression of human tumors: implications for management strategy. Radiother Oncol 1986; 6:167–84.

25. Nicolson GL. Tumor cell instability, diversification, and progression to the metastatic phenotype: from oncogene to oncofetal expression. Cancer Res 1987; 47:1473–87.

26. Berendsen HH, De Leij L, Poppema S, et al. Clinical characterization of non-small cell lung cancer and tumors showing neuroendocrine differentiation features. J Clin Oncol 1989; 7:1614–20.

27. Kibbelaar RE, Moolenaar KEC, Michalides RJAM, et al. Neural cell adhesion molecule expression, neuroendocrine differentiation and prognosis in lung carcinoma. Eur J Cancer 1991; 27:431–5.

28. Pujol JL, Simony J, Demoly P, Charpentier R, Laurent JC, Daurès JP, Lehmann M, Guyot V, Godard P, Michel FB. Neural cell adhesion molecule and prognosis of surgically resected lung cancer. Am Rev Respir Dis 1993; 148:1071–1075.

29. Broers JLV, Klein Rot M, Oostendorp M, Belpler G, De Leij L, Carney DN, Vooijs GP, Raemakers FCS. Spontaneous changes in intermediated filament protein expression patterns in lung cancer cell lines. J Cell Sci 1988; 91:91–100.

30. Doyle LA, Borges M, Hssain A, Elias A, Tomiyasu T. An adherent sub-line of a unique small cell lung cancer cell line down regulates antigens of the neural cell adhesion molecule. J Clin Invest 1991; 86:1848–1854.

31. Mabry M, Nakagawa R, Nelkin BD, McDowell E, Gesell M, Eggleston JC, Casero RAJ, Baylin SB. v-Ha-ras-oncogene insertion: a model for tumor progression of human small cell lung cancer. Proc Natl Acad Sci (Wash.) 1988; 85:6523–6527.

32. Scheidegger PE, Sternberg LR, Roth J, Lowe JB. A human STX cDNA confers polysialic acid expression in mammalian cells. J Biol Chem 1995; 270:22685–22688.

33. Yang P, Major D, Rutishauser U. Role of charge and hydration in effects of polysialic acid on molecular interactions on and between cell membranes. J Biol Chem 1994; 269:23039–23044.

34. Carbone DP, Koros AMC, Linnoila RI, Jewett P, Gazdar AF. Neural cell adhesion molecule expression and messenger RNA splicing patterns in lung cancer cell lines are correlated with neuroendocrine phenotype and growth morphology. Cancer Res 1991; 51:6142–49.

35. Takamatsu K, Auerbach B, Gerardy-Schahn R, Eckhardt M, Jacques G, Madry N. Characterization of tumor-associated neural cell adhesion molecule in human serum. Cancer Res 1994; 54:2598–2603.

27

Tumor Markers: Clinical Meaning and Use

GIANFRANCO BUCCHERI

Azienda Ospedaliera "S.Croce e Carle"
Cuneo, Italy

I. Introduction

Neoplastic cells produce and release several substances. Some molecules are tumor-specific and can be produced by few or several types of cancer. Other substances are produced by tumor cells in larger amounts than normal cells. Occasionally, normal cells release abnormal quantities of their products in response to the invasion of cancer cells. Independent of the mechanism of production, an array of biological substances "marks" the existence, response, or progression of certain types of cancer. Such substances are called "tumor markers."

Although the term tumor marker is sometimes more broadly defined to include any tumor cell-surface antigen, intracellular protein, and even chromosomal and genetic abnormalities detectable in a tumor pathologic specimen, in this chapter the word "tumor marker" refers to substances that are present in the blood of patients with cancer and suitable for an easy and inexpensive serum test.

Several characteristics define an ideal tumor marker:

It should be produced preferentially by tumor cells and readily detectable in body fluids.
It should not be present in health or in benign diseases.

It should be present frequently enough and early enough in the development of a malignancy to be useful in screening for that cancer.

Its quantity in the blood should directly reflect the bulk of the tumor and yet be detectable when the tumor is in a subclinical phase.

It should correlate with the results of anticancer therapy and the ultimate prognosis.

Tumor markers are of significance not only to the researcher in developing theories concerning the biology of the malignant process, but also to the clinician in the management of patients with cancer. For example, they may be useful in the diagnosis and histopathologic classifications, as well as in staging, prognostication, and therapy monitoring (including the evaluation of tumor response and early relapse). Well-known examples of clinically useful markers are amines in carcinoids and pheochromocytomas, and the M-component in myeloma. In recent years, human chorionic gonadotropin and α-fetoprotein have contributed significantly to the diagnosis and treatment of germ cell tumors, including testicular cancer.

II. Roles of Lung Tumor Markers

The expression of lung tumor markers has been known for many years (1–3). However, new information produced during the last decade has radically changed our knowledge and practice (4–7). Lung tumor markers fall into several categories including oncofetal proteins, structural proteins, enzymes, membrane antigens, peptide and nonpeptide hormones, and other tumor-associated antigens. Table 1 outlines a possible classification and a list of the most popular markers for lung cancer.

Essentially, lung tumor markers play four potential roles in clinical practice: screening, diagnosis, assessing the stage of disease and prognosis, and monitoring anticancer therapy.

A. Screening

Screening involves the search for disease in asymptomatic individuals. The low frequency of patients with cancer in any asymptomatic population requires high validity of the measurement method. The value of a screening test for cancer involves an evaluation of its sensitivity. Because the prevalence of any one cancer in any one individual at a specific time is low, a marker that is found in a small percentage of patients with cancer is unlikely to be useful. The ideal marker is elevated in virtually all cases and in the early stages of malignancy. Most current markers are rarely elevated in early stages and cannot be used in this way. The specificity of a marker is also important. False-positive results appear unacceptable from the ethical and economical point of view because the clinical confirmation of positive results is usually invasive. Unfortunately, no tumor marker is sensitive enough or reliably specific enough to be used as a screen. A follow-up study of lung cancer occurrence was done in individuals who had health examinations during a large-scale Finnish health

Table 1 Working Classification of Lung Tumor Markers

Classification	Tumor marker	Refs.
Oncofetal proteins	Carcinoembryonic antigen (CEA)	8–25
Structural proteins (cytokeratins)	Tissue polypeptide antigen (TPA)	10–12,14,23,26–35
	Cytoketarin 19 fragment (Cyfra 21–1)	23,24,33,36–46
	Tissue polypeptide-specific antigen (TPS)	33,42,47
Enzymes	Neuron-specific enolase (NSE)	8,16–19,23,24,34,48–59
	Lactate dehydrogenase (LDH)	10,18,19,59–61
	Creatin-phosphokinase isoenzyme BB (CPK-BB)	16,48,62
Membrane antigens	Neural cell adhesion molecule (NCAM)	62
	Soluble interleukin-2 receptors (sIL2-R)	63–68
Hormones	β-HCG	10,25
	Gastrin-releasing peptide (GRP)	69
Other tumor-associated antigens	Squamous cell carcinoma antigen (SCC-Ag)	9,13,21,23,24,70–73
	CA 125	13,74–77
	CA 19–9	
	CA 242	78
	CA 15–3	24
	Chromogranin A	18,79–81
	Ferritin	14,82,83

survey (17). Four lung tumor markers were measured in serum specimens collected. Assuming a cancer prevalence of 1%, the best results would include 50 false-positive results, 8 false-negative results, and only 2 true-positive results (17). Since the real prevalence of lung cancer in a population of healthy smokers is definitely lower, these figures show the inefficiency and impracticability of measuring markers in screening.

B. Diagnosis

The identification of a tumor marker that is highly sensitive and specific and that can be used reliably to support the diagnosis of lung cancer remains an important goal of clinical research on tumor markers. The definite diagnosis of bronchogenic carcinoma is cytological or histopathological. However, one could ask: Is the elevation of any one marker so specific for lung cancer that its presence is highly suggestive for the diagnosis? Is any combination of markers diagnostic? In only a very few narrowly defined clinical settings is the answer yes. Clearly, the presence of suspect clinical signs, appropriate radiological evidence, and highly elevated levels of certain tumor markers in the blood is strongly suggestive for malignancy and recommends further clinical testing. Gail et al. (84,85) used eight tumor markers in an attempt to distinguish subjects with chronic pulmonary obstructive disease from those affected by lung cancer. Taking into account a disease prevalence of 30%, the best combination of markers (CEA, ferritin, and sialic acid) yielded an acceptable positive predictive value (60%), a sensitivity of 36%, and an almost absolute specificity. These data confirm that the pathological elevation of one or more markers, in an appropriate clinical setting, may be virtually diagnostic of lung cancer.

C. Staging and Prognosis

The third recurrent question, and perhaps the most important, is whether the level of the marker correlates with the stage and prognosis. Lung tumor markers will most likely be elevated in patients with advanced stages of disease. In some cases, the correlation is too close to allow excluding the surgical cure if the plasmatic level of the marker exceeds a given threshold (28). Therefore, while lung tumor markers are poor tools for screening of asymptomatic patients and may be moderately useful in the differentiation between cancer and nonmalignant lung disorders, their elevation is particularly useful in the evaluation of the extent of disease, leading to a more intense search for metastatic disease. In this sense, those markers whose level of elevation directly reflects tumor mass are mostly useful. At least three classes of tumor markers [CEA, the cytokeratin-derived markers TPA and Cyfra 21–1 in non–small-cell lung cancer (NSCLC), and NSE in small-cell lung cancer (SCLC)] respond to the above-mentioned prerequisite (5–7).

Marker elevations may correlate with the prognosis, but this is usually inseparable from tumor mass. However, there are examples in which the correlation with the prognosis reflects directly the malignant potential of the marker-producing population of cells (86).

D. Monitoring Therapy

The fourth issue concerning the clinical use of lung tumor markers is postsurgical surveillance or the follow-up of patients undergoing medical treatments. Marker elevations may correlate with patients' posttreatment status, as a reflection of their correlation with tumor mass. Because all the markers reported have both false-negative and false-positive results, they cannot be completely relied on when used to monitor the course of disease. Difficulties are due to the heterogeneity of marker expression among different tumors and, additionally, among cancer cells within the same tumor. All studies of markers include subsets of patients whose tumors do not or will never produce the marker. At the time of cancer recurrence, that population is included and may contribute to the false-negative rate. In addition, variations in marker expression between primary and metastatic lesions may develop because of the multiclonal process of cancer progression. Finally, the efficacy of therapy is as important in determining the value of a tumor marker as its sensitivity and specificity. If therapy is entirely inadequate, then it is irrelevant that a tumor marker may help to discover clinically silent postoperative recurrences or to recognize rare and short-lasting responses to chemotherapy. This occurs often (but not always) in lung cancer (87–90).

In monitoring therapy, however, CEA, cytokeratin degradation products, and NSE are the most useful markers (5–7).

III. Main Tumor Markers

In this section, the focus will be on tumor markers whose clinical utility is certain and quantitatively important.

A. Carcinoembryonic Antigen

Carcinoembryonic antigen (CEA) is an oncofetal protein normally found in the embryonic and fetal gut and sometimes produced by malignant cells. CEA was discovered in 1965 by Gold and Freedman in patients with adenocarcinoma of the colon (91,92). Carcinoembryonic antigen is normally present in the body fluids during the fetal life, occurs at low concentrations in adults, and circulates in high concentrations in patients with epithelial tumors (93). Abnormally elevated values of CEA are usually observed in malignant tumors of the gastrointestinal tract and of other sites, including breast, bronchus, urethelium, ovary, uterus and cervix (5). Soon after its discovery, a role of CEA as a nonspecific marker for malignancy was postulated and soon recognized. A consensus conference held at the National Institute of Health in 1980 (94) concluded its work with the following statements:

1. The use of plasma CEA assays in cancer screening of an asymptomatic population is unjustified.
2. In symptomatic patients, grossly raised values, greater than 5–10 times the upper limit of the normal range, should be considered strongly suspected for the presence of cancer and should suggest further diagnostic tests.
3. A preoperative plasma CEA value should be obtained in patients with either colorectal or bronchial carcinoma because of its correlation with the stage of disease and the prognosis.
4. The role of regular and sequential assays of plasma CEA in the postoperative and therapeutic monitoring of patients with other cancers is less convincing than it is for colorectal cancer. However, in patients with lung cancer it may be of value in reflecting response to chemotherapy.

Raised CEA concentrations may be detected in cigarette smokers, in patients with benign neoplasms, and in 15–20% of subjects with inflammatory disorders such as ulcerative colitis, pancreatitis, liver disease, and pulmonary infections (94). When measured in healthy asymptomatic individuals, CEA does not provide adequate means for lung cancer screening (17). In patients affected by lung cancer, abnormally elevated values of the marker can be found in 30–70% of the sample, with the lower sensitivity in early stage cancers (10–12,16,19,20,23,32). Elevated CEA levels are particularly common in adenocarcinoma cell types (8,21,32), however, they can be found in any histologic type, including 20–60% of patients with SCLC (16,19,20). Therefore, the practical use of this marker for diagnosis of cancer and histological discrimination is limited.

Studies published in the last decade have offered additional support to increased CEA levels occurring more frequently in advanced cancers (10,20), although reported differences were not always statistically significant (11,18). Also the correlation between plasmatic CEA and the response to treatment was further confirmed both in SCLC (18,20) and NSCLC (10). Today, the prognostic significance of CEA is almost certain (thousands of patients and six large studies provide corroborating information on the antigen), rather weak (not confirmed in any study with limited statistical power), and probably not independent of other prognostic factors (the marker was never found significant in any multivariate analysis using more than six variables) (86).

CEA is currently used as the "gold standard" or the "historic reference" for the evaluation of new potentially useful marker substances, or, within panels of markers, to increase the diagnostic yield of a single marker determination.

B. Tissue Polypeptide Antigen

The cytoskeleton is a complex network of cytoplasmic filaments that influence the dynamic morphology of all eukaryotic cells in their tissue environment (95). The cytoskeleton is composed of three types of filamentous structures: microfilaments (7–9.5 nm in diameter), microtubules (25 nm), and intermediate filaments (10–12 nm) (95). Cytokeratins are the major components of the intermediate filaments (96). Cytokeratins may be divided into 20 different types, according to molecular weight and isoelectric point (97). The cytokeratin family is expressed by all epithelial cells and might be a useful marker of epithelial differentiation (97–100). The expression of a single cytokeratin or a combination of certain cytokeratins is typical of a specific tissue. For example, cytokeratins 7 and 8 are highly expressed in the epithelium of the trachea and urethelium (33). Cytokeratin fragments are soluble and can be measured in serum and in other body fluids.

Nearly half a century ago, Björklund, moving from the observation that different tumor tissues resemble each other as they progress, supposed that all malignant tumors might contain a common antigenic principle. The antigen could be obtained by mixing many different tumors and by producing an immune serum against the mixture (101–103). With the introduction of cell culture techniques in vitro and the development of cytotoxicity inhibition methods, the idea of a common cancer antigenicity was experimentally verified (102). This property was found associated with an insoluble part of the cancer cells, from which a purified protein complex was isolated. The substance, tissue polypeptide antigen (TPA), was stereochemically characterized and detected in the serum, urine, and other human body fluids by hemoagglutination inhibition techniques and then by radioimmunological methods (104). Experimental data by Luning and Nilsson (105) helped to clarify the possible origin of TPA, being consistent with a sequence homology between TPA and the cytokeratins (105). Today, TPA is identified in a complex of fragments of the cytokeratins 8, 18, and 19 (106).

As a clinical marker of malignancy, TPA has never been as popular as the simultaneously discovered CEA. After its discovery and characterization (101–103), interest declined. Most review papers in the early 1980s did not include this complex substance in the list of the potentially useful markers (107). Only during the last decade has the interest in TPA been vitalized and several relevant studies published (Table 1).

TPA has been found in practically every tested human malignant tumor (autopsy) (104). Elevated concentrations of serum TPA have been observed in patients with different types of cancer and found to correlate with important clinical parameters, such as the burden of tumor, its proliferating activity, and the consequent prognosis (12,31,108–111). In lung cancer, studies of large and nonselected populations showed sensitivity rates between 51 and 85%, with no clear preference for a specific cell type (112). The incidence of false-positive tests in patients affected by benign diseases was between 2 and 10% (112). In patients with confirmed lung cancer, the pretreatment level of TPA correlated positively with either the primary tumor characteristics, the nodal involvement, or the type and grade of the metastatic spread (113–116). During the follow-up, sequential measurements of TPA correlated well with the clinical status of patients as assessed by the categories of response to treatment (115–117). TPA was also an effective prognostic indicator: eight studies with several hundred patients showed that this marker correlated with the clinical outcome, even when many other prognostic factors were taken into account (86).

Between 1986 and 1987, a clinical evaluation of a panel of serum markers including CEA, TPA, human chorionic gonadotropin β-subunit, lactate dehydrogenase, and the carbohydrate antigenic determinant 19–9 was reported (10,11). It was concluded that TPA was of real clinical utility, even more useful than CEA and the other measured substances (11). Measurements of TPA were continued in any patient with lung cancer, and this made it possible to reevaluate and periodically confirm the earlier findings (12,26–29,118). Recently, the clinical yield of TPA was determined in either the pretreatment assessment of operability (28) or the follow-up evaluation of the status of disease (29). The diagnostic yield of TPA was compared with either a baseline clinical-radiological evaluation or a multiorgan computed tomographic assessment. Using appropriate threshold values of TPA, surgical resectability (28) and objective responses to treatment (29) could be predicted with the same accuracy as the most conventional techniques.

C. Cytokeratin 19 Fragments

Cytokeratin 19 fragments (Cyfra 21–1) is a new cytoskeleton marker. Cytokeratin 19 is an acidic (type I) subunit with a low molecular weight (40 kDa) (99). It is expressed and immunohistochemically detectable in the cytoplasm of epithelial tumor cells, including bronchial cancer (98,99). Cytokeratin 19 fragments may be released in the blood because of cell lysis and tumor necrosis. They can be measured by a new immunoradiometric assay, using two mouse monoclonal antibodies, KS 19–1 and BM 19–21 (119).

The Cyfra 21–1 test is less than 5 years old, but the evidence concerning its clinical significance is already abundant (Table 1). Eventually, it could be recognized as the best lung tumor marker available (6,7). Cyfra 21–1 is closely related to TPA, sharing with this marker a common antigenic determinant (i.e., cytokeratin 19) (35). Such a close relationship has been confirmed clinically in a series of 50 lung cancer patients assayed simultaneously for TPA and Cyfra 21–1, in which the amazing index of correlation of 0.81 was reported (35). Therefore, like TPA, Cyfra 21–1 has been found:

1. Elevated in all cell types of lung cancer (although it is more sensitive in NSCLC, and especially in squamous cell cancer) (24,33,36,38,39,43,77)
2. More sensitive in the advanced stages of disease because of its correlation with tumor mass (24,33,36,39,43,77)
3. Useful in monitoring the course of disease and in the surveillance of post-surgical relapse (35,39)

The plasmatic levels of both Cyfra 21–1 and TPA were determined in 50 normal subjects and in 118 lung cancer patients (120). All patients had pathologically diagnosed lung cancer and different anatomical involvement (ranging from stage I to stage IV, UICC classification) (121).

Marker assays were performed using commercial kits provided by the CIS Bio-international, Gif/Yvette, France (Cyfra 21–1) and the AB Sangtec Medical Co., Bromma, Sweden (TPA). Reference values were up to 1.02 ng/ml (Cyfra 21–1) and 100 U/L (TPA).

In patients with NSCLC, the overall sensitivity of Cyfra 21–1 and TPA was identical (67%). Figure 1 shows the sensitivity of Cyfra 21–1 and TPA according to the cell type (squamous cell vs. adenocarcinoma) and the stage of disease. TPA was somewhat more sensitive than Cyfra 21–1 in squamous cell types (79% vs. 72%). In stage I, the sensitivity of Cyfra 21–1 was 47% and the sensitivity of TPA 57%; in stage II, Cyfra 21–1 and TPA sensitivity rates were 60% and 72%, respectively; in stage IIIa, corresponding figures were 62% and 53%; in stage IIIb, 91% and 75%; and in stage IV, 80% and 82%. All of these differences were not statistically significant. Tables 2 and 3 show the median values of Cyfra 21–1 and TPA, respectively, according to the cell type and the stage of disease. Cyfra 21–1 and TPA levels were higher in squamous cell cancer than in adenocarcinoma as well as in stages IIIb and IV (all differences were statistically significant).

Sixty-four patients had a concurrent determination of TPA and Cyfra 21–1. As previously observed (35), the correlation between the two markers was high (Fig. 2).

Univariate analyses of survival showed that patients with values of Cyfra 21–1 higher than 1.02 ng/ml (Fig. 3) and TPA above 100 U/L had reduced survivals. The prognostic significance of the two markers was further confirmed when patients

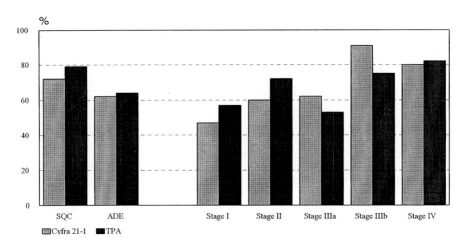

Figure 1 Sensitivity rates of Cyfra 21–1 and TPA in different cell types and stages of disease. (SQL = squamous cell lung cancer; ADE = adenocarcinoma.)

were stratified by stage of disease. In correlation with the Cyfra 21–1 levels, survival probabilities were significantly different for patients with limited disease (stage I, II, IIIa; $p = 0.01$) and also for subjects with metastatic or locally advanced cancers (stage IIIb, IV; $p = 0.007$). Similar differences were observed for TPA (stage I, II, IIIa; $p = 0.02$ and stage IIIb, IV; $p = 0.005$). Using Cox's multivariate analysis, however, only the stage of disease emerged as an independent factor of prognosis.

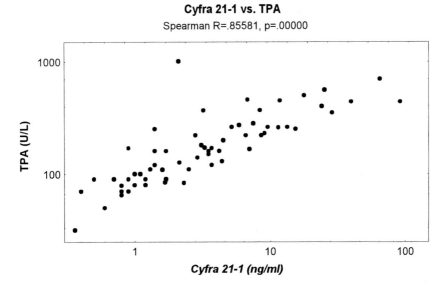

Figure 2 Correlation between Cyfra 21–1 and TPA.

Table 2 Median Values of Cyfra 21–1 and TPA in Different Cell Types

Isotype	No.	Cyfra*21–1 (ng/ml)		TPA** (U/L)	
		Median	Range	Median	Range
Unclassified	10	1.1	0.9–1.5	125	90–184
Squamous	53	6.7	0.9–11	250	123–340
Small-cell	12	2.5	1–3.5	120	84–160
Adenocarcinoma	37	2.1	0.7–2.4	160	80–325
Large-cell	6	1	0.5–1.2	110	100–125

Kruskall-Wallis $*p = 0.02$, $**p = 0.04$; range = interquartile range.

In conclusion, Cyfra 21–1 and TPA are closely related markers. Both provide similar if not identical information. Given its recent introduction, little information is available concerning the value of Cyfra 21–1 in long-term evaluations, especially in assessment of the prognosis. Because of this limitation, there is no justification in choosing Cyfra 21–1 assay rather than TPA, for which a body of knowledge exists covering any possible clinical application. Reformulating of conclusions may be necessary as mature data on Cyfra 21–1 become available.

D. Neuron-Specific Enolase

Enolases are glycolytic enzymes that convert 2-phopshoglycerate into phosphoenol-pyruvate. They occur as a series of dimeric isoenzymes made of three immunologi-cally distinct subunit (α, β, γ) (122,123). The α subunit is widely distributed. The β subunit is found mainly in the heart and other striated muscles. The γ subunit is called neuron-specific enolase (NSE) (124). NSE is restricted to neurones, periph-eral neuroendocrine tissue, and tumor of the APUD (amine precursor uptake and degradation system) cell series, the most important of which are small-cell lung can-cer and neuroblastoma (125–128).

Table 3 Median Values of Cyfra 21–1 and TPA in Different Stages of Disease

Stage	No.	Cyfra*21–1 (ng/ml)		TPA**(U/L)	
		Median	Range	Median	Range
I	24	1.3	0.5–2.1	90	80–143
II	25	1.4	0.6–4.9	160	60–260
IIIa	30	1.7	0.8–3.3	90	79–200
IIIb	14	3.5	2–12.5	165	120–300
IV	25	5.5	1.1–5.4	250	105–325

Kruskall-Wallis $*p = 0.002$, $**p = 0.04$; range = interquartile range.

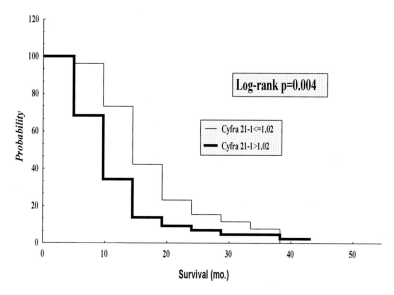

Figure 3 Probability of survival with normal and elevated levels of Cyfra 21–1.

It has been 15 years since Carney et al. (129) suggested NSE as a marker for SCLC, and considerable experience with this marker has been gained (Table 1). Cumulatively, an elevated pretreatment level of serum NSE has been reported in 10–20% of patients with NSCLC, 50–60% of patients with SCLC and limited disease, and 75–90% of patients with extensive SCLC. With cutoff levels of 10–15 ng/ml, the overall specificity is 75–95%, when series containing a large number of patients are included. Like CEA, TPA, and Cyfra 21–1, the real value of NSE resides in its capability to assess the extension of disease, to follow (and sometimes predict) the clinical course of disease, and to give important prognostic insights. NSE is an intracellular enzyme involved in energy production, and therefore the serum concentration of NSE may be a reflection of the cell turnover and death rate (19). NSE levels correlate positively with the pretreatment tumor mass (56,129,130), fall with the clinical response to chemotherapy, and rise again during tumor progression or relapse (57,129,130). Falling most often within the normal range, the levels of NSE seem unable to discriminate between complete and partial remissions (57). Sequential measurement of this marker may anticipate the clinical recognition of relapses (130,131). Daily serum determinations of NSE revealed a transient increase immediately after the start of the cytotoxic drug administration (tumor lysis syndrome), followed by a decrease to the normal level in complete or partial responders (57,132,133). This phenomenon seems to indicate tumor sensitivity to chemotherapy (48). In NSCLC, an initially raised NSE might be a predictor of response to chemotherapy (59).

With few exceptions (31,34), many studies suggest that NSE is an effective prognostic indicator in SCLC (16,31,49–52,58). However, data concerning the possible independence of this marker from other prognostic factors are still limited (86).

IV. Conclusion

Although computerized tomography (CT) scans provide excellent staging and follow-up data, they are expensive and time-consuming. Tumor markers that could be measured by blood tests would be highly desirable. In 1985 no such test was generally available, although neuron-specific enolase in small-cell lung cancer and carcinoembryonic antigen for all types of lung cancer were regarded as potential candidates (1). Today, both CEA and NSE, along with the new class of cytokeratin-derived markers, are convincible tools for staging and monitoring lung cancer. For one of these markers (i.e., TPA), the equivalence with CT has been proven (28,29). In future, the combined use of the single most useful markers (e.g., CEA and TPA in NSCLC and TPA and NSE in SCLC) should be optimized. Guidelines should also be elaborated for the clinical interpretation of results. It is time for a mandatory use of one or more of such markers in national and international therapy protocols.

References

1. Minna JD, Higgins GA, Glatstein EJ. Cancer of the lung. In: De Vita VT, Jr., Hellman S, Rosemberg SA, eds. Cancer. Principles and Practice of Oncology. 2d ed. Philadelphia: J.B. Lippincott Co., 1985:507–597.
2. Rasmuson T, Bjork GR, Dambe L. Tumor markers in bronchogenic carcinoma. Acta Radiol Oncol 1983; 22:209–214.
3. Yamaguchi K, Abe K, Adachi I. Peptide hormone production in primary lung tumors. Rec Res Cancer Res 1985; 99:107–116.
4. Reeve JG. Clinical and biological relevance of lung tumour markers. Diagn Oncol 1990; 1:305–315.
5. Ferrigno D, Buccheri G, Biggi A. Serum tumour markers in lung cancer: history, biology and clinical applications. Eur Respir J 1994; 7:186–197.
6. Niklinski J, Furman M. Clinical tumour markers in lung cancer. Eur J Cancer Prev 1995; 4:129–138.
7. Ferrigno D, Buccheri G. Clinical applications of serum markers for lung cancer. Respir Med 1995; 89:587–597.
8. Bergman B, Brezicka F-T, Engström C-P, Larsson S. Clinical usefulness of serum assays of neuron-specific enolase, carcinoembryonic antigen and CA-50 antigen in the diagnosis of lung cancer. Eur J Cancer [A] 1993; 29A:198–202.
9. Body JJ, Sculier JP, Raymakers N, Paesmans M, Ravez P, Libert P, et al. Evaluation of squamous cell carcinoma antigen as a new marker for lung cancer. Cancer 1990; 65:1552–1556.
10. Buccheri G, Violante B, Sartoris AM, Ferrigno D, Curcio A, Vola F. Clinical value of a multiple biomarker assay in patients with bronchogenic carcinoma. Cancer 1986; 57:2389–2396.
11. Buccheri G, Ferrigno D, Sartoris AM, Violante B, Vola F, Curcio A. Tumor markers in bronchogenic carcinoma: superiority of tissue polyptide antigen to carcinoembryonic antigen and carbohydrate antigenic determinant 19–9. Cancer 1987; 60:42–50.

12. Buccheri G, Ferrigno D, Vola F. Carcinoembryonic antigen (CEA), tissue polyptide antigen (TPA), and other prognostic indicators in the squamous cell carcinoma of the lung. Lung Cancer 1993; 10:21–33.
13. Diez M, Torres A, Maestro ML, Ortega MD, Gómez A, Pollán M, et al. Prediction of survival and recurrence by serum and cytosolic levels of CEA, CA125 and SCC antigens in resectable non-small-cell lung cancer. Br J Cancer 1996; 73:1248–1254.
14. Ferrigno D, Buccheri G. A comprehensive evaluation of serum ferritin levels in lung cancer patients. Lung Cancer 1992; 8:85–94.
15. Icard P, Regnard J-F, Essomba A, Panebianco V, Magdeleinat P, Levasseur P. Preoperative carcinoembryonic antigen level as a prognostic indicator in resected primary lung cancer. Ann Thorac Surg 1994; 58:811–814.
16. Jaques G, Bepler G, Holle R, Wolf M, Hannich T, Gropp C, et al. Prognostic value of pretreatment carcinoembryonic antigen, neuron-specific enolase, and creatine kinase-BB levels in sera of patients with small cell lung cancer. Cancer 1988; 62:125–134.
17. Järvisalo J, Hakama M, Knekt P, Stenman U-H, Leino A, Teppo L, et al. Serum tumor markers CEA, CA 50, TATI, and NSE in lung cancer screening. Cancer 1993; 71:1982–1988.
18. Johnson PWM, Joel SP, Love S, Butcher M, Pandian MR, Squires L, et al. Tumour markers for prediction of survival and monitoring of remission in small cell lung cancer. Br J Cancer 1993; 67:760–766.
19. Jorgensen LGM, Hansen HH, Cooper EH. Neuron specific enolase, carcinoembryonic antigen and lactate dehydrogenase as indicators of disease activity in small cell lung cancer. Eur J Cancer Clin Oncol 1989; 1:123–128.
20. Laberge F, Fritsche HA, Umsawasdi T, Carr DT, Welch S, Murphy WK, et al. Use of carcinoembryonic antigen in small cell lung cancer. Prognostic value and relation to the clinical course 1. Cancer 1987; 59:2047–2052.
21. Niklinski J, Furman M, Laudanski J, Kozlowski M. Prognostic value of pretreatment CEA, SCC-Ag and CA 19–9 levels in sera of patients with non-small cell lung cancer. Eur J Cancer Prev 1992; 1:401–406.
22. Picardo AL, Torres AJ, Maestro M, Ortega D, Garcia-Asenjo JA, Mugüerza JM, et al. Quantitative analysis of carcinoembryonic antigen, squamous cell carcinoma antigen, CA 125, and CA 50 cytosolic content in non-small cell lung cancer. Cancer 1994; 73:2305–2311.
23. Plebani M, Basso D, Navaglia F, De Paoli M, Tommasini A, Cipriani A. Clinical evaluation of seven tumour markers in lung cancer diagnosis: Can any combination improve the results? Br J Cancer 1995; 72:170–173.
24. Stieber P, Hasholzner U, Bodenmüller H, Nagel D, Sunder-Plassmann L, Dienemann H, et al. CYFRA 21–1: a new marker in lung cancer. Cancer 1993; 72:707–713.
25. Walop W, Chrétien M, Colman NC, Fraser RS, Gilbert F, Hidvegi RS, et al. The use of biomarkers in the prediction of survival in patients with pulmonary carcinoma. Cancer 1990; 65:2033–2046.
26. Buccheri G, Ferrigno D. Usefulness of tissue polypeptide antigen in staging, monitoring, and prognosis of lung cancer. Chest 1988; 93:565–569.
27. Buccheri G, Ferrigno D. Prognostic value of the tissue polyptide antigen in lung cancer. Chest 1992; 101:1287–1292.
28. Buccheri G, Ferrigno D. The tissue polypeptide antigen serum test in the preoperative evaluation of non-small cell lung cancer: Diagnostic yield and comparison with conventional staging methods. Chest 1995; 107:471–476.
29. Buccheri G, Ferrigno D. Monitoring lung cancer with tissue polyptide antigen: an ancillary, profitable serum test to evaluate treatment response and posttreatment disease status. Lung Cancer 1995; 13:155–168.
30. Correale M, Arnberg H, Blockx P, Bombardieri E, Castelli M, Encabo G, et al. Clinical profile of a new monoclonal antibody-based immunoassay for tissue polypeptide antigen. Int J Biol Markers 1994; 9:231–238.
31. Gronowitz JS, Bergstrom R, Nou E, Pahlman S, Brodin O, Nilsson S, et al. Clinical and serologic markers of stage and prognosis in small cell lung cancer. Cancer 1990; 66:722–732.

32. Mizushima Y, Hirata H, Izumi S, Hoshino K, Konishi K, Morikage T, et al. Clinical significance of the number of positive tumor markers in assisting the diagnosis of lung cancer with multiple tumor marker assay. Oncology 1990; 47:43–48.

33. Stieber P, Dienemann H, Hasholzner U, Fabricius PG, Schambeck C, Weinzierl M, et al. Comparison of CYFRA 21–1, TPA and TPS in lung cancer, urinary bladder cancer and benign diseases. Int J Biol Markers 1994; 9:82–88.

34. Van der Gaast A, Van Putten WL, Oosterom R, Cozijnsen M, Hoekstra R, Splinter TAW. Prognostic value of serum thymidine kinase, tissue polypetide antigen and neuron specific enolase in patients with small cell lung cancer. Br J Cancer 1991; 64:369–372.

35. Van der Gaast A, Kok TC, Kho GS, Blijenberg BG, Splinter TAW. Disease monitoring by the tumour markers Cyfra 21.1 and TPA in patients with non-small cell lung cancer. Eur J Cancer [A] 1995; 31A:1790–1793.

36. Bombardieri E, Seregni E, Bogni A, Ardit S, Belloli S, Busetto A, et al. Evaluation of cytokeratin 19 serum fragments (CYFRA 21–1) in patients with lung cancer: results of a multicenter trial. Int J Biol Markers 1994; 9:89–95.

37. Lai RS, Hsu HK, Lu JY, Ger LP, Lai NS. CYFRA 21–1 enzyme-linked immunosorbent assay—evaluation as a tumor marker in non-small cell lung cancer. Chest 1996; 109:995–1000.

38. Muraki M, Tohda Y, Iwanaga T, Uejima H, Nagasaka Y, Nakajima S. Assessment of serum CYFRA 21–1 in lung cancer. Cancer 1996; 77:1274–1277.

39. Niklinski J, Furman M, Chyczewska E, Chyczewski L, Rogowski F, Laudanski J. Diagnostic and prognostic value of the new tumour marker CYFRA 21–1 in patients with squamous cell lung cancer. Eur Respir J 1995; 8:291–294.

40. Niklinski J, Furman M, Burzykowski T, Chyczewski L, Laudanski J, Chyczewska E, et al. Preoperative CYFRA 21–1 level as a prognostic indicator in resected primary squamous cell lung cancer. Br J Cancer 1996; 74:956–960.

41. Pujol JL, Grenier J, Daures JP, Daver A, Pujol H, Michel FB. Serum fragment of cytocheratin subunit 19 measured by CYFRA 21–1 immunoradiometric assay as a marker of lung cancer. Cancer Res 1993; 53:61–66.

42. Pujol JL, Grenier J, Parrat E, Lehmann M, Lafontaine T, Quantin X, et al. Cytokeratins as serum markers in lung cancer: a comparison of CYFRA 21–1 and TPS. Am J Respir Crit Care Med 1996; 154:725–733.

43. Rastel D, Ramaioli A, Cornillie F, Thirion B. CYFRA 21–1, a sensitive and specific new tumour marker for squamous cell lung cancer. Report of the first European multicentre evaluation. Eur J Cancer [A] 1994; 30A:601–606.

44. Sugama Y, Kitamura S, Kawai T, Ohkubo A, Hasegawa S, Kuriyama T, et al. Clinical usefulness of CYFRA assay in diagnosing lung cancer: measurement of serum cytokeratin fragment. Jpn J Cancer Res 1994; 85:1178–1184.

45. Van der Gaast A, Schoenmakers CHH, Kok TC, Blijenberg BG, Cornillie F, Splinter TAW. Evaluation of a new tumour marker in patients with non-small-cell lung cancer: CIFRA 21–1. Br J Cancer 1994; 69:525–528.

46. Wieskopf B, Demangeat C, Purohit A, Stenger R, Gries P, Kreisman H, et al. Cyfra 21–1 as a biologic marker of non-small cell lung cancer: evaluation of sensitivity, specificity, and prognostic role. Chest 1995; 108:163–169.

47. Marino P, Buccheri G, Preatoni A, Ferrigno D, Luporini AC, Pravettoni G. Tissue polypeptide specific antigen (TPS) and objective response to treatment in solid tumors. Int J Biol Markers 1992; 7:65–67.

48. Ariyoshi Y, Kato K, Ueda R. Biological and clinical implication of neuron-specific enolase and creatine kinase BB in small cell lung cancer. Jpn J Clin Oncol 1986; 16:213–221.

49. Ferrigno D, Buccheri G, Cecchini C, Marchetti G. Clinical value of a multiple biomarker assay (CEA, TPA, NSE) in patients with SCLC. G I M T 1990; 44:135–140.

50. Harding M, McAllister J, Hulks G, Vernon D, Monie R, Paul J, et al. Neurone specific enolase (NSE) in small cell lung cancer: a tumour marker of prognostic significance? Br J Cancer 1990; 61:605–607.

51. Jorgensen LG, Osterlind K, Hansen HH, Cooper EH. The prognostic influence of serum neuron specific enolase in small cell lung cancer. Br J Cancer 1988; 58:805–807.
52. Jorgensen LG, Hirsch FR, Skov BG, Osterlind K, Cooper EH, Larsson LI. Occurrence of neuron specific enolase in tumour tissue and serum in small cell lung cancer. Br J Cancer 1991; 63:151–153.
53. Jorgensen LGM, Osterlind K, Hansen HH, Cooper EH. Serum neuron-specific enolase (S-NSE) in progressive small-cell lung cancer (SCLC). Br J Cancer 1994; 70:759–761.
54. Jorgensen LGM, Osterlind K, Genollá J, Gomm SA, Hernández JR, Johnson PWM, et al. Serum neuron-specific enolase (S-NSE) and the prognosis in small-cell lung cancer (SCLC): A combined multivariable analysis on data from nine centres. Br J Cancer 1996; 74: 463–467.
55. Milleron B, Cadranel J, Dominique S, Rosencher L, Akoun G. L'enolase neurono-specifique serique au cours des cancers bronchiques α petites cellules. Rev Mal Respir 1990; 46: 161–165.
56. Quoix E, Charloux A, Popin E, Pauli G. Inability of serum neuron-specific enolase to predict disease extent in small cell lung cancer. Eur J Cancer [A] 1993; 29A:2248–2250.
57. Splinter TAW, Cooper EH, Kho GS, Osterom R, Peake MD. Neuron specific enolase as a guide to the treatment of small cell lung cancer. Eur J Cancer Clin Oncol 1987; 23:171–176.
58. Szturmowicz M, Roginska E, Roszkowski K, Kwiek S, Filipecki S, Rowinska-Zakrzewska E. Prognostic value of neuron-specific enolase in small cell lung cancer. Lung Cancer 1993; 8:259–264.
59. Van Zandwijk N, Jassem E, Bonfrer JMG, Mooi WJ, Van Tinteren H. Serum neuron-specific enolase and lactate dehydrogenase as predictors of response to chemotherapy and survival in non-small cell lung cancer. Semin Oncol 1992; 19(suppl. 2):37–43.
60. Kohno N, Hamada H, Fujioka S, Hiwada K, Yamakido M, Akiyama M. Circulating antigen KL-6 and lactate dehydrogenase for monitoring irradiated patients with lung cancer. Chest 1992; 102:117–122.
61. Sagman U, Feld R, Evans WK, Warr D, Shepherd FA, Payne D, et al. The prognostic significance of pretreatment serum lactate dehydrogenase in patients with small-cell lung cancer. J Clin Oncol 1991; 9:954–961.
62. Jaques G, Auerbach B, Pritsch M, Wolf M, Madry N, Havemann K. Evaluation of serum neural cell adhesion molecule as a new tumor marker in small cell lung cancer. Cancer 1993; 72:418–425.
63. Buccheri G, Marino P, Preatoni A, Ferrigno D, Moroni GA. Soluble interleukin 2 receptor in lung cancer. An indirect marker of tumor activity? Chest 1991; 99:1433–1437.
64. Chan CHS, Ho J, Lai CKW, Leung JCK, Lai KN. Elevated serum levels of soluble interleukin-2 receptors in lung cancer and the effect of surgery. Respir Med 1993; 87: 383–385.
65. Ginns LC, Hoyos AD, Brown MC, Gaumond BR. Elevated concentrations of soluble interleukin-2 receptors in serum of smokers and patients with lung cancer. Am Rev Respir Dis 1990; 142:398–402.
66. Yamaguchi K, Nishimura Y, Kiyokawa T. Elevated serum levels of soluble interleukin-2 receptors in small cell lung cancer. J Lab Clin Med 1990; 116:457–461.
67. Poulakis N, Sarandakou A, Rizos D, Phocas I, Kontozoglou T, Polyzogopoulos D. Soluble interleukin-2 receptors and other markers in primary lung cancer. Cancer 1991; 68:1045–1049.
68. Tisi E, Lissoni P, Angeli M, Arrigoni C, Corno E, Cassina E, et al. Postoperative increase in soluble interleukin-2 receptor serum levels as predictor for early recurrence in non-small cell lung carcinoma. Cancer 1992; 69:2458–2462.
69. Takada M, Kusunoki Y, Masuda N, Matui K, Yana T, Ushijima S, et al. Pro-gastrin-releasing peptide(31–98) as a tumour marker of small-cell lung cancer: Comparative evaluation with neuron-specific enolase. Br J Cancer 1996; 73:1227–1232.
70. Sanchez De Cos J, Masa F, De la Cruz JL, Disdier C, Vergara C. Squamous cell carcinoma antigen (SCC Ag) in the diagnosis and prognosis of lung cancer. Chest 1994; 105:773–776.

71. Ebert W, Leichtweis B, Bulzebruck H, Drings P. The role of IMx SCC assays in the detection and prognosis of primary squamous-cell carcinoma of the lung. Diagn Oncol 1992; 2:203–210.

72. Ebert W, Muley T, Drings P. Does the assessment of serum markers in patients with lung cancer aid in the clinical decision making process? Anticancer Res 1996; 16:2161–2168.

73. Mino N, Atsushi I, Hamamoto K. Availability of tumor-antigen 4 as a marker of squamous cell carcinoma of the lung and other organs. Cancer 1988; 62:730–734.

74. Diez M, Cerdan FJ, Ortega MD, Torres A, Picardo A, Balibrea JL. Evaluation of serum CA 125 as a tumor marker in non-small cell lung cancer. Cancer 1991; 67:150–154.

75. Diez M, Torres A, Pollán M, Gomez A, Ortega D, Maestro ML, et al. Prognostic significance of serum CA 125 antigen assay in patients with non-small cell lung cancer. Cancer 1994; 73:1368–1376.

76. Kimura Y, Fujii T, Hamamoto K, Miyagawa N, Kataoka M, Iio A, et al. Serum CA125 level is a good prognostic indicator in lung cancer. Br J Cancer 1993;

77. Molina R, Agusti C, Mañe JM, Filella X, Jo J, Joseph J, et al. CYFRA 21–1 in lung cancer: Comparison with CEA, CA 125, SCC and NSE serum levels. Int J Biol Markers 1994; 9:96–101.

78. Pujol J-L, Cooper EH, Lehmann M, Purves DA, Dan-Aouta M, Midander J, et al. Clinical evaluation of serum tumour marker CA 242 in non-small cell lung cancer. Br J Cancer 1993; 67:1423–1429.

79. Bergh J, Arnberg H, Eriksson B, Lundquist G. The release of chromogranin A and B like activity from human lung cancer cell lines: a potential marker for a subset of small cell lung cancer. Acta Oncol 1989; 5:651–654.

80. O'Connor DT, Deftos LJ. Secretion of chromogranin A a by peptide-producing endocrine neoplasms. N Engl J Med 1986; 314:1145–1151.

81. Sobol RE, O'Connor DT, Addison J, Suchocki K, Roiston I, Deftos LJ. Elevated serum chromogranin A concentration in small-cell lung carcinoma. Ann Intern Med 1986; 105:698–700.

82. Cox R, Gyde OH, Leyland MJ. Serum ferritin levels in small cell lung cancer. Eur J Cancer Clin Oncol 1986; 22:831–835.

83. Muller T, Marshall RJ, Cooper EH, Watson DA, Walker DA, Mearns AJ. The role of serum tumour markers to aid the selection of lung cancer patients for surgery and the assessment of prognosis. Eur J Cancer Clin Oncol 1985; 21:1461–1466.

84. Gail MH, Muenz L, McIntire KR. Multiple markers for lung cancer diagnosis: validation of models for advanced lung cancer. J Natl Cancer Inst 1986; 76:805–816.

85. Gail MH, Muenz L, McIntire KR. Multiple markers for lung cancer diagnosis: validation of models for localized lung cancer. J Natl Cancer Inst 1988; 80:97–101.

86. Buccheri G, Ferrigno D. Prognostic factors in lung cancer: tables and comments. Eur Respir J 1994; 7:1350–1364.

87. Haraf DJ, Devine S, Ihde DC, Vokes EE. The evolving role of systemic therapy in carcinoma of the lung. Semin Oncol 1992; 19(suppl. 11):72–87.

88. Ihde DC. Drug therapy: Chemotherapy of lung cancer. N Engl J Med 1992; 327:1434–1441.

89. Shepherd FA. Current review: induction chemotherapy for locally advanced non-small cell lung cancer. Ann Thorac Surg 1993; 55:1585–1592.

90. Edelman MJ, Gandara DR, Roach M, Benfield JR. Multimodality therapy in stage III non-small cell lung cancer. Ann Thorac Surg 1996; 61:1564–1572.

91. Gold P, Freedman SO. Demonstration of tumor-specific antigenin in human colonic carcinomata by immunological tolerance and absorption techniques. J Exp Med 1965; 121:439–462.

92. Gold P, Freedman SO. Specific carcinoembryonic antigens of the human digestive system. J Exp Med 1965; 122:457–481.

93. Fletcher RH. Carcinoembryonic antigen. Ann Intern Med 1986; 104:66–73.

94. N.H.I. Carcinoembryonic antigen: its role as a marker in the management of cancer. Br Med J 1981; 282–373.

95. Luna EJ, Hitt AL. Cytoskeleton-plasma membrane interactions. Science 1992; 258: 955–963.
96. Lazarides E. Intermediate filaments as mechanical integrators of cellular space. Nature 1980; 283:249–256.
97. Debus E, Moll R, Franke WW, Weber K, Osborn M. Immunohistochemical distinction of human carcinomas by cytocheratin typing with monoclonal antibodies. Am J Pathol 1984; 114:121–130.
98. Moll R, Franke WW, Geiber B, Krepler R. The catalog of human cytocheratins: patterns of expression in normal epithelia, tumors and cultured cells. Cell 1982; 31:11–24.
99. Broers JLV, Ramaekers FCS, Rot MK, Oostendorp T, Huysmans A, Muijen GNP, et al. Cytocheratins in different types of human lung cancer as monitored by chain-specific monoclonal antibodies. Cancer Res 1988; 48:3221–3229.
100. Osborn M, Weber K. Intermediate filaments: cell-type-specific markers in differentiation and pathology. Cell 1982; 21:303–306.
101. Bjorklund B. Serological analysis of human cancer antigen. In: Anonymous Proceedings: VI Internat. Congres. Microbiol. Rome: 1953:344.
102. Bjorklund B, Bjorklund V. Antigenicity of pooled human malignant and normal tissues by cytoimmunological technique: presence of an insoluble, heat-labile tumor antigen. Int Arch Allergy 1957; 10:153–184.
103. Bjorklund B, Lundblad G, Bjorklund V. Antigenicity of pooled human malignant and normal tissues by cytoimmunological technique: II. Nature of tumor antigen. Int Arch Allergy 1958; 12:241–261.
104. Bjorklund B, Bjorklund V, Wiklund B, Lundstrom R, Ekdahl PH, Harbard L, et al. A human tissue polypeptide related to cancer and placenta: I. preparation and properties, II. Assay technique, III. Clinical studies of 1483 individuals with cancer and other conditions. In: Bjorklund B, editor. Immunological Techniques for Detection of Cancer. Stockholm: Bonniers, 1973:133–187.
105. Luning B, Nilsson U. Sequence homology between tissue polypeptide antigen (TPA) and intermediate filament (IF) proteins. Acta Chem Scand 1983; B 37:731–733.
106. Bjorklund B. Tissue polypeptide antigen (TPA): biology, biochemistry, improved assay methodology, clinical significance in cancer and other conditions, and future outlook. In: Schonfeld H, ed. Laboratory Testing for Cancer. Vol. 22. Basel: Karger, 1978:16–31.
107. Coombes RC, Powels TJ. Tumour markers in the management of human cancer. In: Deeley TJ, ed. Topical Reviews in Radiotherapy and Oncology. Bristol: Wright PGS, 1982:39.
108. Buccheri G, Parachini F, Perroni D, Bumma C. Tissue polypeptide antigen (TPA) correlates with tumor load in breast cancer (BC). Cancer Chemother Pharmacol 1989; 23 (suppl 1):C 53 Abstract.
109. Nemoto T, Constantine R, Chu TM. Human tissue polypeptide antigen in breast cancer. J Natl Cancer Inst 1979; 63:1347–1350.
110. Adolphs HD, Oher P. Significance of plasma tissue polypeptide antigen determination for the diagnosis and follow-up of urethelial bladder cancer. Urol Res 1984; 12:125–128.
111. Kew MC, Berger EL. The value of serum concentrations of tissue polypeptide antigen in the diagnosis of hepatocellular carcinoma. Cancer 1986; 58:868–872.
112. Rapellino M, Pecchio F, Baldi S, Scappaticci E, Cavallo A. Clinical utility of tissue polypeptide antigen determination in lung cancer management. Anticancer Res 1995; 15:1065–1070.
113. De Angelis G, Cipri A, Flore F, Munno R, Pau F, Pigorini F. Valutazione dei titoli plasmatici dell'antigene carcinoembrionario (CEA) e dell'antigene polipeptidico tissutale (TPA) in 158 soggetti normali e in 140 pazienti con carcinoma polmonare primitivo (summary in english). Min Pneumol 1985; 24:31–33.
114. Pau F, De Angelis G, Antilli A, Cruciani AR, Cipri A, Pigorini F. Valore prognostico dell'antigene carcinoembrionario (CEA) e dell'antigene polipeptidico tissutale (TPA) nel cancro polmonare primitivo 'non-small cell' (summary in English). Min Pneumol 1985; 24:27–29.

115. Volpino P, Cangemi V, Caputo V. Clinical usefulness of serum TPA (tissue polypeptide antigen) in postsurgical diagnosis, prognosis, and follow-up of lung cancer. J Nucl Med Allied Sci 1985; 29:241–244.

116. Luthgens M, Schlegel M. Verlaufskontrolle bei Bronchialkarzinomen mit Tissue Polypeptide Antigen und carcinoembrionalem Antigen (summary in English). Tumor Diagn Therap 1985; 6:1–7.

117. Schultek T, Wiessmann KJ, Braun J, Wood WG. Karzinoembryonales antigen (CEA) und Tissue Polypeptide Antigen (TPA) in der Diagnose des kleinzelligen und nicht-kleinzelligen Bronchialkarzinoms (summary in English). Prax Klin Pneumol 1985; 39:962–966.

118. Ferrigno D, Buccheri G, Rendine S. The prognostic value of CEA and TPA in the initial evaluation of lung cancer: results of a multivariate analysis of 312 patients. In: Motta G, ed. Lung Cancer: Advanced Concepts and Present Status. Genova: IASLG, 1989:179–188.

119. Bodenmuller H, Banauch D, Ofenloch B, Jaworek D, Dessauer A. Technical evaluation of a new automated tumor marker assay: the Enzymun-Test CYFRA 21–1. In: Klapdor R, ed. Tumor Associated Antigens, Oncogenes, Receptors, Cytokines in Tumor Diagnosis and Therapy. Zuckschwerdt Verlag 1992:137–138.

120. Lequaglie C, Ravasi G, Buccheri G, Ferrigno D, Maioli C, Marino P. Cyfra 21–1 compared with TPA in lung cancer—Results of a multicentric study. Chest 1995; 108 (suppl):198s Abstract.

121. UICC. TNM Classification of Malignant Tumours. 4th ed. Berlin: Springer-Verlag, 1987.

122. Rider CC, Taylor CB. Enolase isoenzyme in rat tissue. Electrophoretic, chromatographic, and kinetic properties. Biochim Biophys Acta 1974; 365:285–300.

123. Fletcher R, Rider CC, Taylor CB. Enolase isoenzymes. III. Chromatographic and immunological characteristics of rat brain enolase. Biochim Biophys Acta 1976; 452:245–252.

124. Schmechel D, Marangos PJ, Zis AP, Brightman M, Goodwin FK. The brain enolases as specific markers of neural and glial cells. Science 1978; 199:313–315.

125. Rider CC, Taylor CB. Evidence for a new form of enolase in rat brain. Biochim Biophys Res Commun 1975; 66:814–820.

126. Schmechel D, Marangos PJ, Brightman M. Neuron specific enolase is a molecular marker for peripheral and central neuroendocrine cells. Nature 1978; 276:834–836.

127. Warton J, Polak JM, Cole GA, Marangos PJ, Pearse AGE. Neuron-specific enolase as an immunocytochemical marker for the diffuse neuroendocrine system in human fetal lung. J Histochem Cytochem 1981; 29:1359–1364.

128. Tapia FJ, Polak JM, Barbosa AJA. Neuron-specific enolase is produced by neuroendocrine tumors. Lancet 1981; 1:808–811.

129. Carney DN, Marangos PJ, Ihde DC, Bunn PAJ, Cohen MH, Minna JD, et al. Serum neuron-specific enolase: a marker for disease extent and response to therapy of small-cell lung cancer. Lancet 1982; 1:583–585.

130. Johnson DH, Marangos PJ, Forbes JT. Potential utility of serum neuron-specific enolase levels in small cell carcinoma of the lung. Cancer Res 1984; 44:5409–5414.

131. Cooper EH, Splinter TAW, Brown DA, Muers M, Peake M, Pearson S. Evaluation of a radioimmunoassay for neuron specific enolase in small cell lung cancer. Br J Cancer 1985; 52:333–338.

132. Esscher T, Steinholz L, Bergh J, Nou E, Nilsson K, Pahlman S. Neuron specific enolase: a useful diagnostic serum marker for small cell carcinoma of the lung. Thorax 1985; 40:85–90.

133. Fukuoka M, Takada M, Kamei T. Serial measurements of serum carcinoembryonic antigen (CEA) and neuron-specific enolase (NSE) during chemotherapy of patients with inoperable lung cancer. Gan To Kagaku Ryoho 1987; 14:871–880.

28

The p53 Tumor Suppressor Gene: From Molecular Biology to Clinical Investigation

THIERRY SOUSSI

Institut Curie
Paris, France

I. Introduction

Mammalian cells respond to DNA-damaging agents by activating cell cycle checkpoints. These control mechanisms determine temporary arrest at a specific stage of the cell cycle to allow the cell to correct possible defects (1). At least two checkpoints monitor DNA damage: one at the G1/S transition and the other at the G2/M transition. The G1 checkpoint prevents replication of damaged DNA, whereas the G2/M transition is triggered by damaged and/or incompletely replicated DNA. Several findings have demonstrated that the product of the p53 tumor suppressor gene is responsible for the G1 checkpoint (2,3), and recent observations suggest that it may also play a role in regulating G2/M transition (4,5). In response to genotoxic stress, the levels of p53 protein increase and this increase either determines a transient arrest of cell cycle progression in the G1 phase or triggers apoptosis.

The arrest in G1 is thought to give the cells time to repair critical damage before DNA replication occurs, thereby avoiding the propagation of genetic lesions to progeny cells. The cell cycle can resume once the damage has been repaired. This growth arrest is, at least in part, mediated by transcriptional activation of p21WAF1/CIP1, which binds and inactivates the cyclin-dependent kinases required for cell progression (6). Accordingly, homozygous deletion of p21 in mouse embryonic fibroblasts or in human colon cancer cells partially or completely abrogates radiation-induced G1 arrest mediated by p53 (7,8).

The mechanism by which p53 stimulates apoptosis is largely unknown. Several genes linked to apoptosis, including bax (9) and Fas/APO-1 (10), are transactivated following p53 expression in some cell types, but whether the apoptotic properties of p53 are dependent on its sequence specific transcriptional activation properties is controversial (11,12).

The biochemical and genetic determinants that dictate which of the two pathways, death or arrest, will be chosen by a particular cell following p53 expression remain largely obscure.

In cells with no or mutated p53, DNA replication proceeds in the presence of a damaged template, thereby generating clones of genetically aberrant cells from which malignant clones may arise. Loss of the G1 checkpoint also results in genomic instability, as seen by the increase in the frequency of gene amplification in p53-defective cells (13,14). Based on such findings, it has been proposed and is now largely accepted that the main function of normal p53 is to preserve genome integrity by acting as the "guardian of the genome" (15).

Further insights into the role of p53 have come from the study of null animals that lack endogenous p53 genes as a result of targeted gene disruption (16). Mice homozygous for p53 null alleles have increased cancer predisposition, but are otherwise developmentally normal.

II. Association Between p53 Mutation and Human Cancer

Point mutations in the p53 gene have been found in most human cancers (17,18). More than 10,000 different tumors of various types have been analyzed for p53 alteration and have led to the identification of mutations in many cancer types (19). Their frequency varies from one type to another, but it is on the order of 45–50% for all cancer types (19). In general, these mutations are associated with a loss of the second allele of the gene. In certain specific types of cancer, p53 inactivation can be achieved through an epigenetic mechanism (see Ref. 20 for review). In cervical carcinoma, where the frequency of the p53 mutation is very low, p53 inactivation is considered to be due to the association of this cancer with human papillomavirus, which induces p53 protein degradation (21). In soft tissue sarcoma, overexpression of the cellular protein mdm-2 leads to functional inactivation of p53 via the formation of a p53-mdm-2 inactive complex (22).

Another potential mutation-independent mechanism of p53 inactivation involves abnormal cytoplasmic sequestration of wild-type p53 with concomitant nuclear exclusion. This phenotype is present in 37% of inflammatory breast carcinomas and over 97% of undifferentiated neuroblastomas (23,24). Recently, it has been shown that this translocation compromises the suppressor function of p53, suggesting that it plays a role in the tumorigenesis of these tumors (25).

III. Analysis of Alterations in the p53 Gene

A. Molecular Analysis

PCR followed by sequence analysis enables direct study of the type of mutational event that altered the gene. In over 90% of cases, this event is a point mutation that alters a single nucleotide among the 23,000 in the gene. Unlike the ras gene, for which only 3 of the 189 codons are targets of oncogenic mutations, in the p53 gene, mutations may occur in 90 of the 393 codons required for the synthesis of the protein. This high degree of heterogeneity makes diagnosis more difficult because the region to be analyzed extends over almost the entire gene. Thus, the molecular analysis of the p53 gene is somewhat tricky, and unsuited for routine diagnostic analysis. It is nonetheless essential for molecular epidemiological analyses in which it is important to determine the relationship between the type of cancer and the type of mutational event. Semidirect detection methods such as SSCP (single strand conformation polymorphism), DGGE (denaturant gradient gel electrophoresis), and CDGE (constant denaturant gel electrophoresis) may enable selection of the region of the gene to be analyzed. However, these methods are not 100% reliable (see Ref. 26 for comparison between SSCP and DGGE).

In the not-so-distant future, it is possible to imagine that new technical advances in sequencing methods (such as sequencing by hybridization on solid support) or in screening point mutations (such as ligase detection reaction) and associated techniques will permit routine molecular analysis.

B. Immunohistochemical Approach

One of the significant properties of mutant p53 proteins is their extended half-life. In normal cells, p53 is undetectable because it has an extremely short half-life (15–20 min). In transformed cells, the mutant protein is much more stable, with a half-life of 4–12 hours, and it accumulates in the nucleus. It is therefore possible to perform an immunocytochemical diagnosis (coupled with a histological analysis) in tumor tissue to directly visualize this nuclear accumulation. Such an approach has been used in many different types of cancer with a generally good correlation between molecular analysis (presence of a mutation) and immunohistochemical analysis (overexpression of the mutant protein) (27,28). The advantage of this approach is that it can be routinely used in histology laboratories. However, there are also a number of disadvantages, including the fact that any mutations that abolish p53 expression (splicing signal mutations, nonsense mutations, insertions, or deletions) do not produce the protein and therefore give a negative result. These types of mutations are found in 5–10% of cases. On the other hand, it is now known that tumors can accumulate p53 in the complete absence of mutations in any part of the gene. Since this accumulation is specific to tumor cells and does not affect normal tissue, this result is generally considered to result from an alteration of p53 by unknown mechanisms. The problems of evaluating p53 accumulation in tumors have been addressed in several recent reviews (28).

In the past 2 years, new monoclonal antibodies against human p53 have been produced by several laboratories (29–33). Their advantage is that they can be used for immunohistochemical diagnosis in highly varied conditions, such as detection of p53 in paraffin-embedded sections after fixation in formal or Bouin's solution (33).

C. Serological Analysis

Ten percent of breast cancer patients have anti-p53 antibodies in their serum (34). This percentage reaches 20% in children with B lymphomas, while it is zero in patients with T lymphomas (35). These studies, conducted during a lull in scientific interest in p53, were reviewed more recently in light of new knowledge on p53 inactivation and stabilization. Anti-p53 antibodies have been found in most human cancers (36–40). There is generally a good correlation between their frequency and that of p53 gene alterations (41). In lung cancer, which has a high rate of p53 mutation, the frequency of these anti-p53 antibodies is high (24%) (42). In prostate cancer, where the p53 mutation rate is low, or in mesotheliomas where it is nil, the incidence of seropositivity is very low. Several multifactorial studies show a very good correlation between the presence of anti-p53 antibodies, overexpression of the mutant protein in the tumor, and the presence of a mutation in the gene (36,38,43). In breast cancer, the prognostic value of p53-Ab was studied in 353 primary breast cancer patients. p53-Ab were detected in 42 cases (12%) and were negatively related to estradiol and progesterone receptors (44). The median duration of follow-up for patients was 5.3 years. In actuarial analyses, overall survival was worse in patients with p53-Ab ($p < 10^{-4}$); in Cox multivariate analysis, p53-Ab was an independent prognostic parameter (44).

Detailed analysis of these antibodies indicates that accumulation of the p53 protein in tumor cells is responsible for the appearance of auto-antibodies (32,37,42,43). Serological analysis has the following advantages: (1) simplicity of analysis (ELISA); (2) no need for tumor tissue; (3) the possibility of following the fate of the antibodies during treatment of the patient. In addition, evaluation of p53-Ab could represent a very powerful tool for detecting infraclinical tumor lesions (see below).

D. Functional Assay

A functional assay for p53 mutations has been described (45). Mutations are detected by assaying the transactivational activity of p53 protein in yeast. This test was used for detection of germline p53 mutations (46), but recent improvement in the test has led to its use in analysis of surgical specimens of tumor tissue (47).

IV. p53 Mutations: A Model for Molecular Epidemiology

Analysis of types of mutation in different types of tumors defines the mutational spectra according to the cancer being studied. Generally speaking, there are two types of genetic alteration, those derived from endogenous processes resulting from errors occurring during the various biological processes linked to DNA metabolism and those of exogenous origin involving environmental factors. The location and type of substitution occurring as a result of these two types of alterations are different. It is therefore possible to use the spectra of these mutations to study the etiology of a cancer (see Ref. 48 for review).

A. Endogenous Mutations

Analysis of all mutational events affecting the p53 gene shows that 42% are $G:C \rightarrow A:T$ transitions, 60% of which affect a CpG dinucleotide. It is well known that spontaneous deamination of 5-methylcytosine at these nucleotides may be an important cause of this type of transition. In fact, the three hot spot codons 175, 248, and 273 contain such a dinucleotide. More than 90% of the mutational events in these codons are compatible with a deamination phenomenon. This observation is confirmed by various studies showing that codons 248 and 273 are methylated in vivo (49). Analysis of the mutational events in cancers such as colon cancer, malignant hemopathies, or brain cancer (cancers known to be unrelated to exogenous carcinogens) shows that the mutation rate at the CpG dinucleotide is very high, suggesting that most of the mutations that alter the p53 gene in these cancers are due to endogenous processes related to the deamination of 5-methylcytosine.

B. Hepatocarcinoma and Aflatoxin B1

In 1990, there were two reports of mutations in the p53 gene in hepatocarcinomas (HCC), with a predominance of the $G:C \rightarrow T:A$ transversion at the third base of codon 249 (Arg $\rightarrow$ Ser) (50,51). In one case, the patient series was from Mozambique, while the second was from the Qidong province in China. These two regions are known for their consumption of food contaminated by the fungus *Aspergillus flavus*, producer of aflatoxin B1, which is a very potent hepatic carcinogen implicated in the development of HCC and known to interact synergistically with the hepatitis B virus. A worldwide epidemiological study showed that the mutation in codon 249 is strictly specific to countries in which the food is contaminated by aflatoxin B1 (52). In Mozambique, for example, more than 50% of the mutations were found in codon 249, while in Transkei, which borders on Mozambique (and has a similar rate of chronic HBV infection), the mutation rate at codon 249 is less than 10%. In fact, in countries that do not consume contaminated food (including Europe and the United States), the rate of p53 mutations in HCC is low.

It has been demonstrated in vitro and in vivo that this phenomenon is due to a very high sensitivity of codon 249 to the action of aflatoxin B1 (53,54). This observation, along with the fact that this mutation is quite deleterious for p53 function, explains the existence of this mutational hot spot (55).

C. Skin Cancer and Ultraviolet Radiation

Brash et al. (56,57) showed that, in skin spinocellular cancer, $C \rightarrow T$ mutations predominate in pyrimidine dimers. It is well known that ultraviolet radiation, an etiological agent of most skin cancers, acts directly on these dimers. A particular characteristic of the action of UV radiation is the occurrence of tandem mutations such as CC $\rightarrow$ TT, observed in Brash's series but also in other skin cancer series such as basocellular cancers (58). In patients with genetic DNA repair deficiencies, such as xeroderma pigmentosum (XP), the phenotype is much more marked (59,60). All mutations found in skin cancers are located on the pyrimidine dimers and 55% are tandem mutations CC $\rightarrow$ TT (61). This type of mutation is only very rarely found in internal cancers (less than 1%). In skin cancers from XP patients, more than 95% of the mutations are located on the noncoding strand of the p53 gene, while in other skin tumors and in internal cancers, no special trends are observed. This result suggests that there is preferential repair of the coding strand, which has been confirmed by Tornaletti and Pfeifer (62), who showed that the repair rate of pyrimidine dimers in the p53 gene is highly variable, with an especially low rate in the codons that are often mutated in skin cancer. Such p53 mutations seem to be very early events as they can be found both in precancerous lesions such as actinic keratosis (63) and in normal skin exposed to UV (64).

These results taken together (predominance of CC $\rightarrow$ TT lesions on the noncoding strand) were experimentally confirmed in animals carrying UV-induced tumors (65).

D. Bronchopulmonary Cancers, Smoking, and p53 Mutations

Numerous investigations have consistently reported increased occurrence of lung cancer among smokers. All investigations have shown a clear-cut dose-response relationship between the amount of tobacco smoked daily and the subsequent risk of lung cancer (66). It is now thought that cigarette smoking is responsible for 90% of lung cancers. In experimental animals, cigarette smoke induces tumors of the respiratory tract. This smoke is a complex mixture of several hundred different molecules, including well-characterized carcinogens such as polycyclic aromatic hydrocarbons (benzo(*a*)pyrene) and N-nitrosamines. Benzo(*a*)pyrene, a highly carcinogenic compound, was one of the molecules found in coal tar, which was implicated in the scrotal cancer identified during the nineteenth century. Exposure to coal tar is no longer a public health hazard, but benzo(*a*)pyrene from sources such as cigarette smoke and automobile exhaust fumes is highly prevalent in the environment.

The total frequency of p53 mutation in lung cancer is around 70%. They are found in 70–100% of small-cell lung cancer (SCLC) (67–71) and 45–75% of non–small-cell lung cancer (SCLC) (72–74). These mutations are mostly G:C $\rightarrow$ T:A transversions, with a rate of transition mutations lower than in other cancers (Fig. 1). A strong correlation has been detected between the frequency of these G:C $\rightarrow$ T:A transversions and lifetime cigarette smoking. This high frequency of transversions has not been detected for other cancers such as colon, breast, ovary, or brain cancer, which are not directly associated with smoking (Fig. 1). This observation is compatible with the role of exogenous carcinogens such as benzo(*a*)pyrene in lung cancer.

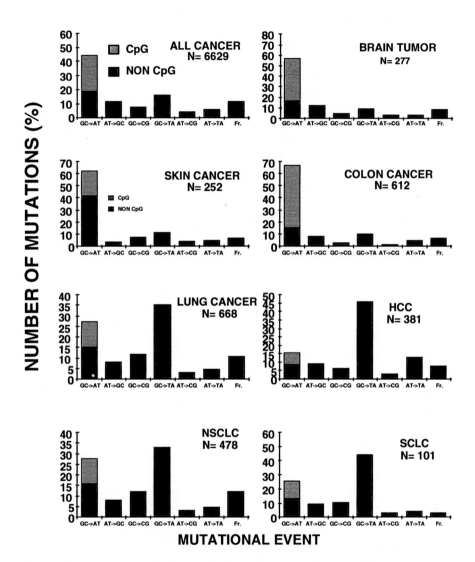

Figure 1 The spectrum of p53 mutations in various types of tumors. All cancer types correspond to the mutations found in more than 50 types of cancer (48,110). $G:C \rightarrow A:T$ mutations at CpG dinucleotide are the consequence of spontaneous deamination of 5-methylcytosine, whereas $G:C \rightarrow T:A$ mutations are strongly indicative of exposure to exogenous carcinogens.

Experimentally, it has been shown that after metabolic activation, one of the derivative products of benzo(*a*)pyrene binds predominantly to guanine and gives rise to specific transversions. A recent study has shown that exposure of cells to benzo-(*a*)pyrene leads to the formation of adducts at codons 157, 248, and 273 in the p53 gene (75). These positions are the major mutational hot spots in human lung cancer. Thus, these studies clearly show that the p53 gene is one of the targets of carcinogens found in tobacco (Fig. 2).

Another study on bronchial cancers in radon miners revealed a mutational hot spot in codon 249 (16 of 29 mutations) (76). The mutation differs from that seen in HCC because it affects the second base of codon 249 (codon AGG → ATG). This suggests that radon is responsible for this particular signature, since this mutation is found in less than 1% of other lung cancers. Nonetheless, this result should be interpreted with caution since some authors have suggested that this mutation is due to a mycotoxin synthesized by a fungus often found in the bronchi of radon miners (77).

E.   p53 Mutation in Breast Cancer

Analyses of the pattern of p53 mutations in breast cancer have led to the discovery of substantial diversity of the mutational pattern among cohorts from various areas in the world (78). This heterogeneity concerns (1) the frequency of p53 mutations, (2) the frequency of frameshift mutation (deletions and insertion), and (3) the frequency of transversions.

The frequency of the p53 mutation could reflect the sensitivity of the various methods used in these studies. Nevertheless, different frequencies and patterns were found among six populations analyzed by the same laboratory using the same methodology, suggesting that other factors could be involved (78). Blaszyk et al. reported some striking differences in mutation frequency within Japanese populations, but the reasons for such observations are unclear (79). The unusually high frequency of deletions and insertions in rural Caucasian Midwestern women compared to other populations is also difficult to explain, and could reflect exposure to particular environmental carcinogens (80). A similar explanation can be advanced for the heterogeneous frequency of transition and transversions.

The pattern of p53 mutations in breast cancer is highly complex. The differences in these patterns of mutation in geographically and/or racially diverse populations reflect an intrinsic (endogenous) pattern of mutation plus exposure to particular environmental carcinogens.

F.   p53 Gene: A Model for Molecular Epidemiology?

In order for a particular gene to be used in the study of origin of mutagenesis in the human population, it must exhibit the following properties: (1) it must be mutated in a large number of cancers; (2) the mutation rate must be high; (3) it must be altered mainly by point mutations; and (4) molecular analysis of the gene must be relatively easy to carry out (small-size gene). At present, these characteristics are

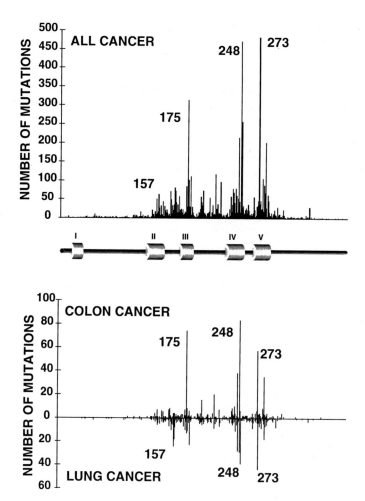

Figure 2 Distribution of p53 mutation in cancer. The evolutionarily conserved regions of the p53 protein (I to V) are indicated in the schematic representation of the p53 protein in each diagram. In colon cancer, hot spot mutations are found at codons 175, 248, and 273. A similar situation is found in various other cancers such as breast, brain, and bladder cancer or leukemia and lymphoma. The hot spot at codon 157 is specific for lung cancer. All data are taken from the last issue of the p53 database, which are available on the internet (http://perso. curie.fr/tsoussi/p53__mutation.html).

found in two genes, the Ha-ras oncogene and the p53 gene. One of the disadvantages of ras is the small number of codons (3) that are the target of mutations. In contrast, more than 100 of the 393 codons in the p53 gene can be modified. Moreover, the p53 gene is mutated in more than 50% of cancers. It is therefore possible to undertake molecular epidemiological studies with the aim of seeking specific signatures of certain carcinogens and demonstrating their role in the development of neoplasia (48).

V. Heterogeneity of p53 Mutant Behavior: Clinical Implications

p53 gene mutations are not random and are localized in the central region of the p53 protein. The importance of this region in p53 function has been suggested by several observations: (1) the presence of four of the five evolutionarily conserved blocks (81); (2) the high concentration of mutations in this region (17); and (3) the fact that it is the binding site of SV40 T antigen (82,83). The finding that p53 is never mutated in SV40-transformed cells suggests that its alteration occurs through interaction with AgT.

X-ray crystallography of p53 has been an important step in the understanding of the structure of this protein (84). The central region (amino acids 102 to 292) has been crystallized in the form of a protein-DNA complex. This core region has been shown to include the following motifs: (1) two antiparallel β sheets composed of four and five β-strands, respectively (these two sheets form a kind of compact sandwich that holds the other elements); (2) a loop-sheet-helix motif (LSH) containing three β-strands, an α-helix, and the L1 loop; (3) an L2 loop containing a small helix; and (4) an L3 loop mainly composed of turns. It is quite remarkable to note the very good agreement between these various structural elements and the four evolutionarily conserved blocks (II to V). The LSH motif and the L3 helix are involved in direct DNA interaction (LSH with the major groove and L3 with the minor groove). The L2 loop is presumed to provide stabilization by associating with the L3 loop. These two loops are held together by a zinc atom tetracoordinated to the following amino acids: Cys^{176} and His^{179} on the L2 loop and Cys^{278} and Cys^{242} on the L3 loop (84).

Analysis of the distribution of mutations in p53 shows a high concentration in the central region of the protein, and especially in the four blocks II–V which have been identified as the DNA-binding region. In view of the three-dimensional structure of the protein, it has been proposed that two classes of mutations can be predicted: class I mutations, which affect the amino acids directly involved in the protein-DNA interaction (residues in the LSH and L3), and class II mutations, which affect the amino acids involved in stabilization of the three-dimensional structure of the protein (residues in L2).

In fact, as described above, it has been established that mutant p53 can undergo conformational changes leading to its interaction with the heat shock protein hsp70, but also to altered accessibility to certain monoclonal antibodies such as PAb1620, which recognizes a specific conformational epitope of wild-type p53, or PAb240, which recognizes a cryptic epitope revealed in mutant p53 (85). In reality the situation is not so simple, and there have been various reports of a certain degree of heterogeneity in the behavior of different p53 mutants (see Ref. 86 for review). With the aim of analyzing a possible correlation between conformational changes and loss in activity, Ory et al. (87) studied a library of 23 p53 proteins mutated in the three hot spot codons Arg^{175}, Arg^{248}, and Arg^{273}. The results show that these mutants may be classified into two different phenotypes, corresponding to the two classes discussed above. The phenotype PAb1620−/PAb240+/hsp70+ corresponds to all mutations found in codon 175 and to a single mutant in codon 273 (Arg → Pro), while phenotype PAb1620+/PAb240−/hsp70− corresponds to mutations in codons 248 and 273. No intermediate cases were found, and each of these mutant p53 proteins had lost its transactivation and growth inhibition activities (87). In fact, the conformational changes in p53 were dissected by a new battery of monoclonal antibodies directed against the central region of the protein (88). All these antibodies recognize different epitopes in the central region of p53. Like PAb240, none of these antibodies was able to recognize native, wild-type p53. On the other hand, they were all able to recognize the category I mutants described above, suggesting that these mutants all undergo an overall conformational change that loosens up the compact structure of the protein (88).

Moreover, the analysis of the properties of the different mutant p53 proteins shows that not all mutations are equivalent (89–91). Analysis of a series of p53 point mutants has revealed the potential for selection of the ability to transactivate some, but not all cellular p53-response promoters. p53 mutant Pro^{175} and Leu^{181} are tumor-derived mutants which have retained the ability to activate expression of the cyclin-dependent kinase inhibitor p21Waf1/Clp1, but Pro^{175} is defective in activation of the p53-responsive sequence derived from the bax promoter and the insulin-like growth factor binding protein 3 gene (IGF-BP3) promoter, while Leu^{181} shows loss of the ability to activate a promoter containing IGF-BP3 box B sequences (90). These specific defects are correlated with the impaired apoptotic function displayed by these mutants, whereas they display a normal ability to induce G1 cell cycle arrest (90).

These observations are of key importance because they predict that tumors may behave differently according to the localization of the mutation. In fact, recent works have associated a poor prognosis for breast (92) or colon cancer (93) with specific p53 mutations.

VI. p53 Antibodies in Cancer Patients: Application to Lung Tumors

One of the most promising future applications of p53-Ab concerns their detection in the sera of people with high risk for cancer such as lung cancer or workers exposed to carcinogens. As stated above p53 alteration is an early event in lung cancer, occurring several years before clinical diagnosis of the tumor (Fig. 3). Recently, p53-Ab were detected in sera of two patients who were heavy smokers

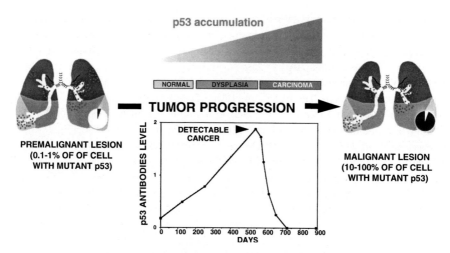

Figure 3 p53 alteration in lung cancer. Using molecular analysis, several groups demonstrate that a small number of tumoral cells harbor a p53 mutation in early neoplastic lesion of the lung (111–113). During tumor progression, cells with p53 mutations are selected and correspond to the majority of tumoral cells in the primary tumor. Immunohistochemistry identified the accumulation of mutant as early as dysplastic cells (114). Serological analysis indicates that p53-Ab can be detected several years before clinical diagnosis of the tumor (94).

without diagnosed lung malignancy (94). Both of these patients developed invasive squamous lung cancer 5 and 15 months, respectively, after detection of serum p53-Ab. In one patient, the level of serum antibodies directed against different epitopes of p53 protein was shown to progressively increase during the 15 months of follow-up before the diagnosis. In this patient, p53 overexpression was detected in tumoral cells from bronchial biopsy specimens. Since p53 alterations represent an early genetic change in lung carcinogenesis, it is suggested that p53-Ab detection represents a new and sensitive tool for detection of preneoplastic and microinvasive bronchial lesions in patients with a high risk of lung cancer, i.e., heavy smokers. This finding was confirmed by Trivers et al. (95) using three types of assays to detect p53-Ab. They were able to find p53-Abs before diagnosis in several patients with chronic obstructive pulmonary disease. This is also supported by the recent observation that p53-Ab can be detected in the sera of workers exposed to vinyl chloride and highly susceptible to developing angiosarcoma of the liver (96).

It should be emphasized that assay of p53-Ab corresponds to a global approach to assessing p53 alterations and does not depend on sampling of the tumor, the composition of which may be very heterogeneous. Molecular analysis of tumor tissues or biopsies corresponds to local analysis of p53 status and may be erroneous if the tumor is too heterogeneous or highly contaminated by normal tissue. Furthermore, mutation is not necessary for p53 accumulation (23,97), and p53 antibodies can be detected in such patients.

VII. p53 and Response to Therapy

It has long been known that some antitumor agents such as fluorouracil and ionizing radiation act by inducing apoptosis in tumor cells. Lowe et al. (98) showed that cells expressing mutant p53 are totally resistant to apoptosis upon treatment, whereas cells expressing wild-type p53 are sensitive to these therapeutic agents. This finding was extended to other tumor cell types and to various DNA-damaging agents (99–101). This observation is of major interest as knowledge of the state of the p53 gene in a tumor makes it possible to make a suitable treatment choice. Recently, it has been shown that specific p53 mutations are associated with de novo resistance to doxorubicin in breast cancer patients (102). In lung cancer, Rusch et al. showed that aberrant p53 expression predicts clinical resistance to cisplatin-based chemotherapy in locally advanced NSCLC (103), whereas Safran et al. showed that p53 mutations do not predict response to paclitaxel/radiation for NSCLC (104). More studies are needed to confirm these observations, and time will tell if p53 status is a good predictor of response to therapy.

VIII. p53 and Therapy

The observations described above suggest that the reintroduction of wild-type p53 in tumor cells or the conversion of mutant p53 to a wild-type conformation could induce apoptosis in these cells. In fact, this hypothesis proved correct, as it was shown that infection of a cisplatin-resistant NSCLC tumor with a recombinant adenovirus expressing wild-type p53 induced a return to chemosensitivity of the tumor, which is destroyed by apoptosis (105). A similar result was obtained in a SCLC cell line (106). Phase I retrovirus-mediated wild-type p53 gene therapy of lung cancer has recently been reported (107). No clinically significant vector-related toxicity was noted. Local tumor regression was reported in three of nine lung cancer patients who had previously failed conventional therapy. These results suggest that combination of p53 gene therapy and chemotherapy could be a promising approach for lung cancer therapy (108). New therapeutic approaches using a defective adenovirus which replicates selectively in p53-deficient cancer cells are also very promising (109).

IX. Conclusions and Perspectives

In addition to our knowledge of the p53 status of the patient and its clinical consequences, all our studies provide considerable information and material concerning p53 function. It is clear at present that not all of these mutations are equivalent in terms of biological activity. It is now necessary to perform more basic research to elucidate such p53 mutant activity and its relationship to the transformed phenotype. All these efforts highlight one of the most exciting aspects of p53 studies, i.e., the constant exchange between basic research and clinical studies. It is expected that this knowledge will be of future benefit to the patient by enabling earlier, more precise diagnosis and by generating new therapeutic approaches.

References

1. Hartwell L, Weinert T, Kadyk L, Garvik B. Cell cycle checkpoints, genomic integrity, and cancer. Cold Spring Harb Symp Quant Bio 1994; 59:259–263.
2. Kastan MB, Onyekwere O, Sidransky D, Vogelstein B, Craig RW. Participation of p53 protein in the cellular response to DNA damage. Cancer Res 1991; 51:6304–6311.
3. Kuerbitz SJ, Plunkett BS, Walsh WV, Kastan MB. Wild-type p53 is a cell cycle checkpoint determinant following irradiation. Proc Natl Acad Sci USA 1992; 89:7491–7495.
4. Guillouf C, Rosselli F, Krishnaraju K, Moustacchi E, Hoffman B, Liebermann DA. p53 involvement in control of G2 exit of the cell cycle: role in DNA damage-induced apoptosis. Oncogene 1995; 10:2263–2270.
5. Stewart N, Hicks GG, Paraskevas F, Mowat M. Evidence for a second cell cycle block at G2/M by p53. Oncogene 1995; 10:109–115.
6. El-Deiry WS, Tokino T, Velculescu VE, Levy DB, Parsons R, Trent JM, Lin D, Mercer WE, Kinzler KW, Vogelstein B. WAF1, a potential mediator of p53 tumor suppression. Cell 1993; 75:817–825.
7. Waldman T, Kinzler KW, Vogelstein B. p21 is necessary for the p53-mediated g(1) arrest in human cancer cells. Cancer Res 1995; 55:5187–5190.
8. Deng CX, Zhang PM, Harper JW, Elledge SJ, Leder P. Mice lacking p21(C/P1/WAF1) undergo normal development, but are defective in g1 checkpoint control. Cell 1995; 82: 675–684.
9. Miyashita T, Reed JC. Tumor suppressor p53 is a direct transcriptional activator of the human bax gene. Cell 1995; 80:293–299.
10. Owenschaub LB, Zhang W, Cusack JC, Angelo LS, Santee SM, Fujiwara T, Roth JA, Deisseroth AB, Zhang WW, Kruzel E, Radinsky R. Wild-type human p53 and a temperature-sensitive mutant induce Fas/APO-1 expression. Mol Cell Biol 1995; 15:3032–3040.
11. Haupt Y, Rowan S, Shaulian E, Vousden KH, Oren M. Induction of apoptosis in HeLa cells by trans-activation-deficient p53. Gene Dev 1995; 9:2170–2183.
12. Sabbatini P, Lin JY, Levine AJ, White E. Essential role for p53-mediated transcription in E1A-induced apoptosis. Gene Dev 1995; 9:2184–2192.
13. Livingstone LR, White A, Sprouse J, Livanos E, Jacks T, Tlsty TD. Altered cell cycle arrest and gene amplification potential accompany loss of wild-type p53. Cell 1992; 70:923–935.
14. Yin YX, Tainsky MA, Bischoff FZ, Strong LC, Wahl GM. Wild-Type p53 restores cell cycle control and inhibits gene amplification in cells with mutant p53 alleles. Cell 1992; 70: 937–948.
15. Lane D. p53, guardian of the genome. Nature 1992; 358:15–16.
16. Donehower LA, Harvey M, Slagle BL, McArthur MJ, Montgomery CA, Butel JS, Bradley A. Mice deficient for p53 are developmentally normal but susceptible to spontaneous tumours. Nature 1992; 356:215–221.
17. Caron de Fromentel C, Soussi T. TP53 Tumor suppressor gene: a model for investigating human mutagenesis. Genes Chrom Cancer 1992; 4:1–15.
18. Hollstein M, Sidransky D, Vogelstein B, Harris CC. p53 mutations in human cancers. Science 1991; 253:49–53.

19. Greenblatt MS, Bennett WP, Hollstein M, Harris CC. Mutations in the p53 tumor suppressor gene: clues to cancer etiology and molecular pathogenesis. Cancer Res 1994; 54:4855–4878.

20. Soussi T. The p53 tumour suppressor gene: from molecular biology to clinical investigation. In: Cowell JK, ed. Molecular Genetics of Cancer, 1995:135–178.

21. Crook T, Wrede D, Tidy JA, Mason WP, Evans DJ, Vousden KH. Clonal p53 mutation in primary cervical cancer—association with human-papillomavirus-negative tumours. Lancet 1992; 339:1070–1073.

22. Cordon-Cardo C, Latres E, Drobnjak M, Oliva MR, Pollack D, Woodruff JM, Marechal V, Chen JD, Brennan MF, Levine AJ. Molecular abnormalities of mdm2 and p53 genes in adult soft tissue sarcomas. Cancer Res 1994; 54:794–799.

23. Moll UM, Riou G, Levine AJ. Two distinct mechanisms alter p53 in breast cancer—mutation and nuclear exclusion. Proc Natl Acad Sci USA 1992; 89:7262–7266.

24. Moll UM, Laquaglia M, Benard J, Riou G. Wild-type p53 protein undergoes cytoplasmic sequestration in undifferentiated neuroblastomas but not in differentiated tumors. Proc Natl Acad Sci USA 1995; 92:4407–4411.

25. Moll UM, Ostermeyer AG, Haladay R, Winkfield B, Frazier M, Zambetti G. Cytoplasmic sequestration of wild-type p53 protein impairs the G(1) checkpoint after DNA damage. Mol Cell Biol 1996; 16:1126–1137.

26. Moyret C, Theillet C, Laurant-Puig P, Moles JP, Thomas G, Hamelin R. Relative efficiency of denaturing gradient gel electrophoresis and single strand conformation polymorphism in the detection of mutations in exons 5 to 8 of the p53 gene. Oncogene 1994; 9:1739–1743.

27. Dowell SP, Wilson POG, Derias NW, Lane DP, Hall PA. Clinical utility of the immunocytochemical detection of p53 protein in cytological specimens. Cancer Res 1994; 54:2914–2918.

28. Hall PA, Lane DP. P53 in tumour pathology—can we trust immunohistochemistry—revisited. J Pathol 1994; 172:1–4.

29. Vojtesek B, Bartek J, Midgley CA, Lane DP. An immunochemical analysis of the human nuclear phosphoprotein-p53—new monoclonal antibodies and epitope mapping using recombinant-p53. J Immunol Methods 1992; 151:237–244.

30. Midgley CA, Fisher CJ, Bartek J, Vojtesek B, Lane D, Barnes D. Analysis of p53 expression in human tumors: an antibody raised against human p53 expressed in E. coli. J Cell Sci 1992; 101:183–189.

31. Legros Y, Lacabanne V, D'Agay MF, Larsen CJ, Pla M, Soussi T. Production of human p53 specific monoclonal antibodies and their use in immunohistochemical studies of tumor cells. Bull Cancer 1993; 80:102–110.

32. Legros Y, Lafon C, Soussi T. Linear antigenic sites defined by the B-cell response to human p53 are localized predominantly in the amino and carboxy-termini of the protein. Oncogene 1994; 9:2071–2076.

33. Tenaud C, Negoescu A, Labatmoleur F, Legros Y, Soussi T, Brambilla E. Methods in pathology—p53 immunolabeling in archival paraffin-embedded tissues: optimal protocol based on microwave heating for eight antibodies on lung carcinomas. Modern Pathol 1994; 7:853–859.

34. Crawford LV, Pim DC, Bulbrook RD. Detection of antibodies against the cellular protein p53 in sera from patients with breast cancer. Int J Cancer 1982; 30:403–408.

35. Caron de Fromentel C, May-Levin F, Mouriesse H, Lemerle J, Chandrasekaran K, May P. Presence of circulating antibodies against cellular protein p53 in a notable proportion of children with B-cell lymphoma. Int J Cancer 1987; 39:185–189.

36. Davidoff AM, Iglehart JD, Marks JR. Immune response to p53 is dependent upon p53/HSP70 complexes in breast cancers. Proc Natl Acad Sci USA 1992; 89:3439–3442.

37. Schlichtholz B, Legros Y, Gillet D, Gaillard C, Marty M, Lane D, Calvo F, Soussi T. The immune response to p53 in breast cancer patients is directed against immunodominant epitopes unrelated to the mutational hot spot. Cancer Res 1992; 52:6380–6384.

38. Winter SF, Minna JD, Johnson BE, Takahashi T, Gazdar AF, Carbone DP. Development of antibodies against p53 in lung cancer patients appears to be dependent on the type of p53 mutation. Cancer Res 1992; 52:4168–4174.

39. Hassapoglidoi S, Diamandis EP. Antibodies to the p53 tumor suppressor gene product quantified in cancer patients serum with a time-resolved immunofluorometry technique. Clin Biochem 1992; 25:445–449.

40. Angelopoulou K, Diamandis EP, Sutherland DJA, Kellen JA, Bunting PS. Prevalence of serum antibodies against the p53 tumor suppressor gene protein in various cancers. Int J Cancer 1994; 58:480–487.

41. Lubin R, Schlichtholz B, Teillaud JL, Garay E, Bussel A, Wild C, Soussi T. p53 antibodies in patients with various types of cancer: assay, identification and characterization. Clin Cancer Res 1995; 1:1463–1469.

42. Schlichtholz B, Tredaniel J, Lubin R, Zalcman G, Hirsch A, Soussi T. Analyses of p53 antibodies in sera of patients with lung carcinoma define immunodominant regions in the p53 protein. Br J Cancer 1994; 69:809–816.

43. Lubin R, Schlichtholz B, Bengoufa D, Zalcman G, Tredaniel J, Hirsch A, Caron de Fromentel C, Preudhomme C, Fenaux P, Fournier G, Mangin P, Laurent-Puig P, Pelletier G, Schlumberger M, Desgrandchamps F, Leduc A, Peyrat JP, Janin N, Bressac B, Soussi T. Analysis of p53 antibodies in patients with various cancers define B-Cell epitopes of human p53—distribution on primary structure and exposure on protein surface. Cancer Res 1993; 53:5872–5876.

44. Peyrat JP, Bonneterre J, Lubin R, Vanlemmens L, Fournier J, Soussi T. Prognostic significance of circulating p53 antibodies in patients undergoing surgery for locoregional breast cancer. Lancet 1995; 345:621–622.

45. Ishioka C, Freburg T, Yan Y, Vidal M, Friend SH, Schmidt S, Iggo R. Screening patients for heterozygotous p53 mutations using a functional assay in yeast. Nature Genetics 1993; 5:124–129.

46. Flaman JM, Frebourg T, Moreau V, Charbonnier F, Martin C, Chappuis P, Sappino AP, Limacher JM, Bron L, Benhattar J, Tada M, Vanmeir EG, Estreicher A, Iggo RD. A simple p53 functional assay for screening cell lines, blood, and tumors. Proc Natl Acad Sci USA 1995; 92:3963–3967.

47. Tada M, Iggo RD, Ishii N, Shinohe Y, Sakuma S, Estreicher A, Sawamura Y, Abe H. Clonality and stability of the p53 gene in human astrocytic tumor cells: quantitative analysis of p53 gene mutations by yeast functional assay. Int J Cancer 1996; 67:447–450.

48. Soussi T. The p53 tumour suppressor gene: a model for molecular epidemiology of human cancer. Mol Med Today 1996; 2:32–37.

49. Rideout WM, Coetzee GA, Olumi AF, Jones PA. 5-Methylcytosine as an endogenous mutagen in the human LDL receptor ans p53 gene. Science 1990; 249:1288–1290.

50. Hsu IC, Metcalf RA, Sun T, Welsh JA, Wang NJ, Harris CC. Mutational hotspot in the p53 gene in human hepatocellular carcinomas. Nature 1991; 350:427–428.

51. Bressac B, Kew M, Wands J, Ozturk M. Selective G-mutation to T-mutation of p53 gene in hepatocellular carcinoma from southern Africa. Nature 1991; 350:429–431.

52. Ozturk M, Other. p53 mutation in hepatocellular carcinoma after aflatoxin exposure. Lancet 1991; 338:1356–1359.

53. Aguilar F, Hussain SP, Cerutti P. Aflatoxin-B(1) induces the transversion of G→T in codon 249 of the p53 tumor suppressor gene in human hepatocytes. Proc Natl Acad Sci USA 1993; 90:8586–8590.

54. Puisieux A, Lim S, Groopman J, Ozturk M. Selective targeting of p53 gene mutational hotspots in human cancers by etiologically defined carcinogens. Cancer Res 1991; 51:6185–6189.

55. Ponchel F, Puisieux A, Tabone E, Michot JP, Froschl G, Morel AP, Frebourg T, Fontaniere B, Oberhammer F, Ozturk M. Hepatocarcinoma-specific mutant p53-249Ser induces mitotic activity but has no effect on transforming growth factor beta 1-mediated apoptosis. Cancer Res 1994; 54:2064–2068.

56. Ziegler A, Leffell DJ, Kunala S, Sharma HW, Gailani M, Simon JA, Halperin AJ, Baden HP, Shapiro PE, Bale AE, Brash DE. Mutation hotspots due to sunlight in the p53 gene of non-melanoma skin cancers. Proc Natl Acad Sci USA 1993; 90:4216–4220.

57. Brash DE, Rudolph JA, Simon JA, Lin A, Mckenna GJ, Baden HP, Halperin AJ, Ponten J. A role for sunlight in skin cancer—UV-induced p53 mutations in squamous cell carcinoma. Proc Natl Acad Sci USA 1991; 88:10124–10128.

58. Rady P, Scinicariello F, Wagner RF, Tyring SK. p53 Mutations in basal cell carcinomas. Cancer Res 1992; 52:3804–3806.

59. Sato M, Nishigori C, Zghal M, Yagi T, Takebe H. Ultraviolet-specific mutations in p53 gene in skin tumors in xeroderma-pigmentosum patients. Cancer Res 1993; 53:2944–2946.

60. Dumaz N, Drougard C, Sarasin A, Dayagrosjean L. Specific UV-induced mutation spectrum in the p53 gene of skin tumors from DNA-repair-deficient xeroderma-pigmentosum patients. Proc Natl Acad Sci USA 1993; 90:10529–10533.

61. Dumaz N, Stary A, Soussi T, Dayagrosjean L, Sarasin A. Can we predict solar ultraviolet radiation as the causal event in human tumours by analysing the mutation spectra of the p53 gene? Mutat Res 1994; 307:375–386.

62. Tornaletti S, Pfeifer GP. Slow repair of pyrimidine dimers at p53 mutation hotspots in skin cancer. Science 1994; 263:1436–1438.

63. Ziegler A, Jonason AS, Leffell DJ, Simon JA, Sharma HW, Kimmelman J, Remington L, Jacks T, Brash DE. Sunburn and p53 in the onset of skin cancer. Nature 1994; 372: 773–776.

64. Jonason AS, Kunala S, Price GJ, Restifo RJ, Spinelli HM, Persing JA, Leffell DJ, Tarone RE, Brash DE. Frequent clones of p53-mutated keratinocytes in normal human skin. Proc Natl Acad Sci USA 1996; 93:14025–14029.

65. Kress S, Sutter C, Strickland PT, Mukhtar H, Schweizer J, Schwarz M. Carcinogen-specific mutational pattern in the p53 gene in ultraviolet-B radiation-induced squamous cell carcinomas of mouse skin. Cancer Res 1992; 52:6400–6403.

66. IARC. IARC monographs on the evaluation of the carcinogenic risk of chemicals to human. Tobacco Smoking 1985; 38:Lyon.

67. Takahashi T, Takahashi T, Suzuki H, Hida T, Sekido Y, Ariyoshi Y, Ueda R. The p53 gene is very frequently mutated in small-cell Lung cancer with a distinct nucleotide substitution pattern. Oncogene 1991; 6:1775–1778.

68. Sameshima Y, Matsuno Y, Hirohashi S, Shimosato Y, Mizoguchi H, Sugimura T, Terada M, Yokota J. Alterations of the p53 gene are common and critical events for the maintenance of malignant phenotypes in small-cell lung carcinoma. Oncogene 1992; 7:451–457.

69. D'Amico D, Carbone D, Mitsudomi T, Nau M, Fedorko J, Russell E, Johnson B, Buchhagen D, Bodner S, Phelps R, Gazdar A, Minna JD. High frequency of somatically acquired p53 mutations in small-cell lung cancer cell lines and tumors. Oncogene 1992; 7:339–346.

70. Lohmann D, Putz B, Reich U, Bohm J, Prauer H, Hofler H. Mutational spectrum of the p53 gene in human small-cell lung cancer and relationship to clinicopathological data. Am J Pathol 1993; 142:907–915.

71. Hensel CH, Xiang RH, Sakaguchi AY, Naylor SL. Use of the single strand conformation polymorphism technique and PCR to detect p53 gene mutations in small cell lung cancer. Oncogene 1991; 6:1067–1071.

72. Kishimoto Y, Murakami Y, Shiraishi M, Hayashi K, Sekiya T. Aberrations of the p53 tumor suppressor gene in human non-small cell carcinomas of the lung. Cancer Res 1992; 52:4799–4804.

73. Chiba I, Takahashi T, Nau MM, d'Amico D, Curiel DT, Mitsudomi T, Buchhagen DL, Carbon D, Piantadosi S, Koga H, Reissman PT, Slamon DJ, Holmes EC, Minna JD. Mutations in the p53 gene are frequent in primary, resected non-small-cell lung cancer. Oncogene 1990; 5:1603–1610.

74. Shipman R, Schraml P, Colombi M, Raefle G, Dalquen P, Ludwig C. Frequent TP53 gene alterations (mutation, allelic loss, nuclear accumulation) in primary non-small cell lung cancer. Eur J Cancer 1996; 32A:335–341.

75. Denissenko MF, Pao A, Tang MS, Pfeifer GP. Preferential formation of benzo[a]pyrene adducts at lung cancer mutational hotspots in P53. Science 1996; 274:430–432.
76. Taylor JA, Watson MA, Devereux TR, Michels RY, Saccomanno G, Anderson M. P53 mutation hotspot in radon-associated lung cancer. Lancet 1994; 343:86–87.
77. Venitt S, Biggs PJ. Radon, mycotoxins, p53, and uranium mining. Lancet 1994; 343:795.
78. Hartmann A, Blaszyk H, Kovach JS, Sommer SS. The molecular epidemiology of P53 gene mutations in human breast cancer. Trends Genet 1997; 13:27–33.
79. Blaszyk H, Hartmann A, Tamura Y, Saitoh S, Cunningham JM, McGovern RM, Schroeder JJ, Schaid DJ, Ii K, Monden Y, Morimoto T, Komaki K, Sasa M, Hirata K, Okazaki M, Kovach JS, Sommer SS. Molecular epidemiology of breast cancers in northern and southern Japan: The frequency, clustering, and patterns of p53 gene mutations differ among these two low-risk populations. Oncogene 1996; 13:2159–2166.
80. Sommer SS, Cunningham J, McGovern RM, Saitoh S, Schroeder JJ, Wold LE, Kovach JS. Pattern of p53 gene mutations in breast cancers of women of the midwestern United States. J Nat Cancer Inst 1992; 84:246–252.
81. Soussi T, Caron de Fromentel C, May P. Structural aspects of the p53 protein in relation to gene evolution. Oncogene 1990; 5:945–952.
82. Tan TH, Wallis J, Levine AJ. Identification of the protein p53 domain involved in formation of the simian virus 40 large T-antigen-p53 protein complex. J Virol 1986; 59:574–583.
83. Jenkins JR, Chumakov P, Addison C, Stürzbzecher HW, Wade-Evans A. Two distinct regions of the murine p53 primary amino acid sequence are implicated in stable complex formation with simian virus 40 T antigen. J Virol 1988; 62:3902–3906.
84. Cho YJ, Gorina S, Jeffrey PD, Pavletich NP. Crystal structure of a p53 tumor suppressor DNA complex: understanding tumorigenic mutations. Science 1994; 265:346–355.
85. Milner J. A conformation hypothesis for the suppressor and promoter functions of p53 in cell growth control and in cancer. Proc R Soc Lond [Biol] 1991; 245:139–145.
86. Soussi T, May P. Structural aspects of the p53 protein in relation to gene evolution: a second look. J Mol Biol 1996; 260:623–637.
87. Ory K, Legros Y, Auguin C, Soussi T. Analysis of the most representative tumour-derived p53 mutants reveals that changes in protein conformation are not correlated with loss of transactivation or inhibition of cell proliferation. EMBO J 1994; 13:3496–3504.
88. Legros Y, Meyer A, Ory K, Soussi T. Mutations in p53 produce a common conformational effect that can be detected with a panel of monoclonal antibodies directed toward the central part of the p53 protein. Oncogene 1994; 9:3689–3694.
89. Rowan S, Ludwig RL, Haupt Y, Bates S, Lu X, Oren M, Vousden KH. Specific loss of apoptotic but not cell-cycle arrest function in a human tumor derived p53 mutant. EMBO J 1996; 15:827–838.
90. Ludwig RL, Bates S, Vousden KH. Differential activation of target cellular promoters by p53 mutants with impaired apoptotic function. Mol Cell Biol 1996; 16:4952–4960.
91. Friedlander P, Haupt Y, Prives C, Oren M. A mutant p53 that discriminates between p53-responsive genes cannot induce apoptosis. Mol Cell Biol 1996; 16:4961–4971.
92. Bergh J, Norberg T, Sjogren S, Lindgren A, Holmberg L. Complete sequencing of the p53 gene provides prognostic information in breast cancer patients, particularly in relation to adjuvant systemic therapy and radiotherapy. Nature Med 1995; 1:1029–1034.
93. Goh HS, Yao J, Smith DR. p53 point mutation and survival in colorectal cancer patients. Cancer Res 1995; 55:5217–5221.
94. Lubin R, Zalcman G, Bouchet L, Trédaniel J, Legros Y, Cazals D, Hirsh A, Soussi T. Serum p53 antibodies as early markers of lung cancer. Nature Med 1995; 1:701–702.
95. Trivers GE, De Benedetti VMG, Cawley HL, Caron G, Harrington AM, Bennet WP, Jett JR, Colby TV, Tazelaar H, Pairolero P, Miller RD, Harris CC. Anti-p53 antibodies in sera from patients with chronic obstructive pulmonary disease can predate a diagnosis of cancer. Clin Cancer Res 1996; 2:1767–1775.
96. Trivers GE, Cawley HL, Debenedetti VMG, Hollstein M, Marion MJ, Bennett WP, Hoover ML, Prives CC, Tamburro CC, Harris CC. Anti-p53 antibodies in sera of workers occupationally exposed to vinyl chloride. J Natl Cancer Inst 1995; 87:1400–1407.

97. Andersen TI, Holm R, Nesland JM, Heimdal KR, Ottestad L, Borresen AL. Prognostic significance of TP53 alterations in breast carcinoma. Br J Cancer 1993; 68:540–548.
98. Lowe SW, Ruley HE, Jacks T, Housman DE. p53-Dependent apoptosis modulates the cytotoxicity of anticancer agents. Cell 1993; 74:957–967.
99. Xia F, Wang X, Wang YH, Tsang NM, Yandell DW, Kelsey KT, Liber HL. Altered p53 status correlates with differences in sensitivity to radiation-induced mutation and apoptosis in two closely related human lymphoblast lines. Cancer Res 1995; 55:12–15.
100. Eliopoulos AG, Kerr DJ, Herod J, Hodgkins L, Krajewski S, Reed JC, Young LS. The control of apoptosis and drug resistance in ovarian cancer: influence of p53 and bcl-2. Oncogene 1995; 11:1217–1228.
101. Fan SJ, El-Deiry WS, Bae I, Freeman J, Jondle D, Bhatia K, Fornace AJ, Magrath I, Kohn KW, O'Connor PM. p53 gene mutations are associated with decreased sensitivity of human lymphoma cells to DNA damaging agents. Cancer Res 1994; 54:5824–5830.
102. Aas T, Borresen AL, Geisler S, Smithsorensen B, Johnsen H, Varhaug JE, Akslen LA, Lonning PE. Specific p53 mutations are associated with de novo resistance to doxorubicin in breast cancer patients. Nature Med 1996; 2:811–814.
103. Rusch V, Klimstra D, Venkatraman E, Oliver J, Martini N, Gralla R, Kris M, Dmitrovsky E. Aberrant p53 expression predicts clinical resistance to cisplatin-based chemotherapy in locally advanced non-small cell lung cancer. Cancer Res 1995; 55:5038–5042.
104. Safran H, King T, Choy H, Gollerkeri A, Kwakwa H, Lopez F, Cole B, Myers J, Tarpey J, Rosmarin A. p53 mutations do not predict response to paclitaxel/radiation for nonsmall cell lung carcinoma. Cancer 1996; 78:1203–1210.
105. Fujiwara T, Grimm EA, Mukhopadhyay T, Zhang WW, Owenschaub LB, Roth JA. Induction of chemosensitivity in human lung cancer cells in vivo by adenovirus-mediated transfer of the wild-type p53 gene. Cancer Res 1994; 54:2287–2291.
106. Gjerset RA, Turla ST, Sobol RE, Scalise JJ, Mercola D, Collins H, Hopkins PJ. Use of wild-type p53 to achieve complete treatment sensitization of tumor cells expressing endogenous mutant p53. Mol Carcinogen 1995; 14:275–285.
107. Roth JA, Nguyen D, Lawrence DD, Kemp BL, Carrasco CH, Ferson DZ, Hong WK, Komaki R, Lee JJ, Nesbitt JC, Pisters KMW, Putnam JB, Schea R, Shin DM, Walsh GL, Dolormente MM, Han CI, Martin FD, Yen N, Xu K, Stephens LC, Mcdonnell TJ, Mukhopadhyay T, Cai D. Retrovirus-mediated wild-type p53 gene transfer to tumors of patients with lung cancer. Nature Med 1996; 2:985–991.
108. Roth JA. Modification of tumor suppressor gene expression and induction of apoptosis in non-small cell lung cancer (NSCLC) with an adenovirus vector expressing wildtype p53 and cisplatin. Hum Gene Ther 1996; 7:1013–1030.
109. Bischoff JR, Kim DH, Williams A, Heise C, Horn S, Muna M, Ng L, Nye JA, Sampson-Johannes A, Fattaey A, McCormick F. An adenovirus mutant that replicates selectively in p53-deficient human tumor cells. Science 1996; 274:373–376.
110. Hainaut P, Soussi T, Shomer B, Hollstein M, Greenblatt M, Hovig E, Harris CC, Montesano R. Database of p53 gene somatic mutations in human tumors and cell lines: Updated compilation and future prospects. Nucleic Acids Res 1997; 25:151–157.
111. Sundaresan V, Ganly P, Hasleton P, Rudd R, Sinha G, Bleehen NM, Rabbits P. p53 and chromosome 3 abnormalities, characteristic of malignant lung tumours, are detectable in preinvasive lesions of the bronchus. Oncogene 1992; 7:1989–1997.
112. Sozzi G, Miozzo M, Donghi R, Pilotti S, Cariani CT, Pastorino U, Dellaporta G, Pierotti MA. Deletions of 17p and p53 mutations in preneoplastic lesions of the lung. Cancer Res 1992; 52:6079–6082.
113. Mao L, Hruban RH, Boyle JO, Tockman M, Sidransky D. Detection of oncogene mutations in sputum precedes diagnosis of lung cancer. Cancer Res 1994; 54:1634–1637.
114. Bennett WP, Colby TV, Travis WD, Borkowski A, Jones RT, Lane DP, Metcalf RA, Samet JM, Takeshima Y, Gu JR, Vahakangas KH, Soini Y, Paakko P, Welsh JA, Trump BF, Harris CC. p53 protein accumulates frequently in early bronchial neoplasia. Cancer Res 1993; 53:4817–4822.-

29

Endoscopic Detection of Preneoplastic Lesions

STEPHEN C. LAM and CALUM MacAULAY

University of British Columbia
British Columbia Cancer Agency
Vancouver, British Columbia,
Canada

I. Introduction

Despite a great deal of effort, the overall cancer mortality has only recently pla-teaued after decades of steady increase (1,2). The increase was mainly due to a lack of significant improvement in the treatment of lung cancer. The prevalent attitude is that by stopping tobacco smoking, the lung cancer problem will be solved. While eliminating tobacco smoking must be our highest priority, we have to consider an additional strategy if we are going to see a significant decrease in lung cancer mor-tality in the next several decades. Although the risk of lung cancer is reduced with smoking cessation, former smokers retain a significant risk, especially those who give up smoking later in life (3). This is reflected in the proportion of former versus current smokers who are diagnosed with lung cancer. Approximately 50% of pa-tients with lung cancer are now former smokers (4). In Canada and the United States, there are approximately 50 million former smokers in addition to 50 million current smokers. Approximately 50% of former smokers are above 45 years of age and hence are prime targets for lung cancer. With this large reservoir of current and former smokers who are at risk of lung cancer and the progressive increase in the incidence of lung cancer among women, it is projected that overall lung cancer mor-tality will continue to rise until approximately the year 2010 and will gradually start

Table 1 Efficacy of Screening

Method	Detection rate (%)
Pap smear	0.1–0.3
Mammography	0.4–0.6
Sputum cytology	0.2–1.7

decreasing around the year 2030 (5). However, because of a larger population base, the absolute number of lung cancer cases will actually continue to rise. Examination of the age-standardized cancer mortality rate shows an interesting difference between men and women (1). While the cancer mortality rate, excluding lung cancer, has remained relatively unchanged among men in the last two decades, until very recently there has been a gradual decline in the mortality rate among women. This is thought to be due to improvements in the detection of intraepithelial (preinvasive/preneoplastic) lesions by means of the Papanicolaou smear for cervical cancer (6) and screening mammography for breast cancer (7,8) followed by the subsequent removal of these lesions. For example, in British Columbia, Canada, as the rate of detection of carcinoma in situ of the cervix increased with the introduction of a cervical cytology program approximately 40 years ago, there was a significant concurrent reduction in the incidence of invasive cancer of the cervix as well as mortality from this disease (6).

The detection rate of sputum cytology examination versus cervical cytology and screening mammography is shown in Table 1. The detection rates for cervical cytology and screening mammography are for the British Columbia Programs (9,10). Even using the sputum cytology examination methods practiced more than two decades ago (11), which would be considered suboptimal at present, the detection rate of lung cancer was only slightly lower than that of screening mammography but comparable to cervical cytology screening, although the latter includes both new and previously screened individuals. By redefining the high-risk population as those with a smoking history of ≥40 pack-years with the presence of airflow obstruction along with adherence to better sputum cytology examination techniques, a recent study by Kennedy and coworkers in Denver, Colorado, showed that the lung cancer detection rate can be as high as 1.7% (12). This is substantially higher than the detection rate of cervical cancer or breast cancer of existing cervical cytology or screening mammography programs. The Lung Health Study in North America also showed that lung cancer is the number one cause of death in a similar high-risk population (13). Almost 1% of the volunteers in the Lung Health Study died of lung cancer within 5 years of the study. The ability to identify a high-risk population among current and former smokers suggests that we should reconsider early detection of intraepithelial (preneoplastic) lesions in the overall management of lung cancer.

Table 2 Natural History of Carcinoma In Situ

Tissue	Progression to invasive cancer (%)	Cure rate of invasive cancer (%)	CIS detection treatment
Bladder	40–80	70	Yes
Breast	15–75	72	Yes
Cervix	50–80	71	Yes
Lung	?40–80	15	No???

II. Rationale for Detection and Treatment of Intraepithelial Bronchial Neoplasia

One problem encountered in the detection and treatment of intraepithelial neoplasia is the uncertainty of the natural history of these lesions. Even carcinoma in situ has been reported to regress spontaneously (14,15). However, several prospective sputum cytology studies show that 40–80% of patients with severe atypia will progress to invasive cancer (16–18). The rate of progression of carcinoma in situ has not been studied because, until now, there has been no tool to detect a significant number of patients with these lesions. The degree of uncertainty of the natural history of bronchial intraepithelial neoplasia is not different from that of other tumor sites, such as the urinary bladder, breast, and cervix (19–22) (Table 2). In these other sites, detection and treatment of carcinoma in situ lesions are accepted as standard clinical practice. Considering the much higher mortality rate of invasive lung cancer compared to cancer of the bladder, breast, or cervix and the fact that the discomfort and potential harm of a diagnostic bronchoscopy is not any higher than cystoscopy (urinary bladder), colposcopy (cervix), needle aspiration, or open biopsy (breast), the conservatism towards detection and treatment of preneoplastic lung lesions is probably not justified.

III. White-Light Bronchoscopy

Although a number of endobronchial treatment modalities, such as photodynamic therapy (23,24), electrocautery (25), cryotherapy (26), or thermoablation with laser (27), have been developed for the curative treatment of small intraepithelial neoplastic lesions, identifying individuals harboring these lesions and localizing their exact sites remains problematic. Recent advances in computer-assisted image analysis of exfoliated sputum cells (28,29), the development of monoclonal antibodies (30), as well as molecular biology techniques (31,32) provide promise of a significant improvement in the sensitivity of sputum cytology examinations to detect intraepithelial neoplastic lesions beyond what has been achieved by conventional sputum cytology examination. However, the improved sensitivity of these newer screening methods may also mean that the size of the underlying bronchial lesions, from which the exfoliated sputum cells are derived, will be smaller and even more difficult to localize with conventional white-light bronchoscopy.

In general, flat or superficially spreading lesions 2 cm or greater in surface diameter and nodular/polypoid lesions greater than 2 mm in size produce obvious changes in the bronchial mucosa visible on conventional white-light examination. Approximately 75% of carcinoma in situ are superficial or flat. The remaining 25% are nodular (23,33). On average, flat lesions 5 mm or smaller are usually invisible on white-light bronchoscopy. Lesions around 10 mm in diameter usually produce nonspecific thickening, redness, or a mild increase in granularity, which are difficult to distinguish from inflammation or squamous metaplasia (34).

In the last decade, there has not been a significant improvement in the use of conventional white-light bronchoscopy for the localization of intraepithelial neoplasia. In a study reported by Cortese and coworkers in 1983 (35), approximately one-third of the patients with sputum cytology–positive x-ray occult lung cancer required more than one bronchoscopy to localize the source of the malignant cells in their sputum specimens. Ten years later, despite a better understanding of the bronchoscopic appearance of early lung cancer, a study by Bechtel and coworkers showed that a similar proportion of these patients required more than one bronchoscopy for localization (36). This is despite the fact that, on average, only a small proportion of these x-ray occult lung cancers were in situ carcinomas (33% and 14%, respectively) while the remaining cancers were invasive and hence larger and easier to be visualized bronchoscopically. If a lesion is not seen, the standard procedure for localization is to perform multiple segmental bronchial brushings and blind spur biopsies (37,38). Clearly, the task of localizing intraepithelial lesions would be much easier if they could be made observable by other means for direct biopsy.

IV. Fluorescence Bronchoscopy

When the bronchial surface is illuminated by light, the light can be reflected, back-scattered, absorbed, or induce tissue fluorescence. Conventional white-light bronchoscopy makes use of the first three optical phenomena. The tissue autofluorescence is not visible because the intensity is very low and overwhelmed by the background illuminating light. However, with suitable instrumentation, the tissue autofluorescence can be made visible to enhance our ability to localize areas of intraepithelial neoplasia in the tracheal bronchial tree.

When the bronchial surface is illuminated by violet or blue light (400–440 nm), normal tissues have a significantly higher fluorescence intensity compare to dysplastic lesions or carcinoma in situ especially in the green region of the emission spectrum (39). The reasons for the decrease in autofluorescence in preneoplastic and neoplastic tissues are shown in Table 3. Optical measurements of the bronchial tissue show that less than 5% of the overall detected fluorescence is contributed by the

Table 3 Reasons for Decrease in Autofluorescence in Preinvasive and Invasive Lung Cancer

1. Decrease in fluorophore amount or quantum yield, e.g., decrease in extracellular matrix from metalloproteinases
2. Changes in tissue architecture, e.g., increased thickness of epithelial layer
3. Increased blood volume from increase in microvascular density

epithelial layer (40,41). The major bulk of the fluorescence signal comes from the submucosa. A decrease in the extracellular matrix in the submucosa, such as from the secretion of metalloproteinases by preneoplastic or neoplastic tissues (42), will result in a decrease in the amount of fluorophores or the quantum yield of these molecules. Recently it was observed that the microvascular density is increased even in dysplastic lesions and in situ carcinoma (43). Due to the increased absorption of the excitation blue light and the emitted autofluorescence light by a larger blood volume, the fluorescence intensity of these lesions is decreased. A third reason for the decrease in autofluorescence in dysplastic tissues and carcinoma in situ is the increase in thickness of the epithelial layer. This thickening impedes transmission of the excitation light to the submucosa and the fluorescence light from the submucosa to the bronchial surface. These effects are particularly pertinent to the green region of the autofluorescence spectra because the absorption characteristics of bronchial tissue and blood favor the absorption of green light (40). These differences in the autofluorescence properties of normal, preneoplastic, and neoplastic tissues were used in the development of the light induced fluorescence endoscopy (LIFE) device (Xillix LIFE Lung Fluorescence Endoscopy System, Xillix Technologies Corp., Richmond, B.C., Canada) for the detection and localization of intraepithelial neoplasia. The features of the LIFE device are shown in Table 4. It is designed as an adjunct to white-light bronchoscopy. The procedure is similar to standard fiberoptic bronchoscopy except the illuminating light is different and a special camera is used. The fluorescence examination adds an average of 10 minutes to the diagnostic bronchoscopic procedure under a local anesthetic (44).

Several studies have shown that fluorescence bronchoscopy, when used as an adjunct to standard white light bronchoscopy enhances the bronchoscopist's ability to localize small lesions especially intraepithelial lesions severalfold (45–47). Fluorescence bronchoscopy has been found to be useful in the localization of sputum cy-

Table 4 Features of the LIFE-Lung System

1. Real-time video image
2. Based on native tissue fluorescence
3. True fluorescence image providing contextural information
4. Adjunct to white-light bronchoscopy
5. Guide to biopsy similar to white-light bronchoscopy

Table 5   Management of Early Lung Cancer

1. Detection: Exfoliated cells in sputum
2. Localization: White-light and fluorescence bronchoscopy
3. Treatment: KTP/YAG laser, electrocautery, PDT, cryotherapy, ?gene therapy

tology positive, x-ray negative lung cancer. It is also useful in preoperative assessment to determine the extent of endobronchial spread and the presence of synchronous cancers. As a tool for clinical investigation, the ability to sample intraepithelial neoplastic lesions sequentially for biomarker studies, before and after chemoprevention, may allow a more rapid identification of promising agents for population studies. Cross-sectional and longitudinal sampling of intraepithelial neoplastic lesions *in vivo* would also provide valuable material to study the pathogenesis of lung cancer and the natural history of these lesions (48–50). Fluorescence bronchoscopy has become an integral part in the overall strategy in the management of early lung cancer (Table 5).

While it is important for us to continue our fight against tobacco smoking, especially among young people, the lung cancer problem must be attacked on two fronts because changing the public's smoking behavior is a gradual process. One must, therefore, deal with the population already at risk in addition to stopping the inflow of new people into the reservoir.

References

1. National Cancer Institute. Canadian Cancer Statistics 1996. Toronto: National Cancer Institute, 1996.
2. Bailar III JC, Gornik HL. Cancer undefeated. N Engl J M 1997; 336:1569–1574.
3. Halpern M, Gillespie B, Warner K. Patterns of absolute risk of lung cancer mortality in former smokers. J Natl Cancer Inst 1993; 85:457–464.
4. Strauss G, De Camp M, Dibbicaro E, Richards W, et al. Lung cancer diagnosis is being made with increasing frequency in former cigarette smokers. Proc ASCO 1995; 14:362.
5. National Cancer Institute of Canada, unpublished work.
6. Anderson GH, Boyes DA, Benedet JL, et al. Organization and results of the cervical cytology screening program in British Columbia, 1955–85. Br Med J 1988; 296:975–978.
7. Nyström L, Rutqvist LE, Wall S, et al. Breast cancer screening with mammography: overview of Swedish randomized trials. Lancet 1993; 341:973–978.
8. Kerlikowske K, Grady D, Rubin S, et al. Efficacy of screening mammography. JAMA 1995; 273:149–154.
9. Screening Mammography Program, Annual Report. British Columbia Cancer Agency, 1996.
10. Cervical Cytology Screening Program, Annual Report. British Columbia Cancer Agency, 1996.
11. The National Cancer Institute. Cooperative early lung cancer detection programme. Summary and conclusions. Am Rev Respir Dis 1984; 130:565–567.
12. Kennedy TC, Proudfoot S, Franklin WA, et al. Cytopathological analysis of sputum in patients with airflow obstruction and significant smoking histories. Cancer Res 1996; 56:4673–4678.

13. Anthonisen E, Pukkala E, Timonen T, et al. Effects of smoking intervention and the use of an inhaled anticholinergic bronchodilator on the rate of decline of FEV_1: the Lung Health Study. JAMA 1994; 272:1497–1505.
14. Auer G, Ono J, Nasiell M, et al. Reversibility of bronchial cell atypia. Cancer Res 1982; 42:4241–4247.
15. Kato H, Konaka C, Hayata Y, et al. Lung cancer histogenesis following in vivo bronchial injections of 20-methylcholanthrene in dogs. Rec Res Cancer Res 1982; 82:69–86.
16. Frost JK, Ball WC Jr, Levin MI, et al. Sputum cytology: use and potential in monitoring the workplace environment by screening for biological effects of exposure. J Occup Med 1986; 28:692–703.
17. Band P, Feldstein M, Saccomanno G. Reversibility of bronchial marked atypia: implication for chemoprevention. Cancer Detect Treat 1986; 9:157–160.
18. Risse EKJ, Vooijs GP, van't Hof MA. Diagnostic significance of "severe dysplasia" in sputum cytology. Acta Cytol 1988; 32:629–634.
19. Frykberg ER, Bland KI. Overview of the biology and management of ductal carcinoma *in situ* of the breast. Cancer 1994; 74:350–361.
20. Koss G. Diagnostic Cytology. Vol. 1. 4th ed. Philadelphia: J.B. Lippincott, 1992:371.
21. Hudson MA, Herr HW. Carcinoma in situ of the bladder. J Urol 1995; 153:564–572.
22. Wolf H, Melson F, Pedersen SE, Nielsen KT. Natural history of carcinoma in situ of the urinary bladder. Scand J Urol Nephrol 1994; 157:147–151.
23. Kato H, Okunaka T, Shimatani H. Photodynamic therapy for early stage bronchogenic carcinoma. J Clin Laser Med Surg 1996; 14:235–238.
24. Furuse K, Fukuoka M, Kato H, et al. A prospective phase II study of photodynamic therapy with Photofrin II for centrally located early-stage lung cancer. J Clin Oncol 1993; 11:1852–1857.
25. Sutegdja TG, Schreurs AJ, Vanderschueren RG, et al. Bronchoscopic therapy in patients with intraluminal typical bronchial carcinoid. Chest 1995; 107:556–558.
26. Ozenne G, Vergnon JM, Roulier A, et al. Cryotherapy of in-situ or microinvasive bronchial carcinoma. Chest 1990; 98:105S.
27. Cavaliere S, Foccoli P, Toninelli C, et al. Nd:YAG laser therapy in lung cancer: an 11 year experience with 2,253 applications in 1,585 patients. J Bronchol 1994; 1:105–111.
28. McKinnon M, Payne P, MacAulay C, et al. Optimal sputum cytology collection method. Chest 1996; 100:1S.
29. Garner D, Gerguson G, Palcic B. The Cyto-Savant™ System, In: Grohs HK, Husain OAN, eds. Automated Cervical Cancer Screening. Hong Kong: Igaku-Shoin Medical Publishers, Inc., 1994:305–317.
30. Tockman MS, Erozan YS, Gupta P, et al. The early detection of second primary lung cancer by sputum immunostaining. Chest 1996; 106:385–390.
31. Mao L, Hruban RH, Boyle Jo, et al. Detection of oncogene mutations in sputum precedes diagnosis of lung cancer. Cancer Res 1994; 54:1634–1637.
32. Mao L, Schoenberg MP, Scicchitano M, et al. Molecular detection of primary bladder cancer by microsatellite analysis. Science 1996; 271:659–662.
33. Nagamoto N, Saito Y, Imai T, et al. Roentgenographically occult squamous cell carcinoma: location in the bronchi, depth of invasion and length of axial involvement of the bronchus. Tohoku J Exp Med 1986; 148:241–256.
34. Usuda K, Saito Y, Nagamoto N, et al. Relation between bronchoscopic findings and tumor size of roentgenographically occult bronchogenic squamous cell carcinoma. J Thorac Cardiovasc Surg 1993; 106:1098–1103.
35. Cortese DA, Pairolero PC, Bergsralh EJ, et al. Roentgenographically occult lung cancer: a 10 year experience. J Thorac Cardiovasc Surg 1983; 86:373–380.
36. Bechtell JJ, Kelly WR, Petty TL, et al. Outcome of 51 patients with roentgenographically occult lung cancer detected by sputum cytologic testing: a community hospital program. Arch Intern Med 1994; 154:975–980.

37. Sato M, Saito Y, Nagamoto N, et al. Diagnostic value of differential brushing of all branches of the bronchi in patients with sputum-positive or suspected positive for lung cancer. Acta Cytol 1993; 37:879–883.

38. Sagawa M, Saito Y, Sato M, et al. Localization of double, roentographically occult lung cancer. Acta Cytol 1993; 38:392–397.

39. Hung J, Lam S, LeRiche J, et al. Autofluorescence of normal and malignant bronchial tissue. Lasers Surg Med 1991; 11:99–105.

40. Qu J, MacAulay C, Lam S, Palcic B. Optical properties of normal and carcinoma bronchial tissue. Appl Optics 1991; 11:99–105.

41. Qu J, MacAulay C, Lam S, Palcic B. Laser induced fluorescence spectroscopy at endoscopy; tissue optics; Monte Carlo modeling and in-vivo measurements. Optical Eng 1995; 34:3334–3343.

42. Bolon I, Brambilla E, Vandenbunder B, et al. Changes in the expression of matrix proteases and of the transcription facter c-Ets 1 during progression of precancerous bronchial lesions. Lab Invest 1996; 75:1–13.

43. Gontaninin G, Vignati S, Bigini D, et al. Neoangiogenesis: a putative marker of malignancy in non-small-cell lung cancer (NSCLS) development. Int J Cancer 1996; 67:615–619.

44. Lam S, Profio AE. Fluorescence tumor detection. In: Hetzel MR, ed. Minimally Invasive Techniques in Thoracic Medicine and Surgery. London: Chapman & Hall, 1995; 179–191.

45. Lam S, MacAulay C, LeRiche LC, et al. Early localization of bronchogenic carcinoma. Diagn Ther Endosc 1994; 1:75–78.

46. Yokomise H, Yanagihara K, Fukuse T, et al. Clinical experience of lung-imaging fluorescence endoscope (LIFE) on lung cancer patients. J Bronchol (in press).

47. Ikeda N, Kim K, Okunaka T, et al. Early localization of bronchogenic cancerous/precancerous lesions with lung imaging fluorescence endoscope. Diagnostic Ther Endosc 1997; 3: 197–201.

48. Hung J, Kashimoto Y, Sugio K, et al. Allele-specific chromosome 3p deletions occur at an early stage in the pathogenesis of lung carcinoma. JAMA 1995; 273:558–563.

49. Thiberville L, Payne P, Vielkind J, et al. Evidence of cumulative gene losses with progression of premalignant epithelial lesions to carcinoma of the bronchus. Cancer Res 1995; 55:5133–5139.

50. Mitsudomi T, Lam S, Shirakusa T, Gazdar A. Detection and sequencing of p53 gene mutations in bronchial biopsy samples in patients with lung cancer. Chest 1993; 104:362–365.

30

Advances in Lung Cancer Imaging

GILBERT R. FERRETTI, JEAN-PHILIPPE VUILLEZ, and MAX COULOMB

Institut Albert Bonniot
Centre Hospitalier Universitaire de Grenoble
Grenoble, France

I. Introduction

Lung cancer is a devastating disease in developed countries with a 5-year survival rate of 13%, regardless of the stage of the disease. Imaging plays a major role at each stage of management of patients with suspected or known lung cancer (1,2): in early diagnosis, in assessing the extent of the disease before surgery or before medical treatment, in guiding biopsies, and in monitoring the treatment response. Advances in imaging should bring answers to some of the questions crucial to the management of patients with lung cancer that have not yet been accurately answered, such as early diagnosis of lung cancer; noninvasive differential diagnosis of solitary pulmonary nodule; initial preoperative staging of the tumor, nodes, and metastases; demonstration of recurrences; treatment follow-up.

In this review, we will discuss the major advances in imaging and their usefulness in patients with suspected or known lung cancer.

II. Chest Radiography/Digital Chest Radiography

Frontal and lateral high-voltage chest radiography remains the main tool for screening and following patients with lung cancer. Digital chest radiography (3) using storage phosphor systems or selenium detectors (4) is now commercially available. Although phantom studies have shown that these techniques are promising for detection of pulmonary abnormalities (3), few clinical studies have assessed these techniques, and they have not demonstrated any statistically significant differences in the performance of radiologists in detecting thoracic abnormalities using conventional or digital radiography (4).

Yankelevitz and Henschke (5) have pointed out that the dogma "two-year stability implies that pulmonary nodules are benign" must be taken with caution. They showed that this concept is based on a study conducted in the 1950s. Using the original data, they calculated that the predictive value for benignity using this criterion was only 65%. Moreover, it can be difficult to precisely measure the growth of small malignant tumors with long doubling time on radiographs for technical reasons.

III. CT/Spiral CT

A. Technical Aspects

Spiral or helical or volumetric computed tomography (CT), a major development in CT technology introduced in the 1990s (6–10), allows an uninterrupted volume acquisition to be acquired during a single breath-hold. Helical CT (HCT) has many advantages compared with conventional incremental CT, such as elimination of respiratory misregistration, decrease in cardiac and respiratory motion artifacts, optimization of contrast enhancement, and reduced radiation doses under certain conditions. As overlapped axial images can be reconstructed prospectively or retrospectively at arbitrary levels within the acquired volume without additional radiation exposure, high-quality two- and three-dimensional reconstructions may be created (9).

As a result, CT protocols of the thorax have been totally altered since the introduction of HCT in routine.

B. Assessment of Pulmonary Nodules

HCT improves the detection and characterization of pulmonary nodules in comparison with conventional incremental CT. Detection of nodules benefits from the ability of HCT to acquire the entire lung in one breath-hold, which eliminates misregistration resulting from repeated breath-holds, and to reconstruct overlapped images. Rémy-Jardin et al. (11) showed that HCT with 10-mm sections without overlapping and 1:1 pitch [defined as the ratio of table speed during 360° rotation (mm/sec) to the slice collimation] increased the detection of pulmonary nodules compared with incremental 10-mm sections (705 vs. 497 nodules, respectively). HCT increased both the number of nodules detected in each patient and nodules smaller than 5 mm. A controversy exists about the best protocol (slice thickness, pitch, increment of reconstruction, radiation dose) to be chosen to optimize the detection of pulmonary nodules (12). Wright et al. (13) recommended not using a pitch greater than 1.5, demonstrating that doing so increased the risk of understaging the disease in patients with solitary pulmonary nodules. More recent studies emphasized the fact that reconstruction of overlapped images, whatever the figure of slice collimation or pitch, is more important than using thin collimation or a pitch of 1 (14).

Chest radiography has a better sensitivity than sputum cytology for screening lung carcinoma in patients with high risk of developing lung cancer (15). Recently, low-dose HCT has been used as a screening procedure for detection of early lung cancer. In a study including 1369 patients followed for 18 months, Kaneko et al. (16) compared frontal and lateral chest radiographs with low-dose spiral CT (120 kvP, 50 mA, 10-mm collimation, 2:1 pitch) for the detection of small peripheral lung cancers. Spiral CT detected 15 cases of cancer out of 3457 examinations, 11 of which were not seen on chest radiographs. Among the 15 cases, 14 were stage I, and therefore potentially surgically curable. However, the cost-effectiveness of HCT was not assessed in the study.

Densitometry of pulmonary nodules has been facilitated by the use of HCT (17,18). Because of the ability of HCT to reconstruct overlapped images, the densitometry of small nodules can always be measured in the centers of the nodules, thus eliminating the effects of partial volume averaging. HCT could have potential value in distinguishing malignant from benign pulmonary nodules (17). In a study including 107 patients with solitary pulmonary nodules (malignant, 52; granulomas, 51; benign, 4), Svensen et al. (17) demonstrated that contrast enhancement of malignant nodules (median, 46.5 HU; range, 11–110 HU) is significantly higher than enhancement of granulomas and benign nodules (median, 8 HU; range, -10 to 94 HU), due to the increased vasculature of malignant nodules. A sensitivity of 98%, a specificity of 73%, and an accuracy of 85% were obtained in discriminating malignant from benign nodules when using a threshold of 20 HU.

HCT allows precise morphologic evaluation of pulmonary nodules. HCT with thin collimation sections has been found of great value in evidencing the relationship between the nodules and the adjacent airways (Fig. 1). Therefore, HCT may help to choose the optimal sampling method to obtain a histological specimen of the nodule.

C. Assessment of Central Airways Using HCT

Conventional CT has been largely appraised for the diagnosis of tumoral and inflammatory diseases of the airways (19). CT is an accurate technique for depicting focal abnormalities of the central airways, but due to the continuous acquisition, HCT with 3- or 5-mm-thick sections allows a more precise evaluation of the central airways. Central bronchi up to the segmental bronchus are constantly identified with HCT, which allows great potentials in evaluating patients with hemoptysis.

Multiplanar reconstructions (MPRs) and three-dimensional imaging have been rated to assess the central airways in patients with centrally located lung cancers. Padhani et al. (20) showed that MPRs are of interest in patients with central lung cancer to reveal more precisely the involvement of the airways. MPRs in fron-

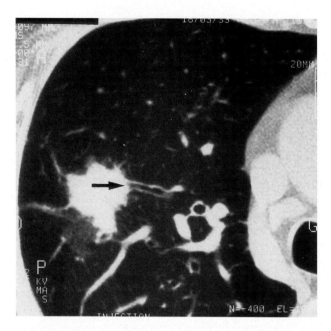

Figure 1 Pulmonary nodule: evaluation with high-resolution CT (1.5 mm section). CT demonstrates peripheral lobulated and spiculated nodule in the right upper lobe and the relationships between the tumor and the lateral subsegmental bronchus (arrow) of the anterior segmental bronchus of this lobe.

tal or coronal plane can help to assess aorto-pulmonary window (Fig. 2) or subcarinal regions. Coronal or oblique reconstructions are useful in evaluating tracheal tumors and localized bronchial tumors before surgery as these reconstructions allow precise representations and measurements of the extension of the tumor (9).

Thanks to advances in computer techniques, virtual endoscopy simulations can be created, derived from spiral CT data (21). The virtual bronchoscopy (VB) technique gives a bronchoscopist's view of the inner surface of the major bronchi and allows one to "fly" through the airways. Endoscopic simulations of the airways produce remarkably high-quality reproductions of major endoluminal abnormalities (Fig. 3) (21,22). VB is a noninvasive technique that can provide endoscopic simulations of the airways even below a nonpassable stenosis. Endobronchial anatomical landmarks shown by VB are the same as those shown by FOB, which has a great potential for improved preprocedural planning of endobronchial interventional techniques, such as transbronchial needle aspiration (23) or stenting of a bronchial stricture. However, VB images should be always interpreted with axial images or MPRs (24). In the series by Ferretti et al. (24), VB showed 39 of the 41 (95%) stenoses of the central airways evidenced by FOB. However, evaluation of the thickness of the airway walls at the level of stenoses required simultaneous display of MPRs. With the technique used (24), the airway walls cannot be rendered transparent; therefore,

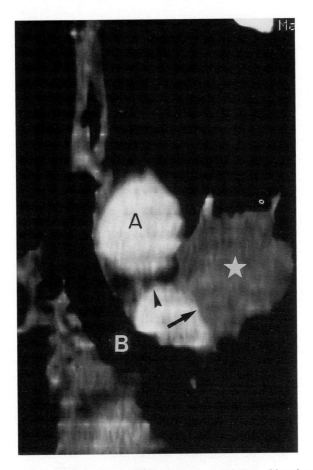

Figure 2 Centrally located left upper lobe carcinoma in 58-year-old patient. Coronal reformation of contrast enhanced helical CT (5-mm collimation) through the aorto-pulmonary window shows the tumor (star) abutting the upper part of the left pulmonary artery (arrow). The aorto-pulmonary window is well demonstrated without adenopathy (arrow-head). At surgery this tumor was resected by left pneumonectomy. Aorta (A), main left bronchus (B).

evaluation of the surrounding tissues required simultaneous display of MPRs. Vining et al. (21) developed a specific software program to display the segmented structures located beyond the airway walls, such as enlarged lymph nodes within the mediastinum.

VB may improve the diagnostic performance of CT and may assist in planning for bronchoscopy, surgery, and endobronchial brachytherapy. However, VB has some limitations that reduce the spectrum of indications. VB does not depict mucosal abnormalities. Therefore, conventional FOB remains the technique of choice for

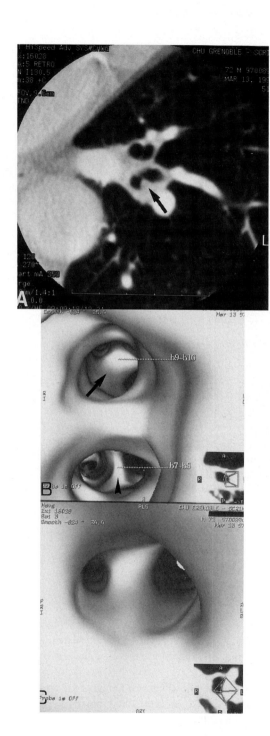

assessing patients with suspected bronchial disease, as it shows the mucosa and permits biopsy.

Further studies are needed to evaluate the diagnosis potential of VB and its usefulness in planning various interventional procedures.

D. Staging Lung Cancer

The prognosis of patients with lung carcinoma depends on both the extent of the disease as evaluated using the TNM system (25) and the histopathologic cell-type, i.e., non–small-cell carcinoma (NSCC) and small-cell carcinoma (SCC). In patients with NSCC, surgery remains the only hope to definitively cure the patient. However, 40–50% of patients with NSCC have unresectable tumors at exploratory thoracotomy. Therefore, imaging should ideally differentiate preoperatively patients who may benefit from surgical resection because the disease is localized from those with unresectable cancers because of local, nodal, or distant extensions. One of the results of the introduction of CT has been a decrease in exploratory thoracotomies from 25 to 10% in the last 15 years (25).

After plain chest radiography, CT is used in most institutions as a standard part of the initial workup of patients with known or suspected lung cancer, although CT disagrees with postoperative TNM staging in about 40% of patients (27). Nowadays, HCT is the technique of choice in assessing the initial staging of lung cancer. Staging lung cancers requires intravenous contrast infusion using a power injector with 80–120 mL of contrast media at a rate of 2–3 mL/sec and a delay of 15–25 sec. Slice thickness and pitch vary from one institution to another. We use a 7.5 mm/sec table feed and 5-mm collimation (pitch: 1.5) with an interval of reconstruction at 5 mm. Two acquisitions are usually needed to cover the entire lung and the adrenals. Resulting from the high quality of vascular enhancement, the capability of reconstructing overlapped slices, and multiplanar or three-dimensional reconstructions, HCT provides a more accurate evaluation of mediastinal and hilar lymph nodes as well as direct mediastinal extension than incremental CT (9).

Evaluation of Primary Tumors

Chest Wall Invasion

Localized chest-wall invasion is not a contraindication to surgery, as surgeons can perform en-bloc resection and thoracic wall reconstruction. Patients with "T3-walls"

Figure 3 Small bronchial carcinoma in a 70-year-old patient. (A) Contrast enhanced helical CT with 1-mm collimation and 1.4:1 pitch shows a small nodule in the division of B9 and B10 bronchus (arrow). (B) Virtual endoscopy at the level of the left lower lobe bronchus demonstrates the enlargement of the division of B9 and B10 (arrow) as compare to the division of B7 and B8 bronchus (arrow head). (C) Close-up of the division of B9 and B10. Left lower lobe lobectomy confirmed a squamous cell carcinoma.

have a 5-year survival rate of about 30% if there is no mediastinal adenopathy or distant metastasis (28,29). As such resections are associated with increased morbidity and mortality, it is worth knowing preoperatively the presence of such invasion. Unfortunately, CT imaging assessment of direct extension of lung cancer to the thoracic wall is disappointing, with sensitivity ranging from 38 to 87% and specificity ranging from 40 to 90%, respectively (30,31). The only reliable CT signs with high positive predictive values are the destruction of a vertebral body or a rib adjacent to the soft tissue mass (30–33), but CT was found less accurate than focal chest pain for the detection of chest wall invasion (30). A contact of more than 3 cm of the tumor with the pleura or obtuse angles of the tumor with the pleura are not reliable signs. Pleural thickening, obliteration of the extrapleural fat plane, or discrete chest-wall soft tissue mass are unreliable signs of cancer infiltration to the chest wall as they may be related to inflammatory changes or desmoplastic reactions (Fig. 4). On the contrary, the tumoral infiltration can be microscopic with respect to the fat plane (29) and therefore be underestimated on CT images.

Acquiring CT after induced pneumothorax has been suggested to recognize chest-wall or mediastinal invasion. In the study including 43 patients by Yokoi et al. (34), sensitivity of pneumothorax CT was 100%, but specificity was only 80% because of inflammatory adhesions between the two layers of pleura. Moreover, the technique is quite invasive.

HCT with thin collimation has been evaluated in 42 patients with peripheral carcinoma (35). At surgery, these patients had pleural invasion in 12 cases, parietal invasion in 5 cases, and no pleural invasion in 25 cases. Three-dimensional surface shaded display (3D SSD) was more accurate than axial images to demonstrate visceral pleural extension (11 vs. 2) and parietal pleural invasion (3 vs. 2) with a sensitivity of 92% and a specificity of 76% for 3D SSD images.

Dynamic spiral CT during the respiratory cycle has been appraised in staging peripheral lung carcinoma (36). HCT can show a lack of respiratory motion between the tumor and the parietal pleura or the chest wall, which indicates extension of the tumor to the parietal pleura or thoracic wall, indicating a T3 lesion (36). Comparison between CT images acquired at inspiration and those acquired at exhalation were of value in determining extension of lung cancer to the middle and lower lobes (37), but the technique was less valuable for evaluating the upper-lobe cancers because of the limited respiratory amplitude.

Mediastinal Invasion

Limited tumoral invasion into mediastinal pleura, pericardium, or even mediastinal fat is not a contraindication to surgery, although direct extension to the great vessels, heart, trachea, esophagus, or vertebral body is usually an obstacle to surgery. Consequently, imaging should distinguish between resectable (T3) and unresectable (T4) cancers.

CT can disclose extensive mediastinal invasion (T4) when showing the mediastinal vessels, main bronchus, trachea, or esophagus completely surrounded by the tumor, which precludes surgery. However, subtle invasion of the mediastinum is dif-

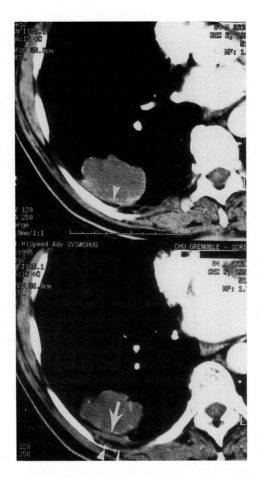

Figure 4   A 5-cm peripheral carcinoma of the right lower lobe abutting the pleura, which is thickened (arrow). The subpleural fat is preserved (arrow head). Extension to the pleural is highly suspected on CT images. Absence of extension to the pleura at pathology indicating a T2.

ficult to diagnose. Simple contact of the tumor with the mediastinum is not a reliable criterion of extension, and neither is the loss of fat planes (Fig. 5). In a study by Glazer et al. (38), the presence of less than 3 cm of tumor contact with the mediastinum, less than 90° tumor contact with the aorta, and a visible fat plane between the tumor and mediastinal structure was associated with a technical resectability in 36 out of 37 tumors (97%). However, defining criteria for unresectable disease (T4) is harder, providing a sensitivity as low as 50% and a specificity between 82 and 89% for CT in evaluating mediastinal invasion (39–41). Therefore, patients with indeterminate mediastinal invasion at CT should not be contraindicated for surgery, only on the basis of CT findings.

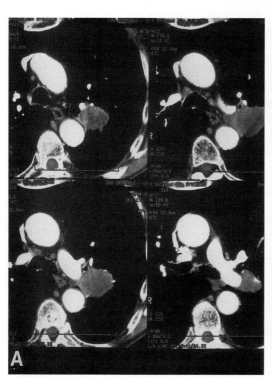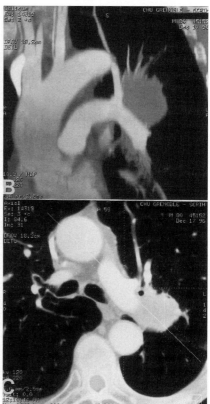

Figure 5 Contrast enhanced helical CT with 5-mm collimation in a patient with left upper lobe cancer demonstrates perfectly (A) the tumor and its relationships with the descending aorta and the left pulmonary artery. Note the respect of the aortic wall. (B) Maximum intensity projection in a sagittal oblique plane (C) shows the mass abutting the left pulmonary artery.

In order to increase the sensitivity of CT, as with chest-wall invasion, multiple-section dynamic CT during respiratory cycles (42,43) and pneumothorax CT (34) have been used to assess the extension to the mediastinum. Although these techniques have yielded promising results, they have not been widely used yet.

Lymph-Node Staging

Ideally, imaging techniques should be able to separate metastatic from uninvolved nodes. The only sign of tumoral spreading to lymph nodes is nodal enlargement. None of the other CT signs such as node attenuation, central necrosis, nodal enhancement, and nodal shape have any value.

Using a 10-mm short-axis diameter cutoff figure and a gold standard consisting of extensive mediastinal dissection, recent studies have reported a low accuracy for CT scanning, with both a low sensitivity and a specificity ranging from 50 to 65% (44–46). Such disappointing results of CT imaging have raised doubts as to the exact role of CT in mediastinal lymph node staging. In practice, mediastinoscopy or alternative biopsy techniques of the mediastinal nodes is recommended in patients with enlarged mediastinal lymph nodes shown on CT images, to prove nodal metastasis that would preclude surgical resection (47). Mediastinoscopy allows sampling of lymph nodes that are adjacent to the trachea (i.e., 2D, 4D, 4G, 2G, and anterior subcarinal nodes), while anterior mediastinal nodes (i.e., 5, 6, 2G) can be assessed with anterior mediastinotomy. Video-assisted thoracoscopy is a new technique of direct visualization of the mediastinum and sampling (48–50). Transbronchial needle biopsy (TBNA) guided by CT images permits the sampling, during FOB, of mediastinal nodes that are difficult to biopsy using mediastinoscopy (i.e., 4G, 7). In patients with enlarged nodes, CT is useful in selecting the optimal technique of biopsy according to the location of the enlarged nodes and in directing the sampling to a specific nodal station (23,51). In patients without nodal enlargement on CT images, the need for preoperative mediastinoscopy is more controversial as the nodes are unlikely to yield metastases, and even though the nodes are microscopically invaded, the patients may benefit from thoracotomy and extensive nodal dissection in terms of survival rate (52).

However, no study has been published to our knowledge that evaluates the sensitivity, specificity, and accuracy of HCT for the assessment lymph nodes in comparison with surgical findings. Unfortunately, because of the morphological nature of CT criteria, little improvement is to be expected from HCT in distinguishing benign from malignant nodes.

IV. Magnetic Resonance Imaging

Magnetic resonance imaging (MRI) has been extensively evaluated in comparison to CT for staging lung cancer (40,46,53–55). The advantages of MRI include multiplanar imaging capability and intrinsic blood flow sensitivity. The basic technique used to investigate the mediastinum and hila has not changed over the last decade and consists in cardiac gated axial, coronal, and sagittal T1-weighted and T2-weighted images. MRI offers limited additional staging information to CT images so that MRI has not replaced CT in the initial evaluation of lung cancer.

Because of its better contrast resolution, multiplanar imaging capabilities, and high-resolution images provided by surface coils, MRI should provide better results than CT in evaluating the chest-wall invasion, as reported by early evaluations (54,56). Criteria for parietal invasion was presence of soft tissue with signal identical to that of the tumor extending into the extrapleural fat on T1-weighted images (Fig. 6). On T2-weighted images, soft tissue mass is of high signal intensity.

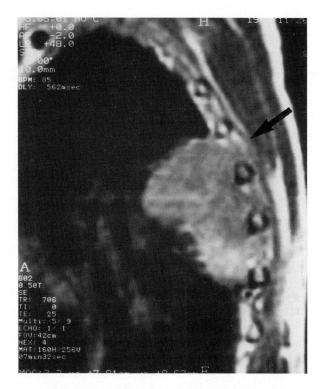

Figure 6   A 62-year-old patient with peripheral lung mass. T1-weighted MR imaging in sagittal plane demonstrates a lobulated lung tumor with extension to chest wall (arrow).

However, MRI has the same limitations as CT to differentiate inflammatory changes from tumoral extension into the chest wall, since the signal intensity of both conditions can be identical (46). In a recent prospective study including 34 patients with surgical proof, Padovani et al. (57) found T1-weighted images (sensitivity, 85%; specificity, 100%) more accurate than both T2-weighted images (sensitivity, 65%; specificity, 100%) and contrast enhanced T1-weighted images (sensitivity, 85%; specificity, 85%). The overall sensitivity of MR images was 90% and specificity was 86%.

MRI is the technique of choice in evaluating superior sulcus tumors (Pancoast) (58). T1-weighted images acquired in coronal and sagittal planes provide highly contrasted anatomical images (Fig. 7). Patients without tumoral extension to vertebral bodies, brachial plexus, or vessels may benefit from aggressive surgery.

The contrast enhancement of solitary pulmonary nodules 30 mm or smaller has been studied in 28 patients using snapshot gradient-echo sequences that allow dynamic measurements of nodule density (59).

The accuracy of CT and MRI are similar for staging mediastinal nodes (40,46,53,55). In specific situations, MRI in coronal or sagittal planes may complete

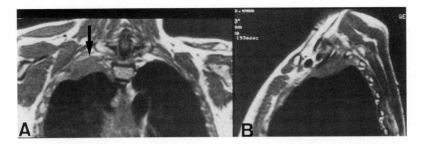

Figure 7   MR imaging of superior sulcus tumor (T1-weighted images). (A) Invasion of extrapleural fat line of right apex is well demonstrated on coronal view (arrow). (B) Sagittal plane shows the absence of extension of the tumor to the right subclavian artery and vein.

the CT scan to assess nodal metastases to the aortopulmonary window or subcarinal nodes (60). However, spiral CT offers the same reformatted planes as MRI with better spatial resolution, which can help in distinguishing small adjacent nodes from enlarged nodes. Dynamic MRI with fast gradient-echo sequences following intravenous gadolinium may help to distinguish benign from metastatic enlarged nodes (61).

V.   Ultrasonography

Transthoracic sonography is applicable for assessment of chest-wall invasion by lung cancer and showed promising results (62,63). Chest-wall invasion is best depicted as a disruption of the pleural surface, tumoral extension through the chest wall, and lack of motion of the tumor during respiration. In a study including 120 patients, 19 of whom had surgically proved chest-wall invasion, Suzuki et al. (63) reported a sensitivity of 100% and a specificity of 98% for ultrasonography (US).

Transesophageal US has been described to assess mediastinal nodes (64,65), to guide aspiration biopsy (66,67), and to estimate cardiac invasion (68). Miniaturized ultrasound probes can be introduced through a flexible bronchoscope port to assess the mediastinum and to guide TBNA of mediastinal nodes (69,70). Miniaturized US probes can be used during videothoracoscopy to assess the aortopulmonary window (71).

VI.   Nuclear Medicine

Although morphological images are limited in some instances for assessing the extension of lung cancer, as previously emphasized in this section, recent nuclear medicine techniques show promise. These techniques take advantage of abnormal functional metabolism in tumoral tissue. Many tracers have been tested, such as gallium-67 (72), thallium-201 (73), SestaMIBI, HMPAO (74), or DMSA (75).

Fluorine-18 fluorodeoxyglucose (FDG) PET assesses the metabolic activity and consumption of glucose in cells. The field of view of PET systems has been increased and reaches 25 cm now, allowing whole-body acquisitions, which are essential for oncological applications (76). Additionally, it is now possible to use dual-head large field of view single-photon emission tomographic (SPECT) cameras with coincidence detection (77).

FDG PET has been widely applied to the noninvasive characterization of pulmonary nodules, with a sensitivity ranging from 93 to 100% and a specificity ranging from 78 to 88% for diagnosis of malignancy (78–82). The specificity is lowered by the incidence of granulomatous diseases responsible for false-negative results.

FDG PET has been used preoperatively for staging patients with known lung cancer for assessing mediastinal lymph nodes and metastases. The sensitivity and specificity for mediastinal lymph node metastases ranged from 78 to 100% and 73 to 100%, respectively (83–85). FDG PET has shown higher accuracy than CT scan for nodal staging as shown by Steinert et al. (86), who reported an accuracy of 96% for PET and 85% for CT for staging N2 and N3 mediastinal nodes (Fig. 8). Whole-body FDG PET has great potential to disclose unknown distant metastases as reported in the study by Lewis et al. (84). Ten unknown metastases were disclosed in the 34 patients included in this study; management of patients was altered in 14 cases because of PET results. PET appears particularly suitable for noninvasive diagnosis of adrenal masses.

FDG PET has proved helpful in several studies for early detection of recurrences (87,88). Abe et al. (89) demonstrated that FDG uptake is useful for the evaluation of therapeutic effects and efficacy of radiotherapy and chemotherapy. Knopp et al. (90) showed that follow-up PET results were the most reliable indicators of patient survival, as compared to clinical evaluation without PET and tumor markers studies.

[11]C-methionine is another usable tracer for PET studies, although its availability is much lower, because of the very short period of carbon 11 (6 min vs. 40 min for fluorine 18). Miyazawa et al. (91) found that the tumor uptake of ^{11}C-methionine was representative of tumor growth rate.

Although not yet fully validated from a clinical point of view, FDG PET appears to be a very interesting technique complementary of morphological imaging and promising for the management of lung cancer. Because of its ability to differentiate benign from malignant processes in the lung, PET should be recommended, if available, prior to invasive procedures such as biopsy or thoracoscopy in patients with a solitary pulmonary nodule less than 3 cm in diameter, especially when biopsy is risky or when the estimated risk for malignancy is low, based on clinical and radiological data. A negative PET scan would preclude the need for biopsy, whereas positive results would confirm the necessity of biopsy. PET should also be helpful for the preoperative staging, avoiding unindicated thoracotomies, and will probably become a criterion for the evaluation of treatment response.

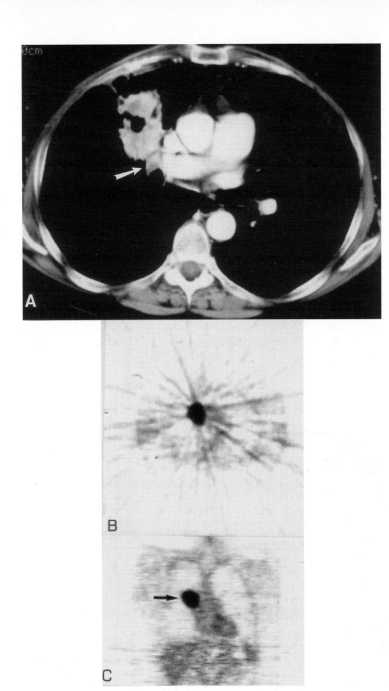

Figure 8 (A) Axial CT scan in a 60-year-old patient showing a 5 × 3 cavitary mass within the right upper lobe and a 1.1-cm node in the right hilum (11R) (Arrow). Axial (B) and coronal (C) positron emission tomography with fluoro-2-deoxyglucose images show intense uptake just superior and anterior to the right hilum (arrow) but no uptake within the mediastinum. Confirmation at surgery. (Images courtesy of R. Chin and C. Chiles, Bowman Gray School of Medicine, Winston-Salem, NC.)

Radiolabeled antibodies, used for radioimmunodetection (mostly immunoscintigraphy), are another interesting class of radiopharmaceuticals for cancer management. These results are detailed in another section.

VII. Conclusion

Currently, conventional chest radiography is the technique of choice for early diagnosis of lung cancer. CT with volume acquisition, although not perfect, is the standard technique for staging lung cancer. MRI has some selected and rare indications when CT is inconclusive. FDG PET is promising but needs to be validated on large population studies. Sonography may play a role in some cases.

In the future, early detection of lung cancer should be the priority as it may increase the percentage of patients who could benefit from surgery. Many techniques have potential value, such as digital chest radiography with computer-aided diagnosis of small nodules (92), dual-energy chest radiography (93), or HCT. Imaging may play a role in assessing the local extension of small lung cancers detected using FOB with fluorescence.

References

1. Quint LE, Francis IR, Walsh RL, Gross BH, Glazer GM. Preoperative staging of non-small-cell carcinoma of the lung: imaging methods. AJR 1995; 164:1350–1357.
2. Hanson JA, Amstrong P. Staging intrathoracic non-small-cell lung cancer. Eur Radiol 1997; 7:161–172.
3. Glazer HS, Muka E, Sagel SS, Jost RG. New techniques in chest radiography. Radiol Clin North Am 1994; 32:711–729.
4. Van Heesewijk HPM, Van Der Graaf Y, De Valois JC, Vos JA, Feldberg MAM. Chest imaging with a selenium detector versus conventional film radiography: a CT-controlled study. Radiology 1996; 200:687–690.
5. Yankelevitz DF, Henschke CI. Does 2-year stability imply that pulmonary nodules are benign? AJR 1997; 168:325–328.
6. Heiken JP, Brink JA, Vannier MW. Spiral (helical) CT. Radiology 1993; 189:647–656.
7. Naidich DP, Gruden JF, McGuiness G, McCauley DI, Bhalla M. Volumetric (helical/spiral) CT (VCT) of the airways. J Thorac Imag 1997; 12:11–28.
8. Naidich DP. Helical computed tomography of the thorax. Clinical applications. Radiol Clin North Am 1994; 32:759–74.
9. Touliopoulos P, Costello P. Helical (spiral) CT of the thorax. Radiol Clin North Am 1995; 33:843–61.
10. Leung AN. Spiral CT of the thorax in daily practice: optimization of technique. J Thorac Imag 1997; 12:2–10.
11. Remy-Jardin M, Remy J, Giraud F, Pulmonary nodules: detection with thick-section spiral CT versus conventional CT. Radiology 1993; 187:513–520.
12. Buckley JA, Scott WW Jr, Kuhlman JE, Urban BA, Bluemke DA, Fishman EK. Pulmonary nodules: effect in increased data sampling on detection with spiral CT and confidence in diagnosis. Radiology 1995; 196:395–400.
13. Wright AR MA, Collie DA, Williams JR, Hashemi-Malayeri B, Stevenson AJM, Turnbull CM. Pulmonary nodules: effect on detection of spiral CT pitch. Radiology 1996; 199: 837–841.

14. Schaeffer-Prokop C, Prokop M, Tohnebohn A, Kolher A, Jorgrnsen M, Palvlicek R, Galanski M. Impact of slice thickness, reconstruction interval, and cine-mode on the visualization of small pulmonary nodules in spiral CT. Eur Radiol 1997; 7:S123.
15. Bragg DG. Imaging in primary lung cancer: the roles of detection, staging, and follow-up. Semin Ultrasound CT MRI 1989; 10:453–466.
16. Kaneko M, Eguchi K, Ohmatsu H, Kakinuma R, Naruke T, Suemasu K, Moriyama N. Peripheral lung cancer: screening and detection with low-dose spinal CT versus radiography. Radiology 1996; 201:798–802.
17. Svensen SJ, Brown LR, Colby TV, Weaver Al, Midthun DE. Lung nodule enhancement at CT: prospective findings. Radiology 1996; 201:447–455.
18. Yamashita K, Matsunobe S, Takahashi R, Nemoto T, Matsumoto K, Miki H, Konishi J. Solitary pulmonary nodule: preliminary study of evaluation with incremental dynamic CT. Radiology 1995; 194:399–405.
19. Naidich DP, Harkin TJ. Airways and lung: correlation of CT with fiberoptic bronchoscopy. Radiology 1995; 197:1–12.
20. Padhani AR, Fishman EK, Heitmiller RF, Wang KP, Wheeler JH, Kuhlman JE. Multiplanar display of spiral CT data of the pulmonary hila in patients with lung cancer. Preliminary observations. Clin Imaging 1995; 19:252–257.
21. Vining DJ, Liu K, Choplin RH, Haponik EF. Virtual bronchoscopy: relationships of virtual reality endobronchial simulations to actual bronchoscopic findings. Chest 1996; 109: 549–553.
22. Ferretti GR, Vining DJ, Knoplioch J, Coulomb M. Tracheobronchial tree: three-dimensional spiral CT with bronchoscopic perspective. J Comput Assist Tomogr 1996; 20:777–81.
23. Wang K-P. Staging of bronchogenic carcinoma by bronchoscopy. Chest 1994; 106: 588–593.
24. Ferretti G, Knoplioch J, Bricault I, Brambilla C, Coulomb M. Central airway stenoses: preliminary results of spiral-CT-generated virtual bronchoscopy simulations in 29 patients. Eur Radiol 1997; 7:854–859.
25. Stitik FP. The new staging of lung cancer. Radiol Clin North Am 1994; 32:635–648.
26. Riquet M, Manac'c D, Dupont P, Dujon A, Hidden G, Debesse B. Anatomic basis of lymphatic spread of lung carcinoma to the mediastinum: anatomo-clinical correlations. Surg Radiol Anat 1994; 16:229–238.
27. Lewis JW, Pearlberg JL, Beaute GH. Can computed tomography of the chest stage lung cancer? Yes and no. Ann Thorac Surg 1990; 49:591–596.
28. Allen MS, Mathisen DJ, Grillo HC, Wain JC, Moncure AC, Hilgenberg AD. Bronchogenic carcinoma with chest wall invasion. Ann Thorac Surg 1991; 51:948–951.
29. Ratto GB, Piacenza G, Frola C, Musante F, Serrano I, Gina R, Salio M, Jacovani P, Rovida S. Chest wall involvement by lung cancer: computed tomographic detection and results of operation. Ann Thorac Surg 1991; 51:182–188.
30. Glazer HS, Duncan-Meyer J, Aronberg DJ, Moran JF, Levitt RG, Sagel SS. Pleural and chest wall invasion in bronchogenic carcinoma: CT evaluation. Radiology 1985; 157: 191–194.
31. Pennes DR, Glazer GM, Wimbish KJ, Gross BH, Long RW, Orringer MB. Chest wall invasion by lung cancer: limitations of CT evaluation. AJR 1985; 144:507–511.
32. Scott IR, Muller NL, Miller RR, Evans KG, Nelems B. Resectable stage III lung cancer: CT, surgical and pathologic correlation. Radiology 1988; 166:75–79.
33. Pearlberg JL, Sandler MA, Beute GH, Lewis JR Jr, Madrazo BL. Limitations of CT in evaluation of neoplasms involving chest wall. J Comput Assist Tomogr 1987; 11:290–293.
34. Yokoi K, Mori K, Miyazawa N, Saito Y, Okuyama A, Sasagawa M. Tumor invasion of the chest wall and mediastinum in lung cancer: evaluation with pneumothorax CT. Radiology 1991; 181:147–152.
35. Kuriyama K, Tateishi R, Kumatani T RT, Kodama K, Doi O, Hosomi N, Sawai Y, Inoue E, Kadota T, Narumi Y, Fujita M, Kuroda C. Pleural invasion by peripheral bronchogenic carcinoma: assessment with three-dimensional helical CT. Radiology 1994; 191: 365–369.

36. Murata K, Takahashi M, Mori M, Shimoyam K, Morita R. Multiple section dynamic CT during expiration for the evaluation of thoracic wall invasion of lung cancer. Radiology 1992; 185(suppl):131–132.

37. Shirakawa T, Fukuda K, Miyamoto Y, Tanabe H, Tada S. Parietal pleural invasion of lung masses: evaluation with CT performed during deep inspiration and expiration. Radiology 1994; 192:809–811.

38. Glazer HS, Kaiser LR, Anderson DJ, Molina PL, Emami B, Roper CL, Sagel SS. Indeterminate mediastinal invasion in bronchogenic carcinoma: CT evaluation. Radiology 1989; 173:37–42.

39. White PG, Adams H, Crane MD, Butchart EG. Preoperative staging of carcinoma of the bronchus: can computed tomographic scanning reliably identify stage III tumours? Thorax 1994; 49:951–957.

40. Grenier P, Dubray B, Carette MF, Frija G, Musset D, Chastang C. Preoperative thoracic staging of lung cancer: CT and MR evaluation. Diagn Intervent Radiol 1989; 1:23–28.

41. Primak SL, Lee KS, Logan PM, Miller RR, Müller NL. Bronchogenic carcinoma: utility of CT in the evaluation of patients with suspected lesions. Radiology 1994; 193:795–800.

42. Minami M, Kawauchi N, Matsuoka Y, Amou K, Shindou T, Araki T. Cine CT with electrocardiography and respiratory gating in the evaluation of structures surrounding lung and mediastinal tumors. Radiology 1992; 185(suppl):132.

43. Murata K, Takahashi M, Mori M, Shimoyam K, Mishina A, Fujino S, Itoh H, Morita R. Chest wall and mediastinal invasion by lung cancer: evaluation with multisection expiratory dynamic CT. Radiology 1994; 191:251–255.

44. McLoud TC, Bourgouin PM, Greenberg RW, Kosiuk JP, Templeton PA, Shepard JA, Moore EH, Wain JC, Mathisen DJ, Grillo HC. Bronchogenic carcinoma: analysis of staging in the mediastinum with CT by correlative lymph node mapping and sampling. Radiology 1992; 182:319–323.

45. McKenna RJ Jr, Libshitz HI, Mountain CE, McMurtrey MJ. Roentgenographic evaluation of mediastinal nodes for preoperative assessment in lung cancer. Chest 1985; 88: 206–210.

46. Webb WR, Gatsonis C, Zerhouni EA, Heelan RT, Glazer GM, Francis IR, McNeil BJ. CT and MR imaging in staging non-small-cell bronchogenic carcinoma: report of the radiologic diagnostic oncology group. Radiology 1991; 178:705–713.

47. Naidich DP. Staging of lung cancer: computed tomography versus bronchoscopic needle aspiration. J Bronchol 1996; 3:69–73.

48. Landreneau RJ, Hazelrigg SR, Mack MJ, Fitzgibbon LD, Dowling RD, Acuff TE, Kennan RJ, Ferson PF. Thoracoscopic mediastinal lymph node sampling: useful for mediastinal lymph node stations inaccessible by cervical mediastinoscopy. J Thorac Cardiovasc Surg 1993; 106:554–558.

49. Rendina EA, Venuta F, Giacomo T, Ciriaco PP, Pescarmona EO, Francioni F, Pulsoni A, Malagnino F, Ricci C. Comparative merits of thoracoscopy, mediastinoscopy, and mediastinotomy for mediastinal biopsy. Ann Thorac Surg 1994; 57:992–995.

50. Roviaro G, Varoli F, Rebuffat C, Vergani C, Maciocco M, Scalambra SM, Sonnino D, Gozi G. Videothoracoscopic staging and treatment of lung cancer. Ann Thorac Surg 1994; 59: 971–974.

51. Epstein DM, Stephenson LW, Gefter WB, Voorde F, Aronchik JM, Miller WT. Value of CT in the preoperative assessment of lung cancer: a survey of thoracic surgeons. Radiology 1986; 161:423–427.

52. Daly BDP, Mueller JD, Faling LJ, Diehlo JT, Bankoff MS, Karp DD. N2 lung cancer: outcome in patients with false-negative computed tomographic scans of the chest. J Thorac Cardiovasc Surg 1993; 105:904–911.

53. Martini N, Heelan R, Westcott J, Bains MS, McCormack P, Caravelli J, Watson R, Zaman M. Comparative merits of conventional, computed tomographic, and magnetic resonance imaging in assessing mediastinal involvement in surgically confirmed lung carcinoma. J Thorac Cardiovasc Surg 1985; 90:639–648.

54. Musset D, Grenier P, Carette MF, Frija G, Hauuy MP, Desbleds MT, Girard P, Bigot JM, Lallemand D. Primary lung cancer staging: prospective comparative study of MR imaging with CT. Radiology 1986; 160:607–611.
55. Coulomb M, Escolano E, Rose-Pittet l, Blanc-Jouvan F, Lebas JF, Brambilla E, Sarrazin R, Brambilla C, Brichon PY. L'extension ganglionnaire médiastinale dans le cancer primitif des bronches: corrélations entre la tomodensitométrie, l'imagerie par résonance magnétique et la médiastinoscopie. J Radiol 1987; 68:549–553.
56. Haggar AM, Pearlberg JL, Froelich JW, Hearshen DO, Beute GH, Lewis JW Jr, Schkudor GW, Wood C, Gniewek P. Chest wall invasion by carcinoma of the lung: detection by MR imaging. AJR 1987; 148:1075–1078.
57. Padovani B, Mouroux J, Seksik L, Chanalet S, Sedat J, Rotomondo C, Richelme H, Serres JJ. Chest wall invasion by bronchogenic carcinoma: evaluation with MR imaging. Radiology 1993; 187:33–38.
58. Rapoport S, Blair DN, McCarthy SM, Desser TS, Hammers LW, Sostman HD. Brachial plexus: correlation of MR imaging with CT and pathologic findings. Radiology 1988; 167:161–165.
59. Gücket C, Schnabel K, Deimling M, Steinbrich W. Solitary pulmonary nodules: MR evaluation of enhancement patterns with contrast-enhanced dynamic snapshot gradient-echo imaging. Radiology 1996; 200:681–686.
60. Bara P, Brown K, Steckel RJ, Collins JD, Ovenfors CO, Aberle D. MR imaging of the thorax: a comparison of axial, coronal and sagittal imaging planes. J Comput Assist Tomogr 1988; 12:75–81.
61. Laissy JP, Gay-Depassier P, Soyer P, Dombret MC, Murciano G, Sautet A, Aubier M, Menu Y. Enlarged mediastinal lymph nodes in bronchogenic carcinoma: assessment with dynamic contrast-enhanced MR imaging. Radiology 1994; 191:263–267.
62. Sugama Y, Kobayashi H, Kitamura S, Kira S. Ultrasonographic evaluation of pleural and chest wall invasion of lung cancer. Chest 1988; 94:1271–1275.
63. Suzuki N, Saitoh T, Kitamura S. Tumor invasion of the chest wall in lung cancer: diagnosis with US. Radiology 1993; 187:39–42.
64. Hawes RH, Gress F, Kesler KA, Cummings OW, Conces DJ Jr. Endoscopic ultrasound versus computed tomography in the evaluation of the mediastinum in patients with non-small cell lung cancer. Endoscopy 1994; 26:784–787.
65. Jakob H, Lorenz J, Clement T, Borner M, Schweden F, Erbel R, Oelert H. Mediastinal lymph node staging with transesophageal echography in cancer of the lung. Eur J Cardiothorac Surg 1990; 4:355–358.
66. Pedersen BH, Vilmann P, Milman N, Folke K, Hancke S. Endoscopic ultrasonography with guided fine needle aspiration biopsy of a mediastinal mass lesion. Acta Radiol 1995; 36: 326–328.
67. Wiersema MJ, Kochman ML, Cramer HM, Wiersema LM. Preoperative staging of non-small cell lung cancer: transoesophageal US-guide fine-needle aspiration biopsy of mediastinal lymph nodes. Radiology 1994; 190:239–242.
68. Tatsumura T. Preoperative and intraoperative ultrasonographic examination as an aid in lung cancer operations. J Thorac Cardiovasc Surg 1995; 110:606–612.
69. Goldberg BB, Steiner RM, Liu JB, Merton DA, Articolo G, Cohn JR, Gottlieb J, McComb BL, Spirn PW. US-assisted bronchoscopy with use of miniature transducer-containing catheters. Radiology 1994; 190:233–237.
70. Shannon JJ, Bud RO, Jonathan BO, Becker FS, Whyte RI, Rubin JM, Quint LE, Martinez FJ. Endobronchial ultrasound-guided needle aspiration of mediastinal adenopathy. Am J Respir Crit Care Med 1996; 153:1424–30.
71. Janssen JP, Staal R, Cuesta MA, Tan TP, Postmus PE. Thoracoscopic ultrasonography of the aortopulmonary window. Chest 1994; 1927–1928.
72. McKenna RJ, Haynie TP, Libshitz HI, Mountain CS, McMurtrey MJ. Critical evaluation of the Ga 67 scan for surgical patients with lung cancer. Chest 1985; 87: 428–431.

73. Takekawa H, Takaoka K, Tsukamoto E, Kanegae K, Miller F, Kawakami Y. Thallium-201 single photon emission computed tomography as an indicator of prognosis for patients with lung carcinoma. Cancer 1997; 80:198–203.
74. Oshima M, Itoh K, Okae S, Tadokoro M, Kodama Y, Sakuma S. Evaluation of primary lung carcinoma using technetium 99m-hexamethylpropylène amine oxime: preliminary clinical experience. Eur J Nucl Med 1990; 16:859–864.
75. Hirano T, Otake H, Yoshida I, Endo K. Primary lung cancer SPECT imaging with pentavalent technetium-99m-DMSA. J Nucl Med 1995; 36:202–220.
76. Dadhlbom M, Hoffman EJ, Hoh CK, Schiepers C, Rosenqvist G, Hawkins RA, Phelps ME. Whole-body positron emission tomography: part I. Methods and performance characteristics. J Nucl Med 1992; 33:1191–1199.
77. Glass EC, Nelleman P, Hines H. Initial coincidence imaging experience with a SPECT/PET dual-head camera. J Nucl Med 1996; 37:53P.
78. Kubota K, Matsuzawa T, Fujiwara T, Ito M, Hatazawa J, Ishiwata K, Iwata R, Ido T. Differential diagnosis of lung tumor with positron emission tomography: a prospective study. J Nucl Med 1990; 31:1927–1933.
79. Rege SD, Hoh CK, Glaspy JA, Aberle DR, Dahlbom M, Razavi MK, Phelps ME, Hawkins RA. Imaging of pulmonary mass lesions with whole-body positron emission tomography and fluorodeoxyglucose. Cancer 1993; 72:82–90.
80. Bury T, Dowlati A, Paulus P, Corhay JL, Benoit T, Kayembe JM, Limet R, Rigo P, Rademecker M. Evaluation of the solitary pulmonary nodule by positron emission tomography imaging. Eur Respir J 1996; 9:410–414.
81. Hübner KF, Buoconore E, Gould HR, Thie J, Smith GT, Stephens S, Dickey J. Differentiating benign from malignant lung lesions using "quantitative" parameters of FDG PET images. Clin Nucl Med 1996; 21:941–949.
82. Knight SB, Delbeke D, Stewart JR, Sandler MP. Evaluation of pulmonary lesions with FDG-PET. Comparison of findings in patients with and without a history of prior malignancy. Chest 1996; 109:982–988.
83. Bury T, Dowlati A, Paulus P, Hustinx R, Radermecker M, Rigo P. Staging of non-small-cell lung cancer by whole-body fluorine-18 deoxyglucose positron emission tomography. Eur J Nucl Med 1996; 23:204–206.
84. Lewis P, Griffin S, Mardsen P, Gee T, Nunan T, Malsey M, Dussek J. Whole-body ^{18}F-fluorodeoxyglucose positron emission tomography in preoperative evaluation of lung cancer. Lancet 1994; 344:1265–1266.
85. Chin R, Ward R, Keyes JW, Choplin RH, Reed JC, Wallenhaupt S, Hudspeth AS, Haponik EF. Mediastinal staging of non-small-cell lung cancer with positron emission tomography. Am J Respir Crit Care Med 1995; 152:2090–2096.
86. Steinert HC, Hauser M, Allemann F, Engel H, Berthold T, von Schulthess GK, Weder W. Non-small cell lung cancer: nodal staging with FDG PET versus CT with correlative lymph node mapping and sampling. Radiology 1997; 202:441–446.
87. Frank A, Lefkowitz D, Jaeger S, Gobar L, Sunderland J, Gupta N, Scott W, Mailliard J, Lynch H, Bishop J, Thorpe P, Dewan N. Decision logic retreatment of asymptomatic lung cancer recurrence based on positron emission tomography findings. Int J Radiat Oncol Biol Phys 1995; 32:1495–1512.
88. Patz EF, Lowe VJ, Hoffman JM, Paine SS, Harris LK, Goodman PC. Persistent or recurrent bronchogenic carcinoma: detection with PET and 2-[18F]-2-deoxy-D-glucose. Radiology 1994; 191:379–382.
89. Abe Y, Matsuzawa T, Fujiwara T, Itoh M, Fukuda H, Yamaguchi K, Kubota K, Hatazawa J, Tada M, Ido T, Watanuki S. Clinical assessment of therapeutic effects on cancer using 18F-2-fluoro-2-deoxy-D-glucose and positron emission tomography: preliminary study of lung cancer. Int J Radiat Oncol Biol Phys 1990; 19:1005–1010.
90. Knopp MV, Bishoff H, Rimac A, Doll J, Oberdorfer F, Lorentz WJ, van Kaick G. Clinical utility of positron emission tomography with FDG for chemotherapy response monotoring—a correlative study of patients with small cell lung cancer. J Nucl Med 1994; 35:75P.

91. Miyazawa H, Arai T, Iio M, Hara T. PET imaging of non-small-cell lung carcinoma with carbon-11-methionine: relationship between radioactivity uptake and flow-cytometric parameters. J Nucl Med 1993; 34:1886–1891.

92. Kobayashi T, Xu X-W, MacMahon H, Metz CE, Doi K. Effect of a computer-aided diagnosis scheme on radiologist's performance in detection of lung nodules on radiographs. Radiology 1996; 199:843–848.

93. Ho JT, Kruger RA. Comparison of dual-energy and conventional chest radiography for nodule detection. Invest Radiol 1989; 24:861–868.

31

Radioimmunodetection and Radioimmunotherapy in Lung Cancer

JEAN-PHILIPPE VUILLEZ and DENIS MORO

Institut Albert Bonniot
Centre Hospitalier Universitaire de Grenoble,
Grenoble, France

In vivo targeting of tumoral cells using radiolabeled molecules specifically retained by these cells, has appeared for several years to be a promising new technique complementary to morphological imaging.

Morphological imaging, based on the detection of anatomical abnormalities, cannot be used when a disease does not lead to anatomical modifications, e.g., infiltrative lesions, inframillimetric lesions, or isodense or isoechogenic lesions. In these cases, detection of neoplastic cells is theoretically feasible using a scintigraphic approach. Indeed, radiotracer imaging is based on the detection of functional abnormal properties of cancer cells. This "magic bullet" approach has been proved successful in many cancers; for lung cancer, several radiopharmaceutical agents have been studied (1): gallium 67, thallium 201, SestaMIBI, and receptor binding peptides [mainly somatostatin analogs (2)], HMPAO (3), DMSA (4), and more recently fluorine 18-labeled fluoro-deoxy-D-glucose (^{18}F-FDG).

Immunoscintigraphy offers the theoretical advantage of better oncospecificity, considering the properties of the antigen-antibody recognition. In addition, internal radiotherapy, which uses radiolabeled molecules specifically recognizing tumor cells, is an interesting new therapeutic modality that targets tumor cells with β-emitting and, possibly in the future, α-emitting radionuclides. In this way, radio-

503

immunotherapy using labeled monoclonal antibodies opens a very interesting field of investigation.

I.   Diagnostic Applications of Radiolabeled Monoclonal Antibodies

A.   Theoretical Aspects

Immunodetection of lung cancer is limited by the absence of sufficiently specific antigen. The choice of the targeted antigen is very important, since no antigen is either specific for bronchogenic cancers or 100% expressed in all tumors as shown by immunohistochemistry data.

Many antibodies raised against non–small-cell lung carcinoma (NSCLC) have been produced and studied; a detailed review can be found in Stein and Goldenberg (5). Few of these antibodies have been used for clinical studies. Although other antibodies have been used with different but encouraging results (6–10), anti-CEA is the most commonly used antibody for this application, and the best results have been obtained with anti-CEA antibody. CEA is a logical choice as target antigen since it is expressed in 60–70% of bronchial NSCLC cases (11,12), as also confirmed in our study (14/21 cases), not always shown by a concomitant increase in circulating CEA (13). Anti-CEA is used whole (14–16) or as F(ab′)2 fragments (13,17–20), a form reported to be superior in terms of the tumor:nontumor ratio. Moreover, indium 111–labeled F(ab′)2 anti-CEA has also been proven effective in imaging colon (21) and medullary thyroid (22) cancers.

For small cell lung cancer (SCLC), anti-CEA antibodies could be used as well, since CEA is expressed by these tumors. Among the numerous SCLC-related antigens (23,24), other targets have been tested for radioimmunodetection, such as ganglioside antigen fucosyl-GM1 (25), NCAM (26), glioma-specific antibody [GA-17 raised against the glioblastoma cell line GI1, (27)], MOC-31 [raised against a 38 kDa pan-carcinoma membrane antigen (28)].

Lung cancers are very often poorly vascularized and perfused, resulting in poor accessibility of tumor cells for radiolabeled antibodies. This explains limited tumor uptake and subsequent poor contrast of scintigraphic images. The higher the blood pool activity, the lower is this contrast, which is especially problematic in the mediastinum because of heart and large vessels.

B.   Immunoscintigraphy in Non–Small-Cell Lung Carcinoma

Different studies on radioimmunodetection of NSCLC have been reported in animals (29) and humans (6–10,13–20), showing that this method should be suitable but needs some technical improvements before being clinically useful in lung cancer. Several situations are indicated for which immunoscintigraphy is more suitable than other techniques, particularly morphological imaging: initial diagnosis (to confirm malignancy of a lung lesion), loco-regional staging and metastasis workup, appreciation of treatment response, detection of residual disease, and early detection of recurrences (14–17,20).

Diagnosis of the Primary Tumor

Immunoscintigraphy has been proposed to be helpful in distinguishing between malignant and nonmalignant lesions and in avoiding unnecessary invasive diagnostic procedures. Results are at present, however, still preliminary (see Table 1).

Considering the published data, and no matter what underlying mechanism might cause the partial failure of anti-CEA immunoscintigraphy, this technique seems to have little or no place in the histologic confirmation of a suspected lung cancer. The insufficient accuracy (only 90%) is explained, in some cases, by the absent or heterogeneous expression of the antigen, anomalies in tumor angioarchitecture with consequent limitations (or increase) of blood access, greater than normal leaking of tumor capillaries, cross-reactivity with nontarget antigens, and nonspecific ^{111}In uptake by transferrin receptors of tumor cells (18).

Invasive procedures cannot be avoided on the sole basis of a potentially false-negative anti-CEA immunoscintigraphy. In its present form, immunoscintigraphy is unlikely to be a practical or robust screening method for early lung cancer detection (35).

Presurgical Staging

Since the only effective treatment for NSCLC is complete surgical excision, preoperative staging is a major goal (36) in order to reduce the number of unnecessary thoracotomies (37) without excluding surgery for patients who stand a chance of being cured by this technique.

Contiguous mediastinal involvement is difficult to establish. CT is of limited value in the assessment of chest wall, mediastinal, pleural, or pericardial tumor extension (38,39).

The presence of involved mediastinal lymph nodes in NSCLC has a very bad signification for prognosis with very few long-term survivors overall (40). One of the most important aspects of preoperative staging of patients with NSCLC, therefore, is the evaluation of the mediastinum for the possible presence and extent of metastatic disease. The number of lymphatic sites involved is also a problem for prognosis (41).

Structural imaging modalities such as computed tomography (CT) or magnetic resonance imaging (MRI) provide excellent anatomic detail, but, although mediastinal nodes larger than 1 cm in diameter are likely to be involved with tumor, node enlargement seen on CT scan can be due to reactive hyperplasia or other nonmalignant conditions. On the other hand, CT cannot depict involvement of normal-sized lymph nodes. Thus there is a need for a new method of assessing accurately the extent of tumor in patients with lung cancer, aiming to avoid unnecessary thoracotomies and limit the number of staging mediastinoscopies (42).

Table 1   Results of Clinical Trials with Immunoscintigraphy for the Diagnosis of Primary Lung Tumor

Author	Ref.	Antibody (radionuclide)	Number of tumors vizualized	Comments
Perkins et al.	30	791/T36 (^{131}I or ^{111}In)	3/8 with ^{131}I 9/13 with ^{111}In	5 NSCLC; 16 SCLC.
Kalonofos et al.	6	HMFG1 F(ab′)2 (^{111}In)	14/14	Observable tumor localization could also be achieved with nonspecific indium-labeled antibody F(ab′)2 fragments.
Aronen et al.	16	BW431/26	9/12	
Kairemo et al.	31	BW431/26	19/25	
Krishnamurthy et al.	14	Whole anti-CEA (^{111}In)	12/16	20 patients before surgical resection of lung cancer. Surgery confirmed the diagnosis of cancer in 16 patients. IS results were 12 TP, 4 FN, 3 VN and 1 FP (in the case of resolutive pneumonia). Overall sensitivity was 75%, better for squamous cell carcinomas (8/9) than for adenocarcinomas (4/7).
Bourguet et al.	9	Po66 (^{131}I)	22/27	Of the negative cases, four were also negative by immunohistochemistry, and in two cases, the tumor was less than 2 cm.
Biggi et al.	17,18	Anti-CEA FO23C5 F(ab′)2 (^{111}In)	57/63	This study did not include SPECT. 57 NSCLC and 6 SCLC. 6 false-positive cases among 11 cases of benign disease.
Biggi et al.	19			All tumors but one (corresponding to an in situ carcinoma) were visualized.

Table 1 Continued

Author	Ref.	Antibody (radionuclide)	Number of tumors vizualized	Comments
Divgi et al.	10	MoAb225 (anti-EGF-R) (^{111}In)		All tumors were visualized in patients who were injected with the radiolabeled antibody.
Kazumoto et al.	32	Anti-CEA F(ab')2 (^{131}I)		Antibody uptake was related to the number of tumor cells and the blood perfusion.
Vansant et al.	33	NR-LU-10 (^{99m}Tc)	33/33	33 patients with proved lung cancer (12 SCLC, 21 NSCLC).
Rusch et al.	34	NR-LU-10 (^{99m}Tc)	22/22	A benign lesion didn't retain the radiolabeled antibody.

Immunoscintigraphy, because of the specificity of antigen/antibody recognition, is here best indicated, at least theoretically. An underestimation of lymph node involvement has been reported even by pathological studies as long as immunohistochemistry is performed (43).

Few studies have attempted evaluate mediastinal involvement with immunoscintigraphy (IS). Some preliminary studies concerning limited series of patients have shown low sensitivity and specificity using ^{131}I-labeled Po66 monoclonal antibody (9), ^{99m}Tc-labeled anti-CEA monoclonal antibody BW 431/26 (15), or the anti-CEA MA FO23C5 F(ab')2 labeled with indium 111 (20).

Buccheri et al. (18) used anti-CEA MA FO23C5 F(ab')2 labeled with indium 111. In their study of 63 patients (including 6 SCLC), with planar imaging only, the sensitivity of anti-ACE IS compared to histology was 73% for stages N1, 71% for stages N2, and 100% for stages N3; the specificity was 73, 80, and 67%, respectively. This led to a weak positive predictive value (PPV), except for N3 stages (respectively, 67, 56, and 83%) and a good negative predictive value (NPV) (respectively, 79, 89, and 100%).

In another series of 45 patients (including 2 SCLC) combining anti-CEA MA FO23C5 F(ab')2 labeled with indium 111 and SPECT, the same authors found a 75% sensitivity and a 79% specificity in stages N2, and 100% and 100% in stages N3 (combining planar and SPECT images), better than that obtained with CT (respectively, 75 and 66%, 43 and 40%) (19). The PPV was weak for N2 prediction (50%), but better than CT, and excellent for predicting N3 stages (100%); likewise,

NPV was >80% in all cases. The authors concluded that IS improved the selection of patients for a more invasive staging procedure (i.e., mediastinoscopy) or for direct thoracotomy.

In our study (13) with 28 patients we reached similar conclusions, using SPECT with anti-CEA F6 F(ab′)2 labeled with indium 111 and simultaneous visualization of blood pool using ^{99m}Tc-labeled albumin. We found that IS was very complementary to CT, since among 17 patients for whom results agreed with CT, surgery had confirmed the preoperative staging. In contrast, in four cases of discrepancies, IS was correct two times and CT two times. Figure 1 shows a demonstrative case of involved lymph nodes depicted by IS despite their normal size on CT.

When the IS results are concordant with the initial clinical staging, there is very low probability of error and mediastinoscopy can thus be excluded. Mediasti-

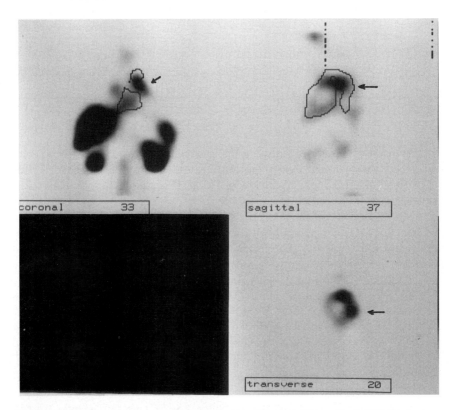

Figure 1   Tomographic sections showing uptake of the anti-CEA antibody F(ab′)2 fragment labeled with indium 111 in mediastinal lymph nodes of a patient with lung squamous cell carcinoma. A focus (arrow) was clearly visible and concordant on the coronal, sagittal, and transversal sections. This focus was located under the aortic arch visualized by ^{99m}Tc-albumin distribution, here represented by delimited area. The CT scan was normal, but surgery confirmed involvement of the aortico-pulmonary lymph nodes.

noscopy should be proposed when there is discordance between the initial clinical staging and the IS results. Thus, IS staging could be of potential clinical use in guiding therapy. These results are more encouraging than previous conclusions (6).

Three studies using the antibody NR-LU-10 Fab fragment labeled with technetium 99m and concerning, respectively, 44, 33, and 24 patients led to a preliminary but encouraging conclusion (7,33,34). Another anti-CEA fragment labeled with technetium 99m (IMMU-4 Fab′ fragment) gave similar results (44).

Results of a study by Boilleau et al. in 17 patients were rather disappointing (45). Lack of specificity and insufficient sensitivity led to the conclusion that IS adds only weak information to a CT scan in the noninvasive mediastinal staging of lung cancer. But in this study, a cocktail of two different antibodies (anti-CEA and anti-CA 19-9) labeled with iodine 131 was used, probably leading to a lower tumor:nontumor ratio.

Detection of Metastases

Very few studies have addressed this question. Torres et al. (20) with the anti-CEA MA FO23C5 F(ab′)2 labeled with indium 111, have been able to visualize 9 out of 13 metastases (2/3 adrenal metastases, 3/3 lymph nodes, 1/3 in liver, 2/2 skull, 1/2 brain metastases).

In our study (13), the detection of an adrenal metastasis was possible (Fig. 2). Although we rarely noted contralateral or distant lung uptake, indicating metastasis, it was favored in a few cases. This uptake could be an essential parameter for guiding complementary examinations, since if metastasis is confirmed (classifying the patient as M1), the patient could be exempted from undergoing an unnecessary thoracotomy.

Diagnostic of Recurrences

The diagnosis of recurrences may be difficult with CT or MRI. IS has not yet been used in this situation, and studies in this area are necessary.

C. Immunoscintigraphy in Small-Cell Lung Cancer

Small-cell lung cancer tumors are not surgically treated, and staging is indicated for prognosis or indication of radiotherapy after chemotherapy. Several preliminary studies have been performed in vitro (25) or in animal models (e.g., xenografts in the nude mouse) (26–28) showing the feasibility of the method.

Initial Diagnosis

Once more, results are still preliminary, but encouraging. Perkins et al. (30) investigated 16 patients with SCLC using antibody 791T/36. The tumor was visualized on planar scintigraphy in 11 (69%) cases (SPECT was performed in only a few cases). The series of Chan et al. included 7 SCLC, all of which were visualized with CT 14 antibody (raised against oncogene c-*myc*) labeled with iodine 131 (46).

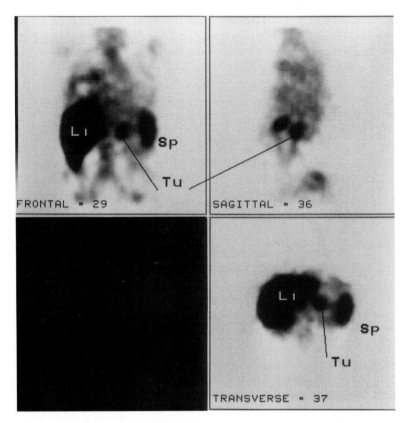

Figure 2 Tomographic sections showing uptake of the anti-CEA antibody F(ab')2 fragment labeled with indium 111 in a left adrenal metastasis of a lung squamous cell carcinoma. The tumoral site (Tu) is clearly visible despite liver (Li) and spleen (Sp) nonspecific activity.

Staging

Only very preliminary studies involving few patients but with encouraging results have been performed. Antibodies used were ^{131}I-labeled antibodies to vasopressin-associated human neurophysin (VP-HNP) (47), technetium-99m monoclonal antibody fragment (Fab) (48), ^{131}I SWA11 (recognizing the cluster w4 antigen) (49), anti-CEA labeled with indium 111 or technetium 99m (50), anti-GD2 ganglioside monoclonal antibody 3F8 labeled with iodine 131 (51), or 111-DTPA-MOC-31 (52). Most of these studies were undertaken with a preradioimmunotherapeutic purpose.

D. Remaining Problems

Insufficient Contrast

In all previous studies, that contrast between specific activity retained in the tumor and nonspecific background activity is not sufficient, even with SPECT, to allow a routine use of IS in lung cancer. This is due to the limited accessibility of targeted antigen on tumor cells (because of a poor vascularization and an elevated interstitial pressure due to the absence of lymphatic vessels) and poor tumor uptake, together with a still high background activity in blood and normal tissues, especially the liver. Therefore it is necessary to improve the tumor:nontumor ratio of antibody uptake.

Human Anti-Mouse Antibodies

Human immune response to injected monoclonal antibodies (53) is one of the major drawbacks of immunoscintigraphy. It occurs in 20–40% of cases on average, depending on the antibody used and the injected form (whole antibody or fragments). Human anti-mouse antibodies (HAMA) preclude repetition of immunoscintigraphy, and most radioimmunotherapy, since after a new injection, complexes between HAMA and murine antibody are rapidly formed and eliminated by the reticuloendothelial system. Another problem is the interference with tumor marker assays and the risk of false-positive results (54). Several approaches, some of which are already under clinical evaluation, will make it possible to reduce the frequency of HAMA occurrence. These include short Fab or Fv fragments, chimeric antibodies, reshaped or human antibodies, and synthetic peptides.

Discrepancies Between IS Results and Immunostaining Data

The presence or absence of an IS focus can only be interpreted relative to CEA expression, as determined by immunohistochemistry, and to vascularization and the extent of necrosis at each tumoral site. Nonetheless, discrepancies between IS results and immunohistochemistry have been observed.

In a study by Krishnamurthy et al. (14), IS was positive in two patients whose tumors were negative for CEA by immunostaining and negative in three cases of tumors expressing CEA. In a study by Biggi et al. (17), in 89% of lung cancer patients the accumulation of radiolabeled anti-CEA MAb by the tumor was related to the presence of positive CEA cells as detected by immunostaining. But a discrepancy between immunoscintigraphy and immunostaining was observed in 11% of patients. A positive IS was observed despite negative immunostaining as well as negative IS despite positive immunostaining for CEA.

In our study of 28 patients (13), there was no anti-CEA uptake in the primary tumor in 7 cases (25%), in agreement with previous studies (8,16,18). Four of these 7 patients were positive for CEA by immunohistochemistry and were actually false negatives. These cases might be explained by poor Ag accessibility (tumoral vascularization) or by the small size of the tumors (8). On the other hand, 6 of the 21 IS-positive tumors showed negative immunohistochemical staining. This phenomenon had been noted previously (16,18). Dienhart et al. (8) found no correlation between prestudy immunohistochemical staining intensity or the percentage of positive tumor cells and imaging results. Several hypotheses may explain these discrepancies.

The first hypothesis is that the tumoral uptake of the radiolabeled antibody may be due not to immunologically specific recognition, but to nonspecific mechanisms. In support of this hypothesis, Kalofonos et al. (6) demonstrated that nonspecific immunoglobulins are taken up by tumors in 71% of cases. In five patients, Torres et al. (20) also found that primary tumors could be imaged with a nonspecific immunoglobulin [F(ab')2 fragments of 4C4 monoclonal antibody directed against hepatitis B surface antigen]. However, the index for tumoral anti-ACE uptake was higher than nonspecific immunoglobulin in all cases. Use of human polyclonal immunoglobulins for scintigraphic tumor detection (55) has shown quite poor results. Thus, nonspecific uptake seems relatively limited.

Another hypothesis relates to immunohistochemistry of tumor specimens, which should be considered as an incomplete gold standard unless the complete tumor, not just a sample, is studied, since a clear vision of the presence of CEA in the tumor can only be obtained in this way (16,20). Moreover, immunohistochemistry techniques do not have 100% sensitivity. Therefore, even if some nonspecific uptake of anti-CEA F(ab')2 does occur, discordance between the IS-positive and immunohistochemical-negative results could be better explained by intratumoral heterogeneity in CEA expression. Tissue specimens and, moreover, biopsies used for the immunohistochemical analysis only represented parts of tumors expressing little or no CEA, although this antigen was expressed in other parts as shown by uptake of radiolabeled antibody. This heterogeneous antigen reactivity has already been noted (11).

E. Improvements and Perspectives

Improving tumor uptake of the radiolabeled antibody by external beam irradiation (56) to improve tumor perfusion, or cytokines to improve the antigen expression (57,58), seems difficult to propose for diagnosis procedures. Technical progress should be mainly obtained through methods lowering the nonspecific activity.

Whole antibodies or F(ab')2 or Fab fragments directly labeled with iodine 131, indium 111, or technetium 99m generate a high nonspecific activity in the blood pool and in tissues. The first possibility of overcoming this problem consists in labeling the antibody through a metabolizable linker, which will be cut in tissues but not in the tumor (59).

The most impressive progress has been obtained with two-step methods. The general principle is to first inject a nonlabeled antibody (or derived molecule) coupled to a "binding" site, and then inject a radiolabeled small molecule that is specifically recognized by this binding site. The cold antibody will accumulate in the tumor, while being eliminated after uptake from normal tissues, particularly the liver and the kidneys. The radiotracer will be recognized and retained only in the tumor, and not in other tissues (60). Clinical studies have already been performed with the *avidin-biotin* system in lung cancer (61–63).

Another approach uses cold *bispecific antibodies*, which are built with an antitumor Fab fragment, and another Fab raised against a small hapten, which is coupled to the radionuclide; this approach was introduced by Goodwin et al. (64). It initially generated important blood pool activity, because of binding between bispecific antibody and radiolabeled hapten in the blood. This technique has been

improved upon by Le Doussal et al. (65,66) using a bispecific antibody and a divalent hapten, which allows low binding in blood, but very strong binding in the tumor
because of binding of the hapten with two antibodies retained by the tumor (Fig. 3).
This affinity enhancement system (AES) allows much better contrast and has already been used in clinical studies (67,68). It must be noted that the low uptake in
the liver allows the detection of hepatic metastasis, not possible with directly labeled
antibodies.

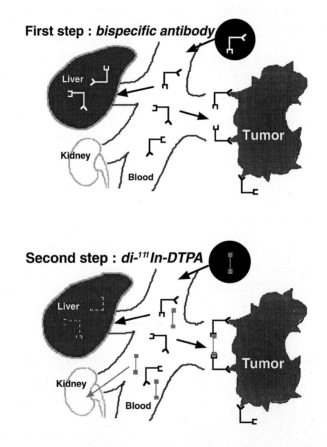

Figure 3 Diagram of the AES method. (A) During the first step a cold bispecific anti-CEA/
anti-DTPA antibody is injected and distributed throughout the body. It is specifically retained
by tumor cells through recognition and binding. (B) Four days later, the second step consists
of injecting the di-DTPA-tyrosyl-lysine bivalent hapten labeled with indium 111. There is
no accumulation of activity in the liver because the bispecific antibody has been catabolized
in this organ. The blood activity decreases rapidly because monovalent binding between
DTPA and bispecific antibody is weak, so that radiolabeled haptens are quickly cleared
through the kidneys. In the tumor, bivalent haptens exhibit an enhanced affinity for tumor
cell–bound bispecific antibody as the result of formation of stable cyclic complexes on the
cell membrane.

We conducted a preliminary study on mediastinal involvement using the AES technique in 12 patients with NSCLC (69). To avoid surgical treatment delay, the same patients could not be investigated successively using directly labeled antibodies and the AES technique. Thus, the results were compared to those of the previous study, which used an indium 111–labeled F(ab′)2 fragment of the same antibody (22). The AES method seems promising for at least two reasons. The main advantage is clearly the great improvement in contrast of images, allowing easier delineation of tumors. Le Doussal et al. (68) have shown that the wider distribution and the accelerated clearance of the hapten [when compared to F(ab′)2] led to a decrease in the radioactivity in normal tissues, followed by an increase in uptake ratio. Moreover, indium 111 uptake by the liver was dramatically reduced. Our results were in agreement with these observations; indeed, when positive, the tumor activity was clearly visualized, without the need for image processing, while liver activity was rather low, especially in tomographic sections (Fig. 4). The hepatic activity that persisted on planar images was much lower and likely due to circulating activity. Furthermore, this sharper contrast was obtained within 24 hours following the injection of the radiolabeled hapten, whereas 72 hours were necessary to reach a sufficient contrast following the injection of directly labeled antibodies.

The other main advantage of the AES method is the improvement of immunospecificity. In our study, 4 of 11 patients in whom IHC was performed were to-

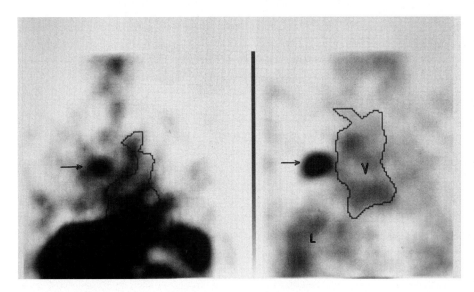

Figure 4 (Right) Frontal tomographic section obtained in a patient with squamous cell carcinoma of the right upper lobe, injected with the "AES" two-step system. It shows tumor uptake with excellent contrast (arrow), whereas liver (L) and vascular (V) activities were very low. (Left) Frontal section obtained in a patient with a similar tumor who received the anti-CEA antibody as the F(ab′)2 fragment directly labeled with indium 111. The tumor (arrow): liver (L) ratio is clearly less favorable. Both tumors strongly expressed CEA (>80% of the cells).

tally CEA negative and CEA expression was very low (<40%) in two other patients. In only two cases did 100% of tumor cells strongly express CEA. In this context, the immunospecificity of AES seemed excellent, better than that obtained with directly labeled antibodies. Indeed, we noted a relationship between tumor expression of CEA and tumor contrast in scintigraphic images. Although such data concerned a relative low number of patients, they are in agreement with those obtained under other pathological conditions (67,68) and support the idea that the AES technique is associated with a decrease in nonspecific uptake. However, nonspecific uptake is not totally eliminated, as we have noticed in three cases an uptake in the tumor area whereas Immunohistochemistry of the tumor was negative. A nonspecific uptake of the antibody or of the radiolabeled hapten in a pneumonia area or nonspecific uptake in the tumor itself (e.g., through activated macrophages) are possible explanations. On the other hand, heterogeneity and large necrosis of the tumor make false negatives by immunohistochemistry possible.

The next step will be the synthesis of small antibody–derived peptides by biomolecular techniques (70). These would be less or not at all antigenic and not induce HAMA.

It appears that combining morphological imaging (i.e., CT and MRI) and immunoscintigraphy and fusion between images of the two modalities would be interesting (71).

II. Radioimmunotherapy

External radiation beam therapy is one efficient modality of cancer treatment, in addition to surgery and chemotherapy; however, its indications are limited. Its efficiency is maximal for tumoral targets that are both radiosensitive and anatomically well delimited, so that a good ballistic and dosimetric characterization is feasible. In contrast, disseminated and tumor targets are not relevant for external beam treatments. However, such disseminated lesions could be accessible to radiopharmaceutical agents, labeled with β-emitting radionuclides, which, after systemic administration, would be specifically retained by tumoral cells (i.e., internal radiotherapy). Internal radiotherapy has been proved efficient for many years and is routinely performed with iodine 131 for differentiated thyroid carcinomas: complete remission rate at 15 years is more than 50% in the case of pulmonary diffuse metastatic spread and 90% in the case of micronodular metastases not detectable by techniques other than iodine 131 body scanning (72).

More recently, malignant pheochromocytomas or neuroblastomas have been treated using iodine 131–labeled metaiodobenzylguanidine (mIBG) (73,74). Such a therapeutic approach has been proposed in various cancers using monoclonal antibodies labeled with β-emitting radionuclides, e.g., iodine 131; this approach defined radioimmunotherapy. High activities have been injected intravenously, but initial results have been disappointing, which was predictable because of low tumor uptake (generally <0.01% of injected dose per gram of tumor).

However, significant and encouraging results have been obtained for non-Hodgkin's malignant lymphomas using repeated injections of ^{131}I-anti-CD20 antibody, with 40% responses, especially in low-grade cases in which 77% of patients have had a response during until 31 months (75). Another study showed similar results with unique injection of high activity of ^{131}I-anti-CD20 antibody (up to 777 mCi) and autologous bone marrow transplant support (76,77).

In fact, for radioimmunotherapy two conditions are mandatory: good radiosensitivity and small size tumoral lesions, i.e., less than a few millimeters. Dosimetric estimations have shown tumor doses no more than 40–50 Gy (usually in the range of 10–40 Gy) for activities of 3.7–18.5 GBq (100–500 mCi) (78,79). These doses are inadequate to destroy most solid tumors, but could be efficient for highly radiosensitive targets like lymphomas. On the other hand, it has been showed that penetration of antibodies in tumors (80) is very weak in lesions larger than 5 mm, which precludes any significant therapeutic effect of radiolabeled antibodies, as has been shown in peritoneal residues of ovarian cancers (81). Behr et al. showed a linear correlation between the tumor mass and the logarithm of tumor uptake (in % of ID/g) or the logarithm of the tumor dose in cGy/mCi (78).

Small-cell lung carcinoma appears to be a good target for clinical trials of radioimmunotherapy, since it is a highly metastatic disease with good radiosensitivity and rapid evolution. Several experimental studies have been undertaken for this purpose (82–85).

Preliminary clinical results have already been reported. Behr et al. (78) treated 57 patients with ^{131}I-labeled anti-CEA NP4, 9 of whom had lung carcinoma, in a phase I/II trial involving advanced tumor stages; no response was observed, but in all cases tumor burden was too large to deliver a sufficient radiation dose to the tumor without unacceptable myelotoxicity. Until now, however, no trial has been published concerning lung cancer itself. We are currently participating in a multicenter phase I/II trial using the two-step approach (AES), i.e., bispecific anti-CEA/anti-di-DTPA and iodine 131–labeled di-DTPA for SCLC radioimmunotherapy. With this approach it may be possible to overcome one of challenges of radioimmunotherapy, i.e., nonspecific uptake in nontumor tissue. Preliminary dosimetric studies in patients with NSCLC have shown a possibly favorable dose rate delivery (86). Some interesting results have already been obtained; we observed some stabilization of the disease for more than 6 months in at least two cases. However, it will probably turn out that this treatment is more efficient in earlier stages of disease, after initial chemotherapy has reduced the tumor, in order to eradicate residual small tumoral clusters. Radioimmunotherapy will probably be complementary to other modalities and in some cases may contribute to the cure of some otherwise incurable malignancies (79).

III. Conclusion

The use of radiolabeled monoclonal antibodies in nuclear medicine is a still in development but appears promising for both diagnosis and therapeutic purposes. Progress will result from the best tumor:nontumor ratios, the best methodological approaches, and the comprehension of the mechanisms of uptake, penetration, and distribution of the antibodies in the tumors (87,88) as well as reduced immunogenicity of the antibodies used. The future of immunoscintigraphy and radioimmunotherapy will depend on technological advances and the real impact of these techniques on the strategy of therapeutic decision and patient survival; this impact is beginning to be apparent but must still be confirmed.

References

1. Abdel-Dayem HM, Scott A, Macapinlac H, Larson S. Tracer imaging in lung cancer. Eur J Nucl Med 1994; 21:57–81.
2. Leitha T, Meghdadi S, Studnicka M, Wolzt M, Marosi C, Angelberger P, Neumann M, Schlick W, Kletter K, Dudczak R. The role of iodine-123-Tyr-3-octreotide scintigraphy in the staging of small-cell lung cancer. J Nucl Med 1993; 34:1397–1402.
3. Oshima M, Itoh K, Okae S, Tadokoro M, Kodama Y, Sakuma S. Evaluation of primary lung carcinoma using technetium 99m-hexamethylpropylene amine oxime: preliminary clinical experience. Eur J Nucl Med 1990; 16:859–864.
4. Hirano T, Otake H, Yoshida I, Endo K. Primary lung cancer SPECT imaging with pentavalent technetium-99m-DMSA. J Nucl Med 1995; 36:202–220.
5. Stein R, Goldenberg DM. Prospects for the management of non-small-cell carcinoma of the lung with monoclonal antibodies. Chest 1991; 99:1466–1476.
6. Kalofonos HP, Sivolapenko GB, Courtenay-Luck NS, Snook DE, Hooker GR, Winter R, MacKenzie CG, Taylor-Papadimitriou JJ, Lavender PJ, Epenetos AA. Antibody guided targeting of non-small cell lung cancer using ^{111}In-labeled HMFG1 F(ab')$_2$ fragments. Cancer Res 1988; 48:1977–1984.
7. Friedman S, Sullivan K, Salk D, Nelp WB, Griep RJ, Johnson DH, Blend MJ, Aye R, Suppers V, Abrams PG. Staging non-small cell carcinoma of the lung using technetium-99m-labeled monoclonal antibodies. Hematol/Oncol Clin North Am 1990; 4:1069–1078.
8. Dienhart DG, Schmelter F, Lear JL, Miller GJ, Glenn SD, Bloedow DC, Kasliwal R, Moran P, Seligman P, Murphy JR, Kortright K, Bunn PA. Imaging of non-small cell lung cancers with a monoclonal antibody, KC-4G3, which recognizes a human milk fat globule antigen. Cancer Res 1990; 50:7068–7076.
9. Bourguet P, Dazord L, Desrues B, Collet B, Ramee MP, Delava LP, Martin A, Logeais Y, Pelletier A, Toujas L, Bourel D, Kernec J, Saccavini JC, Kremer M, Herry JY. Immunoscintigraphy of human lung squamous cell carcinoma using an iodine-131 labelled monoclonal antibody (Po66). Br J Cancer 1990; 61:230–234.
10. Divgi CR, Welt S, Kris M, Real FX, Yeh SDJ, Gralla R, Merchant B, Schweighart S, Unger M, Larson SM, Mendelsohn J. Phase I and imaging trial of indium 111-labeled anti-epidermal growth factor receptor monoclonal antibody 225 in patients with squamous cell lung carcinoma. J Natl Cancer Inst 1991; 83:97–104.
11. Battista P, Murano R, Mammarela S, Curia MC, Colasante A, Rosini S, Lesti G, Sacco R, French D, Frati L, Costantini RM. Complementary reactivities of anti-carcinoembryonic antigen and antitumor-associated glycoprotein 72 monoclonal antibodies in lung carcinomas. Cancer Res 1990; 50:6987–6994.
12. Said JW, Nash G, Tepper G, Banks-Schlegel S. Keratin proteins and carcinoembryonic antigen in lung carcinoma: an immunoperoxydase study of fifty-four cases, with ultrastructural correlations. Human Path 1983; 14:70–76.
13. Vuillez JP, Moro D, Brambilla E, Brichon PY, Feretti G, Saccavini JC, Brambilla C. Immunoscintigraphy using ^{111}In-labelled F(ab')2 fragments of anti-carcinoembryonic antigen (CEA) monoclonal antibody for staging of non-small cell lung carcinoma. Eur J Cancer 1994; 30A:1089–1092.

14. Krishnamurthy S, Morris JF, Antonovic R, Ahmed A, Galey WT, Duncan C, Krishnamurthy GT. Evaluation of primary lung cancer with indium 111 anti-carcinoembryonic antigen (type ZCE-025) monoclonal antibody scintigraphy. Cancer 1990; 65:458–465.

15. Leitha T, Walter R, Schlick W, Dudczak R. ^{99m}Tc-anti-CEA radioimmunoscintigraphy of lung adenocarcinoma. Chest 1991; 99:14–19.

16. Aronen HJ, Paavonen T, Heikkonen J, Virkkunen P, Mäntyla M, Mäki-Hokkonen H, Kairemo KJK. Imaging of non-small cell lung cancer with Tc-99m-labeled monoclonal anti-CEA antibody with a comparison to immunohistochemistry. Antibody Immun Radiopharm 1991; 4:569–575.

17. Biggi A, Buccheri G, Ferrigno D, Vigliett IA, Chiara Farinelli M, Comino A, Leone A, Quaranta M, Taviani M. Detection of suspected primary lung cancer by scintigraphy with indium-111-anti-carcinoembryonic antigen monoclonal antibodies (type FO23C5). J Nucl Med 1991; 32:2064–2068.

18. Buccheri G, Biggi A, Ferrigno D, D'Angeli B, Vassallo G, Leone A, Taviani M, Comino A. Imaging lung cancer by scintigraphy with indium 111-labeled F(ab')2 fragments of the anti-carcinoembryonic antigen monoclonal antibody FO23C5. Cancer 1992; 70:749–759.

19. Buccheri G, Biggi A, Ferrigno D, D'Angeli B, Leone A, Taviani M, Quaranta M. Anti-CEA immunoscintigraphy might be more useful than computed tomography in the preoperative thoracic evaluation of lung cancer. Chest 1993; 104:734–742.

20. Torres M, Jimenez-Hefferman A, Valverde A, Gonzalez FM, Latre JM, Llamas JM, Baamonde C, Lopez-Rubio F, Mateo A. Immunoscintigraphy of lung cancer using ^{111}In-labelled antiCEA FO23C5-F(ab')2 fragments. Nucl Med Commun 1991; 12:937–950.

21. Chatal JF, Saccavini JC, Fumoleau P, Douillard JY, Curtet C, Kremer M, Le Mevel B. Immunoscintigraphy of colon carcinoma. J Nucl Med 1984; 25:307–314.

22. Vuillez JP, Peltier P, Carave LJP, Chetanneau A, Saccavini JC, Chatal JF. Immunoscintigraphy using ^{111}In-labeled F(ab')2 fragments of anticarcinoembryonic antigen monoclonal antibody for detecting recurrences of medullary thyroid carcinoma. J Clin Endocrinol Metab 1992; 74:157–163.

23. Okabe T, Kaizu T, Fujisawa M, Watanabe J, Kojima K, Yamashita T, Takaku F. Monoclonal antibodies to surface antigens on small cell lung carcinoma of the lung. Cancer Res 1984; 44:5273–5278.

24. Takahashi T, Ueda R, Song X, Nishida K, Shinzato M, Namikawa R, Ariyoshi Y, Ota K, Kato K, Nagatsu T, Imaizumi M, Abe T, Takahashi T. Two novel cell surface antigens on small cell lung carcinoma defined by mouse monoclonal antibodies NE-25 and NE-35. Cancer Res 1986; 46:4770–4775.

25. Vangsted AJ, Zeuthen J. Monoclonal antibodies for diagnosis and potential therapy of small cell lung cancer-the ganglioside antigen fucosyl-GM$_1$. Acta Oncol 1993; 32:845–851.

26. Kwa HB, Wesseling J, Verhoeven AHM, van Zandwijk N, Hilkens J. Immunoscintigraphy of small-cell lung cancer xenografts with anti neural cell adhesion molecule monoclonal antibody, 123C3: improvement of tumor uptake by internalisation. Br J Cancer 1996; 73: 439–446.

27. Kobayashi H, Sakahara H, Hosono M, Shirato M, Kondo S, Miyatake SI, Kikuchi H, Namba Y, Endo K, Konishi J. Scintigraphic detection of neural-cell-derived small-cell lung cancer using glioma-specific antibody. J Cancer Res Clin Oncol 1994; 120:259–262.

28. de Jonge MWA, Kosterink JGW, Bin YY, Bulte JWM, Kengen RAM, Piers DA, The TH, de Leij L. Radioimmunodetection of human small cell lung carcinoma xenografts in the nude rat. Eur J Cancer 1993; 29A:1885–1890.

29. Stein R, Sharkey RM, Goldenberg DM. Monoclonal antibody targeting of human non-small cell carcinoma of the lung. Cancer Res 1990; 50:866s–868s.

30. Perkins AC, Pimm MV, Morgan DAL, Wastie ML, Reynolds JR, Baldwin RW. ^{131}I and ^{111}In-labelled monoclonal antibody imaging of primary lung carcinoma. Nucl Med Commun 1986; 7:729–739.

31. Kairemo KJA, Aronen HJ, Liewendahl K, Paavonen T, Heikkonen JJ, Virkkunen P, Mäki-Hokkonen H, Karonen SL, Brownell AL, Mäntylä MJ. Radioimmunoimaging of non-small cell lung cancer with ^{111}In and 99mTc-labeled monoclonal anti-CEA-antibodies. Acta Oncol 1993; 32:771–778.

32. Kazumoto T, Mitsuhashi N, Hayakawa K, Yonome I, Niibe H. Radioimmunodetection of lung cancer with IMACIS-1, I-131 labeled monoclonal antibodies to CEA and CA19-9. Comparison of accumulations in irradiated and non-irradiated site. Ann Nucl Med 1993; 7:39–44.

33. Vansant JP, Johnson DH, O'Donnel DM, Stewart JR, Sonin AH, McCook BM, Powers TA, Salk DJ, Frist WH, Sandler MP. Staging lung carcinoma with a Tc-99m labeled monoclonal antibody. Clin Nucl Med 1992; 17:431–438.

34. Rusch V, Macapinlac H, Heelan R, Kramer E, Larson S, McCormack P, Burt M, Martini N, Ginsberg R. NR-LU-10 monoclonal antibody scanning. A helpful new adjunct to computed tomography in evaluating non-small-cell lung cancer. J Thor Cardiovas Surg 1993; 106: 200–204.

35. Greene R. Immunoscintigraphy for lung cancer: reality testing (editorial). J Nucl Med 1991; 32:2069–2070.

36. Naruke T, Goya T, Tsuchiya R, Suemasu K. Prognosis and survival in resected lung carcinoma based on the new international staging system. J Thor Cardiovas Surg 1988; 96: 440–447.

37. Goldstraw P. The practice of cardiothoracic surgeons in the perioperative staging on non-small cell lung cancer (editorial). Thorax 1992; 47:1–2.

38. Scott IR, Müller NL, Miller RR, Evans KG, Nelems B. Resectable stage III lung cancer: CT, surgical, and pathologic correlation. Radiology 1988; 166:75–79.

39. Glazer HS, Kaiser LR, Anderson DJ, Molina PL, Amami B, Roper CL, Sagel SS. Indeterminate mediastinal invasion in bronchogenic carcinoma: CT evaluation. Radiology 1989; 173:37–42.

40. Shields TW. The significance of ipsilateral mediastinal lymph node metastasis (N2 disease) in non-small cell carcinoma of the lung. J Thor Cardiovas Surg 1990; 99:48–63.

41. Conill C, Astudillo J, Verger E. Prognostic significance of metastases to mediastinal lymph node levels in resected non-small cell lung carcinoma. Cancer 1993; 72:1199–1202.

42. Brown JS, Rudd R. New staging investigations for lung cancer: What will they have to offer to be clinically useful? Eur J Nucl Med 1995; 22:497–498.

43. Chen ZL, Perez S, Homes EC, Wang HJ, Coulson WF, Wen DR, Cochran AJ. Frequency and distribution of occult micrometastases in lymph nodes of patients with non-small-cell lung carcinoma. J Natl Cancer Inst 1993; 85:493–498.

44. Kramer EL, Noz ME, Liebes L, Murthy S, Tiu S, Goldenberg DM. Radioimmunodetection of non-small cell lung cancer using technetium-99m-anticarcinoembryonic antigen IMMU-4 Fab' fragment. Preliminary results. Cancer 1994; 73:890–895.

45. Boilleau G, Pujol JL, Ychou M, Faurous P, Marty-An EC, Michel FB, Godard P. Detection of lymph node metastases in lung cancer: comparison of ^{131}I-anti-CEA-anti-CA 19-9 immunoscintigraphy versus computed tomography. Lung Cancer 1994; 11:209–219.

46. Chan S, Evan G, Ritson A, Watson J, Wraight P, Sikora K. Localisation of lung cancer by a radiolabelled monoclonal antibody against the c-*myc* oncogene product. Br J Cancer 1986; 54:761–769.

47. North WG, Hirsh V, Lisbona R, Schulz J, Cooper B. Imaging of small cell carcinoma using ^{131}I-labelled antibodies to vasopressin associated human neurophysin (VP-HNP). Nucl Med Commun 1989; 10:643–651.

48. Morris JF, Krishnamurthy S, Antonovic R, Duncan C, Turner FE, Krishnamurthy GT. Technetium-99m monoclonal antibody fragment (Fab) scintigraphy in the evaluation of small cell lung cancer: a preliminary report. Nucl Med Biol 1991; 18:613–620.

49. Ledermann JA, Marston NJ, Stahel RA, Waibel R, Buscombe JR, Ell PJ. Biodistribution and tumour localisation of ^{131}I SWA11 recognising the cluster w4 antigen in patients with small cell lung cancer. Br J Cancer 1993; 68:119–121.

50. Macmillan CH, Perkins AC, Wastie ML, Leach IH, Morgan DAL. Immunoscintigraphy of small-cell lung cancer: a study using technetium and indium labelled anti-carcinoembryonic antigen monoclonal antibody preparations. Br J Cancer 1993; 67:1391–1394.

51. Grant SC, Kostakoglou L, Kris MG, Yeh SDJ, Larson SM, Finn RD, Oettgen HF, Cheung NKV. Targeting of small-cell lung cancer using the anti-GD2 ganglioside monoclonal antibody 3F8: a pilot trial. Eur J Nucl Med 1996; 23:145–149.

52. Kosterink JGW, de Jonge MWA, Smit EF, Piers DA, Kengen RAM, Postmus PE, Shochat D, Groen HJM, The HT, de Leij L. Pharmacokinetics and scintigraphy of indium-111-DTPA-MOC-31 in small-cell lung carcinoma. J Nucl Med 1995; 36:2356–2362.

53. Khazaeli MB, Conry RM, LoBuglio F. Human immune response to monoclonal antibodies. J Immunother 1994; 15:42–52.

54. Kuroki M, Matsumoto Y, Arakawa F, Haruno M, Murakami M, Kuwahara M, Ozaki H, Senba T, Matsuoka Y. Reducing interference from heterophilic antibodies in a two-site immunoassay for carcino-embryonic antigen (CEA) by using a human/mouse chimeric antibody to CEA as the tracer. J Immunol Meth 1995; 180:81–91.

55. Martini N, Heelan R, Westcott J, Bains MS, McCormack P, Caravelli J, Watson R, Zaman M. Comparative merits of conventional, computed tomographic, and magnetic resonance imaging in assessing mediastinal involvement in surgically confirmed lung carcinoma. J Thorac Cardiovasc Surg 1985; 90:639–648.

56. Warhoe KA, DeNardo SJ, Wolkov HB, Doggett EC, Kroger LA, Lamborn KR, DeNardo GL. Evidence for external beam irradiation enhancement of radiolabeled monoclonal antibody uptake in breast cancer. Antibodies Immunoc Radiopharm 1992; 5:227–235.

57. Thakur ML, DeFulvio J, Tong J, John E, McDevitt MR, Damjanov I. Evaluation of biological response modifiers in the enhancement of tumor uptake of technetium-99m labeled macromolecules. A preliminary report. J Immunol Meth 1992; 152:209–216.

58. Greiner JW, Guadagni F, Goldstein D, Borden EC, Ritts RE, Witt P, LoBuglio AF, Saleh MN, Schlom J. Evidence for the elevation of serum carcinoembryonic antigen and tumor-associated glycoprotein-72 levels in patients administered interferons. Cancer Res 1991; 51:4155–4163.

59. Faivre-Chauvet A, Gestin JF, Mease RC, Sai-Maurel C, Thédrez P, Slinkin M, Meinken GE, Srivastava SC, Chatal JF. Introduction of five potentially metabolizable linking groups between ^{111}In-cyclohexyl EDTA derivatives and F(ab')2 fragments of anti-carcinoembryonic antigen antibody-II. Comparative pharmacokinetics and biodistribution in human colorectal carcinoma-bearing nude mice. Nucl Med Biol 1993; 20:763–771.

60. Stoldt HS, Aftab F, Chinol M, Paganelli G, Luca F, Testori A, Geraghty JG. Pretargeting strategies for radio-immunoguided tumour localisation and therapy. Eur J Cancer 1997; 33:186–192.

61. Kalofonos HP, Rusckowski M, Siebecker DA, Sivolapenko GB, Snook D, Lavender JP, Epenetos AA, Hnatowich DJ. Imaging of tumor in patients with indium-111-labeled biotin and streptavidin-conjugated antibodies: preliminary communication. J Nucl Med 1990; 31:1791–1796.

62. Paganelli G, Magnani P, Zito F, Villa E, Sudati F, Lopalco L, Rossetti C, Malcovati M, Chiolerio F, Seccamani E, Siccardi AG, Fazio F. Three-step monoclonal antibody tumor targeting in carcinoembryonic antigen-positive patients. Cancer Res 1991; 51:5960–6966.

63. Dosio F, Magnani P, Paganell IG, Samuel A, Chiesa G, Fazio F. Three-step tumor pre-targeting in lung cancer immunoscintigraphy. J Nucl Biol Med 1993; 37:228–232.

64. Goodwin DA, Meares CF, McCall MJ, McTigue M, Chaovapong W. Pretargeted immunoscintigraphy of murine tumors with indium-111-labeled bifunctional haptens. J Nucl Med 1988; 29:226–234.

65. Le Doussal JM, Gautherot E, Martin M, Barbet J, Delaage M. Enhanced in vivo targeting of an asymetric divalent hapten to double antigen-positive mouse B cells with monoclonal antibody conjugate cocktails. J Immunol 1991; 146:169–175.

66. Le Doussal JM, Gruaz-Guyon A, Martin M, Gautherot E, Delaage M, Barbet J. Targeting of indium 111-labeled divalent hapten to human melanoma mediated by bispecific monoclonal antibody conjugates: imaging of tumors hosted in nude mice. Cancer Res 1990; 50:3445–3452.

67. Peltier P, Curtet C, Chatal JF, Le Doussal JM, Daniel G, Aillet G, Gruaz-Guyon A, Barbet J, Delaage M. Radioimmunodetection of medullary thyroid cancer using a bispecific anti-CEA/anti-indium-DTPA antibody and an indium-111-labeled DTPA dimer. J Nucl Med 1993; 34:1267–1273.

68. Le Doussal JM, Chetanneau A, Gruaz-Guyon A, Martin M, Gautherot E, Lehur PA, Chatal JF, Delaage M, Barbet J. Bispecific monoclonal antibody-mediated targeting of an indium-111-labeled DTPA dimer to primary colorectal tumors: pharmacokinetics, biodistribution, scintigraphy and immune response. J Nucl Med 1993; 34:1662–1671.

69. Vuillez JP, Moro D, Brichon PY, Rouvie E, Brambilla E, Peltier P, Meyer P, Sarrazin R, Brambilla C. Two-step immunoscintigraphy for nonsmall cell lung cancer staging using a bispecific anti-CEA/anti-indium DTPA antibody and an indium-111-labeled DTPA dimer. J Nucl Med 1997; 38:507–511.

70. Williams WV, Kieber-Emmons T, VonFeldt J, Greene MI, Weiner DB. Design of bioactive peptides based on antibody hypervariable region structures. Development of conformationally constrained and dimeric peptides with enhanced affinity. J Biol Chem 1991; 266:5182–5190.

71. Katyal S, Kramer EL, Noz ME, McCauley D, Chachoua A, Steinfeld A. Fusion of immunoscintigraphy single photon emission computed tomography (SPECT) with CT of the chest in patients with non-small cell lung cancer. Cancer Res 1995; 55:5759s–5763s.

72. Schlumberger M, Arcangioli O, Piekarski JD, Tubiana M, Parmentier C. Detection and treatment of lung metastases of differentiated thyroid carcinoma in patients with normal chest X-rays. J Nucl Med 1988; 29:1790–1794.

73. Krempf M, Lumbroso J, Mornex R, Brendel AJ, Wemeau JL, Delisle MJ, Aubert B, Carpentier P, Gobold C, Guyot M, Lahneche B, Marchandise X, Schlumberger M, Charbonnel B, Chatal JF. Use of m-[^{131}I]iodobenzylguanidine in the treatment of malignant pheochromocytoma. J Clin Endocrinol Metab 1991; 72:455–461.

74. Lashford LS, Lewis IJ, Fielding SL, Flower MA, Meller S, Kemshead JT, Ackery D. Phase I/II study of iodine 131 metaiodobenzylguanidine in chemoresistant neuroblastoma: a United Kingdom Children's Cancer Study Group investigation. J Clin Oncol 1992; 10:1889–1896.

75. Kaminski MS, Zasadny KR, Francis IR, Fenner MC, Ross CW, Milik AW, Estes J, Tuck M, Regan D, Fisher S, Glenn SD, Wahl RL. Iodine-131-anti-B1 radioimmunotherapy for B-cell lymphoma. J Clin Oncol 1996; 14:1974–1981.

76. Press OW, Eary JF, Applebaum FR, Martin PJ, Badger CC, Nelp WB, Glenn S, Butchko PJ, Fisher D, Porter B, Matthews DC, Fisher LD, Bernstein ID. Radiolabeled-antibody therapy of B-cell lymphoma with autologous bone marrow support. N Engl J Med 1993; 329:1219–1224.

77. Press OW, Eary JF, Applebaum FR. Phase II trial of 131-I-B1 (anti CD20) antibody therapy with autologous stem cell transplantation for relapsed B cell lymphomas. Lancet 1995; 346:336–340.

78. Behr TM, Sharkey RM, Juweid ME, Dunn RM, Vagg RC, Ying Z, Zhang CH, Swayne LC, Vardi Y, Siegel JA, Goldenberg DM. Phase I/II clinical radioimmunotherapy with an iodine-131-labeled anti-carcinoembryonic antigen murine monoclonal antibody IgG. J Nucl Med 1997; 38:858–870.

79. Wilder RB, DeNardo GL, DeNardo SJ. Radioimmunotherapy: recent results and future directions. J Clin Oncol 1996; 14:1383–1400.

80. Jain RK. Physiological barriers to delivery of monoclonal antibodies and other macromolecules in tumors. Cancer Res 1990; 50(suppl):814s–819s.

81. Chatal JF, Saccavini JC, Gestin JF, Thedrez P, Curtet C, Kremer M, Guerreau D, Nolibe D, Fumoleau P, Guillard Y. Biodistribution of indium 111-labeled OC125 monoclonal antibody intraperitoneally injected into patients operated on for ovarian carcinomas. Cancer Res 1989; 49:3087–3094.

82. Smith A, Groscurth P, Waibel R, Westera G, Stahel RA. Imaging and therapy of small cell carcinoma xenografts using ^{131}I-labeled monoclonal antibody SWA11. Cancer Res 1990; 50:980s–984s.

83. Smith A, Zangemeister-Wittke U, Waibel R, Schenker T, Schubiger PA, Stahel RA. A comparison of ^{67}Cu- and ^{131}I-labelled forms of monoclonal antibodies SEN7 and SWA20 directed against small-cell lung cancer. Int J Cancer 1994; 8(suppl):43–48.

84. Hosono MN, Hosono M, Endo K, Ueda R, Onoyama Y. Effect of hyperthermia on tumor uptake of radiolabeled anti-neural cell adhesion molecule antibody in small-cell lung cancer xenografts. J Nucl Med 1994; 35:504–509.

85. Olabiran Y, Ledermann JA, Marston NJ, Boxer GM, Hicks R, Souhami RL, Spiro SG. The selection of antibodies for targeted therapy of small-cell lung cancer (SCLC) using a human tumour spheroid model to compare the uptake of cluster 1 and cluster w4 antibodies. Br J Cancer 1994; 69:247–252.
86. Bardiès M, Bardet S, Faivre-Chauvet A, Peltier P, Douillard JY, Mahé M, Fiche M, Lisbona A, Giacalone F, Meyer P, Gautherot E, Rouvier E, Barbet J, Chatal J-F. Bispecific antibody and iodine-131-labeled bivalent hapten dosimetry in patients with medullary thyroid or small-cell lung cancer. J Nucl Med 1996; 37:1853–1859.
87. Dazord L, Thomas D, Brichory F, Cavalier A, Meritte H, Desrues B, Caulet-Maugendre S, Bourguet P. The uptake of a monoclonal antibody (Po66) in lung tumour cell aggregates involves a phagocytose-like phenomenon. Int J Oncol 1997; 10:609–613.
88. Rouse MK, Chappell MJ, Bradwell AR. Optimal tumour targeting by antibodies: kinetic considerations. Adv Drug Deliv Rev 1996; 19:469–484.-

32

Photodynamic Therapy for Lung Cancer

ERIC S. EDELL

Mayo Medical School
and Mayo Clinic
Rochester, Minnesota

DENIS A. CORTESE

Mayo Medical School
and Mayo Clinic
Jacksonville, Florida

Bronchogenic carcinoma is currently a leading cause of cancer death in both men and women in several countries of the world. Studies have shown that diagnosis and treatment at an early stage offers the best opportunity for long-term survival. Methods available at this time for early diagnosis include only chest roentgenogram and sputum cytology. Screening studies undertaken at Memorial Sloan-Kettering, Johns Hopkins University, and the Mayo Clinic demonstrated that superficial squamous cell carcinomas can be detected at their earliest stages using sputum cytology. Unfortunately, many of these patients required a pneumonectomy to control the disease. Photodynamic therapy offers a new method for local treatment of superficial squamous cell carcinoma, if these cancers can be detected and localized at a very early stage.

Photodynamic therapy involves a photosensitizing agent, which, when exposed to light of the proper wavelength, forms toxic oxygen radicals that results in cell death. This therapy has been used in several institutions for the past 17 years in the management of early superficial cancers.

I. Historical Background

Photosensitizing agents can absorb photons of appropriate wavelength and become excited to a triplet species. The photon is then transferred to ground-state triplet

523

oxygen to produce the excited singlet oxygen. This is called a type II photo-oxidation reaction. A type I photo-oxidative process is one in which the excited sensitizer initiates a free radical reaction. Both types of reactions have been associated with photodynamic therapy (PDT). However, singlet oxygen is the main agent believed to produce cell death in PDT. Photodynamic therapy, as defined above, was first described in 1900 when the photosensitizer acridine was found to kill paramecia exposed to light (1). The first clinical use of PDT was in the treatment of skin cancer as early as 1903 (2). Porphyrin-based photosensitizers were first used in 1911 and are currently the most widely used in PDT today (3). Hematoporphyrin derivative (HpD) was prepared by Lipson and colleagues in the 1950s. The tumor-localizing properties of crude hematoporphyrin were improved using the supernatant that results from the preparation of hematoporphyrin (4). HpD was found to be retained in a large percentage of squamous and adenocarcinomas (5–8) and did prove to be a better agent for tumor localization than hematoporphyrin. Using multiple sessions of treatment with HpD, a therapeutic response was reported by Lipson in a patient with recurrent breast cancer (9). Although the tumor was not eradicated, there was objective evidence of a cytotoxic effect. In 1975, a patient with bladder carcinoma was treated after intravenous injection of hematoporphyrin derivative (10). Again, a clear cytotoxic effect was documented.

Dougherty and colleagues have maintained a basic science and clinical investigative program since the mid-1970s. These investigators have evaluated the mechanism of action of photodynamic therapy using porphyrin-based photosensitizers (11–15). Through the combined efforts of other investigators, PDT is now being explored in several areas of oncology.

Several photosensitizing agents are currently under investigation. These include chlorins, phthalocyanines, tetraphenylporphine sulfate (TPPS), and cationic sensitizers such as rhodamine 123. By far the most commonly used and evaluated photosensitizers are the porphyrin-based agents, including hematoporphyrin derivative (also known as Photofrin I), and a further refined mixture of hematoporphyrin derivative named dihematoporphyrin ether/ester, DHE (Photofrin II) (13). Both of these agents localize in tumors, but DHE appears to require a slightly lower dose than HpD. The absorption spectra for both porphyrin-based agents are similar, with an absorption peak at 405 nm. The resultant fluorescence enables the chemical to act as a tumor marker. Since this wavelength of light is nearly completely absorbed within a millimeter of penetration, a wavelength of 630 nm is used for therapeutic intervention because it produces deeper tissue penetration.

II. Mechanism of Action

The uptake and retention of porphyrin compounds have been extensively studied in several murine models. Sensitizers accumulate and are retained by vascular endothelium through the mechanism of endocytosis (16–18). This cellular uptake correlates to the lipophilic nature of the compounds (19–22). In murine models, the highest levels have been found in the liver, adrenal glands, and urinary bladder, with lower levels declining in the following order: pancreas, kidney, spleen, stomach, bone, lung, heart, muscle, and brain (16,19,20,23). The serum half-life in humans is 20–30 hours, but a photosensitizing component is retained in the skin for up to 6 weeks (22).

The selective retention of photosensitizer by malignant tissue was first reported by Figge et al. in 1948 (24). Lipson et al. again showed that HpD was retained in tumor tissue to a greater extent than crude hematoporphyrin (4–6). The concentrations of hematoporphyrin were determined from the emitted fluorescence when tumor was irradiated with light of the appropriate wavelength. Subsequently, several other investigators have demonstrated that both HpD and DHE have greater retention in tumor than in normal tissues (25–28). The tumor–to–normal tissue ratio is greatest 24–48 hours after intravenous injection. Lipson et al. did demonstrate that malignant tissue fluoresced within 3 hours of intravenous injection, well before normal tissue (6). The 3-hour time interval has been used for detection and localization (29,30). For purposes of therapy, a time interval of between 48 and 72 hours is commonly used.

The mechanisms involved in tissue selectivity of DHE and HpD are unknown and are the subject of ongoing research. Possible explanations for this phenomenon include variations in the route of delivery, binding to lipoproteins, pH changes within tumor stroma and cells, tumor angiogenesis factors, and poor tumor lymphatic drainage (31).

PDT requires the simultaneous interaction of a sensitizer and light in the presence of oxygen. Any light source that delivers photons of appropriate spectral characteristics will activate these photosensitizers. For bronchogenic carcinoma, the development of endoscopic devices allows for laser light to be transmitted within the bronchial tree. Laser light offers conveniences, such as uniform spectral wavelength and coherence, so that it can be easily focused into a fiberoptic bundle for use with flexible endoscopes. The fiber probes can be tailored to fit most clinical situations. These include cleaved tips for forward light projection, bulbous structures for spherical distribution of light, and coated or scored fibers to allow cylindrical scattering of light that can be inserted into the tumor directly for interstitial delivery in situations of obstructing airway cancers.

The lasers most frequently used for lung cancer therapy include the argon dye pump lasers using rhodamine-B and the excimer laser. Satisfactory therapeutic effects in human bronchogenic carcinoma can be accomplished with power densities between 200 and 300 mW/cm^2 and a total energy density of 200–400 J/cm^2. Greater energy density is associated with greater phototoxicity. Cells may escape PDT toxicity due to their ability to repair sublethal damage if inadequate power densities are used (32,33). On the other hand, undesired thermal effects may exceed the photochemical effects if excessive power densities are used (34).

PDT appears to be a type II photo-oxidative process. In vitro experiments have shown that cells are resistant to PDT in the presence of low oxygen conditions (35,36). In a type II photo-oxidative reaction, energy transfer occurs from the sensitizer in its excited state to molecular oxygen with the generation of singlet oxygen species. This is believed to be the predominant mechanism since PDT-induced cytotoxicity has been reduced in the presence of 1,3-diphenylisobenzofuran (37), a singlet oxygen scavenger (38). Other in vivo murine models have demonstrated the production of singlet oxygen during PDT (39). Several other experiments have demonstrated that oxygen is a key component in PDT. These include a decreased cell sensitivity to PDT in the presence of low oxygen concentration (40–42) and a decreased effect of PDT in a tissue hypoxemia animal model (43). Some studies suggest that areas of local tumor hypoxia account for the nonresponsiveness of some tumors to PDT (44,45).

In vitro experiments have shown that the earliest cellular injury from PDT is to plasma membranes and other cellular membranes. The membranes are thought to be the primary target because of initial binding to the plasma membrane followed by migration of the photosensitizer into intracellular regions (46). Cell culture experiments show that photodynamic therapy causes normal cell movement to cease and the cells become resistant to trypsin removal from plastic plates, implying the membrane proteins are binding to the plastic (25,47–49). Further evidence of cell membrane damage has been shown through the development of blebs protruding from the cell membrane (50–52). Mitochondrial injury has been demonstrated by inhibition of electron transport enzymes, reduction in cellular adenosinetriphosphate levels, and blockage of oxidative phosphorylation (54,54). Nuclear injury with direct damage to DNA is not believed responsible for cellular death, although several studies have shown DNA strand breakage following PDT (55,56).

Several in vivo experiments have suggested that the endothelium of the neovasculature may be the prime target for PDT (57–59). These experiments show stasis of blood flow in both arterioles and venules soon after PDT. Subsequently, aggregation of neutrophils and platelets may allow release of vasoactive compounds. There is increased coagulation and an alteration of the vessel integrity. Experiments using cyclo-oxygenase inhibitors have demonstrated a reduced PDT effect on arterioles (60). PDT may also reduce tumor viability, perhaps due to a combination of change in ATP concentration, acidosis, and increased tumor interstitial pressure (23,61–63).

III. PDT: Treatment of Bronchogenic Carcinoma

Bronchogenic carcinoma continues to be the leading cause of cancer death in both men and women in the United States. Most patients are not candidates for curative resection at the time of diagnosis. Additionally, patients with radiographically occult lung cancer often undergo pneumonectomy and are at slightly increased risk for surgical resection. Patients also have a risk of 5% per year of developing a second primary lung cancer. Photodynamic therapy has been used as an investigational treatment for both advanced and early superficial lung cancer since 1980. Patients can receive this therapy under either local or general anesthesia using a standard flexible bronchoscope. Patients with underlying medical conditions, such as heart disease or chronic lung disease, can be treated safely with this technique. PDT has been used in the treatment of large obstructing cancers of the major airway, but the most useful clinical application of PDT has proven to be in patients with early stage superficial squamous cell carcinoma of the tracheobronchial tree (64). Several studies have indicated that superficial squamous cell carcinomas have demonstrated a complete response (no evidence of residual cancer) after PDT while large obstructing cancers showed, at most, a partial response (65). Reports of hemorrhage within 2 weeks after treatment have also been noted in patients with lung cancer extending beyond the bronchial wall (65). Extensive tumor necrosis in already necrotic carcinoma was suspected to be the cause of hemorrhage and death following PDT. It is felt that superficial tumors that do not erode through a bronchial wall would be safer to treat and more likely to heal completely after treatment. Empirical observations have shown that light doses as high as 600 J/cm^2 and DHE doses of 2 mg/kg are not associated with any serious complications when treating early stage lung cancer (66). Animal experiments using PDT on a normal trachea have showed no damage to the cartilage and suggest that perforation or collapse of major airways is unlikely using PDT (67).

IV. Obstructive Carcinomas

Several studies have reported a large number of patients who have received PDT for advanced obstructing cancers of the tracheobronchial tree. One report noted 17 patients with carcinoma of the trachea and main stem bronchi. No complete responses were reported. However, there was a greater than 50% reduction in the degree of obstruction in 41% of these patients (68). Complications included secretion retention, fever, pneumonia, and abscess formation. Another series of 35 patients described the need for a second bronchoscopy to remove retained secretions and necrotic material approximately 2 days after PDT. This resulted in complete opening of obstructed airways after only one session of PDT in 80% of the patients (69,70). Use of PDT preoperatively has been reported to reduce the extent of surgical resection in some patients (71). PDT can also be used in relief of obstruction involving lobar bronchi, main stem bronchi, and the main carina (72). McCaughan et al. reported on a large series of patients who have undergone PDT for obstructing cancers. Treatment was accomplished with either surface irradiation or implanting cylinder fibers using power densities of 500 mW/cm of fiber and energy densities of 400 J/cm of fiber. They reported a complete response in 16% of patients (73–76).

The use of PDT for obstructing carcinoma of the tracheobronchial tree seems to be most effective in the treatment of polypoid tumors. Several authors have noted a poor response to submucosal and peribronchial disease (77–80). Evaluation of the mean duration of complete response appears to be about 22 weeks if more than 50% of the airway obstruction is due to a mucosal process. The median duration is only 7 weeks if the tumor is predominantly submucosal or peribronchial in nature. Other studies have shown that extraluminal tumor compression as demonstrated by CT scanning indicates a poor response (81,82).

V. Early-Stage Squamous Cell Carcinoma

Surgical resection remains the treatment of choice for early-stage lung cancer. However, some cancers are inoperable because of either high surgical risk or refusal of surgery. In Japan, photodynamic therapy has been used to treat a large number of patients with lung cancer (64,83,84). During the past decade, 196 patients (239 lesions) with central lung cancer, including 56 patients (66 lesions) with early-stage lung cancer, have been treated with PDT at the Tokyo Medical College. The 56 patients with endoscopic findings suggestive of early-stage lung cancer involved predominantly male patients with an age distribution from 36 to 82 years (mean age 65 years). Fifty-five of the lesions were squamous cell carcinoma, and one was an adenocarcinoma. The majority of patients were treated with either an argon laser coupled to a rhodamine-B dye laser or an excimer laser, both generating 630 nm laser light. Treatment was performed via flexible fiberoptic bronchoscope under topical anesthesia and intravenous sedation approximately 48 hours after injection of 2.0 mg/kg body weight of DHE. The laser beam was transmitted via a fiber (400 μm diameter) through the instrument channel of a fiberoptic bronchoscope. Power was adjusted to a range of 80–400 mW using the argon dye laser. When an excimer laser was used, the frequency was set at 30 Hz with an energy adjusted to 4 mJ/pulse. The response to PDT was evaluated endoscopically, roentgenographically, cytologically, and histologically at periodic intervals after treatment. Specimens obtained from surgical resection or at autopsy were examined microscopically and histologically. In 43 of 66 cancers (65%) and 36 of 56 patients (64%), a complete response was obtained. Recurrence was noted in 5 patients (8%). After 140 months of follow-up, 37 patients remained disease-free. In patients in which a complete response was not obtained, the lesions were anatomically difficult to photoradiate or they had evidence of invasion beyond the cartilage. These results indicate that PDT has a potential to treat certain early stage lung cancers.

The use of PDT at the Mayo Clinic is slightly different than the Tokyo experience, but clinical observations are similar and complementary in nature. PDT at the Mayo Clinic uses hematoporphyrin derivative and an argon pump dye laser using rhodamine-B. Photoradiation is usually delivered between 3 and 5 days after intravenous injection of hematoporphyrin derivative. Since 1980, more than 100 patients have been treated with this therapy. The overall experience shows at least a 65% complete response for tumors that fulfill the following criteria: roentgenographically occult, squamous cell carcinoma, appear to be superficial mucosal tumors by bronchoscopic inspection, and are less than an estimated 3 cm^2 in surface area (65,85,86) (Fig. 1).

The above information suggested that PDT may be an alternative to surgical resection in properly selected patients. In a preliminary study of 13 patients, a total

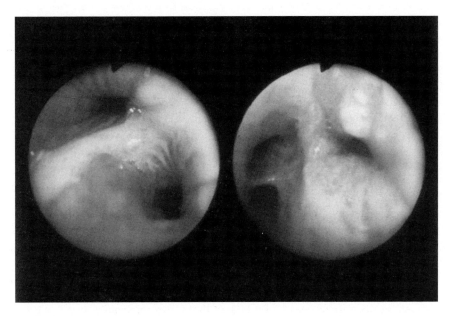

Figure 1 (Left) Superficial squamous cell carcinoma, lingular bronchus. (Right) Nodular squamous cell carcinoma, right upper lobe.

of 14 cancers were identified (87). Patients were treated with the understanding that if residual cancer was found after no more than two sessions of PDT, they would receive standard surgical therapy. A complete response was obtained in 12 of the 13 patients (92%). Ten of the 14 cancers (70%) required a single photodynamic treatment. Three others demonstrated a complete response after the second treatment. Of the 14 cancers, 13 demonstrated a complete response after two treatments. All 13 were superficial and appeared to be spreading over the mucosa at the time of bronchoscopic inspection. The one cancer that failed to show a complete response was bulky and exfoliative by bronchoscopic inspection. Three of the 13 cancers (23%) that demonstrated a complete response recurred within the first 2 years of follow-up. Two were surgically resected, and a third was subsequently treated with a second PDT treatment and has not recurred since. Ten of the 13 cancers that showed a complete response have not recurred for up to 5 years of follow-up. In all, 10 of 13 patients (77%) were spared a surgical resection. The 3 patients that had persistent disease after PDT each underwent surgical resection and had surgical stage T1N0M0.

These preliminary data suggest that photodynamic therapy may be an alternative to surgical resection as a form of local therapy in patients who are properly selected with early superficial squamous cell carcinoma. To evaluate this hypothesis, a single arm, prospective, multicenter trial has been initiated. Because of the small number of patients that present with superficial squamous cell carcinoma, a single arm study was necessary. Patients have been enrolled, treated with PDT, and followed closely for response to treatment. If PDT is unsuccessful, the patients then undergo surgical resection; if there is a complete response to PDT, the patients are followed every 3 months for 2 years and then annually for a total of 5 years. If recurrence is noted, the tumors are resected.

A report of 21 patients with early stage, roentgenographically occult lung cancer has recently been published (88). All patients were surgical candidates prior to PDT and were followed a minimum of 24 months after PDT. There were a total of 23 early stage squamous cell cancers in these 21 patients. Two patients had two simultaneous cancers at the time of their initial PDT treatments. The range of follow-up is from 21 months to 116 months. There were 18 males and 3 females. The age range was 53–81 years with a mean and median age of 65.

Fifteen patients (71%) demonstrated a complete response 3 months after initial PDT (Fig. 2). However, 11 of the 21 patients (54%) maintained a complete response longer than 12 months. Two of these 11 patients had a second primary lung cancer develop in the same lobe as the original endobronchial cancer that was treated with PDT. These patients had surgical resection 12 months and 54 months after PDT. There was no evidence of recurrence of the original tumor treated with PDT and the nodal status was N_0 for both of them. The remaining four patients had

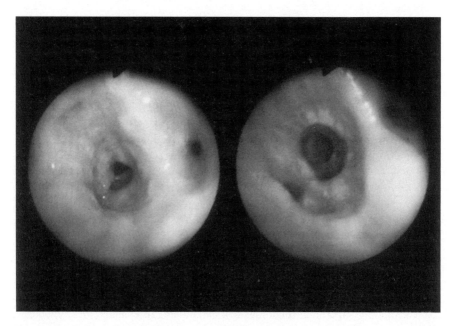

Figure 2   Superficial squamous cell carcinoma before (left) and after (right) photodynamic therapy.

recurrence within 12 months and underwent surgical resection. Therefore, a total of 9 of the original 21 patients (43%) were spared surgery.

VI. Summary

Photodynamic therapy is effective in the management of bronchogenic carcinoma. It can be used in the palliation of obstructing lesions but is best suited for the treatment of superficial squamous cell carcinomas. In properly selected patients, PDT may be an alternative to surgical resection. The challenge is the identification of patients with lesions that are appropriate for this therapy. Early detection studies are important in identifying patients that may be candidates for this local therapy. Studies using biological markers on sputum are in progress. Some of these biological markers show promise in the detection of patients with roentgenographically occult squamous cell carcinoma. New photosensitizers that are more active than the current compounds and have less phototoxicity are being developed.

References

1. Raab O. Über die Wirkung fluoreszierenden Stoffen. Infusoria Z Biol 1900; 39:524.
2. Jesionek A, Tappeiner VH. Zur Behandlung der Hautcarcinoma mit fluorescierenden Stoffen. Muench Med Wochenshr 1903; 47:2042.
3. Hausman W. Die sensibilisierende Wirkung des Hematoporphyrins. Biochem Z 1911; 30:276.
4. Lipson RL, Baldes EJ. The photodynamic properties of a particular hematoporphyrin derivative. Arch Dermatol 1960; 82:508–516.
5. Lipson RL, Baldes EJ, Gray MJ. Hematoporphyrin derivative for detection and management of cancer. Cancer 1967; 20:2254–2257.
6. Lipson RL, Baldes EJ, Olsen AM. The use of a derivative of hematoporphyrin in tumor detection. J Natl Cancer Inst 1961; 26:1–11.
7. Gray M, Lipson RI, Mack JVS. Use of hematoporphyrin derivative in detection and management of cervical cancer. Am J Obstet Gynecol 1967; 9:766.
8. Gregorie HG Jr, Horger EO, Ward JL, Green JF, Richards T, Robertson HC Jr, Stevenson TB. Hematoporphyrin-derivative fluorescence in malignant neoplasms. Ann Surg 1968; 167:820–828.
9. Lipson RI, Gray MJ, Baldes EJ. Hematoporphyrin derivative for detection and management of cancer. Proc 9th International Cancer Congress Tokyo, Japan, 1966, p. 393.
10. Kelly JF, Snell ME, Berenbaum MC. Photodynamic destruction of human bladder carcinoma. Br J Cancer 1975; 31:237–244.
11. Dougherty TJ, Grindley GE, Fiel R, Weishaupt KR, Boyle DG. Photoradiation therapy II. Cure of animal tumors with hematoporphyrin and light. J Natl Cancer Inst 1975; 55:115–121.
12. Dougherty TJ, Kaufman JE, Goldfarb A, Weishaupt KR, Boyle DG, Mittleman A. Photoradiation therapy for the treatment of malignant tumors. Cancer Res 1978; 38:2628–2635.
13. Dougherty TJ, Potter WR, Weishaupt KR. The structure of the active component of hematoporphyrin derivative. In: Doiron DR, Gomer CJ, eds. Porphyrin Localization and Treatment of Tumors. New York: Alan R. Liss, 1984:301.
14. Dougherty TJ. Activated dyes as antitumor agents. J Natl Cancer Inst 1974; 51:1333–1336.
15. Dougherty TJ. Photosensitizers: therapy and detection of malignant tumors. Photochem Photobiol 1987; 45:874–889.
16. Bugelski PH, Porter CW, Dougherty TJ. Autoradiographic distribution of hematoporphyrin derivative in normal and tumor tissue of the mouse. Cancer Res 1981; 41:4606–4612.

17. Selman SH, Kreimer-Birnbaum M, Klaunig JE, Goldblatt PJ, Keck RW, Britton SL. Blood flow in transplantable bladder tumors treated with hematoporphyrin derivative and light. Cancer Res 1984; 44:1924–1927.

18. Star WM, Marijnissen HP, van den Berg-Blok AE, Versteeg JA, Franken KA, Reinhold HS. Destruction of rat mammary tumor and normal tissue microcirculation by hematoporphyrin derivative photoradiation observed in vivo in sandwich observation chambers. Cancer Res 1986; 46:2532–2540.

19. Jori G, Tomio L, Reddi E, Rossi E, Corti L, Zorat PL, Calzavana F. Preferential delivery of liposome-incorporated porphyrins to neoplastic cells in tumour-bearing rats. Br J Cancer 1983; 48:307–309.

20. Barel A, Jori G, Perin A, Perin A, Romandini P, Pagnan A, Biffanti S. Role of high-, low- and very low-density lipoproteins in the transport and tumor-delivery of hematoporphyrin in vivo. Cancer Lett 1986; 32:145–150.

21. Maziere JC, Morliere P, Santus R. The role of the low density lipoprotein receptor pathway in the delivery of lipophilic photosensitizers in the photodynamic therapy of tumours. J Photochem Photobiol B 1991; 8:351–360.

22. Pass HI. Photodynamic therapy for lung cancer. Chest Surg Clin North Am 1991; 1:135–151.

23. Bellnier DA, Henderson BW. Determinants for photodynamic tissue destruction. In: Henderson BW, Dougherty TJ, eds. Photodynamic Therapy. New York: Marcel Dekker, 1992:117.

24. Figge FHJ, Weiland GS, Manganiello LOJ. Cancer detection and therapy. Affinity of neoplastic embryonic and traumatized tissue for porphyrins and metalloporphyrins. Proc Soc Exp Biol Med 1948; 68:640–641.

25. Kessel D. Effects of photoactivated porphyrins at the cell surface of leukemia L 1210 cells. Biochemistry 1977; 16:34–43.

26. Kessel D. Sites of photosensitization by derivatives of hematoporphyrin. Photochem Photobiol 1986; 44:489–493.

27. Gomer CJ, Dougherty TJ. Determination of [^{3}H]- and [^{14}C]-hematoporphyrin derivative distribution in malignant and normal tissue. Cancer Res 1979; 39:146–151.

28. Kaye AH, Morstyn G, Ashcroft RG. Uptake and retention of hematoporphyrin derivative in an in vivo/in vitro model of cerebral glioma. Neurosurgery 1985; 17:883–890.

29. Cortese DA, Kinsey JH, Woolner LB, Sanderson DR, Fontana RS. Hematoporphyrin derivative in the detection and localization of radiographically occult lung cancer. Am Rev Respir Dis 1982; 126:1087–1088.

30. Benson RC Jr, Farrow GM, Kinsey JH, Cortese DA, Zinche H, Utz DC. Detection and localization of in situ carcinoma of the bladder with hematoporphyrin derivative. Mayo Clin Proc 1982; 57:548–555.

31. Tochner Z, Mitchell JB, Smith P, Harrington F, Glatstein E, Russo D, Russo A. Photodynamic therapy of ascites tumours within the peritoneal cavity. Br J Cancer 1986; 53:733–736.

32. Matthews W, Cook J, Mitchell JB, Perry RR, Evans S, Pass HI. In vitro photodynamic therapy of human lung cancer: investigation of dose-rate effects. Cancer Res 1989; 49:1718–1721.

33. Kinsey JH, Cortese DA, Moses HI, Ryan RJ, Branum EL. Photodynamic effect of hematoporphyrin derivative as a function of optical spectrum and incident energy density. Cancer Res 1981; 41:5020–5026.

34. Kinsey JH, Cortese DA, Neel HB. Thermal considerations in murine tumor killing using hematoporphyrin derivative phototherapy. Cancer Res 1983; 43:1562–1567.

35. Mitchell JB, McPherson S, DeGraff W, Gamson J, Zabell A, Russo A. Oxygen dependence of hematoporphyrin derivative-induced photoinactivation of Chinese hamster cells. Cancer Res 1985; 45:2008–2011.

36. Lee See K, Forbes IJ, Betts WH. Oxygen dependency of photocytotoxicity with haematoporphyrin derivative. Photochem Photobiol 1984; 39:631–634.

37. Rizzoni WE, Matthews K, Pass HI. In vitro photodynamic therapy of human lung cancer. Influence of dose rate, hematoporphyrin concentration and incubation, and cellular targets. Surg Forum 1987; 38:452–455.

38. Keller SM, Taylor PD, Weese JL. In vitro killing of human malignant mesothelioma by photodynamic therapy. J Surg Res 1990; 48:337–340.

39. Sery TV, Shields JA, Augsburger JJ, Shah HG. Photodynamic therapy of human ocular cancer. Ophthalmic Surg 1987; 18:413–418.

40. Pope AJ, Masters W, Macrobert AJ. The photodynamic effect of a pulsed dye laser on human bladder carcinoma cells in vitro. Urol Res 1990; 18:267–270.

41. Raab GH, Schneider AF, Eierman W, Gottschalk-Deponte H, Baumgartner R, Beyer W. Response of human endometrium and ovarian carcinoma cell-lines to photodynamic therapy. Arch Gynecol Obstet 1990; 248:13–20.

42. Jamieson CH, McDonald WN, Levy JG. Preferential uptake of benzoporphyrin derivative by leukemic versus normal cells. Leuk Res 1990; 14:209–219.

43. Rogers DW, Lanzafame RJ, Hinshaw JR. Effect of argon laser and Photofrin II on murine neuroblastoma cells. J Surg Res 1991; 50:266–271.

44. Powers WE, Tolmach U. A multicomponent x-ray survival curve for mouse lymphosarcoma cells irradiated in vivo. Nature 1963; 197:710.

45. Thomlinson RH, Gray LH. The histological structure of some human lung cancers and the possible implications for radiotherapy. Br J Cancer 1977; 9:539.

46. Andreoni A, Cubeddu R, DeSilvestri S, Laponta P, Ambesi-Impiombato FS, Esposito M, Mastrocinque M, Tramontano D. Effects of laser irradiation on hematoporphyrin-treated normal transformed thyroid cells in culture. Cancer Res 1983; 43:2076–2080.

47. Belliner DA, Dougherty TJ. Membrane lysis in Chinese hamster ovary cells treated with hematoporphyrin derivative plus light. Photochem Photobiol 1982; 36:43.

48. Moan J, Christensen T, Jacobsen PB. Porphyrin-sensitized photoinactivation of cells in vivo. Prog Clin Bio Res 1984; 170:419–442.

49. Denstaman SC, Dillehay LE, Williams JR. Enhanced susceptibility to HPD-sensitized phototoxicity and correlated resistance to trypsin detachment in SV40 transformed IMR-90 cell. Photobiochem Photobiol 1986; 43:145–147.

50. Volden G, Christensen T, Moan J. Photodynamic membrane damage of hematoporphyrin derivative-treated NHIK 3025 cells in vitro. Photobiochem Photobiophys 1981; 3:105.

51. Jewell SA, Bellomo G, Thor H, Orrenius S, Smith M. Bleb formation in hepatocytes during drug metabolism is caused by disturbances in thiol and calcium ion homeostasis. Science 1982; 217:1257.

52. Borrelli MJ, Wong RSL, Dewey WC. A direct correlation between hyperthermiainduced blebbing and survival in synchronous G, CHO cells. J Cell Physiol 1986; 126:181–190.

53. Hilf R, Smail DB, Murant RS, Leaky PB, Gibson SL. Hematoporphyrin derivative-induced photosensitivity of mitochondrial succinate dehydrogenase and selected cytosolic enzymes of R3230AC mammary adenocarcinomas of rats. Cancer Res 1984; 44:1483–1488.

54. Hilf R, Murant RS, Narayanan U, Gibson SL. Relationship of mitochondrial function and cellular adenosine triphosphate levels of hematoporphyrin derivative-induced photosensitization in R3230AC mammary tumors. Cancer Res 1986; 46:211–217.

55. Gomer CJ. DNA damage and repair in CHO cells following hematoporphyrin photoradiation. Cancer Lett 1980; 11:161.

56. Moan J, Waksvik H, Christensen T. DNA single-stand breaks and sister chromatid exchanges induced by treatment with hematoporphyrin and light or by x-rays in human NHIK 3025 cells. Cancer Res 1980; 40:2915.

57. Reed MW, Schuschke DM, Ackermann JI, Harty JI, Wieman TJ, Miller FN. The response of rat urinary bladder microcirculation to photodynamic therapy. J Urol 1989; 142:865–868.

58. Wieman TJ, Mang TS, Fingar VS, Hill TG, Reed MW, Corey TS, Nguyen VQ, Render ER Jr. Effect of photodynamic therapy on blood flow in normal and tumor vessels. Surgery 1988; 104:512–517.

59. Stern SJ, Flock S, Small S, Thomsen S, Jacques S. Chloraluminum sulphonated phthalocyanine versus dihematoporphyrin ether: early vascular events in the rat window chamber. Laryngoscope 1991; 101:1219–1225.

60. Fingar VH, Wieman TJ, Doak KW. Role of thromboxane and prostacycline release on photodynamic therapy-induced tumor destruction. Cancer Res 1990; 50:2599–2603.

61. Dodd NJ, Moore JV, Poppitt DG, Wood B. In vivo magnetic resonance imaging of the effects of photodynamic therapy. Br J Cancer 1989; 60:164–167.
62. Moore JV, Dodd NJ, Wood B. Proton nuclear magnetic resonance imaging as a predictor of the outcome of photodynamic therapy of tumors. Br J Radiol 1989; 62:869–870.
63. Mattiello J, Evelhoch JL, Brown E, Schaap AP, Hetzel FW. Effect of photodynamic therapy on RIF-I tumor metabolism and blood flow examined by 31 P and 2H NMR spectroscopy. NMR Biomed 1990; 3:64–67.
64. Hayata Y, Kato H, Konaka C, Ono J, Takizawa N. Hematoporphyrin derivative and laser photoradiation in the treatment of lung cancer. Chest 1982; 81(3):269–276.
65. Cortese DA, Kinsey JH. Endoscopic management of lung cancer with hematoporphyrin derivative phototherapy. Mayo Clin Proc 1982; 57:543–547.
66. Hayata Y, Kato H, Konaka C. Photodynamic therapy in early stage lung cancer. Lung Cancer 1993; 9:287–294.
67. Smith SG, Bedwell J, MacRoberts AJ, Griffiths MH, Bown SG, Hetzel MR. Experimental studies to assess the potential of photodynamic therapy for the treatment of bronchial carcinomas. Thorax 1993; 48:474–480.
68. Vincent RG, Dougherty TJ, Rao U, Boyle DG, Potter WR. Photoradiation therapy in advanced carcinoma of the trachea and bronchus. Chest 1984; 85(1):29–33.
69. Balchum OJ, Doiron DR, Huth GC. Photoradiation therapy of endobronchial lung cancers employing the photodynamic action of hematoporphyrin derivative. Lasers Surg Med 1984; 4:13–30.
70. Balchum OJ, Doiron DR. Photoradiation therapy of endobronchial lung cancer. Large obstructing tumors, nonobstructing tumors, and early-stage bronchial cancer lesions. Clin Chest Med 1985; 6(2):255–275.
71. Kato H, Konaka C, Ono J, Kawate N, Nishimiya K, Shinohara H, Saito M, Sakai H, Noguchi M, Kito T. Preoperative laser photodynamic therapy in combination with operation in lung cancer. J Thorac Cardiovasc Surg 1985; 90:420–429.
72. Hugh-Jones P, Gardner WN. Laser photodynamic therapy for inoperable bronchogenic squamous carcinoma. Q J Med, N Ser 1987; 64(243):565–581.
73. McCaughan JS Jr, Hawley PC, Bethel BH, Walker J. Photodynamic therapy of endobronchial malignancies. Cancer 1988; 62(4):691–701.
74. McCaughan JS Jr, Hawley PC, Brown DG, Kakos GS, Williams TE Jr. Effect of light dose on the photodynamic destruction of endobronchial tumors. Ann Thorac Surg 1992; 54(4):705–711.
75. McCaughan JS Jr, Hawley PC, Walker J. Management of endobronchial tumors: a comparative study. Semin Surg Oncol 1989; 5(1):38–47.
76. McCaughan JS Jr, Williams TE Jr, Bethel BH. Photodynamic therapy of endobronchial tumors. Lasers Surg Med 1986; 6(3):336–345.
77. LoCicero J, Metzdorff M, Almgren C. Photodynamic therapy in the palliation of late stage obstructing non-small cell lung cancer. Chest 1990; 98(1):97–100.
78. Pass HI, Delaney T, Smith PD, Bonner R, Russo A. Bronchoscopic phototherapy at comparable dose rates: early results. Ann Thorac Surg 1989; 47:693–699.
79. Delaney TF, Sindelar WF, Tochner Z, Smith PD, Friauf WS, Thomas G, Dachowski L, Cole JW, Steinberg SM, Glatstein E. Phase I study of debulking surgery and photodynamic therapy for disseminated intraperitoneal tumors. Int J Radiation Oncol Biol Phys 1993; 25:445–457.
80. Sutedja T, Baas P, Stewart F, van Zandwijk N. A pilot study of photodynamic therapy in patients with inoperable non-small cell lung cancer. Eur J Cancer 1992; 28A:1370–1373.
81. Lam S, Muller NL, Miller RR, Kostashuk EC, Szasz IJ, Le Riche JC, Lee-Chuy E. Predicting the response of obstructive endobronchial tumors to photodynamic therapy. Cancer 1986; 58:2298–2306.
82. Zwirewich CV, Muller NL, Lam SCT. Photodynamic laser therapy to alleviate complete bronchial obstruction: comparison of CT and bronchoscopy to predict outcome. AJR 1988; 151:897–901.

83. Hayata Y, Kato H, Konaka C, Amemiya R, Ono J, Ogawa I, Kinoshita K, Sakai H, Takahashi H. Photoradiation therapy with hematoporphyrin derivative in early and stage 1 lung cancer. Chest 1984; 86(2):169–177.

84. Kato H, Konaka C, Kawate N, Shinohara H, Kinoshita K, Noguchi M, Ootomo M, Hayata Y. Five-year disease-free survival of a lung cancer patient treated only by photodynamic therapy. Chest 1986; 90:768–770.

85. Cortese DA, Kinsey JH. Hematoporphyrin derivative phototherapy in the treatment of bronchogenic carcinoma. Chest 1984; 86:8–13.

86. Edell ES, Cortese DA. Bronchoscopic phototherapy with hematoporphyrin derivative for treatment of localized bronchogenic carcinoma: a 5-year experience. Mayo Clin Proc 1987; 62:8–14.

87. Edell ES, Cortese DA. Photodynamic therapy in the management of early superficial squamous cell carcinoma as an alternative to surgical resection. Chest 1992; 102:1319–1322.

88. Cortese DA, Edell ES, Kinsey JH. Photodynamic therapy for early stage squamous cell carcinoma of the lung. Mayo Clin Proc 1997; 72:595–602.

33

Endobronchial Brachytherapy

M. TAULELLE, P. VINCENT, B. CHAUVET, R. GARCIA, and FRANÇOIS L. REBOUL

Clinique Sainte Catherine
Avignon, France

I. Introduction

Lung cancer is the leading cause of death from cancer in males. Moreover, its incidence has been steadily increasing in women over the past years. Clinical symptoms due to bronchial obstruction are initially present in 20–30% of cases (1). During the course of the disease, metastatic disease remains a major problem, but local progression is observed in about 31–51% of patients (2). Tumor progression in the proximal bronchial tree is generally responsible for major complications such as hemoptyses, infection, or dyspnea, which are detrimental to quality of life in these patients. These distressing clinical symptoms may also occur after treatment in about 50% of patients (3). External beam radiotherapy is generally active on these complications. However, there is an increasing interest in using endoluminal techniques, such as laser photoresection, cryotherapy, high-frequency thermocoagulation, stent placement, phototherapy and endobronchial brachytherapy to relieve bronchial obstruction. In some cases, these techniques may be combined in order to improve local efficacy.

II. History

The first cases of lung cancer treated with endobronchial brachytherapy were reported in 1922 by Yankauer. The treatment technique consisted of introducing a radon capsule through a rigid bronchoscope under local anesthesia (4). In 1932 Pancoast, and one year later Kernan, reported a similar experience (5,6). In 1961, the use of radon pearls was also reported by Pool in 43 patients treated for malignant tumors of the trachea or local relapses after surgery (7). During the 1960s, Radon was replaced by cobalt-60 because of its higher activity allowing shorter treatment time and better patient tolerance (8). Treatment with radon could require a 5-day exposure as opposed to 3–5 hours with cobalt-60. Limiting factors with this technique were (1) the need for using a rigid bronchoscope, which could not be introduced any further than the trachea and main bronchi (Fig. 1), and (2) the difficulties in dosimetry calculations and in achieving proper radioprotection. This precluded to a widespread use of this technique. In the early 1980s, two major technical developments

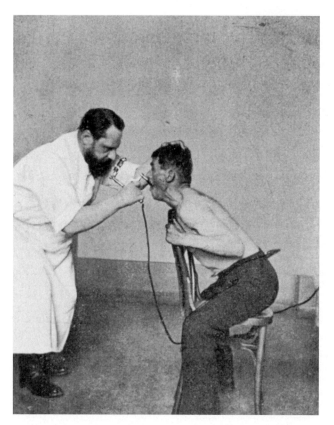

Figure 1   Rigid bronchoscopy at the beginning of the twentieth century.

gave a new impulse to the field of endobronchial brachytherapy: the advent of the flexible fiberoptic bronchoscope, and the availability of miniature iridium-192 radioactive sources. Initially, iridium-192 sources were of low dose rate, inferior to 1 Gy/hr. Only one applicator was used, and it was charged manually. In order to deliver a radiation dose of 10 Gy at 10 mm from the center of the source, treatment time lasted from 30 to 60 hours, which required patient hospitalization (9,10). Due to the length of the treatment, tolerance was poor, the applicator was often dislodged during coughing spells, and treatment had to be interrupted prior to reaching the prescribed dose. In the late 1980s, two additional breakthroughs took place— high-dose rate iridium sources and source projectors—allowing shorter, ambulatory treatments. In addition, optimization of dosimetry and afterloading techniques allowed optimal radioprotection of the medical staff. More recently, treatment techniques were further improved by better accuracy in the placement of the catheters, the advent of new applicators more adapted to the different anatomical situations, the progress made in dosimetry calculations through computerized treatment planning, and increased radiobiological understanding of the biological effects of dose-time-fractionation relationships.

III. Technical Aspects

A. Physical Characteristics of Radioactive Sources

Radioactive sources for high-dose-rate endobronchial brachytherapy are made of an iridium-192 seed placed within a metal capsule welded at the extremity of a small cable. The source is 0.6 mm in diameter and 3.5 mm long. The capsule has a diameter of 1.1 mm and a length of 5 mm. Each source has an initial maximum activity of 370 Gbq (10 Ci), which decreases to about 120 Gbq (3.2 Ci) by the end of its use. Therefore, the source must be replaced every 3 months. The radioactive period of iridium-192 is 74.02 days with a gamma energy of 0.38 MeV. This energy level stands as a good compromise between tissue penetration and radioprotection requirements during transportation, storage, and treatment.

B. Source Projectors

Commercially available source projectors display excellent mechanical and electronic properties as required to ensure maximal treatment accuracy. The radioactive source is attached to the edge of a cable and remains inside a tungsten container. The attenuation through this container allows the staff to work in accordance with radioprotection safety rules (the dose rate is inferior to one μGy/hr at one meter). A second cable projects a dummy source prior to each treatment and makes it possible to check for the safety of the application. Eighteen to 24 channels are available, but endobronchial brachytherapy applications require a maximum of three catheters. Treatment is continuously monitored thanks to a computer located outside the treatment room. The times corresponding to the positions of the source can be set manually or derived from the dose calculations done for each patient. The source can be positioned at various intervals, chosen according to geometrical and dosimetric considerations. During treatment, all safety parameters, such as position of the source, irradiation time at each stopping location, source exit and entrance from the container, etc., can be checked continuously. The walls of the treatment room are equivalent to 4 cm of lead or 40 cm of concrete. The actual dimensions depend on the size of the room and its near environment.

C. Bronchial Catheters

Numerous kinds of catheters are currently available. They can vary in size, caliber, and rigidity, and present with or without radio-opaque tips, inflatable balloons, or sleeved applicators (11). The purpose of these devices is to prevent, or at least reduce, overexposure of the bronchial mucosa in contact with the catheter. However, in the palliative setting, simple catheters are usually sufficient. The caliber of the catheters varies from 5- to 6-French (1.7–2 mm). The 5-French catheters are easy to introduce through the accessory port of the bronchoscope and to position into the distal bronchial tree. They can be curved easily, allowing proper positioning even in such difficult locations as the right upper lobe. The larger 4-mm catheters are semirigid, and their introduction requires oral intubation.

D. Catheter Positioning

The therapeutic endoscopy is carried out after complete clinical and biological workup has been obtained: blood gases, coagulation profile, spirometric and hemodynamic evaluation. A CT scan is also essential prior to making the final treatment decision. The procedure must be performed in a suite fully equipped for endoscopy and general anesthesia. During the entire procedure, the patient is under close monitoring for pulse, arterial blood pressure, and oxyhemoglobin saturation. For patients with severe respiratory impairment, the treatment is delivered under continuous oxygenotherapy by nasal cannula. It is our current practice to deliver the treatment under narcoanalgesia with Hypnovel® (1 mg/10 kg maximum) and Fentanyl® (0.005 mg). Local anesthesia is also necessary to suppress the cough reflex, which may dislodge the catheter. This is generally obtained with instillation of 2% xylocaïne in the nose, the larynx, the trachea, and the main bronchi as the bronchoscope progresses through the airways. Steroids and antitussive drugs may be necessary as well, in the event of chronic bronchitis with major inflammation of the bronchial mucosa. Each treatment must be preceded by a thorough examination of the entire bronchial tree, including the opposite side, in order to accurately assess the location of the endobronchial lesions. We routinely assess the extrinsic component of the endobronchial tumor as well, because of its relevance at the time of response evaluation. This is made on the basis of endoscopic findings and CT scan imaging and the results are scored as follows: limited, 25–30% bronchial obstruction; intermediate, 30–50%; high, greater than 50%. A video camera is useful for pre- and posttherapeutic photographic evaluation. After completion of this workup, the next step is to position one, two, or sometimes three applicators depending upon the extent of the lesions to treat. This is achieved through the accessory port of the bronchoscope and under continuous visual monitoring. The applicators are introduced as distally as possible into the bronchial tree and as far beyond as feasible from the treatment target. This makes it possible to fixate the catheter to the distal bronchial tree, which will limit the risks of displacement during patient transportation and treatment. Moreover, it allows optimal curvature of the catheter alongside the tumor (Fig. 2). The fiberoptic bronchoscope is then withdrawn along the catheter under fluoroscopic monitoring in order to maintain the catheter in place. The applicator is then secured to the nostril. The third step is to perform the dosimetric study. Dummy sources are introduced through the applicator, and orthogonal radiographs are obtained to verify their correct positioning. The location of the lesions, the target volume, the dose to be delivered, and the thickness to be treated are then defined. All parameters are transmitted to the dosimetry computer for calculations. Optimization of the timing of the source at every point is performed in order to eliminate hotspots when catheters are close to each other and to limit any heterogeneity in dose distribution within the treated volume. The patient is then transferred to the treatment room. The applicator is attached to the projector. Treatment may last from 3 to 20 minutes.

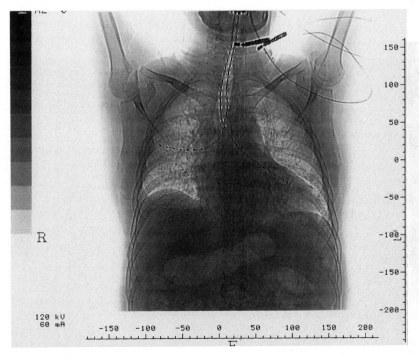

Figure 2 Patient with a tumor of the carina, x-ray radiography, with dummy sources in place.

E. Dose Distribution

The preparation of the treatment is done in the room where the catheter is positioned into the patient. Anterior and lateral radiographs are taken. The use of a frame with radio-opaque markers placed around the patient allows the dose calculation to be made in the exact treatment position. The active region of each catheter is specified on the two orthogonal films by digitizing the discrete positions of the source as well as markers belonging to the frame. As a result, the program is able to determine the exact position of each consecutive position of the source in each catheter. Dose-calculation software uses different methods according to the kind of application. For interstitial brachytherapy, standard geometries exist. This is not the case for endoluminal brachytherapy, where the catheter has to be against the lesion and the source positions optimized for each patient according to lesion and its geometry. The dose distribution is calculated using one or several points where the dose is optimized. Those points are set relative to anatomical points or to the catheters. For endobronchial brachytherapy, the prescription is currently made at 10 mm from the axis of the catheter. The irradiation time for each position of the source in each catheter is calculated by iterations so that the isodose where the dose is prescribed is as close as possible to the optimization points. The dose distribution takes into consideration the CT scanner data of the patient in the treatment area. The patient is positioned on the couch of the scanner in the treatment position with a catheter (Fig. 3). The dose calculation can be made either by digitizing on orthogonal films or by setting the

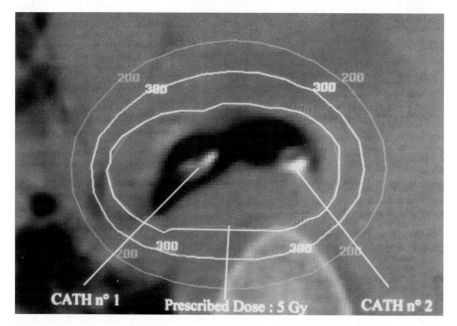

Figure 3   Projection of dosimetry on CT scan image.

source positions as they appear on the transverse slices. Dose distribution can be visualized in different planes (transverse, coronal, sagittal, oblique) or in three dimensions with the patient data. The three-dimensional representation of the tumor and its extensions is very useful in order to adapt the geometry of the irradiation to the target. The target can with that tool be evaluated and correlated to the response to the treatment. The prescription can be adapted to the shape of the tumor and to its modifications after each fraction.

IV. Clinical Indications and Results

Due to the heterogeneity of the patient populations and the diversity of treatment protocols, it remains difficult to make definitive statements about the results of endobronchial brachytherapy from the available data in the literature. However, it is possible to define two main clinical situations where endobronchial brachytherapy has been used with encouraging results. In the palliative setting, endobronchial brachytherapy has as its primary goal relief of symptomatic bronchial obstruction. In the curative setting, endobronchial brachytherapy has been successfully used to treat small endobronchial tumors not amenable to other forms of therapy, especially in patients with severe respiratory impairment. It can also be used as a method of boosting the primary tumor bed after external beam radiotherapy.

A. Endobronchial Brachytherapy in the Palliative Setting

From the start, endobronchial brachytherapy was mainly used for bronchial obstruction relief in two different palliative settings: previously untreated locally advanced endobronchial tumors requiring immediate obstruction relief because of acute respiratory distress secondary to collapse of the lung and/or hemoptyses, and local recurrences following initial therapy. In the former clinical setting, the purpose of endobronchial brachytherapy is to stop hemoptyses and/or to relieve the obstruction in order to rapidly improve the respiratory function. Symptomatic relief is generally achieved, sometimes in combination with LASER photoresection. Treatment duration is usually brief and requires no more than one or two applications, after which a reappraisal strategy has to be defined. A CT scan obtained following disappearance of the atelectasis and reexpansion of the lung will make it possible to define more accurately the local extension of the tumor and the degree of lymph node involvement. In some cases, a curative treatment strategy combining external beam radiotherapy or surgery with or without chemotherapy will then be defined. When patients present with endobronchial recurrence after prior treatment with external beam radiation therapy, and sometimes surgery, endobronchial brachytherapy will often be the only therapeutic option allowing symptomatic relief of dyspnea, cough, or hemoptyses. A new primary endobronchial lesion after pneumonectomy is also a good indication for endobronchial brachytherapy, used either alone or in association with external beam radiotherapy. Endobronchial brachytherapy is a very efficient way of relieving bronchial obstruction, with a clinical and endoscopic response rate

Table 1 Endoscopic Response to Endobronchial Brachytherapy

Year	No. of patients	HDR dose (Gy)	Prescription at (mm)	No. of fractions	Endoscopic response (%)	Ref.
1992	38	6	10	3	76	12
1992	24	15	6	2	88	13
1992	54	5	10	3–5		14
1993	19	15	10	1	89	15
1992	31	4	20	4	78	16
1993	15	5	10	3	100	17
1990	162	15–20		1	58–94	18
1996	189	10–8–7	10	3–4–5	54–79	19
1985	20	10	10	1	94	20
1993	295	10–7.5	10	3	80	21
1992	31	10	10	3	71	22
1993	82	10–4.7	10	1–5	82	23
1994	93	5–7–10	10	3–2–1	85	24
1994	406	10–15–20	10	1–2	70	25
1995	59	7	10	3	85	26

approximating 80% in most series, as shown in Table 1 (12–26). More than 1500 patients were included in 15 series, and endoscopic response was observed in 70–100% of the patients. Gollins et al. reported a clinical response rate of 88% for hemoptyses, 62% for cough, and 60% for dyspnea in a population of 406 patients (25). Our own experience is very similar to the data published in the literature, with a symptomatic response rate of 74% for hemoptyses, 54% for cough, and 54% for dyspnea (19). A few studies have reported a quantitative evaluation of the respiratory function. Goldman et al. have demonstrated a positive effect of endobronchial brachytherapy on pulmonary function tests and ventilation-perfusion scintigraphy in a small series of patients (15). The therapeutic effect is generally obtained within a short period of time for hemoptyses, but many take as long as 10–15 days for obstruction-related dyspnea. In terms of durability of the symptomatic response, published data report an excellent palliative effect, generally lasting several months (25). Upon analyzing prognosis factors for endoscopic response, our experience shows an adverse influence of the extrinsic component with a complete response rate of 62% in the case of limited extrinsic component as compared to 44% when the extrinsic component is greater than 50% (19). However, there is no general agreement on this point since the presence of a predominant extrinsic component is not considered as a contraindication to the method by some authors, especially if external beam radiotherapy can be associated to endobronchial brachytherapy (21,27,28). At any rate, it seems logical to limit the total number of treatment applications in the palliative setting in order to obtain a maximum therapeutic effect without impairing the quality of life. In our institution, patients benefit from one to two 6 Gy fractions delivered at 10 mm from the source axis at 1-week intervals. Although endobronchial brachytherapy clearly has a proven efficacy in the palliative setting, it remains difficult to recommend a standard treatment schedule to define the role of associated external beam radiotherapy and the role of the other procedures of endobronchial obstruction relief without further comparative clinical trials.

B. Endobronchial Brachytherapy in the Curative Setting

The role of endobronchial brachytherapy, particularly in association with external beam radiotherapy, has been considered in a number of studies for the treatment of lung cancer with curative intent (14,17,21,29). However, these studies were inconclusive about the exact role of adjuvant brachytherapy in prolonging patient survival. Speiser and Spratling (21) have proposed to deliver an endobronchial boost after external beam radiation therapy to 60 Gy in 30 fractions in patients with T1-3 N0-3 tumors. However, endobronchial treatment did not appear to confer any additional benefit to external beam radiotherapy alone in terms of local control and survival. On the other hand, Van Bodegon et al. (30) have delineated a small subset of patients that could benefit from this approach. Treatment consisted of combined external beam radiotherapy to 46 Gy and three 5-Gy courses of endobronchial brachytherapy. Median survival was not reached at the time of publication, possibly reflecting a local control benefit when endobronchial treatment was used as a boost. The potential advantage of this approach appears to be confirmed in a randomized trial by Huber et al., comparing external beam radiotherapy with or without endobronchial brachytherapy delivered as two 4.8 Gy fractions at 10 mm from the source axis prior to and following standard radiotherapy (31). Local control was significantly better in the combined treatment group, but there was no significant difference in terms of overall survival. However, there is at least one clinical situation where endobronchial brachytherapy appears to confer a significant benefit—when there is persistent endobronchial tumor and/or positive biopsies at the initial tumor site after full-dose external beam radiotherapy. In this case, additional brachytherapy can potentially make it possible to achieve a complete response, hopefully leading to definitive local control. In selected patients with medical contraindications to surgery or external beam radiotherapy, endobronchial brachytherapy has been used with curative intent to treat small endobronchial tumors limited to the bronchial wall. In the study by Tredaniel et al., treatment protocol consisted of 6 fractions of 7 Gy 10 mm from the source axis (32). Among the 25 evaluable patients, there were 21 complete endoscopic responses with 18 negative biopsies at the initial tumor site. For patients with complete pathological response, median survival exceeded 26 months. Ardiet et al. (33) have also reported encouraging results in the same clinical setting. Twenty-eight patients with a less than 1 cm tumor strictly endobronchial tumor, as assessed by CT scan were entered into this study. Treatment consisted of three to five 7-Gy fractions 10 mm from the source axis. Complete pathologic response rate was 84%, and median follow-up was 11 months. Complications occurred in 14% of the cases and included one fatal hemoptysis and four radiation-induced bronchitis. Our experience with 22 patients treated with a similar protocol as resulted in a median survival of 17.4 months (19). It is therefore legitimate to conclude from these studies that endobronchial brachytherapy has a definite curative potential in this selected group of patients. However, it should be kept in mind that this approach can only be proposed for patients with very limited tumors, whose volume, including a possible extrinsic component, can be fully encompassed in the endobronchial radiation field. In this situation, helical CT scan studies with volumetric acquisition are particularly helpful in accurately defining the target volume. Other investigators have proposed in this case to associate endobronchial brachytherapy to external beam radiotherapy. In the study designed by Yokoyama and Saiko, 40 patients with small 5- to 20-mm tumors were treated with combined external irradiation to 40 Gy and five 5 Gy fractions of endobronchial brachytherapy resulting in prolonged local control in 38 patients (34). At this time, however, it is not possible to make any definitive statement about the potential of endobronchial brachytherapy in improving local control over external beam radiotherapy alone. Well-controlled randomized studies with large numbers of patients are mandatory to assess the definitive role of endobronchial brachytherapy as a boost and to determine the best treatment schedule in terms of dose, timing, and fractionation.

C. Complications

A review of the literature on the tolerance to high-dose rate endobronchial brachytherapy shows excellent feasibility and absence of early toxicity in more than 90% of the cases, as reflected by the satisfactory patients' compliance to treatment (21,25). Late complications, occurring 2 months or later after completion of therapy, are more significant but also more difficult to assess due to the heterogeneity of patient populations, the diversity of treatment protocols, the difficulties in establishing the differential diagnosis between true complications of the treatment and disease progression, the inherent subjectivity of evaluation criteria, and the frequency of early disease-related deaths. Major complications include radiation bronchitis with or without bronchial stenosis, fistula, hemorrhages, and soft tissue necrosis. The incidence of radiation bronchitis is high, but it is considered a complication only in the event of clinical symptoms. Its incidence has been reported with some variation in the literature (Table 2). Although not mentioned in the studies by Bedwinek et al. and Nori et al. (12,17), it was estimated to occur in 12–13% of the cases in the large series ($n = 141$) published by Speiser and Spratling (21). These authors proposed a score for grading radiation bronchitis depending upon the intensity of the symptoms and the endoscopic clinical findings, as shown in Table 3 (35). Grade 1 radiation bronchitis consisted of mild asymptomatic mucosal inflammation with partial fibrinoid nonobstructive membranes requiring no intervention. Grade 2 consisted of a worsening of the former status with moderate obstruction of the bronchial lumen by a thick complete circumferential membrane responsible for cough and/or other obstructive symptoms and requiring local debridement or medical intervention. In grade 3 radiation bronchitis, severe inflammatory reaction was associated with marked pseudomembranous formation and mild fibrosis of the bronchial wall. In

Table 2 Radiation Bronchitis: Review of the Literature

No. of patients	Protocol	%	Ref.
50	15/20 Gy × 1	2	36
141	10/7.5 Gy × 3	12–13	37
38	6 Gy × 3	0	12
65	2.7–10 Gy × 2–4	2	29
49	7 Gy × 4	0	32
189	10/8/6/5 Gy × 3–4–3–6	6.3	19
406	15/20 Gy × 1	0	25

this case, multiple endoscopic maneuvers of debridment were necessary for symptomatic relief. Grade 4 was characterized by major fibrosis with circumferential stenosis requiring major local interventions such as laser photoresection, bougie dilatation, or stent placement. As a rule, grade 1 complications occur earlier in the course of the follow-up than grade 4 toxicity, with a median interval of 16 weeks versus 54 weeks, respectively, from the time of endobronchial brachytherapy. In our study, symptomatic radiation bronchitis occurred in 6.3% of the cases. Fistula are generally due to necrosis of the bronchial wall, with at least two different etiologies. Early fistula are mainly due to massive tumor necrosis or progression, while late-occurring fistula are the ultimate complication of grade 4 radiation bronchitis. It is our current practice to classify these different complications according to the endocopic appearance of the lesions (Table 4). Hemoptyses may be an early- or a late-occurring complication, but are always of extremely poor prognosis because they are fatal in most cases. There is considerable variation in their reported incidence, as shown in Table 5. Furthermore, it is always difficult to assess the respective roles of tumor progression and true treatment toxicity in their pathogenesis. Endobronchial brachytherapy being most commonly performed in patients with massive endobronchial lesions eroding through the bronchial wall and associated with medias-

Table 3 Speiser Score for Radiation Bronchitis

Grade	Clinical findings
1	Mild asymptomatic mucosal inflammation with thin whitish circumferential nonobstructive membrane
2	Symptomatic circumferential membrane with greater thickness reaction requiring therapeutic intervention
3	Severe mucosal inflammation with marked membranous exudate and fibrosis-stenosis of the bronchus requiring multiple interventions
4	No membrane; severe fibrosis and stenosis obliterating the bronchus and requiring multiple interventions

Table 4 The Clinique Sainte Catherine Grading System for Radiation Bronchitis

Grade	Clinical findings
1	Mucosal inflammation without obstruction
2	Mucosal inflammation with whitish discoloration and telangectasia
3	Same as grade 2 + nonobstructive pseudomembranous formation
4A	Obstruction of the lumen by pseudomembranes requiring debridement
4B	True bronchial stenosis
5	Bronchial wall necrosis

tinal involvement, the risk of pulmonary hemorrhage is significant, whatever treatment is delivered. A number of factors appear to increase this risk, including prior high-dose external beam radiotherapy and anatomical location of the tumor. When located in upper lobes, the close proximity of large pulmonary vessels in the mediastinum is a major risk factor. This is in fact a common problem in the field of therapeutic bronchology, not solely related to high dose rate endobronchial brachytherapy. Bedwinek et al. have proposed three different mechanisms to explain pulmonary hemorrhage: tumor progression through the bronchial wall despite endobronchial brachytherapy, effects of local irradiation on anteriorly irradiated tissues, and bronchial-arterial fistula formation due to massive tumor necrosis following treatment (12). It may be necessary to propose a special treatment, such as lower dose per fraction, lower total dose, or prolonged overall treatment time, to previously irradiated patients or with upper lobe tumors, both at higher risk of hemopty-

Table 5 Hemoptyses: Review of the Literature

No. of patients	Protocol	Incidence (%)	Ref.
62	5 Gy × 3/5	15	14
38	6 Gy × 3	32	12
24	15 Gy × 2	4	13
56	7.5 Gy × 3	7	35
31	4 Gy × 3	3	16
31	10 Gy × 1/3	32	22
295	10/7.5 Gy × 3	7	21
50	15/20 Gy × 1	1	36
20	10 Gy × 1	0	20
65	2.7–10 Gy IDR	1.5	29
49	7 Gy × 4	4	32
189	10/8/6/5 Gy × 3/4/3/6	6.9	19
32	5 Gy × 3	0	17
406	15/20 Gy × 1	7.9	25
100	15/20 Gy × 1	4	38

sis. However, in a study by Aygun et al., postmortem evaluation of fatal pulmonary hemorrhage has shown that most patients presented with peribronchial active disease and that there was no evidence of residual tumor in one case only (14). These findings have been confirmed in other autopsy series (21). The unusually high incidence of hemoptyses in the Bedwinek et al. study is probably related to patient selection, since palliative treatments for local recurrences were mainly performed in patients previously treated with high-dose external radiation (12). Sutedja et al. has observed a similar rate of complications in patients treated for local recurrence (22). Our experience has shown a hemoptysis rate very similar to the one reported in the Speiser and Spratling study (6.9% and 7.3%, respectively) (19,21). In a population of patients treated with either laser photoresection or external beam radiotherapy, Macha et al. have shown an hemoptysis rate of 34.5% as opposed to 7% in the latter group (35). On the other hand, when patients are treated with endobronchial brachytherapy for small noninvasive tumors surrounded by a healthy mucosa, they are less likely to develop delayed local toxicity than when treatment is applied to large tumors that have destroyed the normal architecture of the bronchial wall. In the studies reported by Macha et al. (35), as well as Suh et al. (28), the rate of fatal hemoptyses was 33.3% in patients treated by laser photoresection and low dose rate endobronchial brachytherapy. In a recent publication by Gollins et al. (25), high dose per fraction (a single 10–20 Gy fraction in this case), prior laser photoresection, repeated endobronchial brachytherapy on a previously treated site, and synchronous external beam radiotherapy were found to be strongly predictive of subsequent fatal hemoptysis. In addition, the authors report that the fiberoptic endoscopic evaluation preceding the hemorrhage is abnormal as a rule, with findings of either local recurrence or grade 2–3 radiation bronchitis. The relationship between total irradiation dose and rate of delayed toxicity is now clearly established (29). In the experience of Nori et al. (17), toxicity rate has been nil with a 5 Gy dose per fraction for three courses. Average complication rate is in the range of 15–18%. The pathophysiology of fatal pulmonary hemorrhages primarily involves bronchial wall or tumor necrosis, as confirmed by our own experience where follow-up endoscopic examination evidenced major mucosal inflammation with architectural disruption of the bronchial wall prior to the hemorrhagic episode. There is a clear dose-effect relationship in the development of radiation bronchitis. Therefore, it is of major importance to accurately calculate the cumulated dose of irradiation (external beam radiotherapy + endobronchial brachytherapy) in designing future protocols. The current tendency is to customize treatment for each individual clinical setting rather than routinely apply the same treatment protocol to each patient. Protecting the adjacent bronchial mucosa by technical means aimed to increase the distance between the bronchial wall and the radioactive source should decrease the rate of delayed local complications. Only prospective and possibly randomized trials will allow to define the optimal therapeutic strategy.

V. Conclusions

Endobronchial brachytherapy was designed at the turn of the century and has now become a major tool for the treatment of obstructive lung cancer thanks to significant technical improvements. The review of the literature on the subject indicates its excellent efficacy in symptomatic relief of bronchial obstruction, with an approximately 80% response rate. In highly selected patients with small strictly endobronchial tumor, this procedure, used either alone or in combination with external beam radiotherapy, has provided encouraging results in terms of local control. Current developments in dosimetry, particularly CT scan–based conformational techniques, should make it possible to better delineate the target volume and therefore to evaluate a possible integration of this technique into the primary treatment strategy of lung cancer. However, no standard attitude is to date recommended for each specific clinical setting, and additional studies appear warranted.

References

1. Perez CA, Stanley K, Grundy G, et al. Impact of irradiation technique and tumor extent in tumor control and survival of patients with unresectable non-oat cell carcinoma of the lung. Cancer 1982; 50:1091.
2. Minna JD, Higgins GA, Glatstein EJ. Cancer of the lung. In: De Vita VT, Hellman S, Rosenberg SA, eds. Cancer Principles and Practice of Oncology. 2d ed. Philadelphia: JB Lippincott, 1985:518.
3. Moylan D. Overview of endobronchial brachytherapy and review of literature. New Orleans, AERALTS II, 1987.
4. Yankauer S. Two cases of lung tumour treated bronchoscopically. NY Med J 1922; June 21:741.
5. Kernan JD. Carcinoma of the lung and bronchus. Treatment with radon implantation and diathermy. Arch Otolaryngol 1933; 17:457.
6. Pancoast HK. Superior pulmonary sulcus tumor. JAMA 1932; 99:139.
7. Pool JL. Bronchoscopy in the treatment of lung cancer. Ann Otol Rhinol Laryngol 1961; 70:1172–1178.
8. Schlungbaum W, Blum H, Brandt HJ. Ergebnisse der endobronchialen Strahlentherapie des Bronchialkarzinoms. Radiol Aust 1962; XIII/3:201.
9. Roach M, Leidholdt EM, Tatera BS, Joseph J. Endobronchial radiation therapy in the management of lung cancer. Int J Radiat Oncol Biol Phys 1990; 18:1449–1454.
10. Schray MF, McDougall JC, Martinez A, Cortese DA, Brutinel WM. Management of malignant airway compromise with laser and low dose rate brachytherapy. Chest 1988; 93: 264–269.
11. Fritz P, Schraube P, Becker HD, Loeffler MS, Wannemacher M, Pastyr O. A new applicator, positionable to the center of tracheobronchial lumen for HDR Ir192 afterloading of tracheobronchial tumors. Int J Rad Oncol Biol Phys 1991; 20:1061.
12. Bedwinek J, Petty A, Bruton C, Sofield J, Lee L. The use of high dose rate endobronchial brachytherapy to palliate symptomatic endobronchial recurrence of previously irradiated bronchogenic carcinoma. Int J Radiat Oncol Biol Phys 1992; 22:23–30.
13. Gauwitz M, Ellerbroek N, Komaki R, Putnam JB Jr, Ryan MB, DeCaro L, Davis M, Cundiff J. High dose endobronchial irradiation in recurrent bronchogenic carcinoma. Int J Radiat Oncol Biol Phys 1992; 23:397–400.

14. Aygun C, Weiner S, Scariato A, Spearman D, Starck L. Treatment of non small cell lung cancer with external beam radiotherapy and HDR brachytherapy. Int J Radiat Oncol Biol Phys 1992; 23:127–132.
15. Goldman JM, Bulman AS, Rathmell AJ, Carey BM, Muers MF, Joslin CA. Physiological effect of endobronchial radiotherapy in patients with major airway occlusion by carcinoma. Thorax 1993; 48:110–114.
16. Mehta M, Petereit D, Chosy L, Harmon M, Fowler J, Shahabi S, Thomadsen B, Kinsella T. Sequential comparison of low dose rate and hyperfractionated high dose rate endobronchial radiation for malignant airway occlusion. Int J Radiat Oncol Biol Phys 1992; 23: 133–139.
17. Nori D, Allison R, Kaplan B, Samala E, Oslan A, Karbowitz S. High dose rate intraluminal irradiation in bronchogenic carcinoma. Chest 1993; 104:1006–1011.
18. O'Driscoll BR, Burt PA, Notley HM, Stout R, Barber PV. Palliative treatment of lung cancer by high dose rate intraluminal radiotherapy. World Conference on Lung Health, May 20–24, 1990, Boston, A427.
19. Taulelle M, Chauvet B, Vincent P, Felix-Faure C, Bucciarelli B, Garcia R, Reboul F. Curiethérapie endobronchique à haut débit de dose: résultats et complications chez 189 patients. Bull Cancer/Radiother 1996; 83:127–134.
20. Seagren SL, Harrell JH, Horn RA. High dose rate intraluminal irradiation in recurrent endobronchial carcinoma. Chest 1985; 88–86.
21. Speiser BL, Spratling I. Remote afterloading brachytherapy for the local control of endobronchial carcinoma. Int J Radiat Oncol Biol Phys 1993; 25:579–587.
22. Sutedja G, Baris G, Schaake-Koning C, van Zandwijk N. High dose rate brachytherapy in patients with local recurrences after radiotherapy of non-small cell lung cancer. Int J Radiat Oncol Biol Phys 1992; 24:551–553.
23. Zajac AJ, Kohn ML, Heiser D, Peters JW. High-dose-rate intraluminal brachytherapy in the treatment of endobronchial malignancy. Work in progress. Radiology 1993; 187:571–575.
24. Muto P, Ravo V, Panelli G. HDR brachytherapy and external beam radiotherapy in the treatment of stage IIIa/b non small cell lung cancer. A two year experience. Radiother Oncol 1994; 31(suppl 1):97.
25. Gollins S, Burt PA, Barber PV, Stout R. High dose rate intraluminal radiotherapy for carcinoma of the bronchus outcome of treatment of 406 patients. Radiother Oncol 1994; 33: 31–40.
26. Lo TC, Beamis JF. Intraluminal low-dose rate brachytherapy for malignant endobronchial obstruction. Annual Brachytherapy Meeting of the European Society for Therapeutic Radiology and Oncology, May 21–23, 1990. Antwerp, Belgium, p. 37.
27. Miller JI Jr, Phillips TW. Neodymium:yag LASER and brachytherapy in the management of inoperable bronchogenic carcinoma. Ann Thorac Surg 1990; 50:190–195.
28. Suh JH, Dass KK, Mehta AC, Pagliaccio L, Taylor ME, Saxton JP, Higgins P, Saffle P. Use of endobronchial radiation therapy or endobronchial radiation therapy and nd-yag LASER for management of malignant airway obstruction. American Radium Society's 75th Annual Meeting. April 24–28, 1993, Aruba, 1993, p. 23.
29. Cotter GW, Herbert DE, Ellingwood KE. Inoperable endobronchial obstructing lung carcinoma treated with combined endobronchial and external beam irradiation. South Med J 1991; 84:562–565.
30. Van Bodegon PC, Becker HD, Fritz P, Schraube P, Drings P, Wannenmacher M, Vogt-Moykopf I. Long-term palliation of advanced tracheobronchial tumors by HDR brachytherapy in the interdisciplinary concept. Eur Respir J 1992; 5(suppl 15):337–338s.
31. Huber RM, Fischer R, Hautmann H, Pöllinger B, Haussinger K, Wendt T. Does additional brachytherapy improve the effect of external irradiation? A prospective randomized study in central lung tumors. ERS Annu Meet 1996.abst 0165.
32. Tredaniel J, Hennequin C, Zalcman G, Walter S, Homasson JP, Maylin C, Hirsch A. Prolonged survival after high-dose rate endobronchial radiation for malignant airway obstruction. Chest 1994; 105:767–772.

33. Ardiet JM, Perol M, Mornex F, Montbarbon X, Rebattu P, Carrie C, Wagner JP, Zouai ME. Curative irradiation of limited endobronchial epidermoid carcinomas with HDR endolumenal brachytherapy. A pilot study. Ann Oncol 1992; 3(suppl 5):38.

34. Yokoyama A, Saïko M. A phase II study of combined endobronchial brachytherapy and external radiotherapy for centrally located early stage lung cancer. ASCO Proc 1995; 14:1069.

35. Macha HS, Becker KO, Kemmer HP. Pattern of failure and survival in endobronchial LASER resection. A matched pair study. Chest 1994; 105:1668–1672.

36. Burt PA, O'Driscoll BR, Notley HM, Barber PV, Stout R. Intraluminal irradiation for the palliation of lung cancer with the high dose rate micro-selectron. Thorax 1990; 45:765–768.

37. Speiser BL, Spratling L. Radiation bronchitis and stenosis secondary to high dose rate endobronchial irradiation. Int J Radiat Oncol Biol Phys 1993; 25(4):589–597.

38. Stout R, Barber PV, Burt PA, O'Driscoll BR, Notley M. Intraluminal brachytherapy in bronchial carcinoma. Br J Radiol 1990; 63(suppl, Congress):16.

34

Multimodality Therapy in Locally Advanced Non–Small-Cell Lung Cancer (NSCLC Stage IIIB)

JEAN-CHARLES SORIA, THIERRY LE CHEVALIER, CÉCILE LE PÉCHOUX, RODRIGO ARRIAGADA

Institut Gustave-Roussy
Villejuif, France

I. Introduction

Locally advanced non–small-cell lung cancer (NSCLC) without distant metastases (stage III disease) affects a subset of patients considered inoperable at the time of presentation because of unproven benefit from initial surgical resection. Patients are conventionally classified as having stage IIIA disease when the tumor is marginally resectable or stage IIIB when it is definitively unresectable. Classic stage IIIB disease defines lesions found in patients with extensive pulmonary tumors or lymph node invasion (T4 and/or N3 disease). T4 tumors may invade the mediastinal structures (carina, trachea, heart and great vessels, esophagus, and vertebral bodies) and/or cause malignant pleural effusions. N3 disease is observed in patients with metastases to contralateral mediastinal or hilar nodes or ipsilateral or contralateral supraclavicular nodes. In fact, staging is not always an easy task, particularly in patients with bulky N2 disease involving the mediastinal fat, who should be considered as stage IIIB for the therapeutic strategy. Such a borderline situation led us to propose a modified staging system for locally advanced NSCLC (1).

For a long time, thoracic radiotherapy was the standard treatment for stage III patients. While this treatment can play a major role in the control of such tumors, the main reason for reported failures in partially or nonresected tumors is the development of resistance to radiation, which in turn leads to local or distant progression. In fact, in stage IIIB disease, which is almost always considered a definitively unresectable tumor, radiation is unfortunately merely palliative, and the long-term survival rate does not exceed 5% with this treatment modality alone (2–5). Chemotherapy has traditionally been considered of modest benefit for the survival of NSCLC patients, and its activity/toxicity ratio has been extensively debated (6,7). It is therefore important to establish the precise value of chemotherapy in the treatment of stage III patients and not to focus solely on the marginal impact observed in patients with metastatic lesions.

During the last 15 years, several trials have evaluated the role of chemotherapy combined or not with radiotherapy. The different possible combinations of these two treatment modalities, each of which offers a substantial, albeit insufficient benefit, will be developed here. The place of more aggressive strategies and particularly the role of surgery in locally advanced NSCLC will also be discussed in this chapter.

II. Therapeutic Options

A. Radiotherapy

Background

For many years, radiotherapy alone was the treatment of choice for patients with stage IIIB NSCLC. The results obtained, however, were generally disappointing. Many uncontrolled studies have been published showing a 1-year survival rate ranging from 29 to 58% and a 5-year survival rate ranging from 4 to 10% (8).

Only two randomized studies have been conducted in which a group having received irradiation was compared to an untreated group (9,10). Moderate benefit in terms of median survival (although not statistically significant) was achieved only in the large randomized trial conducted by Roswit et al. (10). Some other randomized trials also attempted such a comparison, but all encountered problems in recruiting patients, since withholding any treatment at all in half of the patients, even for symptoms, was not easily accepted by both physicians and patients.

For many years now the dose-time relationship in radiotherapy has aroused considerable interest (11), and many studies have been conducted to assess time-dose factors for radiotherapy in NSCLC. Multiple parameters such as the total dose of radiation, the fraction size, the volume and type of in-field normal tissues, the definition of the target volume, and quality control of the radiotherapy techniques need to be taken into account in the management of stage IIIB NSCLC. These factors are of crucial importance for treatment planning and for the effects of combined approaches. The importance of the quality of radiotherapy has been stressed by many reports, and some have shown a significant impact on long-term local control and a potential benefit for survival with adequate radiation techniques (12–14).

Radiotherapy Parameters

Total Dose

The Radiation Therapy Oncology Group (RTOG) conducted prospective trials to investigate the question of whether incremental or sustained dose intensity had a positive impact on loco-regional control. An initial randomized study suggested that patients treated with a continuous course of 50–60 Gy over 5–6 weeks have better tumor control than those treated with lower doses (5,13).

Since the 1980s, different hyperfractionated radiotherapy schedules allowing incremented total doses have been investigated with no increase in morbidity. No overall difference in survival was observed between the different fractionation regimens. However, a trend for better survival was observed in consecutive pilot studies in favor of the higher-dose groups (14).

Split Course

Split-course radiotherapy, which implies delivery of radiation therapy interrupted by a rest interval, is another possible treatment schedule. It has been criticized by some authors because of the rebound effect of tumor cell proliferation when therapy is discontinued. Nevertheless, it allows patients to benefit from a rest period after 3–4 weeks of treatment, and this is undoubtedly more comfortable for them. Two randomized studies, comparing continuous and split-course therapy, failed to show any difference in survival (15,16). Standard radiotherapy consists in giving 10 Gy per week, e.g., 60 Gy in 6 weeks. Radiation can be hypofractionated (i.e., using a high dose per fraction), given once or twice a week, to obviate discomfort as much as possible for the patient treated with a palliative intent. Some authors believe that there is an advantage to hypofractionated over standard radiotherapy for patients whose life expectancy is short (17).

Fractionation

Several trials have been conducted to examine the effect of fractionating radiation therapy in locally advanced NSCLC (13–22). Two approaches are under evaluation to increase the radiation dose intensity: hyperfractionation, during which several small doses of radiation are delivered to increase the total dose, and accelerated fractionation, with which overall treatment time is shortened.

The objective of hyperfractionation is to provide the best efficacy/tolerance ratio for the few potentially curable patients (11–14). One of the RTOG studies concluded that the greatest benefit, in terms of response, was achieved with a total dose 10% higher than that considered tolerable with standard fractionation (i.e., 69.6 Gy in 5.5 weeks) (14).

Accelerated fractionation seems to yield superior response and control over conventional radiotherapy alone with slightly enhanced survival rates, but more frequent early toxicities and mainly esophagitis (23).

The CHART schedule (Continuous, Hyperfractionated, Accelerated, Radiation Therapy), reported by Saunders and Dische at Mount Vernon Hospital, in which

54 Gy in 36 fractions are given over 12 consecutive days, combines both approaches and appeared to be promising (20). Preliminary results of a randomized, controlled trial comparing conventional fractionated radiotherapy (60 Gy in 30 fractions for 6 weeks) to CHART have recently been published. A significant gain in overall survival has been shown for the CHART strategy with an accrual of 563 patients. At 2 years 30% of the CHART patients were alive compared with 20% in the control group ($p = 0.006$) (24).

B. Chemotherapy

Since approximately half of the patients treated with radiotherapy alone will develop a distant recurrence, the inclusion of chemotherapy in treatment protocols is strongly investigated (2,5). In spite of limited sensitivity to single agents, as reported in the literature, some multidrug regimens can induce partial or complete responses in NSCLC, particularly when a vinca-alkaloid or etoposide is combined with cisplatin. Objective response rates ranging from 25 to 40% have been obtained in inoperable NSCLC with combined regimens, which, nonetheless, are unable to adequately control the primary tumor in the vast majority of cases (6,7,25). When chemotherapy is compared with radiotherapy in locally advanced NSCLC patients, no difference is observed in long-term survival although a better response rate has been obtained with radiotherapy in two randomized trials (26,27).

C. Combined Radiotherapy and Chemotherapy

Thoracic radiotherapy has been considered the standard treatment for locally advanced, inoperable NSCLC. However, when used alone, long-term results are poor with only 15% of patients surviving beyond 2 years, and long-term survival is disappointingly low at 5%.

The rationale for combined chemo-radiotherapy in nonresectable NSCLC is based on several theoretical considerations (28): (1) it decreases the distant metastasis rate by attacking micrometastases already viable at the time of presentation in over 50% of cases, (2) by decreasing loco-regional macroscopic disease it could improve locoregional control. Combined chemo-radiotherapy can be administered either sequentially (i.e., the second modality begins when the previous modality has been concluded), concurrently (i.e., both treatment modalities are given simultaneously), or alternately (i.e., the two modalities are used alternately).

III. Multimodality Treatment

A. Sequential Chemo-Radiotherapy

The sequential chemo-radiotherapy approach is also called induction chemotherapy. It is the most conventional way to combine these modalities in NSCLC in order to avoid additive simultaneous toxicities. Many phase II trials were reported in the 1970s and 1980s, most of which suggested a potential benefit from chemotherapy given prior to radiotherapy (29,30).

Randomized Phase III Studies

Several phase III randomized studies have evaluated the role of chemo-radiotherapy by comparing radiotherapy alone to combination radiotherapy-chemotherapy. We intend to analyze their main findings according to the type of chemotherapy, based on the worldwide meta-analysis performed on individual data of most of these trials (31).

Single-agent trials show that the addition of cytotoxics such as cyclophosphamide, doxorubicin, vindesine, or vinblastine does not improve the results obtained with radiotherapy alone in terms of survival (32–37).

The results of the main six trials with non–cisplatin-containing multidrug regimens show that a multidrug, non–cisplatin-based regimen can enhance the therapeutic effects of radiotherapy, but they are inconclusive in terms of median and long-term survival (38–42).

Trials with cisplatin-based multidrug regimens offer the best results. Although many trials show no statistically significant difference in overall survival between radiotherapy alone and radiotherapy following chemotherapy (43–47), three large randomized trials have shown a gain in survival (48–51) (Table 1). In two of the trials long-term follow-up of patients confirmed survival benefit at 5 years (52,53).

In summary, despite the positive impact of adding chemotherapy to radiotherapy in locally advanced NSCLC, as confirmed in three different randomized trials, overall the profile of the survival curves has not improved substantially. Adding chemotherapy apparently only produces a significant decrease in the rate of distant

Table 1 Positive Randomized Trials of Sequential Cisplatin-Based Regimens Combined with Radiotherapy

| Chemotherapy | Radiotherapy | | | Median survival | Survival at 2 years (%) | p-value | Ref. |
	Total dose	Schedule	N				
Cisplatin-Vinblastine	60	Continuous	78	13.8 months	26	0.0066	49
	60		77	9.7 months	13		
Cisplatin-Vindesine-Cyclophosphamide-Lomustine	60	Continuous	176	12 months	21	<0.02	50
	60		177	10 months	14		
Cisplatin-VP16	56	Continuous	33	52 weeks	30	0.0559	51
	56		33	36 weeks	14		
Cisplatin-Vinblastine	60	Continuous	230	14 months	NA	0.03	48
	60		222	11 months	NA		

metastases with no impact on local control, the main cause of failure in this subset of patients (53).

Results of the Meta-Analysis

The overview conducted jointly by the Institut Gustave Roussy and the British Medical Research Council Cancer Trials Office using updated individual patient data from 52 trials performed between 1961 and 1991 has clarified the role of chemotherapy in NSCLC. Of these trials, 22 involved studies comparing radiotherapy alone to combination chemotherapy-radiotherapy. Trials with drugs used as radiosensitizers were not included in this meta-analysis. Among 17 trials with information on staging, 13 involved more than 70% stage III patients, while the other four had a more uniform distribution of stage I, II, and III inoperable tumors. Results show a statistically significant overall benefit with chemotherapy. The overall hazard ratio (HR) was 0.90 ($p = 0.006$), and the absolute survival benefit was 3% at 2 years and 2% at 5 years. The studies on cisplatin-based chemotherapy provided most of the data (more than 50%) and the most compelling evidence for an effect in favor of chemotherapy. The HR of 0.87 ($p = 0.005$) was equivalent to absolute survival benefits of 4% at 2 years and 2% at 5 years, with a 95% CI of 1–7% and 1–4%, respectively.

The data-based meta-analysis of trials reported in the literature, which enrolled patients with stage IIIA and IIIB disease, showed a 30% reduction in mortality at 2 years in the cisplatin-based group, compared to 18% in the non–cisplatin-based group (54).

B. Concomitant Radiotherapy and Chemotherapy

Simultaneous administration of chemotherapy and radiotherapy is another way to combine them. The additional theoretical benefit of this approach is to increase locoregional control through the direct interaction of the two modalities, which is not the case when they are administered sequentially. An immediate drawback is that toxicity is also increased and suboptimal doses of both modalities are often mandatory. Indeed, concomitant chemoradiotherapy increases toxicities such as myelotoxicity, because the thoracic bone marrow is affected by radiotherapy, esophagitis, and radiation pneumonitis. Several phase II trials have tried to define the best way to administer chemotherapy and radiotherapy concomitantly and the most active drugs for this type of combination. The cytotoxics most frequently used in these trials are cisplatin, carboplatin, and etoposide, as single agents or in combination (55–57).

Phase III randomized trials evaluating concomitant chemotherapy-radiotherapy with single-agent cisplatin or other drugs have largely failed to significantly improve the survival rates of patients with locally advanced NSCLC (58–63) (Table 2). Such a situation is probably due to the lack of systemic activity of low-dose single-agent therapy. The largest available study is the EORTC trial, which conducted a three-arm randomized phase II trial followed by a phase III trial on 331 patients, the results of which were reported by Schaake-Koning et al. (64). Results

Table 2 Randomized Trials of Concomitant Chemoradiotherapy with Cisplatin in Locally Advanced NSCLC

Chemotherapy	Radiotherapy		N	Median survival	Survival at 2 years (%)	*p*-value	Ref.
	Total dose	Schedule					
Cisplatin, weekly	50	Continuous	45	16 months	NA	NS	61
	50	Continuous	50	11 months	NA		
Cisplatin, daily	45	Continuous	83	9.9 months	20	NS	62
	45	Continuous	90	10.3 months	15		
Cisplatin, daily	55	Split	107	NA	26	0.009	58
Cisplatin, weekly	55	Split	110	NA	19		
	55	Split	114	NA	13		
Cisplatin	60	Continuous	104	43 weeks	18	NS	63
	60	Continuous	111	46 weeks	13		

showed that survival was significantly improved in the daily cisplatin group, i.e., 54% at one year, 26% at 2 years, and 16% at 3 years, compared to 46, 13, and 2%, respectively, in the radiotherapy alone group (*p* = 0.009). The benefit obtained for survival with daily combined treatment was through improved local control (*p* = 0.003).

In summary, sequential chemo-radiotherapy has significantly increased survival rates, an objective which has not been clearly attained by concomitant chemoradiotherapy. Nevertheless, the results of trials testing the concomitant approach could be clarified by a meta-analysis on individual data as was the case with phase III trials comparing sequential combinations of radiotherapy and chemotherapy alone. Randomized trials comparing concurrent versus sequential thoracic radiotherapy in combination with chemotherapy are ongoing. In selected patients (unresectable IIIA+B NSCLC including supraclavicular lymph node metastases but excluding T3N0M0 and pleural effusion), a recent report showed that concomitant radiotherapy-chemotherapy yielded significantly better response and survival rates than chemotherapy followed by thoracic irradiation (65).

C. Is There a Place for Adjuvant Surgery?

Patients with stage IIIB disease (T4 or N3 lesions) are usually considered "definitely inoperable." As amply expounded above, the approach applied to treat such patients is combination chemotherapy-radiotherapy but local control with this combined modality is generally poor. Only a small number of stage IIIB patients are technically completely resectable: some patients with T4 tumors (e.g., a tumor with left atrium invasion) and others with N3 disease (e.g., invasion of a right mediastinal lymph node when the primary tumor is in the left lower lobe). The resectability of a tumor depends to a large extent on the experience and attitudes of physicians treating the patient. There are some cases of invasion in which a surgical approach is feasible:

invasion of the trachea, carina, superior vena cava, great vessels, and left atrium. We have therefore proposed, with others, a new staging system in order to distinguish patients with IIIB disease that could undergo a surgical procedure after induction therapy from patients with IIIB lesions in whom surgery is definitively excluded (1).

Induction treatment must achieve elevated response rates to prevent metastatic disease and be compatible with secondary surgery. The majority of studies challenging the role of surgery in locally advanced NSCLC included both stage IIIA and IIIB disease (66–73). Response rates vary from 51 to 84% and resectability rates from 33 to 85%. Comparison of these trials is, however, difficult because chemotherapy doses and radiotherapy schedules differ considerably. These results do, nevertheless, warrant further evaluation.

In summary, there is no consensus about the place of surgery in locally advanced NSCLC. Despite promising results of phase II trials (74), to date, no study has demonstrated that survival can be prolonged by adjuvant surgery.

IV. Future Prospects

With a long-term survival rate of about 5–10%, the prognosis for patients with stage IIIB NSCLC is poor despite recent advances in combined modality treatment.

Improving the management of such patients is therefore a major challenge for the coming years. Chemotherapy has proven useful for inoperable stage III NSCLC, but the gain in survival observed remains modest. Still further investigation is needed to substantially improve long-term control.

Multiple investigational approaches can be explored in the near future:

Developments are foreseen in multifractionated or accelerated fractionated radiation therapy. Major improvements can be expected if fractionation can be tailored to adjust to particular tumor kinetics. It is now established that delayed complications are more strongly related to fractionation than to overall treatment time. Timing must also be better evaluated in chemotherapy-radiotherapy combination protocols.

New promising drugs need to be evaluated in large randomized trials, and new combination regimens may lead to increased complete response rates and thus better control of micrometastases.

Local control may also benefit from aggressive approaches to some stage IIIB NSCLC. Adjuvant surgery may be instrumental in this context, but its role remains to be defined.

Surgical palliation procedures and symptomatic treatments such as laser therapy or cryotherapy can be of great assistance for patients with obstructive tumors.

Local gene therapy is another innovative approach which is in the process of being actively explored (75). The direct transfer of tumor suppressor genes or toxic gene products that specifically promote tumor cell death and spare nonmalignant cells may offer a novel anticancer therapeutic approach. A number of genetic abnormalities, including c-ras and p53 gene alterations, which are associated with lung cancer, have been identified (76).

References

1. Grunenwald D, Le Chevalier T. Stage IIIA category of non-small-cell lung cancer: new proposal. J Natl Cancer Inst 1997; 89:88–89.
2. Stanley K, Cox JD, Petrovich Z, Paig C. Patterns of failure in patients with inoperable carcinoma of the lung. Cancer 1981; 47:2725–2729.
3. Saunders MI, Bennett MH, Dische S, Anderson PJ. Primary tumor control after radiotherapy for carcinoma of the bronchus. Int J Radiat Oncol Biol Phys 1984; 10:499–501.
4. Perez CA, Bauer M, Edelstein S. Impact of tumor control on survival in carcinoma of the lung treated with irradiation. Int J Radiat Oncol Biol Phys 1986; 12:539–547.
5. Perez CA, Pajak TF, Rubin P, Simpson JR, Mohiuddin M, Brady LW, Perez-Tamayo R, Rotman M. Long term observations of the patterns of failure in patients with unresectable non-oat cell carcinoma of the lung treated with definitive radiotherapy. Cancer 1987; 59:1874–1881.
6. Johnson M. Chemotherapy for unresectable non small cell lung cancer. Semin Oncol 1988; 17:20–29.
7. Ihde DC. Chemotherapy of lung cancer. N Engl J Med 1992; 327:1434–1441.
8. Damstrup L, Skovgaard Poulsen H. Review of the curative role of radiotherapy in the treatment of non small cell lung cancer. Lung Cancer 1994; 11:153–178.
9. Durrant KR, Berry RJ, Ellis F, Ridehalgh FR, Black JM, Hamilton WS. Comparison of treatment policies in inoperable bronchial carcinoma. Lancet 1971; i:715–719.
10. Roswit B, Patno ME, Rapp R, Veinbergs A, Feder B, Stulhbarg J, Reid CB. The survival of patients with inoperable lung cancer. A large-scale randomized study of radiation therapy versus placebo. Radiology 1968; 90:688–697.
11. Thames HD, Bentzen SM, Turesson I, Overgaard M, Van den Bogaert W. Time-dose factors in radiotherapy: a review of the human data. Radiother Oncol 1990; 19:219–235.
12. Perez CA. Non-small cell carcinoma of the lung: dose-time parameters. Cancer Treat Symp 1985; 2:131–142.
13. Perez CA, Stanley K, Rubin P, Kramer S, Brady L, Perez-Tamayo R, Brown GS, Concannon JP, Rotman M, Seydel HG. A prospective randomized study of various irradiation doses and fractionation schedules in the treatment of inoperable non-oat cell carcinoma of the lung. Cancer 1980; 45:2744–2753.
14. Cox JD, Azarnia N, Byhardt RW, Skin KH, Ermani B, Pajak TF. A randomized phase I/II trial of hyperfractionated radiation therapy with total doses of 60.0 Gy to 79.2 Gy: possible survival benefit with ≥69.6 Gy in favorable patients with radiation therapy oncology group stage III non-small cell lung carcinoma. Report of radiation therapy oncology group 83–11. J Clin Oncol 1990; 8:1543–1555.
15. Holsti LR, Mattson K. A randomized study of split course radiotherapy of lung cancer: long term results. Int J Radiat Oncol Biol Phys 1980; 6:977–981.
16. Lee RE, Carr DT, Childs DS. Comparison of split-course radiotherapy and continuous radiation therapy for unresectable bronchogenic carcinoma: 5-years results. Am J Roentg Radium Ther Nucl Med 1976; 126:116–121.
17. Slawson RG, Salazar OM, Poussin-Rosillo H, Amin PP, Strohl R, Sewchand W. Once a week vs conventional daily radiation treatment for lung cancer: final report. Int J Radiat Oncol Biol Phys 1988; 15:61–68.
18. Petrovich Z, Stanley K, Cox JD, Paig C. Radiotherapy in the management of locally advanced lung cancer of all cell types. Cancer 1981; 48:1335–1340.
19. Levitt SH, Bogardus CR, Ladd G. Split dose intensive radiation therapy in the treatment of advanced lung cancer: a randomized study. Radiology 1967; 88:1159–1161.

20. Saunders MI, Dische S, Grosch EJ, Fermont DC, Ashford RF, Maher EJ, Makepeace AR. Experience with CHART. Int J Radiat Oncol Biol Phys 1991; 21:871–878.
21. Emami B, Perez CA, Herkovic A, Hederman MA. Phase I/II study of treatment of locally advanced (T3, T4) non-oat cell lung cancer with high dose radiotherapy (rapid fractionation): Radiation Therapy Oncology Study Group. Int J Oncol Biol Phys 1988; 15:1021–1025.
22. Brindle JS, Shaw EG, Su JQ, Mailliard JA, Frank AR, Laurie JA, Mc Lean M, Jackett DM, Owens DT. Pilot study of accelerated hyperfractionated thoracic radiation therapy in patients with unresectable stage III non small cell lung carcinoma. Cancer 1993; 72:405–409.
23. Ginsberg RJ, Vokes EE, Raben A. Non small cell lung cancer. In: De Vita VT, Hellman S, Rosenberg SA, eds. Cancer Principles and Practice of Oncology. Philadelphia: Lippincott, 1996:858–911.
24. Saunders MI, Dische S, Barrett A, Parmar MK, Harvey A, Gibson D. Randomized multicentre trials of CHART vs conventional radiotherapy in head and neck and non-small cell lung cancer: an interim report. CHART Steering Committee. Br J Cancer 1996; 73:1455–1462.
25. Splinter TAW. Chemotherapy in advanced non small cell lung cancer. Eur J Cancer 1990; 10:1093–1099.
26. Johnson D, Einhorn L, Bartolucci A, Birch R, Omura G, Perez CA, Greco FA. Thoracic radiotherapy does not prolong survival in patients with locally advanced unresectable non-small cell lung cancer. Ann Int Med 1990; 113:33–38.
27. Kaasa S, Thorud E, Höst H, Lien HH, Land E, Sjolie I. A randomized study evaluating radiotherapy versus chemotherapy in patients with inoperable non small cell lung cancer. Radiat Oncol 1988; 11:7–13.
28. Vokes EE, Weichselbaum RR. Concomitant chemoradiotherapy: rationale and clinical experience in patients with solid tumors. J Clin Oncol 1990; 8:911–934.
29. Samuels ML, Barkley HT, Holoye PY, Rosenberg PJ, Smith TL. Combination chemotherapy with bleomycin, vincristine, and methotrexate plus split-course radiotherapy in the treatment of non-oat cell bronchogenic carcinoma. Cancer Chemother Rep Part 1 1975; 59:377–383.
30. Le Chevalier T, Arriagada R, Baldeyrou P, Martin M, Duroux P, Jacquotte A, Sancho-Garnier H, Rouessé J. Combined chemotherapy (vindesine, lomustine, cisplatin, and cyclophosphamide), and radical radiotherapy in inoperable nonmetastatic squamous cell carcinoma of the lung. Cancer Treat Rep 1985; 69:469–472.
31. Non Small Cell Lung Cancer Collaborative Group. Chemotherapy in non small cell lung cancer: a meta-analysis using updated data on individual patients from 52 randomized clinical trials. Br Med J 1995; 311:899–909.
32. Bergsagel DE, Jenkin RD, Pringle JF, White DM, Fetterly JC, Klaassen DJ, Mc Dermot RS. Lung cancer: clinical trial of radiotherapy alone vs radiotherapy plus cyclophosphamide. Cancer 1972; 30:621–627.
33. Höst H. Cyclophosphamide as adjuvant to radiotherapy in the treatment of unresectable bronchogenic carcinoma. Cancer Chemother Rep 1973; 4:161–164.
34. Veterans Administration Lung Cancer Study Groups. Preliminary report on non-resectable cancer of the lung. Cancer Chemother Rep 1974; 58:359–364.
35. Simpson JR, Francis ME, Perez-Tamayo R, Marks RD, Rao DV. Palliative radiotherapy for inoperable carcinoma of the lung: final report on a RTOG multi-institutional trial. Int J Radiation Oncol Biol Phys 1985; 11:751–758.
36. Schallier DC, De Neve WJ, De Greve L, Van Belle SP, De Wasch GJ, Dotremont G, Storme GA. Is adjuvant treatment with vinblastine effective in reducing the occurrence of distant metastasis in limited squamous cell lung cancer? A randomized study. Clin Expl Metastasis 1988; 6:39–48.
37. White JE, Chen T, Reed R, Mira J, Stackey WJ, Weatherall T, O'Bryan R, Samson MK, Seydel HG. Limited squamous cell carcinoma of the lung: a Southwest Oncology Group randomized study of radiation with or without doxorubicin chemotherapy and with or without levamisole immunotherapy. Cancer Treat Rep 1982; 66:1113–1120.
38. Anderson G, Deeley TJ, Smith C, Jani J. Comparison of radiotherapy alone and radiotherapy with chemotherapy using adriamycin and 5-fluorouracil in bronchogenic carcinoma. Thorax 1981; 36:190–193.

39. Israel L, Depierre A, Dalesio O. Interim results of EORTC protocol 08742. Comparison after irradiation of locally advanced squamous cell bronchial carcinoma, of abstention, immunotherapy, combination chemotherapy or chemoimmunotherapy. Recent Results in Cancer Research. Berlin-Heidelberg: Springer-Verlag, 1982:214–218.

40. Morton R, Jett JR, Mc Ginnis WL, Earle JD, Therneau TM, Krook JE, Elliott TE, Mailliard JA, Nelimark RA, Maksymiuk AW. Thoracic radiation therapy alone compared with combined chemoradiotherapy for locally unresectable non-small cell lung cancer: a randomized phase III trial. Ann Int Med 1991; 115:681–686.

41. Petrovich Z, Ohanian M, Cox J. Clinical research on the treatment of locally advanced lung cancer. Final report of VALG protocol 13 limited. Cancer 1978; 42:1129–1134.

42. Trovo MG, Minatel E, Veronesi A, Roncadin M, De Paoli A, Franchin G, Magri DM, Tirelli U, Carbone A, Grigoletto E. Combined radiotherapy and chemotherapy vs radiotherapy alone in locally advanced epidermoid bronchogenic carcinoma. Cancer 1990; 65:400–404.

43. Gregor A, Mac Beth FR, Paul J, Cram L, Hansen HH. Radical radiotherapy and chemotherapy in localized inoperable non small cell lung cancer: a randomized trial. J Natl Cancer Inst 1993; 85:997–999.

44. Kim NK, Yang SH, Im YH, Kang KW, Heo DS, Bang YJ. A Phase III randomized comparison of neo-adjuvant chemotherapy with cisplatin, etoposide, and vinblastine (PEV) plus radiation vs radiation alone in stage III NSCLC. Proc Am Soc Clin Oncol 1993; 12:330.

45. Mattson K, Holsti LR, Holsti P, Jackobson M, Kayanti M, Lüffo K, Mantyla M, Niitamo-Korhonen S, Nikkanen V, Nordman E. Inoperable non-small cell lung cancer: radiation with or without chemotherapy. Eur J Cancer Clin Oncol 1988; 24:477–482.

46. Minet P, Bartsch P, Chevalier Ph, Raets D, Gras A, Dejardin-Closon MT, Lennes G. Quality of life of inoperable non-small cell lung carcinoma. A randomized phase II clinical study comparing radiotherapy alone and combined radiotherapy. Radiother Oncol 1987; 8: 217–230.

47. Van Houtte P, Klastersky J, Renaud A, Michel J, Vandermoten G, Nguyen H, Sculier JP, Derriendt J, Mommen P. Induction chemotherapy with cisplatin, etoposide, and vindesine before radiation therapy for NSCLC. Antibiot Chemother 1988; 41:131–137.

48. Sause WT, Scott C, Taylor S, Johnson D, Livingston R, Komaki R, Emami B, Curran WJ, Byhardt RW, Turrissi AT. Radiation Therapy Oncology Group (RTOG) 88–08 and Eastern Cooperative Oncology Group (ECOG) 4588: preliminary results of a phase III trial in regionally advanced, unresectable non-small-cell lung cancer. J Natl Cancer Inst 1995; 87:198–205.

49. Dillman RO, Seagren SL, Propert KJ, Guerra J, Eaton WL, Perry MC, Carey RW, Frei EF 3d, Green MR. A randomized trial of induction chemotherapy plus high-dose radiation versus radiation alone in stage III non-small cell lung cancer. N Engl J Med 1990; 323:940–948.

50. Le Chevalier T, Arriagada R, Quoix E, Ruffié P, Martin M, Tarayre M, Lacombe-Terrier MJ, Douillard JY, Laplanche A. Radiotherapy alone vs combined chemotherapy and radiotherapy in non-resectable NSCLC: first analysis of a randomized trial in 353 patients. J Natl Cancer Inst 1991; 83:417–423.

51. Crino L, Latmi P, Meacci M, Corgna E, Maranzano E, Darwish S, Minotti V, Santucci A, Torato M. Induction chemotherapy plus high dose radiotherapy versus radiotherapy alone in locally advanced unresectable non small cell lung cancer. Ann Oncol 1993; 4:847–851.

52. Dillman RO, Herndon J, Seagren SL, Eaton WL, Green MR. Improved survival in stage III NSCLC: seven year follow-up of Cancer and Leukemia Group B (CALGB) 8433 trial. J Natl Cancer Inst 1996; 88:1210–1215.

53. Arriagada R, Le Chevalier T, Rekacewicz E, Quoix E, De Cremoux H, Douillard JY, Tarayre M, for the CEBI-138 trialists and French Anticancer Centers. Cisplatin based chemotherapy (CT) in patients with locally advanced non small cell lung cancer (NSCLC): late analysis of a French randomized trial. Proc Am Soc Clin Oncol 1997; 16:446.

54. Marino P, Preatoni A, Cantoni A. Randomized trials of radiotherapy alone versus combined chemotherapy and radiotherapy in stages IIIA and IIIB non-small-cell lung cancer. Cancer 1995; 76:593–601.

55. Bedini AV, Tavecchio L, Milani F, Gramayalia A, Spreafico C, Marchiano A, Ravasi G. Non resectable stage III A-B lung carcinoma: a phase II study on continuous infusion of cisplatin and concurrent radiotherapy (plus adjuvant surgery). Lung Cancer 1993; 10:73–84.
56. Belani CP. Multimodality therapy for regionally advanced non-small cell lung cancer. Semin Oncol 1993; 20:302–314.
57. Reboul F, Vincent P, Chauvet B, Brewer Y, Felin-Faure C, Taulelle M, Schrieve DC. Radiation therapy with concomitant continuous infusion cisplatin for unresectable nonsmall cell lung carcinoma. Int J Radiation Biol Phys 1994; 28:1251–1256.
58. Schaake-Koning C, Van Den Bogaert W, Dalesio O, Festen J, Hoogenhout J, Van Houtte P, Kirkpatrick A, Koolen M, Moat B, Nijs A. Effects of concomitant cisplatin and radiotherapy on inoperable non-small cell lung cancer. N Engl J Med 1992; 326:524–530.
59. Ball D, Bishop J, Smith J, Crennan E, O'Brien P, Davis S, Ryan G, Joseph D, Walker Q. A phase III study of accelerated radiotherapy with and without carboplatin in non-small cell lung cancer (NSCLC): interim toxicity analysis. Lung Cancer 1994; 11(suppl. 1):54–55.
60. Kiseleva ES, Pitskhilauri A, Trakhtenberg AK, Daryalova SL, Kosyanenko IV, Zakharchenkov AV, Lebedev VA, Zvekotkina LS. Results of radiotherapy and combined chemotherapy and radiotherapy of inoperable lung cancer. Neoplasia 1983; 30:573–580.
61. Soresi E, Clerici M, Grilli R, Borghini U, Zucali R, Leoni M, Botturi M, Bergari C, Luporini G, Scoccia S. A randomized clinical trial comparing radiation therapy versus radiation therapy plus cis-dichlorodiammine platinum (II) in the treatment of locally advanced non-small cell lung cancer. Semin Oncol 1988; 15(suppl. 7):20–25.
62. Trovo MG, Minatel E, Franchin G, Boccieri MG, Mascinben O, Bolziccio G, Pizzi G, Torretta A, Veronesi A, Gobitti C. Radiotherapy versus radiotherapy enhanced by cisplatin in stage III non small cell lung cancer. Int J Radiat Oncol Biol Phys 1992; 24:11–15.
63. Blanke C, Ansari R, Montravadi, Gonin R, Tokars R, Fisher W, Pennington K, O'Connor T, Rynard S, Miller M. Phase III trial of thoracic irradiation with or without cisplatin for locally advanced unresectable non-small-cell lung cancer: a Hoosier Oncology Group protocol. J Clin Oncol 1995; 13:1425–1429.
64. Schaake-Koning C, Maat B, Van Houtte P, Van den Bogaert W, Dalesio O, Kirkpatrick A, Bartelink H. Radiotherapy combined with low-dose cis-diammine dichloroplatinum (II) (CDDP) in inoperable non-small cell lung cancer (NSCLC): a randomized three arm phase II study of the EORTC Lung Cancer and Radiotherapy Cooperative Groups. Int J Radiat Oncol Biol Phys 1990; 19:967–972.
65. Furuse K, Fukuoka M, Takada Y, Nishikawa H, Katagami N, Ariyosahi Y, for the West Japan Lung Cancer Group. A randomized phase III study of concurrent versus sequential thoracic radiotherapy in combination with mitomycin, vindesine and cisplatin in unresectable stage III non-small-cell lung cancer: preliminary analysis. Proc Am Soc Clin Oncol 1997; 16:459.
66. Grunenwald D, Le Chevalier T, Arriagada R, Baldeyrou G, Dennewald G, Girard P, Bretel JJ, Ruffié P, Tarayre M, Laplanche A. Surgical resection of stage IIIB non-small-cell lung cancer (NSLC) after concomitant induction chemo-radiotherapy. Preliminary results (abstr.). Lung Cancer 1994; 11(suppl. 1):181.
67. Eagan RT, Ruud C, Lee KE, Pairolero PC, Gail MH. Pilot study of induction therapy with cyclophosphamide, doxorubicin, and cisplatin (CAP) and chest irradiation prior to thoracotomy in initially inoperable stage III M0 non-small cell lung cancer. Cancer Treat Rep 1987; 71:895–900.
68. Taylor SG IV, Trybula M, Bonomi PD, Faber LP, Lee MS, Reddy S, Maffey SC, Mathisen DJ, Jensik RJ, Kittle CF. Simultaneous cisplatin fluorouracil infusion and radiation followed by surgical resection in regionally localized stage III, non-small cell lung cancer. Ann Thorac Surg 1987; 43:87–91.
69. Recine D, Rowland K, Reddy S, Lee MS, Bonomi P, Taylor S IV, Faber CP, Warren W, Kittle CF, Hendrick FR. Combined modality therapy for locally advanced non-small cell lung carcinoma. Cancer 1990; 66:2270–2278.
70. Lokich J, Chaffey J, Neptune W. Concomitant 5Fluorouracil infusion and high-dose radiation for stage III non small cell lung cancer. Cancer 1989; 64:1021–1025.

71. Faber LP, Kittle CF, Warren WH, Bonomi PD, Taylor SG IV, Reddy S, Lee MS. Preoperative chemotherapy and irradiation for stage III non-small-cell lung cancer. Ann Thorac Surg 1989; 47:669–675.
72. Albain K, Rusch V, Crowley J, Rice TW, Turrissi AT 3rd, Weick JK, Lonchyna VA, Presant CA, Mc Kenna RJ, Gandara DR. Concurrent cisplatin and etoposide plus chest radiotherapy followed by surgery for stages IIIA (N2) and IIIB non-small-cell lung cancer: mature results of Southwest Oncology Group phase II study 8805. J Clin Oncol 1995; 13:1880–1892.
73. Skarin A, Jochelson M, Sheldon T, Malcolm A, Oliynyk P, Overholt R, Hunt M, Frei 3d. Neoadjuvant chemo-radiotherapy in marginally resectable stage III M0 non-small-cell lung cancer: long term follow-up in 41 patients. J Surg Oncol 1989; 40:266–274.
74. Grunenwald D, Le Chevalier T, Arriagada R, Baldeyrou P, Dennewald G, Girard P et al. Surgical resection of stage IIIB non-small-cell lung cancer after concomitant induction chemo-radiotherapy; preliminary results of a pilot study. Pros Am Soc Clin Oncol 1995; 14:349.
75. Tursz T, Le Cesne A, Baldeyrou P, Gautier E, Opolon P, Schtz C, Pavirani A, Courtney M, Lamy D, Ragot T, Saulnier P, Andremont A, Monier R, Perricaudet M, Le Chevalier T. Phase I study of a recombinant adenovirus-mediated gene transfer in lung cancer patients. J Natl Cancer Inst 1996; 88:1857–1863.
76. Carbone DP, Minna JD. The molecular genetics of lung cancer. Adv Intern Med 1992; 37:153–171.

35

Progress in Chemotherapy in Advanced Non–Small-Cell Lung Cancer

ALAIN DEPIERRE

University Hospital
Besançon, France

I. Introduction

The first trials of combination chemotherapy date from 1965. For many years they were designed with the sole aim of decreasing tumor size, based upon the doctrine that the patient must derive benefit ipso facto.

A therapeutic trial methodology gradually developed. The simple benefit of decreasing tumor size assessed by objective response (OR) was completed by survival duration, survival without recurrence seeking to appreciate the gain offered to the patient by treatment, and, finally, more subjective concepts of quality of life.

II. Superiority of Chemotherapy Over Best Supportive Care Only

The wager of comparing chemotherapy (CT) with the absence of treatment or best supportive therapy (BST) came late in the saga of CT in non–small-cell lung cancer (NSCLC). Cormier et al. (1) were the first to publish a randomized trial. Earlier trials had studied treatments now considered ineffective, such as procarbazine. Cormier et al. chose a MACC (methotrexate-adriblastin-cyclophosphamide-CCNU) regimen. CT gave better results in terms of survival. This trial has been criticized because of the small number of patients (39 in all) and limited survival of its control group. It gave rise to a new trial reported by Rapp et al. (2). Two CT were tested: the combination of vindesine (VDN) and cisplatin (DDP) and the CAP (cyclophosphamide-doxorubicin-cisplatin) combination. Median survivals were as follows: VDN-DPP, 32.6 weeks; CAP, 24.7 weeks; and BST, 17 weeks. Bitherapy was better than tritherapy ($p = 0.01$) and CT better than BST ($p = 0.02$). Eight trials in all were published between 1982 and 1993 (1–8) (Table 1). They are of unequal value, in part because of their date of design, as well as difficulties in maintaining BST from start to finish without recourse to treatment, which might influence survival, in particular radiotherapy (7). As astonishing as it might seem, no randomized trial compared DDP alone with BST. This shows the extent to which the medical community was convinced of the incontrovertible superiority of combination chemotherapy over single-drug therapy. These various trials formed the basis of a meta-analysis (9) conducted by the Medical Research Council (MRC) and the Institut Gustave Roussy (IGR). Of the 1190 patients analyzed, 778 received a DDP-based CT (8 trials, 7 of which also involved a vinca alkaloid). Doses of DPP ranged from 40 to 120 mg/m^2. Trials with DPP showed evidence of a benefit of CT with a hazard ratio of 0.73 (CI 95%: 0.63–0.85; $p \leq 0.0001$), and this 27% reduction in the risk of death was equivalent to a 10% (5–15%) improvement in 1-year survival or a 1.5-month increase in median survival. This meta-analysis confirmed the findings of that undertaken initially by Souquet et al. (10). This gain in survival does not appear to be contested by the community, but its significance in terms of patient management remains controversial. There are two opposing camps: one considers that this gain does not legitimize the routine treatment. The other, more widespread, considers that this slight result has been obtained in patients with the worst prognosis, that CT is the most useful BST for improving clinical symptomatology of cancer (11), and that

Table 1   Randomized Studies of Chemotherapy Compared with Best Supportive Therapy

Authors (Ref.)	Treatment	No. of patients	Median week survival Treatment	BST	*p*-value
Cormier et al. (1)	MACC	39	30.5	8.5	<0005
Rapp et al. (2)	CAP/VDN-DDP	233	32.6/24.7	17	0.02
Woods et al. (3)	VDN-DDP	115	24	21	NS
Ganz et al. (4)	VLB-DDP	48	18.6	14.4	NS
Cellerino et al. (5)	CAP/MEC	89	36.4	21.4	NS
Quoix et al. (6)	VDN/DDP	46	28	10	<0.001
Kaasa et al. (7)	VP 16/DDP	87	21.8	16.5	NS
Cartei et al. (8)	CPM	102	37	17.4	0.0001

MACC: Methotrexate, adriblastine, cyclophosphamide, CCNU; CAP: cyclophosphamide, adriblastine, cisplatin; MEC: methotrexate, etoposide, CCNU; CPM: cyclophosphamide, platine, mitomycin; BST: best supportive therapy.

it is hence now legitimate to treat all patients whose general condition is such that outpatient management is possible.

III. New Drugs

There has been remarkable progress in recent years with the emergence of several drugs active in NSCLC. This began with vinorelbine (Navelbine) (NVB), a new vinca alkaloid. It is less neurotoxic than other vinca alkaloids, apart from producing constipation. Its dose-limiting toxicity is neutropenia. The objective response rate in its first phase II trial was 29% of 78 previously untreated patients (12). This rate was confirmed in a Japanese study (13). The standard dosage is 30 mg/m^2/week. Two other drugs are members of the taxanes group: docetaxel and paclitaxel. This is a new group of drugs which act, like vinca alkaloids, on microtubules. Docetaxel has been used at a well-standardized dosage of 100 mg/m^2 by one-hour infusion every 3 weeks. Response rate in phase II trials was between 23 and 40% (14). Docetaxel also appears to be active in patients treated previously, by cisplatin in particular, with an objective response rate of 20% (14,15). Paclitaxel was used by a short infusion of 3 hours at a dosage of 175 mg/m^2 every 3 weeks. Its objective response rate in NSCLC is 25–35%. Hypersensitivity secondary reactions are usually well controlled by premedication with steroids (16). The fourth drug is gemcitabin, an antimetabolite. The usual suggested dose is 1000 mg/m^2 weekly, 3 weeks out of 4. It has a fairly constant objective response rate of 20%. Its good clinical tolerability seems to be one of its major assets (17). Another agent is at a less advanced stage of development in NSCLC. It is a topoisomerase I inhibitor, topotecan. It is being developed at the fairly standard dosage of 1.5 mg/m^2 given for 5 consecutive days every 3 weeks. It seems to be less active in NSCLC than other drugs, with an OR rate of 12.5% (18). Tirapazamine is a benzotriamine with a marked differential action on hypoxic cells. The maximum tolerated dose has been evaluated at 390 mg/m^2 in combination with DDP (19). Its efficacy is currently being evaluated.

IV. Combinations

The concept of combination chemotherapy emerged in 1965–1970, promoted by Israel et al. (20). Since that time, oncologists have devoted their efforts to discovering effective combinations, although not without difficulty. All combinations are based upon the following theoretical notions: combinations of at least two drugs, without crossover resistance, mode of action at least theoretically different, nonadditive toxicity. The supremacy of DDP, which will be considered later, has led all investigators to first study each new drug in combination with DDP. In phase II trials, addition of cisplatin to another drug leads to a marked increase in OR rates and therefore to the initiation of randomized trials.

    The first stage involved testing one drug versus two drugs (or even three drugs in some instances). All trials included DDP and were based upon two approaches:

DDP + X versus X or DDP + X versus DDP. No consensus exists as to which of these models is the most informative. Twelve trials have been published, which are summarized in Table 2 (21–33). Only six of these were positive in terms of survival. The move to three drugs encountered similar difficulties. Two trials compared single-drug therapy with MVP (32,33), one being favorable to the combination and the other to single-drug therapy. Positive "2 versus 3" trials are lacking. Three authors compared VDN-DDP with classical MVP (34–36). None of these trials was positive. Erkisi et al. (37) compared the combination DDP-VP16 with the triple combination DDP-VP16-ifosfamide. The cohort was small (74 patients), but evidence was found of an improvement in median survival to the advantage of the triple combination. Crino et al., in Italy, compared DDP-VP16 with the triple combination DDP-MTC-ifosfamide and with classical MVP (38). They included 359 patients. Analysis of median survival showed a modest advantage for triple combinations (median of 27 weeks for DDP-VP16 and 42 weeks for triple combinations, $p = 0.05$). Should it be concluded that VP16 (in combination with DPP) is less effective than a vinca alkaloid in the same combination and hence enables the triple combination to make the difference?

In the French study comparing NVB with the combination NVB-DDP (25), in which the combination failed to demonstrate its superiority over single-drug therapy, it is interesting to note that the OR rate was greater with the combination (43 vs. 16%, $p = 0.001$) but that the number of OR lasting more than 9 months was the same in both arms (7 and 6 cases, respectively). The definition of an OR requires a minimum duration of 4 weeks. It might be useful to try to determine a threshold OR

Table 2 Randomized Trials of Single-Drug Compared with Combination Therapy

Authors (Ref.)	Treatment	No. of patients	Response rate (%)	*p*-value	Median survival (weeks)	*p*-value
Klastersky et al. (21)	P-EP	162	19–26	NS	26–22	NS
Crino et al. (22)	P-EP-EPM	150	4–30–26	0.05	18–42–35	0.02
Kawahara et al. (23)	P-VP	160	12–29	0.05	39–45	NS
Wozniak et al. (24)	P-NP	432	10–25	—	24–28	0.001
Depierre et al. (25)	N-NP	240	16–48	0.005	32–33	NS
Le Chevalier et al. (26)	N-NP	412	14–30	<0.001	31–40	0.01
Einhorn et al. (27)	V-MVP	83	14–27	NS	18–26	NS
Sorensen et al. (28)	V-VLCMe	171	22–27	NS	29–34	NS
Elliot et al. (29)	V-VP	105	7–33	<0.01	16–44	0.03
Rosso et al. (30)	E-EP	216	7–26	<0.0001	26–35	NS
Splinter et al. (31)	T-TP	225	6–22	0.001	23–29	0.02
Bonomi et al. (32)	Ca-MVP	264	9–20	0.02	32–22	0.008
Veeder et al. (33)	V-MVP	133	30–43	NS	16–23	NS

C = Cyclophosphamide; Ca = carboplatin; E = etoposide; L = lomustine; M = mitomycin; Me = methotrexate; N = navelbine; NS = nonsignificant; P = cisplatin; T = teniposide; V = vindesine.

duration such that it modifies survival. It has been extensively shown that "responders" exhibited longer survival than "nonresponders" and that this time-dependent variable influences survival in multivariate analysis (39), but no study has integrated response duration in multivariate analysis.

The large number of available new drugs has not enabled clear definition of the potential of each of them. Each drug is currently seen more as a competitor of others in a regimen where everything seems to be interchangeable, with DDP as the pivot. It would be important to seek out strategies where the effects of each are added together. The increasing tendency seems to be that of a more comfortable "niche" approach: docetaxel second-line, gemcitabin in the elderly, etc.

V. The Supremacy of DDP

DDP is credited with a 15% OR rate as single-drug therapy (40). This rate in itself does not place DDP among the most effective drugs when used singly and is not sufficiently convincing, alone, of its supremacy. The idea emerged following a series of analyses, of prognostic factors in particular. The most striking of them was undertaken by Albain et al. (41) on patients included in South West Oncology Group (SWOG) protocols. It provided evidence by multivariate analysis role of the positive influence of having received a DDP-based treatment (hazard ratio: 1.5; CI 95%: 1.0–2.3; $p = 0.05$).

The MRC and IGR meta-analysis (9) included subdivision of trials according to whether they included DDP or not in all the situations studied, i.e., surgery $\pm$ CT, radiotherapy $\pm$ CT, or CT vs. best supportive therapy. CT including DDP were contrasted with earlier alkylating agent–based CT. CT including DDP invariably proved better than those based on alkylating agents. It should nevertheless be noted that the administration of DDP was simultaneous with two other events (almost always associated): addition of a vinca alkaloid (vinblastine, vindesine, and now vinorelbine) and shorter-term treatments. The toxicity of DDP is such that treatment is impossible for 12–18 months, as was commonly the case with cyclophosphamide and doxorubicin. It is difficult to separate these two factors from DDP itself when evaluating its impact on survival in NSCLC.

The dosage of DDP has given rise to many interesting studies, since they raise the problem of dose intensification and optimal dosages. DDP has been used in a range of dosages from 60 to 200 mg/m^2, administered every 3 weeks. Gralla (42) compared two doses of DDP (60 and 120 mg/m^2). The OR rate was the same in both arms, but the durations of response (5.5 months vs. 12 months; $p = 0.05$) and of median survival (10 months vs. 21.7 months; $p = 0.02$) were longer with the high dosage. This was the only study to show superiority of high doses. Klastersky et al. (43), using the same dosages (60 mg/m^2 vs. 120 mg/m^2) but in combination with etoposide, failed to demonstrate any difference in median survival (33 weeks vs. 28 weeks, respectively) or in median response duration (42 weeks vs. 35 weeks, respectively). The SWOG undertook a randomized trial (44) comparing DDP at two dosages (50 and 100 mg/m^2 on days 1 and 8) and the latter dosage in combination with mitomycin. While mitomycin led to an increased OR rate (12, 14, and 27%, respectively; $p = 0.05$), median survival was the same in all three arms (6.9, 5.3, and 7.2 months, respectively). Toxicity becomes prohibitive at 200 mg/m^2. In contrast, no study has been published enabling precise definition of a lower efficacy threshold of DDP below 60 mg/m^2. This concept of a lower efficacy threshold is interesting. It is never looked at because all trials inherently imply the use of maximal doses. It would be useful to choose the dosages of a treatment regimen, drawing a distinction between potentially curative situations (CT in combination with surgery or RT in stage IIIa disease) and palliative situations. It is likely that, in everyday practice, many oncologists avoid using doses which are too toxic and seek to minimize effects by decreasing dosages. However, such an attitude is not free of danger in the absence of precise information about low dosages. Dosage decreases have been shown to be harmful in small-cell lung carcinomas (SCLC) (45,46).

The question of low doses raises the problem of the treatment of elderly patients. Population aging is on the increase in western countries: 10% of the population is over 65 years of age. Life expectancy is 9.7 years at age 75 (47). The incidence of cancer also increases with age. Treatment of the elderly will become an increasingly major preoccupation. While cancer in the elderly does not appear to differ fundamentally from that in a younger person—any differences probably being explained by differences in medical attitudes adopted to them (48)—the same does not apply to the toleration of chemotherapy. Resistance of the kidney, to DDP in particular, seems the same as in younger individuals, at least up to age 75 (48). In contrast, bone marrow aging increases sensitivity to leukopenic drugs (49). However, specific studies in the elderly, and in particular in patients >80 years, remain fragmentary as far as NSCLC is concerned. Gemcitabin has been evaluated in this situation. Response rate and toxicity are similar to those seen with the same drug in younger individuals.

VI. The Challenge of Vinca Alkaloids

This is an old therapeutic group, made up of four analogs: vincristine, vinblastine, vindesine, and, more recently, vinorelbine. The last three are prescribed in NSCLC. Vindesine is accredited with an overall OR rate of 19% (40). The response rate with NVB was 29% in phase II. In two phase III trials comparing NVB alone with its combination with DDP, OR rates were 14% and 16%, respectively (25,26). This decrease in response rates between phase II and phase III is usual, for both single-drug therapy and combinations (50). Only one of these studies (26) revealed a significant gain ($p = 0.01$) in median survival to the advantage of the combination. The combination NVB-DDP was compared with VDN-DPP in Le Chevalier's study (26). A Japanese randomized trial (51) involved, in 210 patients, the comparison of NVB (25 mg/m^2/week) with VDN (3 mg/m^2/week). In case of failure or recurrence, patients were given the other drug combined with DDP on a crossover basis. This approach prevented comparison of survival in the two arms. Response rates (31% vs. 8.9%) were to the advantage of NVB. NVB was also seen to be capable, used as single-drug therapy, of prolonging survival in a study by O'Rourke et al. (52), in which it was compared with 5-fluorouracil. This trial involved 216 patients assigned between two arms: 143 in the NVB arm (30 mg/m^2/week) and 70 in the 5-fluorouracil (425 mg/m^2 × 5 days/3 weeks) and leucovorin (20 mg/m^2 × 5 days/3 weeks) arm. Intent-to-treat analysis revealed an advantage for the NVB arm concerning median survival (29 weeks vs. 21 weeks; $p = 0.02$) and 1-year survival (25 vs. 15%). Vinca alkaloids were first included in combination regimens for NSCLC at the same time as DDP, with which they are combined in all the combinations used in phase III trials but one—combination with VP16. The latter is a notable challenger, and the combination DDP-VP16 has often been suggested as a standard. Unfortunately, in the MRC and IGR meta-analysis, the role of vinca alkaloids was associated in analysis with that of VP16, which may have masked the advantage of one or the other. No trials exist comparing DDP-NVB and DDP-VP16.

VII. Dose Intensification, Maintenance, and Duration of Treatment

While dose intensification in NSCLC has, up to now, not been the object of such intensive research as in SCLC, the approach used when choosing a drug is generally based upon reference to maximum tolerated dose. The optimal duration between two injections is not estimated according to tumor cell kinetics, but rather the time required for recovery from toxic effects, in particular on hematopoietic cells. Some trials have sought to evaluate different timings, in particular weekly (53,54), though without having shown any striking differences in safety and efficacy as yet. In 1986, Hryniuk et al. (55) introduced the concept of dose-intensity, expressing in mg/m^2/week the dose actually received of a given drug in a defined lapse of time. As interesting as this concept may be, it has been little used by investigators. It is a means of detachment from ambitious maximum theoretical doses which the patient does not actually receive. As an example, NVB is administered at the theoretical dose of 30 mg/m^2/week, but calculation of its dose-intensity for the first 9 weeks of treatment showed that the patient actually received, as single-drug therapy, 75% of the theoretical dose, i.e., a mean of 22.5 mg/m^2/week (12) and, in combination with DDP, 63%, i.e., 18.8 mg/m^2/week (25). Gralla et al. suggested an interesting modification of the regimen for administration of NVB combined with DDP-MTC (56), alternating high doses (35 mg/m^2) and low doses (17.5 mg/m^2) so as to increase dose intensity. We did not find the same result, but a decreased dose-intensity of NVB (18.2 mg/m^2/week) because of the frequency of bone marrow aplasia during the administration of high doses of NVB, in particular during weeks 3 and 7 (57). This concept of dose intensity is all the more interesting in that it appears to be correlated with patient survival by multivariate analysis with the introduction of dose intensity as a time-dependent variable (58). The time required to obtain a re-

Table 3 Results of the ECOG Study

Schedule	No. of patients	Response No. (%)	Median survival (weeks)	Median time without progression
MVP	176	36(20)	22.7	
Iproplatin	88	5 (6)	26.1	
Carboplatin	88	8 (9)	31.7	29.0
VP	175	23(13)	25.1	
MVP/CAMP	172	22(13)	25.0	
All			25.4	23.6

MVP vs. All: $p = 0.9$.
Carboplatin vs. All: $p = 0.008$ for median survival, and $p = 0.01$ for median TWP.
Source: Ref. 32.

sponse has not been rigorously defined. It is classically accepted that the first evaluation of response, in a trial, should take place after 9 weeks. Larsen et al. (59) showed, in a cohort of 336 patients with 43 OR, that only 80% of these OR were recorded at 12 weeks, and 24 weeks were required to note more than 95% of the responses. It is possible that long response durations with NVB (4/23 OR lasted more than 18 months in the initial phase II) (12) and with gemcitabin are related to two factors: frequent administration (weekly) and good tolerability (enabling the continuation of treatment in a prolonged initial no change situation). This could explain reports of very long survival durations with NVB as single-drug therapy (60,61). Reference must be made to an article by Bonomi et al. (32) reporting the Eastern Cooperative Oncology Group (ECOG) trial comparing their reference combination at the time, MVP, with the combination VP as well as two DDP derivatives, carboplatin and iproplatin. Results are shown in Table 3. MVP gave a higher response rate (20%) and a shorter median survival (22.7 weeks), while carboplatin, credited with a poor response rate (9%), led to median survival of 31.7 weeks, which was statistically superior. In contrast, and this is an important point, iproplatin did not provide such a result. The medical community does not appear to have drawn all the conclusions necessary from this result.

VIII. Second-Line Chemotherapy

Studies of second-line CT in NSCLC are beginning to appear. Taxanes are being seen as useful in this type of situation, in particular docetaxel, which remains effective even in patients previously treated with DDP (62,63). Their activity rate is between 15 and 20% in patients initially treated with DDP. Activity of a drug used second line depends upon the presence or not of DDP first line, falling overall from 18.4 to 9.4% in a retrospective study of 97 patients treated second line (64). It seems that the influence of first-line DDP is greater than the refractory nature of tumors during first-line treatment. Randomized trials of second-line treatment are an urgent necessity, in particular those testing single-drug therapy versus a BST.

IX. Quality of Life

Measurement of quality of life began to be evaluated in the 1980s, giving rise to a large number of studies. It was first tested in an adjuvant treatment situation, particularly using the Q-TWIST questionnaire (65). It cannot be used in a palliative situation, since it evaluates the time during which the patient experiences no symptoms related to either treatment or disease. This enables calculation of a weighted survival time in which only weeks (or years) without symptoms count fully. A reduction coefficient is attributed to others. Palliative situations required validated questionnaires taking into account the patients' essential subjective and objective feelings, assessed by the patients themselves using self-questionnaires. The questionnaire used most widely, in particular in lung cancer, is the QLQ-C30 of the EORTC (66). FACT (67) and FLIC (68) are two other frequently used questionnaires. It is nevertheless very difficult to assess the degree of patient satisfaction. A wide disparity exists between the perception of the physician and that of the patient. Evaluation itself by the patient is a procedure which may influence feelings in such a way as to make them more acceptable. According to Helson et al.'s (69) degree of adaptation theory, the fact of living a negative experience leads individuals to modify their criteria for evaluation of their quality of life, rendering the judgment they express on their life positive despite everything. Some apparently identical events are accepted totally differently according to the value assigned to them. Vomiting during first-line CT in a patient hoping for a cure is not experienced in the same way as vomiting, of equal intensity, during second-line treatment, at the time of a recurrence when the patient has lost hope of a cure.

Another difficulty encountered in the clinical use of quality-of-life questionnaires is their technical complexity. This creates problems for both patients and physician. For the patients, the questionnaire is long, sometimes difficult to understand, and repetitive since they have to fill it out several times. Its questions may sometimes seem indelicate when the patient's possibilities have slumped to far below those mentioned in the questionnaire or, on the contrary, a source of anxiety when they are still far greater and suggest the possibility of deterioration. It is difficult for the physician to make an immediate assessment of the patient's answers, since software must be used for comparative analysis of the answers to successive questionnaires.

X. Supportive Therapy

Supportive therapy covers two aspects: first, treatment of cancer symptoms and the palliative management of malignant disease, and second, the management of treatment-related symptoms. Only the latter point will be considered here. This aspect has been greatly influenced by the control of nausea and vomiting. This involves three phases: the use of high doses of metoclopramide (70), the addition of intravenous corticosteroids (71), and the introduction of 5HT3 receptor antagonists (72,73). The efficacy of the latter in particular against DDP-induced vomiting has contributed to the increasingly wider acceptance of CT by patients. Their efficacy is enhanced by the addition of intravenous corticosteroids (74,75). Decreased efficacy over the course of time is less with the combination of 5-anti-HT3 and steroids than with 5-anti-HT3 alone. The probability of remaining in total control of nausea and vomiting during subsequent courses is all the greater when complete control has been obtained during the previous course and when a steroid–5-anti-HT3 combination has been used. The result in a given course depends upon that in the previous course, with the phenomenon of "memory of vomiting" potentially leading to earlier vomiting (76). They are active above all on early nausea and vomiting (until 18 hours) and are notably less active on late nausea and vomiting (77).

The management of therapeutic aplasia (leuko-neutropenia), in particular when febrile, has benefited from the availability of cytokines (G-CSF and GM-CSF). No clear consensus exists as yet concerning their routine preventive use, in particular because of their cost. In NSCLC in particular, aplasia is often short-lived (1–4 days) and usually afebrile.

Because of this very control of other toxic effects, fatigue has become the major problem of CT for the patient. This is a complex type of fatigue. It affects muscles, leading to tiring when walking and muscle pains. But it affects all the areas of human activity: mental tiring with lack of interest in activities such as reading, affective tiring with difficulties in human relations (friends, grandchildren), and sexual tiring with decreased libido. Studies are just beginning, but treatment remains problematic (78).

XI. Conclusion

Chemotherapy for NSCLC has progressed. It has resolved a number of points, giving rise to new questions. It has been shown to be effective concerning survival and quality of life. There is better and better mastery of its toxic effects. It nevertheless remains palliative in patients with metastases. But it has not yet taken advantage of the large number of new drugs made available to clinicians. It remains dominated by the omnipresence of DDP and the practice of maximum tolerated dose. Its achievements justify a move into new indications: for elderly patients, second-line chemotherapy.

References

1. Cormier Y, Bergeron D, La Forge J, Lavandier M, Fournier M, Chenard J, Desmeules M. Benefits of polychemotherapy in advanced non-small cell bronchogenic carcinoma. Cancer 1982; 50:845–849.

2. Rapp E, Pater JL, Willan A, Cormier Y, Murray N, Evans WK, Hodson D, Clarck D, Feld R, Arnold P, Ayoub J. Chemotherapy can prolong survival in patients with advanced non-small cell lung cancer—report of a Canadian multicenter randomized trial. J Clin Oncol 1988; 6:633–641.

3. Woods RL, Williams CJ, Levi J, Page J, Bell D, Byrne M, et al. A randomised trial of cisplatin and vindesine versus supportive care only in advanced non-small cell lung cancer. Br J Cancer 1990; 61:608–611.

4. Ganz PA, Figlin RH, Haskell CM, La Soto N, Siau J. Supportive care versus supportive care and combination chemotherapy in metastatic non-small cell lung cancer. Cancer 1989; 63:1271–1278.

5. Cellerino R, Tummarello D, Guidi F, Isidori P, Raspugli M, Biscottini B, Fatati G. A randomized trial of alternating chemotherapy versus best supportive care in advanced non-small cell lung cancer. J Clin Oncol 1991; 9:1453–1461.

6. Quoix E, Dietemann A, Charbonneau J, Boutin C, Meurice JC, Orlando JP, Ducolone JP, Pauli G, Roegel E. La chimiothérapie comportant du cisplatin est-elle utile dans le cancer bronchique non microcellulaire au stade IV? Résultats d'une étude randomisée. Bull Cancer 1991; 78:341–346.

7. Kaasa S, Lund E, Thorud E, Hatevoli R, Host H. Symptomatic treatment versus combination chemotherapy for patients with extensive non-small cell lung cancer. Cancer 1991; 67:2443–2447.

8. Cartei G, Cartei F, Cantone A, Causarano D, Genco G, Tobaldin A, Interlandi G, Giraldi T. Cisplatin-cyclophosphamide-mitomycin combination chemotherapy with supportive care versus supportive care alone for treatment of metastatic non-small cell lung cancer. J Natl Cancer Inst 1993; 85:794–800.

9. Non-small Cell Lung Cancer Collaborative Group. Chemotherapy in non-small cell lung cancer: a meta-analysis using updated data on individual patients from 52 randomised clinical trials. BMJ 1995; 311:899–909.

10. Souquet PJ, Chauvin F, Boissel JP, Cellerino R, Cormier Y, Ganz A, Kaasa S, Pater JP, Quoix E, Rapp E, Tumarello D, Williams J, Woods BL, Bernard JP. Polychemotherapy in advanced non-small cell lung cancer: a meta-analysis. Lancet 1993; 342:19–21.

11. Thatcher, Niven RM, Anderson H. Aggressive vs nonaggressive therapy for metastatic NSCLC. Chest 1996; 109:87S–92S.

12. Depierre A, Lemarié E, Dabouis G, Garnier G, Jacoulet P, Dalphin JC. A phase II study of navelbine (vinorelbine) in the treatment of non-small cell lung cancer. Am J Clin Oncol 1991; 14:115–119.

13. Furuse K, Kubota K, Kawahara M, Ogawara M, Kinuwaki E, Motomiya M, Nishiwaki Y, Niitani H, Sakuma A, the Japan Vinorelbine Lung Cancer Study Group. A phase II study of vinorelbine, a new derivative of vinca alkaloid, for previously untreated advanced non-small cell lung cancer. Lung Cancer 1994; 11:385–391.

14. Le Chevalier T. Docetaxel: meeting the challenge of non-small cell lung cancer management. Anti-Cancer Drugs 1995; 6:13–17.

15. Fossella FV, Lee JS, Shin DM, Calayag M, Huber M, Perez-Soler R, Murphy WK, Lippman S, Benner S, Glisson B, et al. Phase II study of docetaxel for advanced or metastatic platinum-refractory non-small-cell lung cancer. J Clin Oncol 1995; 13:645–651.

16. Weiss RB, Donehover RC, Wiernik PH, Ohnuma T, Gralla R, Trump D, Baker J, Van Echo DA, Von Hoff D, Leyland-Jones B. Hypersensitivity reactions from paclitaxel. J Clin Oncol 1990; 8:1263–1268.

17. Gatzemeier U, Shepherd FA, Le Chevalier T, Weynants P, Cottier B, Groen HJ, Rosso R, Mattson K, Cortes-Funes H, Tonato M, Burkes RL, Gottfried M, Voi M. Activity of gemcitabine in patients with non-small cell lung cancer: a multicentre, extended phase II study. Eur J Cancer 1996; 32A:243–248.

18. Perez-Soler R, Fossella FV, Flisson BS, Lee JS, Murphy WK, Shin DM, Kemp BL, Lee JJ, Kane J, Robinson RA, Lippman SM, Kurie JM, Huber MH, Raber MN, Hong WK. Phase II study of topotecan in patients with advanced non-small-cell lung cancer previously untreated with chemotherapy. J Clin Oncol 1996; 14:503–513.

19. Rodriguez GL, Valdivieso M, Von Hoff DD, Kraut M, Burris HA, Eckardt JR, Lockwood G, Kennedy H, Von Roemeling R. A phase I/II trial of the combination of tirapazamine and cisplatin in patients with non-small cell lung cancer (NSCLC) (abstract). Proc Am Soc Clin Oncol 1996; 15:382.

20. Israel L, Reboul AR, Weil J, Dong P, Bernard E. Essai de polychimiothérapie anticancéreuse dans le traitement des cancers broncho-pulmonaires inopérables. J Franc Med Chir Thor 1965; 17–25.

21. Klastersky J, Sculier JP, Bureau G, Libert P, Ravez P, Vandermoten G, Thiriaux J, Lecomte J, Cordier R, Dabouis G, Brohée D, Thémelin L, Mommen P, for the Lung Cancer Working Party. Cisplatin versus cisplatin plus etoposide in the treatment of advanced non-small-cell lung cancer. J Clin Oncol 1989; 7:1087–1092.

22. Crino L, Tonato M, Darwish S, Meacci ML, Corgna E, Di Costanzo F, Buzzi F, Fornari G, Santi E, Ballatori E, Santucci C, Davis S. A randomized trial of three cisplatin-containing regimens in advanced non-small-cell lung cancer (NSCLC): a study of the Umbrian Lung Cancer Group. Cancer Chemother Pharmacol 1990; 26:52–56.

23. Kawahara M, Furuse K, Kodama N, Yamamoto M, Kubota K, Takada M, Negoro S, Kusunoki Y, Matui K, Takifuji N, M. F. A randomized study of cisplatin versus cisplatin plus vindesine for non-small cell lung carcinoma. Cancer 1991; 68:714–719.

24. Wozniak AJ, Crowley JJ, Balcerzak SP, Weiss GR, Laufman LR, Baker LH, Fisher RI, Bearman SI, Taylor SA, Livingston RB. Randomized phase III trial of cisplatin (CDDP) vs. CDDP plus navelbine (NVB) in treatment of advanced non-small cell lung cancer (NSCLC): report of a southwest oncology group study (SWOG-9308). (abstract). Proc Am Soc Clin Oncol 1996; 15:374.

25. Depierre A, Chastang C, Quoix E, Lebeau B, Blanchon F, Paillot N, Lemarié E, Milleron B, Moro D, Clavier J, Herman D, Tuchais E, Jacoulet P, Bréchot JM, Cordier JF, Solal-Céligny P, Badri N, Besenval M. Vinorelbine versus vinorelbine plus cisplatin in advanced non-small cell lung cancer: a randomized trial. Ann Oncol 1994; 5:37–42.

26. Le Chevalier T, Brisgand D, Douillard JY, Pujol JL, Alberola V, Monnier A, Rivière A, Lianes P, Chomy P, Cigolari S, Gottfried M, Ruffié P, Panizo A, Gaspard MH, Ravaioli A, Besenval M, Besson F, Martinez A, Berthaud P, Tursz T. Randomized Study of Vinorelbine and Cisplatin versus Vindesine and Cisplatin versus Vinorelbine alone in advanced non-small-cell lung cancer: results of a European Multicenter trial including 612 patients. J Clin Oncol 1994; 12:360–367.

27. Einhorn LH, Loehrer PH, Williams SD, Meyers S, Gabrys T, Natta SR, Woodburn RW, Drasga R, Songer J, Fisher W, Stephens D, Hui S. Random prospective study of vindesine versus vindesine plus high-dose cisplatin versus vindesine plus cisplatin plus mitomycin C in advanced non-small-cell lung cancer. J Clin Oncol 1986; 4:1037–1043.

28. Sorensen JB, Hansen HH, P. D, Bork E, Malmberg R, Aabo K, Bodker B, Hansen M. Chemotherapy for adenocarcinoma of the lung (WHO III): a randomized study of vindesine versus lomustine, cyclophosphamide, and methotrexate versus all four drugs. J Clin Oncol 1987; 5:1169–1177.

29. Elliott JA, Ahmedzai S, Hole D, Dorward J, Stevenson RD, Kaye SB, Banham SW, Stack BHR, Calman KC. Vindesine and cisplatin combination chemotherapy compared with vindesine as a single agent in the management of non-small cell lung cancer: a randomized study. Eur J Cancer Clin Oncol 1984; 20:1025–1032.

30. Rosso R, Salvati F, Ardizzoni A, Gallo Curcio C, Rubagotti A, Belli M, Castagneto B, Fusco V, Sassi M, Ferrara G, Pizza A, Pedicini T, Soresi E, Scoditti S, Cioffi R, U. F, Monaco M, Merlano M, Rimoldi R, Tonachella R, Cruciani A, Colantuoni G, Rinaldi M, Portalone L, Bruggi P, Santi L. Etoposide versus etoposide plus high-dose cisplatin in the management of advanced non-small cell lung cancer. Cancer 1990; 66:130–134.

31. Splinter TAW, Sahmoud T, Festen J, Van Zandwijk N, Sörenson S, Clerico M, Burhouts J, Dautzenberg B, Kho GS, Kirkpatrick A, Giaccone G. Two schedules of teniposide with or without cisplatin in advanced non-small-cell lung cancer: a randomized study of the European Organization of research and treatment of Cancer Lung Cancer Cooperative Group. J Clin Oncol 1996; 14:127–134.

32. Bonomi PD, Finkelstein DM, Ruckdeschel JC, Blum RH, Green MD, Mason B, Hahn R, Tormey CD, Harris J, Comis R, Glick J. Combination chemotherapy versus single agents followed by combination chemotherapy in stage IV non-small-cell lung cancer: a study of the eastern cooperative oncology group. J Clin Oncol 1989; 7:1602–1613.

33. Veeder MJ, Jett JR, Su JQ, Mailliard JA, Foley JF, Dalton RJ, Etzell PS, Marschke RF, Kardinal CG, Maksymiuk AN, Ebbert LP, Tazelaar HD, Witrak GA. A phase III trial of mitomycin C alone versus mitomycin C, vinblastine and cisplatin for metastatic squamous cell lung cancer. Cancer 1992; 70:2281–2287.

34. Fukuoka M, Masuda N, Furuse K, Negoro S, Takada M, Matsui K, Takifuji N, Kudoh S, Kawahara M, Ogawara M, Kodama N, Kubota K, Yamamoto M, Kusunoki Y. A randomized trial in inoperable non-small-cell lung cancer: vindesine and cisplatin versus mitomycin, vindesine and cisplatin versus etoposide and cisplatin alternating with vindesine and mitomycin. J Clin Oncol 1991; 9:606–613.

35. Shinkai T, Eguchi K, Sosaki Y. A randomized clinical mitomycin plus vindesine and cisplatin in advanced non-small cell lung cancer. Eur J Cancer 1991; 27:571–576.

36. Dhingra HM, Valdivieso M, Carr DT, Chiuten DF, Farha P, Murphy WK, Spitzer G, Umsawasdi T. Randomized trial of three combinations of cisplatin with vindesine and/or VP-16-213 in the treatment of advanced non-small-cell lung cancer. J Clin Oncol 1985; 3:176–183.

37. Erkisi M, Doran F, Burgut R, Kocabas A. A randomised trial of two cisplatin-còntaining chemotherapy regimens in patients with stade III-B and IV non-small cell lung cancer. Lung Cancer 1995; 12:237–246.

38. Crino L, Clerici M, Figoli L, Barduagni M, Carlini P, Ceci G, Cortesi E, Carpi A, Santini A, Di Costanza F. Superiority of three-drug combination chemotherapy versus cisplatin-etoposide in advanced non-small cell lung cancer: a randomized trial by the Italian Oncology Group for Clinical Research. Lung Cancer 1995; 12:S125–132.

39. O'Connell JP, Kris MG, Gralla RJ, Groshen S., Trust A, Fiore JJ, Kelsen DP, Heelan RT, R.B. G. Frequency and prognostic importance of pretreatment clinical characteristics in patients with advanced non-small-cell lung cancer treated with combination chemotherapy. J Clin Oncol 1986; 4:1604–1614.

40. Joss RA, Cavalli F, Goldhirsch A. New agents in non-small cell lung cancer. Cancer Treat Rev 1984; 11:205–237.

41. Albain K, Crowley J, Leblanc M, Livingston B. Survival determinants in extensive-stage non-small-cell lung cancer: the southwest oncology group experience. J Clin Oncol 1991; 9:1618–1626.

42. Gralla R, Casper E, Kelsen D, Braun D, Dukeman M, Martini N, Young C, Golbey R. Cisplatin and vindesine combination chemotherapy for advanced carcinoma of the lungs: a randomized trial investigating two doses schedules. Ann Intern Med 1981; 95:414–420.

43. Klastersky J, Sculier JP, Ravez P, Libert P, Michel J, Vandermoten G, Rocmans P, Bonduelle Y, Mairesse M, Michiels T, Thiriaux J, Mommen P, Dalesio O, and the EORTC Lung Cancer Working Party. A randomized study comparing a high and a standard dose of cisplatin in combination with etoposide in the treatment of advanced non-small-cell lung carcinoma. J Clin Oncol 1986; 4:1780–1786.

44. Gandara DR, Crowley J, Livingston RB, Perez EA, Taylor CW, Weiss G, Neefe JR, Hutchins LF, Roach RW, Grunberg SM, Braun TJ, Natale RB, Balcerzak SP. Evaluation of cisplatin intensity in metastatic non-small-cell lung cancer: a phase III study of the Southwest Oncology Group. J Clin Oncol 1993; 11:873–878.

45. Souhami RL, Spiro SG, Rudd RM, Ruiz de Evira MC, James LE, Gower NH, Lamont A, Harper PG. Five-day oral etoposide treatment for advanced small-cell lung cancer: randomized comparison with intravenous chemotherapy. J Natl Cancer Inst 1997; 89:577.

46. Arriagada R, Le Chevalier T, Pignon JP, Rivière A, Monnet I, Chomy P, Tuchais C, Tarayre M, Ruffié P. Initial chemotherapeutic doses and survival in patients with limited small-cell lung cancer. N Engl J Med 1993; 329:1848–1852.

47. Souquet PJ, Lombard-Bohas CH, Freyer G, Bombaron P, Gerinière L, Bernard JP. Chimiothérapie des cancers bronchiques des sujets âgés. Rev Mal Respir 1996; 17:327–333.

48. Thiss A, Saudes L, Creisson A, Dassonville O, Schneider M. Renal tolerance of cisplatin in patients more than 80 years old. J Clin Oncol 1994; 12:2121–2125.
49. Begg CB, Elson PJ, Carbone PP. A study of excess hematologic toxicity in elderly patients treated on cancer chemotherapy protocols. In: Verlag S, ed. Cancer in the Elderly. Approach to Early Detection and Treatment. 1989.
50. Bonomi P. Non-small cell lung cancer chemotherapy. In: Pass HI, Mitchell B, Johnson D, Turrisi A. Lung Cancer: Principles and Practice Philadelphia: Lippincott-Raven Publishers 1996:811-824.
51. Kusunoki Y, Furuse K, Yamori S, Negro S, Katagami N, Takada K, Kinuwaki E, Niitani H. Randomized phase II study of vinorelbine (VRB) VS vindesine (VDS) in previously untreated non-small cell lung cancer (NSCLC): Final results (abstract). Proc Am Soc Clin Oncol 1995; 14:353.
52. O'Rourke M, Crawford J, Schiller J, Laufman L, Yanovich S, Ozer H, Langleben A, Barlogie B, Koletscky A, Clamon G, Purvis J, Tuttle R, Hohneker J. Survival advantage for patients with stage IV NSCLC treated with single agent navelbine in a randomized controlled trial (abstract). Proc Am Soc Clin Oncol 1993; 12:343.
53. Jacoulet P, Dubiez A, Depierre A, Pugin JF, Pernet D. One-week versus 3-weeks intervals in the administration of cisplatin in combination with vinorelbine: a randomized study in non small-cell lung cancer (NSCLC) (abstract). Proc Am Soc Clin Oncol 1992; 11:301.
54. Akerley W, Coy H, Glatz M, Safran H, Sikov W, Rege V, Sambandam S, Josephs J, Wittels E, Brown University Oncology Group (BrUOG) Providence R. Phase II trial of weekly paclitaxel for advanced non-small cell lung cancer (NSCLC). Proc Am Soc Clin Oncol 1997; 16:450.
55. Hryniuk W, Levine M. Analysis of dose intensity for adjuvant chemotherapy trials in stade II breast cancer. J Clin Oncol 1986; 4:1162–1170.
56. Gralla RJ, Hesketh PJ, Rittenberg CN, Robertson CL, Bizette GA, Gorman B, Marques CB. Preserving dose-intensity in an active regimen in NSCLC with navelbine + mitomycin + cisplatin (abstract). Proc Am Soc Clin Oncol 1996; 15:377.
57. Westeel V, Jacoulet P, Breton JL, Garnier G, Mercier M, Depierre A. Phase II study of alternating doses of vinorelbine in combination with cisplatin for non-small cell lung cancer (NSCLC): a disappointing experience. Lung Cancer 1996; 16:61–73.
58. Westeel V, Mercier M, Depierre A, Le Chevalier T, Quoix E, Douillard JY, Baud M, Martinez A, Paillot N, Jacoulet P. Dose intensity (DI) of chemotherapy as a survival determinant in advanced non-small cell lung cancer (NSCLC): an analysis of 819 patients from two randomized trials. Proc Am Soc Clin Oncol 1997; 16:487a.
59. Larsen H, Sorensen JB, Nielsen AL, Dombernowsky P, Hansen HH. Evaluation of the optimal duration of chemotherapy in phase II trials for inoperable non-small-cell lung cancer (NSCLC). Ann Oncol 1995; 6:993–997.
60. Jacoulet P, Maheu MF, Loire R, Saugier B, Depierre A. Long-term cure of a non-small-cell lung cancer treated by monochemotherapy. Am J Clin Oncol 1996; 19:260–262.
61. Quoix E, Moro D, Jacoulet P, Miech G, Robinet G, Vaylet F, Vincent M, Grivaux M, Leclerc P, Coudert B, Breton JL, Souquet PJ, Charloux A, on behalf of the 'Groupe d'Oncologie Thoracique de Langue Française." Long term survivors in non resected non small cell lung cancer (NSCLC) patients: a French data base. Proc Am Soc Clin Oncol 1995; 14:368.
62. Fossella FV, Lee JS, Murphy WK, Lippman SM, Calayag M, Pang A, Chasen M, Shin DM, Glisson B, Benner S, Huber M, Perez-Soler R, Hong WK, Raber M. Phase II study of docetaxel for recurrent or metastatic non-small cell lung cancer. J Clin Oncol 1994; 12:1238–1244.
63. Murphy WK, Winn RJ, Huber M, Fossella FV, Goldberg D, Presant CA, Flynn CA, Coldman B, Clements S, Raber M, Hong WK. Phase II study of taxol (T) in patients (pt) with non-small cell lung cancer (NSCLC) who have failed platinum (P) containing chemotherapy (CTX) (abstract). Proc Am Soc Clin Oncol 1994; 13:363.
64. Jacoulet P, Dubiez A, Westeel V, Polio JC, Pernet D, Depierre A. Chimiothérapie de deuxième ligne chez les patients réfractaires et résistants atteints de cancers du poumon non à petites cellules. Rev Mal Respir 1997; 14:29–35.

65. Gelber RD, Goldhirsch A, Castiglione M, Price K, Isley M, Coates AS. Time without symptoms and toxicity (TWIST): a quality-of-life oriented endpoint to evaluate adjuvant therapy. In: SE S, ed. Adjuvant Therapy of Cancer. Philadelphia: Grune Stratton, 1987:455–465.

66. Aaronson NK, Ahmedzai S, Bergman B, for the EORTC study group on quality of life. The EORTC QLQ-C30. A quality of life instrument for use in international clinical trials in oncology. J Natl Cancer Inst 1993; 85:365–376.

67. Cella DF, Tulsky DS, Gray G, Sarafian B, Linn E, Bonomi A, Silberman M, Yellen SB, Winicour P, Brannon J, Eckberg K, Lloyd S, Purl S, Blendowski C, Goodman M, Barnicle M, Stewart I, McHale M, Bonomi P, Kaplan E, Taylor IV S, Thomas CR, Harris J. The functional assessment of cancer therapy scale: development and validation of the general measure. J Clin Oncol 1993; 11:570–579.

68. Shipper H, Clinh J, McMurray A, Lewitt M. Measuring the quality of life of cancer patients. The functional living index-cancer: development and validation. J Clin Oncol 1984; 2: 472–483.

69. Helson H, Bevan W. Contemporary Approaches to Psychology. Princeton: Van Nostrand, 1967.

70. Gralla RJ, Itri LM, Piko SE. Antiemetic efficacy of high-dose metoclopramide: randomized trials with placebo and prochlorperazine in patients with chemotherapy-induced nausea and vomiting. N Engl J Med 1981; 305:905–909.

71. Kris MG, Gralla RJ, Tyson LB, R.A. C, Cirrincione C, Groshen S. Controlling delayed vomiting: double-blind, randomized trial comparing placebo, dexamethasone alone, and metoclopramide plus dexamethasone in patients receiving cisplatin. J Clin Oncol 1989; 7:108–114.

72. Hainsworth J, Harvey W, Pendergrass K. A single-blind comparison of intravenous ondansetron, a selective serotonin antagonist, with intravenous metoclopramide in the prevention of nausea and vomiting associated with high-dose cisplatin chemotherapy. J Clin Oncol 1991; 9:721–728.

73. Marty M, Pouillart P, Scholl S. Comparison of the 5-hydroxytryptamine3 (serotonin) antagonist ondansetron (GR 38032F) with high-dose metoclopramide in the control of cisplatin-induced emesis. N Engl J Med 1990; 322:816–821.

74. Hesketh PJ, Harvey WH, W.G. H. A randomized, double-blind comparison of intravenous ondansetron alone and in combination with intravenous dexamethasone in the prevention of high-dose cisplatin-induced emesis. J Clin Oncol 1994; 12:596–600.

75. Roila F, Tonato M, Cognetti F. Prevention of cisplatin-induced emesis: a double-blind multicenter randomized crossover study comparing ondansetron and ondansetron plus dexamethasone. J Clin Oncol 1991; 9:675–678.

76. Richard A, Chevallier B, Marty M. Construction et validation d'un modèle prédictif du contrôle de l'émésis au fil des cures de chimiothérapies. Cah Oncol 1994; 3:279–283.

77. Olver I, Paska W, Depierre A, Seitz JF, Stewart DJ, Goedhals L, McQuade B, McRae J, Wilkinson JR, on behalf of the Ondansetron Delayed Emesis Study Group. A multicentre, double-blind study comparing placebo, ondansetron and ondansetron plus dexamethasone for the control of cisplatin-induced delayed emesis. Ann Oncol 1996; 7:945–952.

78. Hümy C, Bernhard J, Joss R, Schatzmann E, Cavalli F, Brunner K, Alberto P, Senn HJ, Metzger U, for the Swiss Group for Clinical Cancer Research (SAKK). "Fatigue and malaise" as a quality-of-life indicator in small-cell lung cancer patients. Support Care Cancer 1993; 1:316–320.

36

Prognostic Factors in Unresectable Non–Small-Cell Lung Cancer

E. QUOIX

Hôpitaux Universitaires
Strasbourg, France

Non–small-cell lung cancer represents 75% of all lung cancers. When a diagnosis of non–small-cell lung cancer is established, there are two major questions: Is the tumor resectable and if yes, is the patient operable?

More than 70% of patients with non–small-cell lung cancer are unresectable at the time of diagnosis (1); for these patients the 5-year survival is less than 5%, whereas it is about 35% for operated patients (2). Since resection provides the best chance for cure, it constitutes the major prognostic factor for non–small-cell lung cancer. Thus, studies on prognostic factors in non–small-cell lung cancer are divided into those devoted to resectable and those devoted to unresectable non–small-cell lung cancers.

Correct management decisions in non–small-cell lung cancer depend on prognostic factors; their precise analysis is mandatory in order to evaluate new therapeutic strategies. Comparative clinical trials, especially in advanced non–small-cell lung cancer, lead in general to very small differences (3 or 4% gain in survival at 2 years, for example). This small benefit may be either overestimated or underestimated if prognostic factors are not well balanced in the two arms.

I. Methods of Prognostic Assessment

A. Outcome Is a Delay

This delay may be termed survival, time to progression, duration of response, etc. For purposes of clarity, the term survival will be the only one employed here.

Univariate Analysis of Survival

Censored survival data are explored by the Kaplan-Meier (product limit) or actuarial methods, which are estimators of the survival function (3). Two assumptions must be verified:

> Risk of death is independent of time of entry in the study for each group.
> Homogeneity of distribution of survival time within a group.

The log-rank test (4) assesses differences in survival between two or more groups. For example, one may compare survival of males and females with unresectable non–small-cell lung cancer. This very simple test compares the number of deaths actually observed in each group with the number of deaths expected in each group if the survival were similar in each group.

Multivariate Analysis of Survival

In general, more than one variable summarizes the whole prognosis, and some prognostic factors may actually be confounders.

Stratification is a means of taking into account a factor, for example, age, in order to study the prognostic value of performance status or sex in order to study the prognostic value of weight loss. Stratification may be extended to more than two levels, but obviously by increasing the number of stratas, the number of patients in each stratum will become very small and the survival curves will have wide confidence bands preventing any possible comparisons.

Cox's proportional hazards regression model (5) allows one to test whether a factor or a combination of several factors has any influence on prognosis and provides estimates of the treatment effect adjusted for confounding factors. The extended proportional hazards model is an exponential model in which the risk of an event (death, response, progression, etc) at time t is:

$$h(t,x_i) = h_o (t) \exp (b_1 x_1 + b_2 x_2 + b_3 x_3 + \ldots + b_p x_p)$$

in which $h_o(t)$ is the baseline hazard and h is the hazard at time t of an individual characterized by p variables $(x_1, x_2, x_3, \ldots x_p)$, each of them having an affected coefficient b_i, which is estimated. If b_i is positive, h(t) is greater than $h_o(t)$. If b_i is negative, the instantaneous risk is less than $h_o(t)$. If $b_i = 0$, x_i has no influence on the hazard.

The hazards of two individuals are proportional at any time: in other terms, the hazard ratio is a constant.

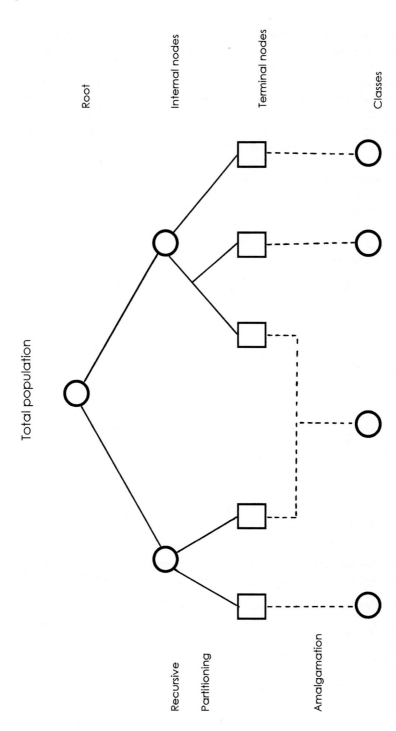

Figure 1 RECPAM model.

More recently, another method of multivariate analysis of survival has been developed: the recursive partition with amalgamation, also called the RECPAM model (6). For clinicians, the RECPAM model has several advantages over Cox's model, the most important being that an arborescent classification is very similar to medical decision analysis. The aim of this method is to identify subgroups of patients with homogeneous outcomes. The initial population, which is the root of the tree (Fig. 1), is split into two groups according to the variable inducing the biggest difference in survival. The two subgroups, which are nodes of the tree, will then be split in the same fashion, until no variable inducing differences of survival can be found. We obtain at this point the terminal nodes. Terminal nodes are then amalgamated (when the log rank test between two of them gives a level of significance > 0.05) to constitute subgroups of patients with homogeneous prognoses.

B. Outcome Is Dichotomic

Examples include response versus no response, toxicity versus no toxicity, 2-year survival versus less than 2-year survival, etc. In this case we may compare the distribution of some variables between two groups: for example, the sex distribution among the patients surviving at least 2 years and among the patients surviving less than 2 years. This can be done by a chi-square test. In most cases, for this purpose, continuous variables are categorized. For example, biological values such as LDH are dichotomized between values less or equal to normal and elevated values.

To take into account more than one variable and to identify those variables which are independently predictive of a response, a toxicity, a response, a 2-year survival, a logistic regression model is performed (7).

The equation of this model is as follows:

$$\text{Log } (p/1 - p) = \text{cst} + b_1x_1 + b_2x_2 + \ldots + b_px_p$$

in which p is the probability of a response, a toxicity, a progression, a long-term survival, and x_i are the predictive factors affected of coefficients b_i.

II. Clinical Prognostic Factors in Unresectable Non–Small-Cell Lung Cancer

A. Patient Characteristics

Performance Status

Performance status (PS) is a major independent prognostic factor consistently found in all multivariate analyses, including this variable, as well in old series (8–10) or in more recent ones (11–19) and whatever the scale used (Karnofsky, WHO, or ECOG)

Weight Loss

Weight loss appears in most studies to be a prognostic factor in univariate analyses (8–11,16,17,19,20) but independently predictive of survival in only five of them (8–10,19,20). This is probably due to the high correlation of this variable with the PS.

Gender

Gender has emerged recently as a discriminating factor in non–small-cell lung cancer patient outcome in North America, with a favorable impact on prognosis for females (11–13,16,18,20). In the latter study, it was suggested that weight loss could play a role in mediating gender-related differences in NSCLC patient survival, as men were more prone to lose weight over the course of their disease. A retrospective study of 478 males and 194 females with primary lung cancer showed that females were diagnosed at a younger age, earlier stage, and had more often adenocarcinoma (21).

While the sex ratio in North America is approximately 2:1 (22), it is higher, between 8 and 12:1 in Belgium, France, Portugal, and other European countries (17,22,23). As a consequence, the possible prognostic role of gender is more difficult to ascertain in those countries.

Age

There are some difficulties in assessing the prognostic role of age. First, elderly patients are often excluded from clinical trials (24); second, the cutoffs are very different according to the studies: 60 years (17,25,26), 70 years (8,10,16), or even 75 years (27). Age was found to be of no prognostic importance in numerous studies (9–14,19,23), while it appeared significant in others (16,17,25,26). In the recent review of the SWOG, age > 70 years was detrimental in the Cox multivariate analysis, but in the RECPAM analysis, within the best prognostic group defined by a good PS and Hb > 11 g/dl, an age cutoff at 47, determined two subgroups, with a better prognosis for those aged over 47 years.

In population-based data of the Surveillance, Epidemiology and End Results (SEER), age proved to be the strongest predictor of survival among the demographic variables, but these data concerned all stages and histologies of lung cancer (27). It is worth noting that for operable non–small-cell lung cancer, age was no longer a prognostic factor when relative survival was estimated (28). However, for unresectable non–small-cell lung cancer, the duration of survival is short and thus estimation of relative survival is probably not mandatory.

Race

The influence of race has not been studied extensively. However, in a series of National Cancer Data Base lung cancer cases, there was a noteworthy poor prognosis among African Americans (29). In the SEER population-based data, white patients survived better than blacks (27). In the SWOG study, however, race had no influence on outcome (16). It appears that socioeconomic status is probably a confounding factor with race (30).

B. Tumor Characteristics

Extent of Disease

Disease extent within unresectable NSCLC is a major prognostic factor (8–11, 14,15,17–19,23,25,26) as well within stage III (15,25) or stage IV versus IIIB (17,23). Single metastasis versus multiple lesions also appears to be an independent favorable factor in recent studies (16,31).

The prognostic role of specific metastatic sites is controversial. However, bone metastases are often found to be predictive of short survival (11,12,14,31), as are skin metastases (12,17) or liver involvement (12,14).

Histology

Histology is a controversial prognostic factor. Even if adenocarcinoma is more prone to develop metastases, histology appears to have no significant influence on survival (8,11,13,17,20,22,23) in most studies. Non–large-cell histology appeared to have a favorable impact in one study (12) and nonsquamous cell histology in another (32). Although histological subtype had no influence on outcome in operated patients, adenocarcinomas other than bronchioloalveolar carcinomas had a pejorative impact on survival, in contrast to bronchioloalveolar carcinoma, which was of better prognosis in unresected NSCLC patients (26). The lack of reproducibility of subtype diagnosis may explain these discrepancies or the fact that if histology has any influence on prognosis, this influence is weak (9).

Neuroendocrine differentiation has been found to be a favorable independent prognostic factor of survival (33), with no increased likelihood of response to chemotherapy, whereas in another study, the presence of two neuroendocrine markers was associated with a higher response rate and longer survival (34).

C. Laboratory Parameters

Their prognostic impact has not been as extensively studied as in small-cell lung cancer. However, LDH has an unfavorable impact on outcome when elevated (11,14,13,23).

Hemoglobin levels appear to be of prognostic importance as well in Cox's regression models or in RECPAM analyses, where the best survival was observed for patients with a good PS and a hemoglobin level > 11 g/dl (16,19).

Both total white blood cell count (9,14,17) and lymphocyte count (9,18,31) have been identified as prognostic factors. The value of neutrophil count has been established in only one study (17).

Thrombocytosis has been shown to correlate strongly with a poor survival in a multivariate analysis of 1115 patients with primary lung cancer (35), but only in the univariate analysis of survival in the European Lung Cancer Working Party (ELCWP) study (17). Platelets had no significant influence on outcome in inoperable adenocarcinoma (14).

Low serum albumin has also been shown to be of bad prognostic value in some studies (18,31), as well as hypercalcemia (16,17).

Among tumor markers, Cyfra 21-1 has proven to be an independent prognostic factor in lung cancer (36) and especially non–small-cell lung cancer (37). In one recent study, NSE level was also identified as an independent prognostic factor (38).

III. Therapeutic Prognostic Factors in Unresectable NSCLC

It is now proven that cisplatinum-based chemotherapy improves survival both in stage IV and in locally advanced NSCLC (39).

A. Is Response to Chemotherapy Predictive of Survival?

It is not easy to answer this question, which gives rise to methodological problems. Indeed, 8–12 weeks of treatment are necessary in order to assess response. Responders, by definition, survive at least this long between the start of treatment and response assessment. The landmark method, which consists of calculating survival starting at the time of response evaluation, dropping patients whose survival is less than this interval, is sometimes used in order to minimize this bias (40). With this methodology, response to chemotherapy was found to be an independent favorable prognostic factor in two studies (11,17). However, response to chemotherapy may only identify patients with a better prognosis, without causal relationship between response and survival (41). In an ECOG study (42), patients who were treated by carboplatin alone had a response rate of only 9%. However, they survived significantly longer than patients treated with a combination of mitomycin, vinblastin, and cisplatin (MVP), for which the response rate was 20%. Also, in a previous study of the same group, the response rate to MVP was the highest, but this was not correlated with a better survival than for the other combinations with lower response rates (43).

B. Is Cisplatinum a Mandatory Compound of Chemotherapy Combinations?

In a recent meta-analysis (39), only cisplatinum-based chemotherapy was associated with a better survival for advanced NSCLC. Whether this is due to cisplatinum itself is not certain, as the cisplatinum combinations were also part of more recent therapies. In the SWOG report (16), cisplatinum-based chemotherapy was an independent prognostic factor of survival. Again, the cisplatinum-based therapy was given in the most recent studies. However, although the year of accrual was a significant prognostic factor in univariate analysis, it was no longer present in the multivariate analysis. This better survival in cisplatinum-based chemotherapy could also be due to the stage migration also known as the Will Rogers phenomenon (44). This issue was also addressed in the SWOG study, and the cisplatin variable was still retained in the model.

In a meta-analysis, Donnadieu et al. found that cisplatinum-based chemotherapy is associated with a higher response rate (45). This was confirmed in two recent trials (46,47) comparing vinorelbin with vinorelbin + cisplatin (within one of them a third arm being vindesin + cisplatin). Response rate in the vinorelbin + cisplatin arm was significantly higher than in the vinorelbin-alone arm in both studies, but this was accompanied by a gain in survival in one only (47).

C. Is Radiotherapy Dose a Prognostic Factor for Survival?

In stage III disease, radiation dose appeared to be an independent prognostic factor (48). This issue has been addressed previously (49) but through univariate analysis, with the same result.

IV. Prediction of Long-Term Survival

Predictive factors of long-term survival have been poorly studied, and results cannot be compared because, depending on the various studies, long-term survival is either 2- and 5-year survival in the review of the trials of the ELCWP (50) devoted to inoperable NSCLC patients regardless of the disease stage or 1- and 2-year survival for the ECOG review of stage IV patients (51). In the ELCWP study (50), the only predictive factor of 2-year survival was limited disease. Independent prognostic factors of a 1-year survival for stage IV patients (51) were a PS = 0, no bone metastasis, female sex, no weight loss, no skin metastasis, non–large-cell histology, no prior symptoms of shoulder or arm pain, and no liver metastasis. Among the 1-year survivors, predictive factors for long-term survival were female sex, no skin metastasis, and a PS = 0.

Taking into account therapy, long-term survival was correlated with the existence of a response to initial chemotherapy (50), but also with the interval before a response was observed (51); the longer the interval, the longer the survival.

V. Prediction of Very Short Survival

To our knowledge there is no specific study devoted to this issue. However, the RECPAM classification tree allows one to identify the subgroups with the worst prognosis. In the SWOG study (16), patients with a PS 2–4, and <45 years had a median survival time of 2.5 months. The results for patients enrolled in recent studies show that patients with a poor PS (2–4) and elevated LDH had the worst prognosis, with only 6% surviving beyond 1 year, whereas all other patients had a 16%

survival ≥ 1 year. In the ELCWP study (17), patients dying within the 12 weeks after diagnosis had significant more frequently skin metastases, neutrophilia > 7500/mm³, and a PS $\leq$ 70 (results of the logistic regression).

As a conclusion, the outcome of a NSCLC patient can be predicted to a certain extent using simple algorithms. However, one must be aware that the prognostic factors have been established from series of patients participating in clinical trials (i.e., selected on inclusion criteria). These patients may not reflect the global population of patients with unresectable non–small-cell lung cancer. Introduction of therapeutic variables implies methodological problems that must be taken into account.

Despite these pitfalls, knowledge of prognostic factors allows the clinician to make the most adequate therapeutic decision for a given patient and for research purposes to optimally distribute significant prognostic factors between two or more randomization arms.

References

1. Vincent RG, Takita H, Lane WW, Guttiriez AC, Pickren JW. Surgical therapy of lung cancer. J Thorac Cardiovasc Surg 1976; 71:581–591.
2. Ginsberg RJ, Goldberg M, Waters PF. Surgery for non-small cell lung cancer. In: Roth JA, Ruckdeschel JC, Weisenburger TH, eds. Thoracic Oncology. Philadelphia: WB Saunders, 1989:177–199.
3. Kaplan EL, Meier P. Non parametric estimation from incomplete observation. J Am Stat Assoc 1958; 53:457–481.
4. Peto R, Peto S. Asymptomatically efficient rank invariant test procedures. JR Statist Soc 1972; A135:185–207.
5. Cox DR. Regression models and life tables (with discussion). JR Stat Soc B 1972; 34: 187–220.
6. Ciampi A, Thiffault J. Recursive partition and amalgamation (RECPAM) for censured survival data: criteria for tree selection. Statistical Software Newsletter 1988; 14:78–81.
7. Hosmer DW, Lemeshow S. Applied Logistic Regression. New York: Wiley, 1989.
8. Lanzotti VJ, Thomas DR, Bayle LE, Smith TL, Gehan EA, Samuels ML. Survival with inoperable lung cancer: an integration of prognostic variables based on simple clinical criteria. Cancer 1977; 39:303–313.
9. Stanley KE. Prognostic factors for survival in patients with inoperable lung cancer. J Natl Cancer Inst 1980; 65:25–32.
10. Pater JL, Lab M. Non-anatomic prognostic factors in carcinoma of the lung. Cancer 1982; 50:326–331.
11. O'Connel JP, Kris MG, Gralla RJ, Groshen S, Trust A, Fiore DP, Kelsen DP, Heelan RT, Golbey RB. Frequency and prognostic importance of pretreatment clinical characteristics in patients with advanced non-small cell lung cancer treated with combination chemotherapy. J Clin Oncol 1986; 4:1604–1614.
12. Ruckdeschel JC, Finkelstein DM, Ettinger DS, Creech RH, Mason BA, Joss RA, Vogl S. A randomized trial of the four most active regimens for metastatic non-small cell lung cancer. J Clin Oncol 1986; 4:14–22.
13. Sakurai M, Shinkai T, Eguchi K, Sasaki Y, Tamura T, Miura K, Fujiwara Y, Otsu A, Horiuchi N, Nakano H. Prognostic factors in non-small cell lung cancer: multiregression analysis in the National Cancer Center Hospital. J Cancer Res Clin Oncol 1987; 113:563–566.
14. Sorensen JB, Badberg JH, Olsen J. Prognostic factors in inoperable adenocarcinoma of the lung: a multivariate regression analysis of 259 patients. Cancer Res 1989; 79:5748–5754.

15. Bonomi P, Gale M, Rowland K, Taylor SG, Purl S, Reddy S, Lee MS, Phillips A, Kittle CF, Wairen W. Pre-treatment prognostic factors in stage III non-small cell lung cancer patients receiving combined modality treatment. Int J Radiol Oncol Biol Phys 1990; 20: 247–252.

16. Albain KS, Crowley JJ, Le Blanc M, Livingston RG. Survival determinants in extensive stage non-small cell lung cancer: the Southwest Oncology Group Experience. J Clin Oncol 1991; 9:1618–1626.

17. Paesmans M, Sculier JP, Libert P, Bureau G, Dabouis G, Thiriaux J, Michel J, Van Cutsem O, Sergysels R, Mommen P, Klastersky J. Prognostic factors for survival in advanced non-small cell lung cancer: uni and multivariate analysis including RECPAM in 1052 patients. J Clin Oncol 1995; 13:1221–1230.

18. Muers MF, Shevlin P, Brown J. Prognosis in lung cancer: physicians' opinions compared with outcome and a predictive model. Thorax 1996; 51:894–902.

19. Takigawa N, Segawa Y, Okahara M, Maeda Y, Takata I, Kataoka M, Fujii M. Prognostic factors for patients with advanced non-small cell lung cancer: univariate and multivariate analysis including recursive partitioning and amalgamation. Lung Cancer 1996; 15:65–77.

20. Palomares MR, Sayre JW, Shekar CK, Lillington LM, Chlebowski RT. Gender influence on weight-less pattern and survival of non-small cell lung carcinoma patients. Cancer 1986; 78:2119–2126.

21. Ferguson MK, Skosey C, Hoffman PC, Golomb HM. Sex-association differences in presentation and survival in patients with lung cancer. J Clin Oncol 1990; 8:6402–6407.

22. Charloux A, Rossignol M, Purohit A, Small D, Wolkove N, Pauli G, Quoix E, Kreisman H. International differences in epidemiology of lung adenocarcinoma. Lung Cancer 1997; 16:133–143.

23. Hespanhol V, Queiroga H, Magalhaes A, Santos AR, Coelho M, Marques A. Survival predictors in advanced non-small cell lung cancer. Lung Cancer 1995; 13:253–267.

24. Trumble EL, Carer CL, Cain D, Freindlin B, Ungerleider RS, Friedman MA. Representation of older patients in cancer treatment trials. Cancer 1994; 74:2208–2214.

25. Jeremic B, Shibamoto Y. Pre-treatment prognostic factors in patients with stage III non-small cell lung cancer. Lung Cancer 1995; 13:21–30.

26. Charloux A, Hedelin G, Dietemann A, Ifoundza TP, Roeslin N, Pauli G, Quoix E. The prognostic value of histology in patients with non-small cell lung cancer. Lung Cancer 1997; 17:123-134.

27. Ries LA. Influence of extent of disease, histology and demographic factors on lung cancer survival in the SEER population-based data. Semin Surg Oncol 1994; 10:21–30.

28. Foucher P, Coudert B, Arveux P, Bouton MC, Kisterman JP, Bernard A, Faivre J, Jeannin L. Age and prognosis of non-small cell lung cancer. Usefulness of relative survival model. Eur J Cancer 1993; 29A:1809–1813.

29. Fry WA, Menck HR, Wincheter DP. The National Cancer Data Base report on lung cancer. Cancer 1996; 7:1947–1955.

30. Graham MV, Geitz LM, Byhardt R, Asbell S, Roach M, Urtasun RC, Cuvean WJ, Lattin P, Russell AH, Cox JD. Comparison of prognostic factors and survival among black patients and white patients treated with irradiation for non-small cell lung cancer. J Natl Cancer Inst 1992; 84:1731.

31. Espinosa E, Felice J, Zamora P, Gonzales Baron M, Sanchez JJ, Ordonez A, Espinosa J. Serum albumin and other prognostic factors related to response and survival patients with advanced non-small cell lung cancer. Lung Cancer 1995: 1:67–76.

32. Rapp E, Pater KL, Willan A, Cormier Y, Huray N, Evans WK, Hodsen DI, Clark DA, Feld R, Arnold AM. Chemotherapy can prolong survival in patients with advanced non-small cell lung cancer: report of a Canadian multicenter randomized trial. J Clin Oncol 1988; 6: 633–641.

33. Schleusener JT, Tazelaar HD, Jung SH, Cha SS, Cera PJ, Myers JL, Creagan FT, Goldberg RM, Marschke RF. Neuroendocrine differentiation is an independent prognostic factor in chemotherapy-treated non-small cell lung carcinoma. Cancer 1996; 77:1284–1291.

34. Graziano SL, Mazid R, Newamn N, Tatum A, Oler A, Mortimer JA, Gullo JJ, DiFino SM, Scalzo AJ. The use of neuroendocrine immunoperoxidase markers to predict chemotherapy response in patients with non-small cell lung cancer. J Clin Oncol 1989; 7:1398–1406.
35. Pedersen LM, Milman N. Prognostic significance of thrombocytosis in patients with primary lung cancer. Eur Respir J 1996; 9:1826–1830.
36. Pujol JL, Grenier J, Daures JP, Daven A, Pujol H, Michel FB. Serum fragment of cytokeratin subunit 19 measured by Cyfra 21–1. Immunoradiometric assay as a marker of lung cancer. Cancer Res 1993; 53:61–66.
37. Wieskopf B, Demangeat C, Purohit A, Stenger R, Gries P, Kreisman H, Quoix E. Cyfra 21–1 as a histological marker of non-small cell lung cancer. Evaluation of sensitivity, specificity and prognostic role. Chest 1995; 108:163–169.
38. Andoh M, Gemma A, Takenaka K, Hisakatsu S, Yamada K, Usuki J, Hasegawa K, Sakonji M, Kudoh S, Tsuboie E. Serum neuron-specific enolase level as a prognostic factor in non-small cell lung cancer. Intern Med 1994; 33:271–276.
39. Non-small cell lung cancer collaboration group. Chemotherapy in non-small cell lung cancer: a meta-analysis using updated data on individual patients from 52 randomised clinical trials. Br Med J 1995; 311:899–909.
40. Anderson JR, Cain KC, Gelber RD. Analysis of survival by tumor response. J Clin Oncol 1983; 1:710–719.
41. Oye RK, Shapiro MF. Does response make a difference in patient survival? JAMA 1984; 252:2722–2725.
42. Bonomi PD, Finkelstein DM, Ruckdeschel JC, Blum RH, Green MD, Mason B, Hahn R, Tormey DC, Harris J, Comis R, Glick J. Combination chemotherapy vesus single agents followed by combination chemotherapy in stage IV non-small cell lung cancer: a study of the Eastern Cooperative Oncology Groups. J Clin Oncol 1989; 7:1602–1613.
43. Ruckdeschel JC, Finkelstein DM, Ettinger DS, Greech RH, Mason BA, Joss RA, Vogl S. A randomized trial of the four most active regimens for metastatic non-small cell lung cancer. J Clin Oncol 1986; 4:14–22.
44. Feinstein AR, Sosin SM, Wells CK. The Will Rogers phenomenon: stage migration and new diagnostic techniques as a source of misleading statistics for survival in cancer. N Engl J Med 1985; 312:1604–1608.
45. Donnadieu N, Paesmans M, Sculier JP. Chemotherapy of non-small cell lung cancer according to disease extent: a meta-analysis of the literature. Lung Cancer 1991; 7:243–252.
46. Depierre A, Chastang C, Quoix E, Lebeau B, Blanchon F, Paillot N, Lemarié E, Milleron B, Moro D, Clavier J, Herman D, Tuchais E, Jacoulet P, Brechot JM, Cordier JF, Solal-Celigny P, Badri N, Besenval M. Vinorelbine versus vinorelbine plus cisplatin in advanced non-small cell lung cancer: a randomized trial. Ann Oncol 1994; 5:37–42.
47. Le Chevalier T, Brisgand D, Douillard JY, Pujol JL, Alberola V, Monnier A Rivière A, Lianes P, Chomy P, Cigolari S, Gottfried M, Ruffié P, Panizo A, Gaspard MH, Ravaioli A, Besenval M, Besson F, Martinez A, Berthaud P, Tursz T. Randomized study of vinorelbine and cisplatin versus vindesine and cisplatin versus vinorelbin alone in advanced non-small cell lung cancer: results of a European multicenter trial including 612 patients. J Clin Oncol 1994; 12: 360–367.
48. Coen V, Van Lancker M, de Neve W, Storme G. Prognostic factors in locoregional non-small cell lung cancer treated with radiotherapy. Am J. Clin Oncol 1995; 18:111–117.
49. Komaki R, Cox JD, Hartz AJ. Characteristics of long-term survivors after treatment for inoperable carcinoma of the lung. Am J Clin Oncol 1985; 8:362–370.
50. Sculier JP, Paesmans M, Libert P, Bureau G, Dabouis G, Thiriaux J, Michel J, Van Cutsen O, Schmerber J, Giner V, Berchier MC, Sergysels R, Mommen P, Klastersky J. Long-term survival after chemotherapy containing platine derivations in patients with advanced unresectable non-small cell lung cancer. Eur J Cancer 1994; 30A:1342–1347.
51. Finkelstein DM, Ettinger DS, Ruckdeschel JC. Long term survivors in metastatic non-small cell lung cancer: an Eastern Cooperative Oncology Group Study. J Clin Oncol 1986; 4: 702–709.

37

Conventional Radiotherapy and New Approaches to Lung Cancer

PAUL VAN HOUTTE

Jules Bordet Institute
Brussels, Belgium

FRANÇOIS MORNEX

Centre Hospitalier Lyon Sud
Pierre-Bénite, France

During recent years, the role and possibilities of radiation in the management of lung cancers have become better understood through the identification of prognostic, biological, and technical factors. In the past, radiation was often regarded more as a palliative form of treatment rather than as a curative modality in spite of an overall 5-year survival rate between 5 and 10%. Indeed, the treatment philosophy varies widely from one country to another based on local tradition. Furthermore, patients referred for radiation are often considered inoperable due either to locoregional tumor extension or to medical contraindication. Therefore, before reviewing the progress made over the last years, it is important to summarize some principles of radiation therapy.

I. Basic Principles

The interaction of ionizing radiation with matter proceeds through a cascade of events from the initial ionization process to the later biological effects. In clinical practice, the radiation cell kill is caused by the loss of capacity for clonogenic cells to proliferate or divide. This explains the delay between the treatment and the clinical signs. Furthermore, the radiation effects on dividing cells are random events: the

595

proportion of surviving cells decreases as the radiation dose increases, but for a given dose of radiation, the proportion of cells destroyed remains constant. Therefore, there is a clear dose-response relationship: the probability of controlling a tumor increases with higher radiation dose. Furthermore, the dose required to control a tumor must increase according to its size or the number of cells present. Those basic principles were identified in the 1960s for head and neck or cervical cancers and have been clearly demonstrated in the well-known Radiation Therapy Oncology Group trial for lung cancer (RTOG 73-01). This trial evaluated three different radiation doses of 40, 50, and 60 delivered with 2 Gy daily fractions; 60 Gy induced a better local control and an improved 3-year survival rate when compared to 40Gy: the 3-year survival rates were, respectively, 6% after 40 Gy, 10% after 50 Gy, and 15% after 60 Gy (1). Several studies including this RTOG trial have also shown the impact of the tumor size on local control and long-term survival (2–4). In the series of Dosoretz including 152 patients with medically inoperable non–small-cell (NSC) lung cancer without lymph node involvement, the 4-year actuarial risk of local relapse was 38% for T1 tumor and 80% for T2 and T3 tumors (3). In the series of Morita including 149 patients, the risk of local failure at 5 years was, respectively, 38% for tumors less than 3 cm, 45% for tumors between 3 and 5 cm, and 68% for tumors larger than 5 cm (4).

The same principle also applies to normal cells and tissues leading to the notion of a therapeutic ratio: the difference between the doses required to control the tumor and the one inducing permanent and severe damage, the limiting factor for radiation. The normal tissues of the body have been divided by their proliferative activities as rapidly proliferating tissues (e.g., bone marrow, esophageal epithelium, skin) and slowly proliferating tissues (e.g., lung, spinal cord, heart). In the former tissues, an active proliferation is seen to maintain a steady state between active progenitor cells and mature functional cells. After irradiation, the number of cells undergoing mitosis is progressively reduced, leading to a nonreplacement of mature cells, which may cause an esophagitis, an erythema, or an epithelitis. A rapid regeneration may take place to compensate for such damage and does occur during a classical radiation course. Damage to rapid proliferating tissues depends on the total dose of radiation and the time interval between fractions. In contrast, slow proliferating tissues do not show any active regeneration process during a radiation course and are more sensitive to the dose per fraction: large fractions lead to more cell deaths and to more late damage.

The quality of the radiation procedure is another important factor. Modern radiation treatment is very complex, requiring the cooperation of many different specialties including radiation oncologists, radiologists, physicists, and technicians. We need to know precisely the tumor limits, the position of normal organs, and their relationship with the target volume to individualize the treatment to achieve the best dose distribution (precise treatment planning based on CT data) and to achieve a good daily reproducibility of each treatment. Any error in this chain of events will necessarily have a negative impact on the treatment results. This has been clearly outlined by several studies performing quality control audit of different radiation protocols. In the already quoted trial of the RTOG, the median survival dropped from 50 weeks for patients treated according to the protocol to 23 weeks for patients with major deviation (the target volume was not well covered by the radiation fields) (2). Interestingly, in the classical Dillman trial, a review has showed that the tumor was not well covered in 22% of the patients: even in a combined approach, a precise radiation technique remains mandatory to take the full benefit from an induction chemotherapeutic program (5).

Studies have also demonstrated the importance of another basic radiobiological property: repopulation may also occur at the tumor level. In 1988, Withers et al. suggested that for head and neck tumors, this mechanism of proliferation may start after 3 weeks of treatment, requiring an additional radiation dose to compensate for an increased number of malignant clonogenic cells (6). The prolongation of the radiation treatment by a few days or a treatment interruption of several weeks, such as the rest period introduced in a split-course schedule, led to a decrease in tumor control or survival: in the RTOG trial evaluating different hyperfractionated schedules, the 2-year survival rate dropped from 33 to 14% if the treatment had been delayed for more than 5 days (7).

Nevertheless, even with the best classical radiation schedule, the results remain disappointing in terms of both survival and local control. In the French trial of Arriagada and Le Chevalier, a precise pattern of failure analysis was performed using repeated fiberoptic bronchoscopies and restaging procedures for stage III disease. This trial compared a course of radiation delivering 65 Gy to an induction chemotherapy program followed by the same radiation schedule. The local control rate at 1 year in the two arms was only 17% (8). This figure differs from several reports but reflects only differences in the definition of local control (e.g., first site of failure, in-field failure, ultimate control, absence of local evolution), in the restaging procedure (e.g., repeated fiberoptic bronchoscopies, CT), and difficulties in differentiating fibrosis from tumor relapse.

Several approaches are under investigation to improve our treatment efficacy: increasing the biological radiation dose (e.g., radiosensitizers, concomitant chemotherapy, modifications of the fractionation) or increasing the physical radiation dose (conformal radiotherapy, brachytherapy, and intraoperative irradiation). In the next pages, we will discuss some of the aspects of these radiation innovations.

II. Increasing the Biological Radiation Dose: Modifications of Fractionation

Fractionation is aimed to take advantage of the four radiobiological principles (reoxygenation, reparation, redistribution, and repopulation). This has led to the classical radiation schedule delivering one fraction per day (usually around 2 Gy), 5 days a week for 3–7 weeks. However, several other fractionation schedules have been developed in the past on an empirical basis and more recently reflecting different radiobiological properties of tumor and normal tissues. In the past, split-course radiation schedules were introduced after the observation that patients tolerated better the treatment after a break of 2–3 weeks, and in case of tumor progression, the second course of radiation may be omitted reducing the number of treatments as well as the workload of busy departments. In fact, split-course radiation schedules use daily fractions for 1–2 weeks followed by a rest period of 2–4 weeks followed by a second radiation course. Nevertheless, this rest period also has a major drawback—allowing a possible tumor repopulation. The use of a daily dose higher than 2 Gy may induce more severe late damage. None of the studies have demonstrated any benefit from a split-course radiation schedule, but some have shown a negative impact on survival or local control (1,2). Such schedules are nowadays reserved for palliation or for experimental protocols including chemotherapy when a break is necessary to overcome excessive toxicity.

The new schedules attempt to take advantage of the most recent radiobiological observations. Indeed, late complications are observed in slowly proliferating tissues where the time factor is not an important parameter but the fraction size has a major influence: large fractions increase the risk of late damage. In contrast, early acute effects are observed in rapidly proliferating tissues and are closely dependent on the daily radiation dose and the weekly dose, rather than the fraction size. Most tumors seems to have a fraction size dependency close to the one of proliferating tissue. The use of several fractions per day each delivering a small dose and separated by a time interval allowing the repair process to take place in normal tissues makes it possible to increase the total radiation dose, which is expected to improve the therapeutic ratio. Classical hyperfractionated schedules delivered two to three fractions per day of 1–1.2 Gy, separated by a 6-hour intervals, 5 days a week for the same duration as a one fraction per day radiation schedule.

The second important radiobiological observation is related to the problem of tumor repopulation: the onset of a repopulation mechanism at the level of the tumor will lead to a loss of efficacy due to a major increase of clonogenic malignant cells. Reducing the duration of the treatment is then the only answer and requires the use of several fractions per day but with doses greater than 1.2 Gy per fraction. The critical issue with those accelerated hyperfractionated radiation schedules is the tolerance of rapidly proliferating tissues and the acute effects: the daily and weekly doses are higher than with a classical one fraction per day schedule. Several approaches have been developed to overcome this problem of acute tolerance: the introduction of a gap during the treatment, the completion of all the treatment before the onset of the acute effect or the use of a concomitant boost to reduce the volume of normal tissue irradiated. Those different schedules will be reviewed in the light of our experience.

A. Clinical Experience in Non–Small-Cell Lung Cancer

Classical Hyperfractionated Schedule

This approach has mainly been investigated by the RTOG. In a large phase II study (RTOG 83-11), two fractions of 1.2 Gy separated by at least 4 hours were delivered to a total dose ranging from 60 to 79.2 Gy. The study was designed to search for the

Table 1 Randomized Trials of Altered Fractionation for Non–Small-Cell Lung Cancer

| Radiation schedule | | | | | 2-year | |
Dose (Gy)	Duration (weeks)	Fraction	No. of patients	Esophageal toxicity (%)	survival rate (%)	Ref.
60	6	30	23	9	No difference	13
60	3	30	26	35		
60	6	30	225	19	20[a]	14
54	2	36	338	49	30	
60	6	30	149		19	10
69.6	6	58	152	1.3[b]	24	
63.9	6	32	51	No difference	No difference	11
69.6	6	38	54			
65	6.5	26	18		31	12
71.5	6.5	52	18		50	

[a]The difference is statistically significant.
[b]Only grade 4 toxicity.

optimal total dose and recruited more than 880 patients. The dose of 69.6 Gy produced the best benefit with a median survival of 13 months compared to 9–10 months in previous RTOG trials with a classical 60 Gy schedule, one fraction per day. This was obtained without an increase in acute or late toxicity (9). This 69.6 Gy hyperfractionated schedule was then tested in a three-arm randomized trial comparing this new experimental schedule to 60 Gy in daily 2 Gy fractions and to an induction chemotherapy program followed by 60 Gy (the combined arm of the CALGB trial)(5). The trial recruited 490 patients, and data are available with a 3-year follow-up. Four grade 4 toxicity were reported in the hyperfractionated arm compared to one in the standard radiation arm: two were directly related to an acute esophagitis. The 1-, 2-, and 3-year survival rates were, respectively, 46, 19, and 6% after a standard radiation course and 51, 24, and 13% after a hyperfractionated schedule (10). Those differences are not statistically significant but suggest a trend in favor of the hyperfractionated schedule. Probably the number of patients included in this trial was too low to show a small difference as expected from the 8% increase in biological total radiation dose. Data from other randomized trials are summarized in Table 1: most trials recruited a limited number of patients (11,12).

Accelerated Hyperfractionated Schedules

This approach has been investigated mainly in several phase II studies. They showed the feasibility of this treatment but also outlined one limiting factor when trying to shortening the treatment duration: the acute tolerance of the esophagus. In a trial conducted in Australia by Ball et al., patients were randomized to receive 60 Gy in 6 weeks and 30 fractions or 60 Gy in 30 fractions over 3 weeks with or without concomitant carboplatin. In an interim analysis including the first 100 randomized patients, the estimated median duration of esophagitis was 1.4 month for the conventional treatment and 3.2 months for the accelerated arm (13). The rate of grade 3 and 4 esophagitis were, respectively, 9 and 0% for the conventional arm and 31 and 4% for the accelerated schedule: six patients required dilatation for an esophageal stricture, and one died from a laryngoesophageal fistula with negative biopsies.

An extreme example of an accelerated program is certainly the CHART (Continuous, Hyperfractionated, Accelerated, Radiation Therapy), a radiation schedule introduced by the Mount Vernon team. The main concept was first not to leave any gap during the treatment by treating every day including the weekend and to complete the treatment before the onset of repopulation or acute effects: patients received three fractions per day of 1.5 Gy separated by a 6-hour intervals for 12 consecutive days. The initial 37.5 Gy were delivered to a large volume including the whole mediastinum, whereas the remaining dose was given to the gross tumor volume. It was felt that the loss of total radiation dose (54 Gy for the CHART vs. 60 Gy for a conventional treatment) would be offset by the gain in tumor repopulation. After a phase II study, this experimental schedule was compared in a randomized trial to a classical treatment of 60 Gy in 6 weeks with one daily fraction of 2 Gy (14). This trial recruited 563 patients in 5 years. Regarding the acute and late effects, moderate or severe dysphagia were seen in 49% of the CHART patients compared to 19% for the conventional arm; esophageal stricture occurred, respectively, in 7% of the CHART patients compared to 4% in the control group. The complete tumor response rates were 34% after the CHART and 29% after a conventional schedule leading, respectively, to 2-year survival rates of 29 and 20% (this difference was statistically significant). The largest benefit was seen in patients with squamous cell carcinoma, with a 34% reduction in the relative risk of death: the 2-year survival rate improved from 19 to 33% for the CHART and the 3-year rate from 10 to 21%. Studies are ongoing to modify this fractionation by omitting treatment during the weekend and by increasing the total dose from 54 to 60 Gy in 3 weeks: CHARTWEL in a phase II trial led to similar results as the CHART schedule (15).

Is 6 hours the optimal interval between two fractions of irradiation? This interval was proposed based on kinetic repair of normal tissue damage (the half-life for most tissues appears to be between 1 and 2 hours) and on clinical experience showing greater damage after shorter intervals: Cox et al. found an increase in late toxicity with intervals less than 4.5 hours for patients treated with two fractions a day for carcinoma of the upper respiratory tract (16). Little information is available on the effect of time interval on the tumor. In a recent paper, Jeremic et al. reviewed their experience in NSC lung cancer treated with two daily fractions of 1.2 Gy to a total of 64.8 Gy with or without chemotherapy (carboplatin and etoposide)(17). In a multivariate analysis, the time interval appeared to be an independent prognostic factor together with the classical factors such as sex, age, performance status, and stage. The 1-, 3-, and 5-year survival rates were, respectively, 71, 30, and 27% for an interval of 5 hours or less and 36, 0, and 0% for an interval of 5.5–6 hours. Additional data are necessary to define the optimal radiation schedule when modifying the classical daily treatment.

The Concomitant Boost

When accelerating a radiation schedule, one main limitation is the esophageal mucosal reaction, as observed in the Ball trial. To avoid this problem, a treatment interruption is often introduced. Another alternative is to use a concomitant boost approach: the second fraction of radiation is limited to the area of known tumor disease. Through this reduction in field size, the large volumes are not treated, reducing the risk of acute and late effects. Several programs have been evaluated in phase II trials varying the total dose, the dose per fraction, and the time interval between the large field and the boost field (Table 2)(18–21). Once again grade 3 or more esophageal toxicity appears to be the main problem. Grade 3 esophageal toxicity implies a severe dysphagia, with a weight loss of more than 15% requiring artificial alimentation. The field size as well as the mean dose were major factors influencing the risk of severe acute and late esophagitis in the Dutch experience; they recommended avoiding an elective field greater than 17 cm in length: one patient developed a late stenosis after receiving 60 Gy with an elective field of 17 cm (18). Those studies showed the feasibility of this approach, but the possible benefit compared to a more classical radiation schedule is unknown. One other possible advantage of the concomitant boost approach is certainly the possibility of delivering the boost at the same time as the large field, avoiding twice-daily treatment, which is always very cumbersome for a radiation department as well as for the patient.

B. Clinical Experience in Small-Cell Lung Cancer

The problem with small-cell lung cancer is slightly different, as the treatment involves combining radiotherapy and chemotherapy taking into account an increasing risk of acute and late effects. A meta-analysis has evaluated the role of thoracic irradiation after chemotherapy on survival and local control: radiation improved the 3-year survival rate by 5.4% and the local control rate by 25.3% (22). Furthermore, Murray carried out a meta-analysis on the optimal timing of radiation: early radiation delivery appeared to be superior in terms of local control and survival (23). The dose response for small-cell lung cancer is certainly not so well-defined as for non–small-cell lung cancer. The data from retrospective studies suggest a dose response with increased local control when increasing the total radiation dose: in the review of Choi and Carey, the 2.5-year local control rates were, respectively, 16% after 30 Gy, 51% after 40 Gy, and 63% after 50 Gy (24). Only one trial addressed the question of the total radiation dose. In the NCI Canada trial, patients were randomized to receive either three courses of cytoxan, doxorubicin, and vincristine followed by three courses of etoposide, cisplatin or an alternating chemotherapy program with the same drugs (25). Responding patients were further randomized to receive either 25 Gy in 10 fractions over 2 weeks or 37.5 Gy in 15 fractions over 3 weeks. The actuarial incidence of local progression rate by 2 years was 80% for 25 Gy and 69% for 37.5 Gy.

Small-cell lung cancer cell lines present interesting radiobiological characteristics: in cell culture, the dose-response curve to radiation presents almost no initial shoulder; this implies a low repair capacity and makes this cell particularly interest-

Table 2 Concomitant Boost Schedules for Non–Small-Cell Lung Cancer

Large field dose/fr (Gy)	Boost field dose/fr (Gy)	Addit.	Interval (hr)	Large field (Gy)	Dose tumor (Gy)	Duration (weeks)	No. of patients	Esophageal toxicity (%)	Ref.
2 × 20	0.5 × 20		6	40	50	4	37	0	19
1.25 × 36	0.35 × 36	1.6 × 10	0	45	73.6	4.5	49	18	20
2 × 20	0.75 × 20		0	40	55	4	33	20	18
1.8 × 25	1.8 × 10		4–6	45	63	5	61		21
1.8 × 28	1.8 × 10		4–6	50.4	70.2	5.5	180	7.2	
1.8 × 25	1.8 × 14		4–6	45	70.2	5	114	14	

ing for a hyperfractionated radiation schedule using doses lower than 2 Gy per fraction. Furthermore, reducing the treatment duration may help avoid the problem of repopulation. In a randomized trial, 45 Gy given daily over 5 weeks was compared to 45 Gy with two fractions per day (1.5 Gy per fraction) over 3 weeks. We should notice that the biological equivalent dose is quite different for both arms (about 40 Gy with conventional fractionation vs. more than 50 Gy with hyperfractionation). In both arms, patients received the same chemotherapy program (cisplatin and etoposide). An increased acute toxicity was observed with two daily fractions. More interestingly, the two survival curves diverged after 2 years with a statistical improvement favoring the two daily fractions: the 2-, 3-, and 5-year survival rates were, respectively, 40.8, 26.7, and 20% for one daily fraction and 46.6, 31, and 28% for two daily fractions. The local failure rate dropped from 52% to 36% (Turrisi, personal communication).

Alternating programs were introduced to keep both chemotherapy and radiotherapy in close temporal proximity but with enough gap to minimize toxicity. In fact chemotherapy is given in "normal" dose and radiation is administered one week after and interrupted one week before the next chemotherapy. This week gap makes it possible to avoid most of the possible toxicity induced by a combined approach. So, radiation is delivered in two to four consecutive courses. The different phase II studies have shown interesting results with 2-year survival rates in the range of 12–40%. This approach was tested by the EORTC Lung Group comparing an alternating schedule to a sequential approach where the radiation was delivered after the six cycles of chemotherapy. No difference was observed in terms of survival or local control, but a higher complication rate was reported for the alternating arm (26). The main criticism of this study is based on the type of chemotherapy used: doxorubicin, cytoxan, etoposide. Currently, the most promising results are observed with a concomitant approach and with early delivery of radiation: 2-year survival rates vary from 40 to 60% (23). The limiting factor is normal tissue toxicity, especially acute esophagitis. Several issues remain unresolved, e.g., the optimal radiation dose, the volume to be treated.

III. Increasing the Physical Radiation Dose

According to a basic principle, increasing the physical radiation dose will make it possible to destroy more clonogenic cells and to control a higher number of tumors leading to a higher cure rate provided that this increase in dose does not induce more severe life-threatening late effects. Several approaches are possible due to recent technical developments: brachytherapy techniques include endoluminal brachytherapy, intraoperative radiotherapy, and conformal radiotherapy.

A. Intraoperative Radiotherapy

Intraoperative radiotherapy (IORT) was introduced to overcome the main limitation of radiation, the tolerance of normal tissues, by delivering the radiation to the target area while keeping the normal tissues outside the radiation field. This approach is very old and has aroused new interest during the last decades, initially in Japan for gastrointestinal tumors and later in several western countries. The use of a cone allows us to keep normal ε structure out of the treated area. The single fraction uses an electron beam to limit the penetration in the tissues. The major drawbacks are certainly this single fraction limiting the total dose due to the absence of possible repair process and the practical organization: the operating rooms are often far away from the radiation department. In animal experiments, the trachea and the main blood vessels tolerate doses in excess of 20 Gy; the critical factor is the limited tolerance of the lung, heart, and esophagus: esophageal fistula were observed for doses in excess of 20 Gy (27). The clinical experience with IORT is very limited due to the technical difficulties but the data available confirmed the feasibility of this approach; the single radiation dose should not exceed 20 Gy (27,28).

B. Conformal Radiotherapy

Three-dimensional conformal radiotherapy is already an old concept which has gained a new interest following the great advances in imaging (CT and MR), computed facilities, and radiotherapeutic equipment. Indeed, the clinical target volume includes the gross tumor volume (GTV) and the microscopic tumor extent (CTV). When planning a radiation course, we must add to this clinical target volume, an area to take into account for uncertainties related to the daily reproducibility of the treatment, the possible displacements (breathing, heart beatings), the characteristics of the radiation equipment (penumbra, shapes of the beam): all those factors contribute to increase the volume of tissue irradiated (planning target volume or PTV). The aim of three-dimensional conformal radiotherapy is to match precisely the borders of the treated volume to the clinical target volume, sparing as much as possible of normal tissues. This reduction of normal tissues irradiated makes it possible to deliver safely an increased dose to the target area. Of course, this new technique seeks to precisely control the chain of events from tumor evaluation to the daily treatment itself and to fulfill several requirements:

> A precise definition of the tumor extent and its relationship to surrounding tissues and organs. For lung cancer, this requires a CT in radiation treatment setup with the possibility of three-dimensional reconstruction.
> A three-dimensional treatment planning aiming to achieve a precise dose distribution by using multiple fields of irradiation including the possibility of dynamic controlled rotation of the linear accelerator and opening of the collimator to modify the field size during the rotation. Furthermore, a digital reconstructed radiography is very helpful in matching the image with the one obtained with an on-line imaging system and so to verify the beam accuracy.
> The linear accelerator should be equipped with a multileaf collimator making it possible to precisely adapt the radiation beam to the treatment require-

ments and an on-line imaging system making it possible to verify the treatment setup.
An accurate patient repositioning during the course of fractionated radiation therapy using immobilization devices.

The data available have clearly demonstrated that three-dimensional conformal radiotherapy makes it possible either to increase the dose above 70 or even 80 Gy while keeping the dose to normal tissues within tolerance limits or to reduce the dose to the normal tissues while keeping the same dose to the target area. The latter is quite interesting when the pulmonary function of the patients is severely altered such as after a pneumonectomy: in the experience of Schraube et al., the dose to the target area was 49 Gy and the biological mean dose to the lung was, respectively, 12 Gy after two-dimensional treatment planning and 9.4 Gy after three-dimensional treatment planning (29). The main limiting factor when escalating the total radiation dose is often the amount of normal lung volume irradiated and not the spinal cord. Dose volume histograms (DVH) have clearly outlined the relation between the volume of lung receiving doses in excess of 25 Gy and the risk of radiation pneumonitis: in a study by Armstrong et al., three patients out of eight developed radiation pneumonitis when more than 30% of the lung received more than 25 Gy, compared to 1 out of 23 for lower irradiated lung volume (30). Graham et al. reported no case of grade 3 pneumonitis when less than 25% of the lung received more than 20 Gy compared to a rate of 19% when the volume of lung irradiated was greater than 37.6% (31). Current protocols are escalating the total dose according to the estimated risk of lung complication based on DVH. Nevertheless, DVH assumes that all parts of the lung have the same biological functions leading to a more favorable estimation, such as in the case of emphysema or lung surgery. Another problem is related to organ displacement due to the breathing. An approach called "gating" is investigating the possibility of performing the radiation during the same phase of the breathing to avoid the problems of displacement and changes in volume. Furthermore, to allow this dose escalation, there is a current trend to reduce the volume treated by not performing an elective nodal irradiation based on the low rate of nodal relapse and to limit the clinical target volume to the gross tumor volume including the enlarged lymph nodes seen on CT. By avoiding this elective nodal irradiation, the sparing of normal lung irradiated allows a dose escalation of about 30% without increasing the probability of radiation pneumonitis (32). Last but not least, the two last limits are related to the ability of CT to define the tumor borders and to the tumor radiosensibility and/or size. The cornerstone for treatment success with conformal radiotherapy is related to the volume treated: when the volume increases due to the size of the tumor or to mediastinal lymph node involvement, the possibility of delivering doses in excess of 70 or 80 Gy is reduced due to the amount of lung volume irradiated.

Several teams have been investigating three-dimensional conformal radiotherapy for lung cancer: the data already available showed the feasibility of such an approach but also the need to deliver higher doses or to better select patients

Table 3 Conformal Radiotherapy for NSC Lung Cancer: Results of Selected Series

No. of patients	Stage I/II (%)	Doses (Gy)	Loc. fail rate (%)	2-year survival rate (%)	Ref.
99	23	60–74	Stage I–II 33%	45 III 11%	31
76	21	64–82	29	Stage I/II 56 IIIa 26 IIIb 9	34
45	13	52–72	46	32	30
37	0	60–70	49	Stage IIIa 49 IIIb 26	35

for this form of treatment (Table 3). In the recent series of Roberston et al. including 48 patients, 10 patients were treated with doses equal or greater than 84 Gy, and local biopsies showed recurrent disease in 3 patients (33). Stage is a poor predictor of tumor volume, whereas the local efficacy of radiation is directly correlated to the tumor size, an important parameter for conformal radiation therapy. In the experience of Martel et al. including 76 consecutive patients, the 2- and 5-year survival rates were correlated to the tumor volume, the nodal status and radiation dose (Table 4)(34).

IV. Conclusions

Progress have been recently made in the treatment of lung cancer with radiation. The knowledge of its limits and the new possibilities using new fractionation schedules and three-dimensional conformal radiotherapy make it important to define the optimal radiation program to be applied to each individual patient either as a single modality or in a multidisciplinary approach with surgery or chemotherapy. The quality of a treatment regardless of the modality remains a major factor for a large benefit of a combined approach: adding modalities to cover a weak technology will never make possible a breakthrough in this dreadful disease.

Table 4 Conformal Radiotherapy for NSC Lung Cancer: 2-Year Survival Rate According to Tumor Volume, Nodal Status, and Tumor Dose

	N0 (%)	N1–3 (%)
Tumor volume < 200 cm^3	59	23
Tumor volume > 200 cm^3	13	16
Isocenter dose > 73 Gy	58	
Isocenter dose < 73 Gy	31	

Source: Adapted from Ref. 34.

References

1. Perez CA, Pajak TF, Rubin P, Simpson JR, Mohiuddin M, Brady LW, Perez-Tamayo R, Rotman M. Long-term observations of the patterns of failure in patients with unresectable non oat-cell carcinoma of the lung treated with definitive radiotherapy. Cancer 1987; 59:1874–1881.
2. Perez CA, Stanley K, Grundy G, Hanson W, Rubin P, Kramer S, Brady L, Marks JE, Perez-Tamayo R, Brown GS, Concannon JP, Rotman M. Impact of irradiation technique and tumor extent in tumor control and survival of patients with unresectable non-oat cell carcinoma of the lung. Report by the Radiation Therapy Oncology Group. Cancer 1982; 50:1091–1099.
3. Dosoretz DE, Katin MJ, Blitzer PH, Rubenstein JH, Salenius S, Rashid M, Dosani RA, Mestas G, Siegel AD, Chadha TT, Chandrahasa T, Hannan SE, Bhat SB, Metke M. Radiation therapy in the management of medically inoperable carcinoma of the lung: results and implications for future treatment strategies Int J Radiat Oncol Biol Phys 1992; 24:3–9.
4. Morita K, Fuwa N, Suzuki Y, Nishio M, Sakai K, Tamaki Y, Niibe H, Chujo M, Wada S, Sugawara T, Kita M. Radical radiotherapy for medically inoperable non-small cell lung cancer in clinical stage I: a retrospective analysis of 149 patients. Radiother Oncol 1997; 42:31–36.
5. Dillman RO, Seagren SL, Propert KJ, Guerra J, Eaton WL, Perry MC, Carey RW, Frei EF, Green MR. A randomized trial of induction chemotherapy plus high-dose versus radiation alone in stage III non-small cell lung cancer N Engl J Med 1990; 323:940–945.
6. Withers HR, Taylor JMG, Maciejewski B. The hazard of accelerated tumor clonogen repopulation during radiotherapy Acta Oncol 1988; 27:131–146.
7. Cox JD, Pajak TF, Asbell S, Russell AH, Pederson J, Byhardt RW, Emami B, Roach M. Interruptions of high-dose radiation therapy decrease long-term survival of favorable patients with unresectable non-small cell carcinoma of the lung: Analysis of 1244 cases from 3 Radiation Therapy Oncology Group (RTOG) trials. Int J Radiat Oncol Biol Phys 1993; 27: 493–498.
8. Arriagada R, Le Chevalier T, Quoix E, Ruffie P, De Cremoux H, Douillard JY, Tarayre M, Pignon JP, Laplanche A for the GETCB, the FNCLCC and the CEBI trials. Effect of chemotherapy on locally advanced non-small lung carcinoma: a randomized study of 353 patients. Int J Radiat Oncol Biol Phys 1991; 20:1183–1190.
9. Cox JD, Axarnia N, Byhardt RW, Shin KH, Emami B, Pajak T. A randomized phase I/II trial of hyperfractionated radiation therapy with total doses of 60.0 to 79.2 Gy—possible survival benefit with 69.6 Gy in favorable patients with Radiation Therapy Oncology Stage III non-small cell lung carcinoma. Report of Radiation Therapy Oncology Group 83-11. J Clin Oncol 1990; 8:1543–1555.
10. Sause W, Scott C, Taylor S, Johnson D, Livingston R, Komaki R, Emami B, Curran WJ, Byhardt RW, Turrisi AT, Dar AR, Cox JD. Radiation Therapy Oncology Group (RTOG) 88-08 and Eastern Cooperative Oncology Group (ECOG) 4588 Preliminary analysis of a phase III trial in regionally advanced unresectable non-small cell lung cancer. J Natl Cancer Inst 1994; 87:198–205.
11. Fu S, Jiang GL, Wang LJ. Hyperfractionated irradiation for non-small cell lung cancer: a phase III clinical trial. Chung-Hua-Chung-Liu-Tsa-Chih 1994; 16:306–309.
12. Kagami Y, Nishio M, Narimatsu N, Ogawa H, Sakurai T. Prospective randomized trials comparing hyperfractionated radiotherapy with conventional radiotherapy in stage III non-small cell lung cancer. Nippon Igaku Hoshasen Gakai Zasshi 1992; 52:1452–1455.
13. Ball D, Bishop J, Smith J, Crennan E, O'Brien P, Davis S, Ryan G, Joseph D, Walker Q. A phase III study of accelerated radiotherapy with and without carboplatin in nonsmall cell lung cancer-an interim toxicity analysis of the first 100 patients. Int J Radiat Oncol Biol Phys 1995; 31:267–272.
14. Saunders MI, Dische S, Barrett A, Parmar MKB, Harvey A, Gibson D on behalf of the CHART Steering Committee. Randomised multicentre trials of CHART vs conventional radiotherapy in head and neck and non-small-cell lung cancer: an interim report. Br J Cancer 1996; 73:1455–1462.

15. Saunders M, Lyn E, Pigott K, Powell M, Goodchild K, Hoskin P, Phillips H. Experience of a dose escalation study using CHARTWEL (continuous hyperfractionated accelerated radiotherapy weekendless) in non-small cell lung cancer. Lung Cancer 1997; 18:123–124.

16. Cox JD, Pajak TF, Marcial VA, Coia L, Mohiuddin M, Fu KK, Selim H, Rubin P, Ortiz H and the Radiation Therapy Oncology Group. Interfraction interval is a major determinant of late effects with hyperfractionated radiation therapy of carcinomas of upper respiratory and digestive tracts: results from Radiation Therapy Oncology Group protocol 8313. Int J Radiat Oncol Biol Phys 1991; 20:1191–1195.

17. Jeremic B, Shibamoto Y. Effect of interfraction interval in hyperfractionated radiotherapy with or without concurrent chemotherapy for stage III nonsmall cell lung cancer. Int J Radiat Oncol Biol Phys 1996; 34:303–308.

18. Schuster-Uitterhoeve ALJ, Hulshof MCCM, Gonzalez DG, Koolen M, Sminia P. Feasibility of curative radiotherapy with a concomitant boost technique in 33 patients with non-small cell lung cancer (NSCLC) Radiother Oncol 1993; 28:247–251.

19. Yu E, Souhami L, Guerra J, Clark B, Gingras C, Fava P. Accelerated fractionation in inoperable non-small cell lung cancer. Cancer 1993; 71:2727–2731.

20. King SC, Acker JC, Kussin PS, Marks LB, Weeks KJ, Leopold KA. High-dose, hyperfractionated, accelerated radiotherapy sing a concurrent boost for the treatment of nonsmall cell lung cancer: unusual toxicity and promising early results. Int J Radiat Oncol Biol Phys 1996; 36:593–599.

21. Byhardt RW, Pajak TF, Emami B, Herskovic A, Doggett RS, Olsen LO. A phase I/II study to evaluate accelerated fractionation via concomitant boost for squamous, adeno, and large cell carcinoma of the lung: report of Radiation Therapy Oncology Group 84-07. Int J Radiat Oncol Biol Phys 1993; 26:459–468.

22. Pignon JP, Arriagada R, Ihde DC, Johnson DH, Perry MC, Souhami RL, Brodin O, Joss RA, Kies MS, Lebeau B, Onoshi T, Osterlind K, Tattersall MH, Wagner H. A meta-analysis of thoracic radiotherapy for small-cell lung cancer. N Engl J Med 1992; 327:1618–1624.

23. Murray N. Treatment of small cell lung cancer: the state of the art. Lung Ca 1997; 17(suppl 1):75–90.

24. Choi NC, Carey RW. Importance of radiation dose in achieving improved loco-regional tumor control in limited stage small-cell lung carcinoma: an update. Int J Radiat Oncol Biol Phys 1989; 17:307–310.

25. Coy P, Hodson I, Payne DG, Evans WK, Feld R, MacDonald AS, Osoba D, Pater JL. The effects of dose of thoracic irradiation on recurrence in patients with limited stage small cell lung cancer: initial results of a Canadian multicenter randomized trial. Int J Radiat Oncol Biol Phys 1988; 14:219–226.

26. Gregor A, Drings P, Burghouts J, Postmus PE, Morgan D, Sahmoud T, Kirkpatrick A, Dalesio O, Giaccone G. Randomized trial of alternating versus sequential radiotherapy/chemotherapy in limited-disease patients with small-cell lung cancer: a European Organization for Research and Treatment of Cancer Lung Cancer Cooperative Group Study. J Clin Oncol 1997; 15:2840–2849.

27. Tochner ZA, Pass HI, Sindelar WF, DeLuca Am, Grisell DL, Bacher JD, Kinsella TJ. Long term tolerance of thoracic organs to intraoperative radiotherapy. Int J Radiat Oncol Biol Phys 1991; 22:65–69.

28. Calvo FA, Ortiz De Urbina D, Abuchaibe O, Azinovic I, Aristu J, Santos M, Escde L, Herreros J, Llorens R. Intraoperative radiotherapy during lung cancer surgery: technical description and early clinical results. Int J Radiat Oncol Biol Phys 1990; 19:103–109.

29. Schraube P, Kampen M, Oetzel D, Sroka G, Wannenmacher M. The impact of 3-D treatment planning after a pneumonectomy compared to a conventional treatment set-up. Radiother Oncol 1995; 37:65–70.

30. Armstrong J, Raben A, Zelefsky M, Burt M, Leibel S, Burman C, Kutcher G, Harrison L, Hahn C, Ginsberg R, Rusch V, Kris M, Fuks Z. Promising survival with three-dimensional conformal radiation therapy for non-small cell lung cancer. Radiother Oncol 1997; 44:17–22.

31. Graham MV, Purdy JA, Harms W, Emami B, Drzymala R. Clinical results of three-dimensional radiation therapy for non-small cell lung cancer. Lung Cancer 1997; 18: 124–125.
32. Belderbos JSA, Lebesque JV, Barillot I. Normal tissue complication probabilities for irradiation of NSCLC patients with and without elective nodal irradiation. Lung Cancer 1997; 18:126.
33. Roberston JM, Ten Haken RK, Hazuka MB, Turrisi AT, Martel MK, Pu AT, Litlles JF, Martinez FJ, Francis IR, Quint LE, Lichter AS. Dose escalation for non-small cell lung cancer using conformal radiation therapy. Int J Radiat Oncol Biol Phys 1997; 37:1079–1085.
34. Martel MK, Strawderman M, Hazuka MB, Turrisi AT, Fraass BA, Lichter AS. Volume and dose parameters for survival of non-small cell lung cancer patients. Radiother Oncol 1997; 44:23–30.
35. Sibley GS, Mundt AJ, Shapiro C, Jacobs R, Chen G, Weichselbaum R, Vijayakumar S. The treatment of stage III nonsmall cell lung cancer using high dose conformal radiotherapy. Int J Radiat Oncol Biol Phys 1995; 33:1001–1007.

38

Chemotherapy in Small-Cell Lung Cancer
Is More Better?

FABRIZIO M. FACCHINI and STEPHEN G. SPIRO

Middlesex Hospital
London, England

I. Introduction

Many treatment strategies have attempted to improve outcomes for patients with small-cell lung cancer (SCLC), but there is still no single standard optimal chemotherapy regime. With present regimes, complete response (CR) is achieved in 45–75% of patients with limited stage disease (LD) and in 20–30% of those with extensive disease (ED). Median response duration is about a year, and the recurrent tumor has become resistant to therapy in most patients. After treatment, only 5.9% of patients are alive at 2 years (1). Overall median survival is about 12 months (8 months in ED and 14 months in LD). The overall 5-year survival rate is 3.5% (4.8% for LD and 2.3% for ED) and at 10 years is 1.8% (2.5% for LD and 1.2% for ED) (2). Although poor, these figures are better than a median survival of 2–4 months and near zero long-term survivors prior to the chemotherapy era (3–5). Active drugs show a single-agent objective response (OR) rate of 20–50% in patients who have never been treated and an OR of 10% or more if given to previously treated patients (Table 1).

Table 1 Response Rates to Single-Agent Chemotherapy in Untreated and Previously Treated Patients

Drug	Naive patients			Previously treated patients		
	No. of patients	OR (CR) %	Ref.	No. of patients	OR (CR) %	Ref.
Cisplatin				143	15(1)	96
Carboplatin	76	59(11)		N/A	17	97
			97	72	13(4)	98
Cyclophosphamide	307	32	99			
Ifosfamide	43[a]	49	100,101	14	43	103
	198	50	102	41	15	98
Mechlorethamine	80	39	99,102			
Hexamethylmelamine	83	26	99,102			
Procarbazine	44	25	99,102	24	0	98
Carmustine (BCNU)	19	21	99,102			
Semustine (MeCCNU)	44	11	99,102			
Lomustine (CCNU)	76	14	99,102			
Fluorouracil				26	12	98
Doxorubicin	86	27	99,102	14	29	98
Epirubicin	40[a]	50	104	14	7	98
	107	49(7.5)	99,102			
Methotrexate	110	26	99,102	17	0	98
Etoposide	61[a]	80	19	388	11	98
	18[b]	100(12)	105			
	59[a]	75(0)	105			
	229	45	99,102			
Teniposide	33	90(30)	106	117	15	98
	48	71(23)	107			
	90	41	99,102			
Vincristine	43	42	99,102	24	21	98
Vindesine	78	8	99,102	100	17	98

[a]ED.
[b]LD.
Source: Modified from Ref. 108.

II. Combination Chemotherapy

Current multiple-agent chemotherapy achieves an OR in 65–100% of patients and a median survival of 7–11 months in patients with ED and 10–14 months in those with LD, with apparent cures in approximately 10% of patients with LD. The most widely used combinations of chemotherapy include cyclophosphamide, doxorubicin, and vincristine (CAV), and etoposide and cisplatin (EP).

A. Epipodophyllotoxins/Platinum Compounds

Sierocki et al. (6) gave two cycles of cisplatin 60 mg/m^2 on day 1 and etoposide 120 mg/m^2 on days 4, 6, and 8. Of the 38 patients with evaluable disease, maximum responses were obtained at the end of the second cycle and did not improve with additional different drug cycles. All 21 LD patients responded with 52% achieving a CR, and 88% of the ED patients responded with 41% achieving a CR. Evans et al. (7) recorded similar response rates (43% of CR and 43% of PR) in 28 previously untreated patients with six cycles of etoposide 100 mg/m^2 on days 1–3 and cisplatin 25 mg/m^2 on days 1–3 given every 21 days. When given as second-line treatment, the EP regime achieved an OR of 40–55% (8,9), with a 17% CR rate in patients with LD. Its efficacy has also been evaluated in randomized trials as induction or consolidation regime or in alternating regimes (10–14). Substitution of etoposide with etoposide phosphate (15) or cisplatin with carboplatin (16–18) has had little additional effect. The scheduling of etoposide and of the combination EP is important. Etoposide 500 mg/m^2 given as a 24-hour continuous infusion gave worse results than the same dose administered as a 2-hour infusion every day for 5 days in 39 previously untreated patients (19). The 5-day schedule achieved an 89% OR versus 10% OR for the 24-hour schedule. Maksymiuk et al. (20) included 552 patients in a four-arm comparison of different duration of i.v. scheduling of EP over 3 days. They found an i.v. bolus of EP to be similar to 24-hour infusion, and it appeared to be superior to the longer infusion scheduling if cisplatin was given as the first drug.

B. Cyclophosphamide/Anthracyclins/Vincristine

The CAV regime is probably the most widely used drug combination in SCLC. Early trials using this combination reported very high response rates, with CR higher than 59% (21–23). Its efficacy has been compared in many randomized trials (24–27).

III. Duration: Short- Versus Long-Course Treatment

Treatment of SCLC in the 1970s was often continued for 18–24 months. Early randomized trials comparing maintenance therapy to short treatment periods were not able to provide an unequivocal answer as to the optimal duration of chemotherapy. However, this question was addressed in several trials during the 1980s. In Birmingham, Cullen et al. (28) gave either no further treatment until relapse or eight further courses of CAV at a lower dosage to 93 patients who had responded to induction therapy with CAV. There was no significant difference for patients with LD in the two study arms. In ED, however, maintenance chemotherapy produced a significantly longer survival than did no further chemotherapy at relapse. In a similar protocol, Byrne et al. (29) gave three courses of EP every 3 weeks followed by three courses of cyclophosphamide, vincristine, methotrexate every 4 weeks plus concomitant thoracic radiotherapy to 68 patients. They were then randomized to no further chemotherapy or six further cycles of cyclophosphamide, vincristine, methotrexate. Patients in complete remission following the induction phase also received PCI. The overall survival of patients randomized to maintenance therapy was significantly worse than those randomized to no maintenance therapy. Subsequent larger randomized trials have proved that first-line chemotherapy beyond six courses has little influence on survival if rescue chemotherapy is given at relapse. The British Medical Research Council Lung Cancer Group randomized 497 patients to receive 6 or 12 cycles of cyclophosphamide, etoposide, methotrexate, and vincristine at 3-week intervals. There was no overall survival advantage to either group, although in 99 patients who achieved a CR there was a suggestion that survival was prolonged in the 12-week arm, but this was not statistically significant. Furthermore, the maintenance chemotherapy was associated with greater toxicity and a poorer quality of life (QOL). Worthwhile clinical advantage was achieved by continuing chemotherapy beyond six courses, except possibly in patients who had a CR to the initial six courses (30). The London Lung Cancer Group compared four with eight cycles of induction chemotherapy in 610 patients with a further randomization to different chemotherapy at relapse compared to no further chemotherapy. Those patients receiving four cycles and no further chemotherapy at relapse had an inferior survival compared to eight courses with or without chemotherapy at relapse and to four courses plus chemotherapy at relapse (31). A joint European trial gave five cycles versus 12 cycles of CAE to 687 patients. All patients received five courses of chemotherapy and the nonprogressing patients were randomized to receive either seven additional cycles of the same chemotherapy or just to follow-up. No difference in survival between the two arms was observed. The patients randomized to the maintenance arm had a progression-free interval approximately 2 months longer than the patients randomized to just follow-up (32). At 2 years after chemotherapy, there was no difference in the survival rates for the longer and shorter regimes in any of the trials described above. The European Lung Cancer Working Party performed a randomized trial to determine if maintenance chemotherapy with 12 courses of etoposide and vindesine could improve progression-free survival. Eighty-four patients who responded to six courses of induction chemotherapy with ifosfamide, etoposide, and an anthracycline (doxorubicin or epirubicin) were randomized to receive or not receive maintenance therapy. Progression-free survival was significantly improved by maintenance therapy, but the overall survival was not increased. This finding has recently been confirmed by other studies. Sculier et al. gave 235 patients etoposide and vindesine as maintenance chemotherapy after induction with ifosfamide, etoposide, and an anthracycline (33). This also showed no survival advantage overall, but a small benefit for patients with LD. Beith et al. (34) studied 129 patients who responded to induction chemotherapy with EP and were randomized to 10 courses of maintenance chemotherapy with CAV or no further treatment. Only 11% completed the maintenance chemotherapy, and 57% developed grade III and IV neutropenia. There was no significant difference in overall survival or disease-free survival in either arm despite the significantly greater toxicity after the induction treatment.

In conclusion, there is no evidence that prolonged chemotherapy offers a better chance of cure or prolongation of survival than short-course chemotherapy. No clear consensus on the duration of chemotherapy in SCLC has been established, but six cycles is now adopted in most current trials.

IV. High-Dose Chemotherapy

It is recognized that conventional dose chemotherapy produces responses below the plateau of the dose-response curve that cytotoxic chemotherapy achieved in tumor models. In fact, combination treatment often necessitates a reduction in the planned dose because of life-threatening toxicity. One problem for high-dose chemotherapy in SCLC is the patients themselves, who are often elderly. The median age in clinical series exceeds 60 years, nearly all of whom are smokers and have coexisting chronic obstructive pulmonary disease and cardiovascular problems. However, despite possible enhanced toxicity and treatment-related deaths, dose escalation might lead to increased rates of long-term survival.

High-dose chemotherapy regimes have been assessed as the first cycle of treatment or as a late intensification in responders. Early randomized studies conducted to determine the efficacy of intensive induction chemotherapy were inconclusive. In one study 32 patients received a high-dose or standard-dose cyclophosphamide, methotrexate, and lomustine regime during the first 6 weeks of treatment. Subsequent maintenance therapy comprised standard doses of cyclophosphamide, methotrexate, lomustine until disease progression. Patients treated with high-dose chemotherapy had an OR of 96% and a 30% CR rate that compared favorably to the 45% PR achieved with the standard chemotherapy (35). In another study 40 patients with ED randomly received either high-dose or low-dose methotrexate with leucovorin rescue in combination with cycles of CAV alternating with cycles of etoposide, vincristine, and hexamethylmelamine. The OR and median survival were similar for the two treatment groups (36). Another trial involving 298 patients with ED received either conventional or high-dose CAV. Vincristine was given at its usual dose in both arms, but cyclophosphamide and doxorubicin doses were increased. Scheduled treatment included six courses, but with the high-dose therapy restricted to the first three cycles. There was significantly greater toxicity in the high-dose arm, and the CR rate was significantly higher, but there was no difference in overall survival (37). Figueredo et al. (38) compared four courses of standard doses of CAV with a regime of increased doses of cyclophosphamide and, but to a lesser extent, doxorubicin in 103 patients. The higher doses of cyclophosphamide and doxorubicin did not improve results, and there were more side effects. Other studies included a multicenter trial which compared cyclophosphamide, etoposide *and* vincristine to high-dose cyclophosphamide and vincristine. Cycles were repeated every 3 weeks. Again no significant differences in response rates, response duration, or survival could be detected in patients with LD. Among patients with ED, response duration and median survival on the normal cyclophosphamide, etoposide, vincristine regime was longer than with high-dose cyclophosphamide and vincristine. The high doses of cyclophosphamide also caused more hemorrhagic cystitis (26). The London Lung Cancer Group gave two cycles of very high-dose cyclophosphamide to untreated patients with LD and demonstrated the rapid emergence of drug resistance. There was no apparent advantage in a similar study in which only one cycle of high-dose cyclophosphamide was given, nor for similar patients treated with conventional chemotherapy in other concurrent studies (39). More optimistic data were reported by Arriagada et al. (40), who increased the dose of cisplatin by 20 mg/m^2 and cyclophosphamide by 75 mg/m^2 in a regime comprising etoposide and doxorubicin with all patients receiving radiotherapy. The 55 patients who received the higher chemotherapy had a better 2-year survival (43%) than those on conventional dose (26%). Disease-free survival at 2 years was 28% in the higher-dose group, compared with 8% in the conventional dose group. Side effects from treatment were not greater in the higher-dose group. In another randomized trial of standard and higher doses of EP in 90 patients with ED, no benefits resulted from increasing the planned doses by 67% for the first two cycles of EP (41). The higher doses were again associated with substantially worse toxicity.

Late intensification has been investigated in phase II trials with disappointingly high rates of toxic deaths and treatment failures (42). The high-dose strategy has also been tested as second-line treatment for nonresponding or relapsing patients, but results were disappointing (43).

In conclusion, the hope that dose escalation would improve survival in SCLC has not found much support and remains controversial.

V. Dose Intensification: Weekly Versus Every-3-Weeks Treatment

As an alternative to high-dose treatment delivered at standard 3-week intervals, a strategy of increasing the dose rate through weekly administration has been investigated. Theoretically, the weekly schedule could administer a greater cumulative dose of chemotherapy over a shorter treatment period, reducing the chance of resistant cell strains emerging. However, the received dose intensity (rDI) may not achieve that planned and the patient may suffer greater toxicity.

The first such randomized trial compared an alternating weekly regime of three combinations (cyclophosphamide, doxorubicin, etoposide; cisplatin, vindesine; and methotrexate, vincristine;) to standard every-3-weeks cyclophosphamide, doxorubicin, and etoposide. There was a significant increase in response rate in the weekly regime for patients with LD, but no improved survival. The weekly regime also had more haematological toxicity and the RDI was significantly lower when compared to the standard treatment arm (44). In another study the weekly schedule of chemotherapy, previously proved to be active and well tolerated in patients with both LD and good prognosis ED (45), was compared to conventional every-3-weeks chemotherapy in a large randomized study. The regime consisted of 12 alternating weekly cycles of ifosfamide, doxorubicin; and EP, with an every-3-weeks treatment of six alternating cycles of CAV and PE. The OR, median survival, and 2-year survival rates were the same in both arms. The rDI was less than intended (71%) with weekly treatment, mainly due to hematological toxicity. This trial showed no benefit in median survival, and no benefit at 2 years with this weekly treatment regime; moreover, QOL measurements indicated that every-3-weeks chemotherapy was preferred to the weekly treatment (46,47).

VI. Dose Reduction: Planned Versus As-Required Treatment

Earl et al. randomized 300 patients (LD and ED) who did not have progressive disease after the first cycle of chemotherapy to receive either regular "planned" chemotherapy or chemotherapy given "as required" (48). All patients received cyclophosphamide, etoposide and vincristine. "Planned" chemotherapy was given regularly every 3 weeks. The "as-required" chemotherapy was given for tumor-related symptoms or for radiological progression of disease. Both groups of patients were assessed every 3 weeks, and a maximum of eight cycles of chemotherapy was given. A detailed QOL assessment was made. Contrary to expectation, in the QOL assessment the "as-required" patients scored themselves as having worse symptoms than patients receiving "planned" treatment. "As-required" treatment resulted in less drug administration for approximately equivalent survival. However, the palliative effect seen with "as-required" treatment was less satisfactory than with "planned" chemotherapy. The trial concluded that conventional every-3-weeks chemotherapy provided better disease control and QOL.

VII. Autologous Bone Marrow Transplant and Stem Cell Support

Autologous bone marrow transplantation (ABMT) and/or hematopoietic stem cell infusions have been used as support to reduce the severity and duration of myelosuppression, hence making it possible to increase the RDI of chemotherapy. Reinfused autologous bone marrow may contain malignant cells, and this is particularly true for SCLC, where about 20% of newly diagnosed patients have bone marrow metastases and where postmortem examinations find bone or bone marrow metastases in at least 35% of LD patients and in 55% of patients with ED (49). Despite this risk, however, there is no proof that the reinfusion of nontreated cells is of clinical importance. Studies in this area often have included only a small number of patients, making interpretation harder. Littlewood et al. treated seven patients with high-dose etoposide (1400–2400 mg/m^2), given as a single course over 3 days, in conjunction with ABMT (50), but the lack of a CR dissuaded the authors from entering further patients into the study. Disappointing results were also obtained in 29 patients who had late intensive combined modality therapy after responsivity to induction chemotherapy (51). A Belgian multicenter randomized trial tested late intensification chemotherapy and ABMT versus conventional chemotherapy. After induction chemotherapy, 45 responding patients were randomized to a final cycle of combined cyclophosphamide, carmustine, and etoposide either at a conventional dose or at a very high dose plus ABMT. In the late intensification group the CR rate and the relapse-free survival were significantly increased. However, since relapse occurred at the primary site (15 out of 16 failures) and toxicity (four deaths with marrow aplasia) was high, overall survival was not significantly improved (52). The London Lung Cancer Group studied a total of 75 patients in four consecutive studies of high-dose chemotherapy with ABMT to assist hematological recovery. In the first study, 25 patients were treated with cyclophosphamide 200 mg/kg as the sole chemotherapy; in the second (26 patients), the cycle of high-dose cyclophosphamide, with or without etoposide, was repeated as induction treatment. In the first study, response rate was high but was not increased by repeating the cycle, and survival was slightly worse in the second trial. In a third study, 15 patients were treated with CEV for two cycles and then with high-dose cyclophosphamide. Although high-dose cyclophosphamide increased the CR rate, the additional responses were short-lived. In their final study, an attempt was made to increase the initial CR rate by combination chemotherapy using cyclophosphamide, etoposide and either high-dose cyclophosphamide or melphalan. Although all nine patients responded, none achieved a CR. The long-term survival does not appear to be different from that in comparably selected cases treated with conventional chemotherapy (53,54). Promising results have been obtained by Elias et al. in 19 LD patients who received combined alkylating agents with ABMT followed by thoracic radiotherapy with a 56% survival at 18 months (55).

The possibility of increasing the rDI by reinfusing haematopoietic progenitors collected at each cycle of chemotherapy has been assessed in a phase II study. Twenty-five patients treated with six cycles of ifosfamide, carboplatin, etoposide received rhG-CSF 300 μg/day subcutaneously on days 4–15 of each cycle. The rDI was increased by shortening the time interval between cycles from the conventional 4 weeks to 3 and 2 weeks. Stem cells were collected as leukapheresis products or as full blood drawn by venesection at day 15 (day 1 of the next cycle in the 2-week arm) and reinfused on day 3 of the next cycle. Toxicity and supportive care requirements were similar to the conventional regime, and rDI was increased to its planned level, i.e., doubled in the 2-week arm (56).

In another study 32 patients with untreated LD received three courses of induction therapy followed by two courses of intensification therapy with ABMT. Patients also received PCI and thoracic irradiation. After induction therapy, 41% of patients were in CR and 53% in PR. After intensification with high-dose chemotherapy and ABMT, the response rates improved with 69% of patients in CR and 31% in PR. Median survival for all patients was 14 months. Of the 13 patients who received intensification therapy when in CR, 5 remained disease-free. Of the 9 patients who achieved a CR with intensification treatment, only one remained disease-free. No patient died during intensification (42).

VIII. Hematopoietic Factors

Myelosuppression and thrombocytopenia frequently are the limiting toxicity of chemotherapy, and theoretically the administration of colony stimulating hematopoietic growth factors might increase our ability to deliver larger RDI of chemotherapy, which in turn may improve clinical outcome.

A. Recombinant Human Granulocyte Colony-Stimulating Factor

Prophylactic treatment with recombinant human granulocyte colony-stimulating factor (rhG-CSF) after chemotherapy reduces both the nadir and duration of granulocytopenia. Two randomized trials, using identical protocols, comparing outcome of treatment with up to six courses of cyclophosphamide, doxorubicin, etoposide, plus placebo or rhG-CSF have been carried out in North America and Europe (57,58). The two trials included 207 and 130 evaluable patients, respectively, with both LD and ED patients. The influence of rhG-CSF was most prominent after the first cycle of chemotherapy, where proportions of patients with neutropenia and fever were reduced from 57 to 28% in the American study and from 41 to 20% in the European study. Overall, number of days of treatment with i.v. antibiotics and days in hospital was 50% less in patients treated with rhG-CSF compared to placebo. In Europe, dose reductions and treatment delays were more frequent in the placebo arm compared to the rhG-CSF arm. Neither of the two trials showed significant differences in CR rates, response duration, or overall survival between the placebo and rhG-CSF arms. Another trial randomized 40 patients to analyze whether rhG-CSF (5 μg/kg subcutaneously) could increase the RDI of EP alternating weekly with ifosfamide, doxorubicin, over a total of 12 courses. As in the previous trials, rhG-CSF significantly decreased dose reductions and treatment delays from neutropenia, but not to a level that would allow an increase in RDI because of hematological and nonhematological toxicity, such as increased creatinine concentration (59). Similar results were obtained in an Australian trial, which verified the role of rhG-CSF administered after the onset of chemotherapy-induced neutropenic infection. They randomized 218 patients in a double-blind placebo-controlled manner. Compared with placebo, rhG-CSF accelerated neutrophil recovery and shortened the duration of febrile neutropenia, but did not reduce days in the hospital (60). The Manchester group randomized 65 patients with newly diagnosed SCLC to receive vincristine, ifosfamide, carboplatin, and etoposide alone or with rhG-CSF 5 μg/kg/day between cycles. Six cycles of chemotherapy were given followed by PCI and thoracic irradiation. There was no fixed dose interval, but no dose reductions were permitted. White blood cell and neutrophil counts were consistently higher in the patients receiving rhG-CSF than in the control group, but there were no differences in the incidence of febrile neutropenia, antibiotic or transfusion requirements, or days in the hospital. The rhG-CSF group received a higher DI than the control group, with the greatest difference in the first three cycles. There were more chemotherapy-related deaths in the rhG-

CSF group than in the control group, but despite this it had a better 2-year survival rate (32% with rhG-CSF, 15% with controls) (61). The same favorable results have been obtained in a recent Japanese trial, where rhG-CSF administration in support of cyclophosphamide, doxorubicin, etoposide, vincristine chemotherapy resulted in increased rDI for all drugs with a significant improvement in survival (62).

Thus, rhG-CSF is well tolerated; it may be useful in supportive care as an adjunct to chemotherapy as it reduces the incidence of fever with neutropenia and culture-confirmed infections, the incidence, duration, and severity of WHO grade IV neutropenia, the total number of days of treatment with i.v. antibiotics, and days of hospitalization; it is still uncertain whether it increases rDI to a level that will improve results obtained with conventional chemotherapy regimes.

B. Recombinant Human Granulocyte-Macrophage Colony-Stimulating Factor

Recombinant human granulocyte-macrophage colony-stimulating factor (rhGM-CSF) is a growth factor also used to induce marrow recovery after chemotherapy. Phase III trials have attempted to address its effective role and safety. A multicenter study randomized 290 newly diagnosed patients to receive six cycles of standard cyclophosphamide, doxorubicin, and etoposide alone or with rhGM-CSF to determine the dose that can safely reduce neutropenia. Adverse events that occurred more frequently in rhGM-CSF–treated patients included injection-site reaction, edema, asthenia, paresthesia, diarrhea, myalgia, musculoskeletal pain, pruritus, and rash. Fever occurred more frequently in the groups receiving 10 and 20 μg/kg rhGM-CSF. RhGM-CSF at 5–10 μg/kg reduced chemotherapy-associated neutropenia and appeared to be the dose range for future studies (63). A Southwest Oncology Group trial assessed whether rhGM-CSF reduced hematological toxicity and morbidity induced by chemoradiotherapy in LD patients. Two hundred and thirty patients were randomized to receive chemotherapy and radiotherapy with or without rhGM-CSF given on days 4–18 of each of six cycles. Patients randomized to rhGM-CSF had more nonhematological toxicity, more days in the hospital, a higher incidence of i.v. antibiotic usage, and more transfusions. There was a significant increase in the frequency and duration of life-threatening thrombocytopenia and toxic deaths. Patients receiving rhGM-CSF had higher WBC and neutrophil nadirs, but no significant difference in the frequency of grade 4 leukopenia or neutropenia (64). RhGM-CSF appears to be associated with many systemic side effects, and so far its clinical profile seems worse than that of rhG-CSF.

C. Polyethylene Glycol Conjugated Recombinant Human Megakaryocyte Growth and Development Factor

Recombinant human megakaryocyte growth and development factor (rhMGDF), a recombinant molecule related to thrombopoietin, specifically stimulates megakaryopoiesis and platelet production and reduces the severity of thrombocytopenia in animals receiving myelosuppressive chemotherapy. So far it has been tested only in a randomized clinical trial for lung cancer and only in patients with non–small-cell lung cancer (65).

D. Recombinant Human Interleukin-3

Recombinant human interleukin 3 (rhIL-3) may be useful for the treatment of chemotherapy-induced thrombocytopenia and its role in SCLC has been evaluated in 41 patients treated with carboplatin and etoposide every 4 weeks. rhIL-3 was administrated subcutaneously at 5 or 10 μg/kg for 10 days following chemotherapy if the platelet count nadir was less than 75,000/μL. There was no difference in the efficacy of the two rhIL-3 dose levels, and both significantly reduced the incidence, duration, and severity of chemotherapy-induced thrombocytopenia and neutropenia. The major side effects were fever (80.5%), headache (24.3%), and fatigue (14.6%). All side effects were tolerable and of less than grade II, but the lowest dose was better tolerated (66).

E. Recombinant Human Erythropoietin

Recombinant human erythropoietin (rhEPO) is an effective anti-anemia medication in untreated patients with cancer. The possibility that rhEPO may also prevent or reduce anemia in patients who receive cytotoxic chemotherapy has been assessed in 36 patients in a three-arm randomized trial. Patients received either 150 IU/kg, 300 IU/kg, or no rhEPO. A maximum of six cycles of ifosfamide, carboplatin, etoposide, and vincristine were given to all patients. Red blood cell or platelet transfusions were given if the hemoglobin fell below 9 g/dL and platelets counts below 20,000/μL. The hemoglobin levels decreased in all patients, but the onset of anemia was delayed in those who received rhEPO. A total of 116 blood units were transfused in the control group, but only 54 and 52, respectively, in patients who were receiving 150 and 300 IU/kg 3 days a week (67).

IX. Sequential and Alternating Chemotherapy

Analogous to antimicrobial therapy, increasing the number of drugs given at the same time would increase the chances of eradicating all neoplastic tumor clones and avoid chemoresistance. This is difficult because of the high toxicity induced by high doses in complex regimes. The sequential use of two hypothetically non–cross-resistant regimes is another approach, and when the EP regime was proved to be as effective as CAV, it was opportune to try them in sequence. The Southeastern Cancer Study Group (11) randomized 160 patients with LD who responded to induction therapy (CAV for six cycles or CAV plus concomitant thoracic irradiation) to consolidation chemotherapy consisting of EP every 4 weeks for two courses versus no further therapy. Consolidation therapy significantly improved the duration of remission (median duration of 49 weeks vs. 28 weeks) and overall survival (median survival 97.7 weeks compared with 68 weeks). Other sequential regimes have been investigated in many phase II studies.

It has been proposed that alternating instead of sequential administration of two initially active treatment regimes will increase the kill of tumor strains and, thus, improve the chances of longer survival or cure (68). The model assumes no cross-resistance between the two alternating therapies, equal efficacy of the regimes, a similar log kill, and equal incidence rates and growth characteristics of emerging clones during the treatment. Trials inspired by this principle failed to demonstrate any advantages for alternating therapy. A German multicenter trial randomized patients to receive either fixed cyclic-alternating treatment with ifosfamide, etoposide, and CAV, or response-oriented treatment with ifosfamide, etoposide therapy to a maximal response and subsequently an immediate switch to CAV (69). Six cycles were given at 3-week intervals in both arms. The cyclic-alternating treatment did not show any advantage to the sequential treatment strategy with the immediate switch to a second-line protocol at the time of no further response to initial therapy. The alternating non–cross-resistant combination, cyclophosphamide, doxorubicin, etoposide versus the same combination alternating with CCNU, methotrexate, vincristine, and procarbazine (109 patients) has not proven useful with respect to response or survival (70).

Many trials have compared sequential CAV with CAV alternating with EP (71–73). A Canadian trial found no difference in patients with LD who also received thoracic irradiation, while the median survival in patients with ED was 1.6 months longer in the alternating arm (74). The difference was significant and worthwhile according to a cost-efficiency study (75), but clearly only very modest. Trials conducted by the Southeastern Cancer Study Group (13) and by Fukuoka et al. (12) included a third arm with EP alone to address the question if the advantage shown in the previous trials could be attributed entirely to the EP combination. In the American trial there were no differences in outcome between any of the three regimes, while the Japanese trial proved CAV, but not EP, to be inferior to the alternating regime. In conclusion, there are no major, clinically useful differences between the effects of CAV, EP, and CAV alternating with EP.

Crossing over to the alternative regime in patients with disease progression on sequential therapy has raised doubt about the lack of cross-resistance between regimes. In the two three-arm trials (12,13) response rates on CAV after EP were 12 and 8%, respectively, and on EP after CAV, 22 and 23%, respectively. The differences between these rates were not significant. The amount of resistance seems to depend on the number of treatment courses given as initial therapy. Thus, response rates on CAV after etoposide plus ifosfamide were 5 out of 10 (1), 11 out of 19 (2), 6 out of 27 (3), 3 out of 13 (4), and 0 out of 9 (5), where the figures in the parentheses represent the number of etoposide plus ifosfamide courses (76). The supposed non–cross-resistance between CAV and EP is also not supported by in vitro investigations (77). Resistance studies in the laboratory may enable composition of more strictly non–cross-resistant regimes—if they exist—and may give ideas how to circumvent resistance; currently, the alternating treatment principle has no definitive clinical importance.

Other alternating regimes have been assessed. The Swiss Group for Clinical Cancer Research performed a randomized phase III trial that enrolled 406 patients to compare six cycles of sequential versus alternating chemotherapy. The two regimes used in the trial were doxorubicin, etoposide, cisplatin and cyclophosphamide, methotrexate, vincristine, CCNU. Cycles were given as frequently as possible. Patients with LD in CR or PR and those with ED in CR received thoracic irradiation and PCI. The overall remission rate, the rate of CR, the median survival, and the rate of long-term survival were similar in the two treatment arms. Patients treated with early alternating chemotherapy rated their tumor symptoms, functional states, fatigue/malaise, and restriction of social activity significantly better, reflecting an improved subjective response (78). The EORTC Lung Cancer Study Group compared the 3-week cyclophosphamide, doxorubicin, etoposide regime with a 3-week alternating cyclophosphamide, doxorubicin, etoposide, and ifosfamide, carboplatin, vincristine regimes in a group of 143 patients with ED. Median survival, time to progression, and median response duration were no better with the alternating non–cross-resistant chemotherapy (43).

Alternating chemotherapy has therefore been extensively studied. Some trials have shown positive results that have not been confirmed in others. In all of the studies, however, the degree of non–cross-resistance in the regimes is probably small.

X. Low-Dose/High-Frequency Chemotherapy

Acute chemotherapy toxicity is related to dose, while survival is correlated to rDI. These statements have brought James et al. (79) to assess whether the widely used every-3-weeks regime was comparable with the same drugs given at half the dose but twice the frequency with the same intended overall DI. One hundred and sixty-seven patients with ED and poor prognostic features were randomized to receive either an every-3-weeks regime of EP alternating with CAV for a maximum of 6 courses or treatment with the same drugs, but with each course comprising half the every-3-weeks dose given every 10 or 11 days for a maximum of 12 courses. Hematological toxicity and treatment delays for infection were more frequent with the 10/11 day regime, but other toxicity was equal. There was a trend for improved QOL on the 10/11 day arm, but there was little difference between the two treatments. The trial showed that a low-dose/high-frequency regime with the same rDI as conventionally scheduled chemotherapy gave similar response rates and survival. This, and other modifications of scheduling, may offer new approaches to palliative treatment of advanced cancer. However, in this trial there was no significant benefit in toxicity or other aspects of QOL (79).

XI. Oral Chemotherapy

There has been some concern about the use of conventional combination chemotherapy in elderly and poor-prognosis patients (80–82). No systematic study has been performed to establish regimes suitable for elderly patients, but results obtained with phase II studies of oral etoposide (83–89) suggested its effect was comparable to that of i.v. combination chemotherapy, and thus feasible, or possibly preferable for elderly and poor-prognosis patients. Moreover, compliance has been not found to be a problem for outpatient-based anticancer treatment (90). Oral ifosfamide plus oral etoposide is probably more efficient than etoposide alone, but central nervous system toxicity in 30% of the patients makes the regime less attractive for elderly patients (91). Similar neurological problems were observed with single-agent oral ifosfamide, and outpatient use of the regime could, therefore, not be recommended (92). However, three recent randomized studies comparing oral etoposide to standard i.v. combination chemotherapy did not favor the use of oral etoposide for palliative treatment, and two have been stopped prematurely on recommendation of independent data monitoring committees (DMC). The Cancer and Leukemia Group B randomized 306 patients with ED and good performance status to receive i.v. etoposide 130 mg/m^2 plus i.v. cisplatin 25 mg/m^2 for three consecutive days for eight 3-week courses versus 21-day 50 mg/m^2 oral etoposide plus i.v. cisplatin 33 mg/m^2 for three days for six 3-week courses. The two schedules showed no differences in outcome for tumor response and survival. However, a significantly greater incidence of severe or life-threatening hematological toxicity was noted on the 21-day oral etoposide treatment schedule (93). The Medical Research Council Lung Cancer Working Party compared single-agent oral etoposide 50 mg twice daily for 10 days for four 3-week cycles to a standard i.v. regime of etoposide, vincristine, or CAV in 339 patients previously untreated and WHO grade performance status 2–4. Interim analysis of the data induced a DMC to advise stopping the enrollment because of poor results in the oral etoposide arm. Toxicity and palliative effects of treatment were similar in the two groups, but patients receiving the i.v. chemotherapy had a higher OR and better survival than with oral etoposide. Median survival was 130 days and 183 days, respectively; survival rates were 35 and 49% at 6 months and 11 and 13% at 12 months in the etoposide group and standard i.v. chemotherapy group, respectively (94). Souhami et al. selected similar patients as the Medical Research Council Lung Cancer Working Party, but they used an oral etoposide schedule of 100 mg twice daily for 5 days for six 3-week cycles compared to the EP/CAV alternating regime (95). When informed of the poor results of the Medical Research Council study, they asked three members of the same DMC to analyze their data. The interim results suggested the study should also stop. Response rate, progression-free survival, and 1-year survival were significantly worse in the oral etoposide arm in addition to a negative trend for the median survival of patients who received oral etoposide.

  Oral etoposide is now considered inferior to standard i.v. multidrug chemotherapy in the palliative treatment, especially for patients with poor performance status, and should no longer be used.

XII. Conclusions

The role of chemotherapy in SCLC has reached a plateau off which it is depressingly slow to move. While combination chemotherapy, at least six courses, seems ideal for the majority of patients with this disease, the intensive effort to improve survival and cure rate, particularly for poor-prognosis patients, has not yet borne fruit. While newer agents show promise, and in some cases better toxicity profiles, a new approach is needed to permit real progress. Current chemotherapy is a compromise between ensuring optimal response, acceptable toxicity, and an improved QOL, at least during the earned remission.

References

1. Souhami R, Law K. Longevity in small cell lung cancer. A report to the Lung Cancer Subcommittee of the United Kingdom Coordinating Committee for Cancer Research. Br J Cancer 1990; 61:584–589.
2. Lassen U, Osterlind K, Hansen M, Dombernowsky P, Bergman B, Hansen H. Long-term survival in small-cell lung cancer: posttreatment characteristics in patients surviving 5 to 18+ years—an analysis of 1,714 consecutive patients. J Clin Oncol 1995; 13:1215–1220.
3. Hyde L, Wolf J, McCracken S, Yesner R. Natural course of inoperable lung cancer. Chest 1973; 64:309–312.
4. Zelen M. Keynote address on biostatistics and data retrieval. Cancer Chemother Rep 1973; 4:31–42.
5. Lanzotti V, Thomas D, Boyle L, Smith T, Gehan E, Samuels M. Survival with inoperable lung cancer: an integration of prognostic variables based on simple clinical criteria. Cancer 1977; 39:303–313.
6. Sierocki J, Hilaris B, Hopfan S, et al. cis-Dichlorodiamineplatinum(II) and VP-16-213: an active induction regimen for small cell carcinoma of the lung. Cancer Treat Rep 1979; 63:1593–1597.
7. Evans W, Shepherd F, Feld R, Osoba D, Dang P, Deboer G. VP-16 and cisplatin as first-line therapy for small-cell lung cancer. Clin Oncol 1985; 3:1471–1477.
8. Evans W, Feld R, Osoba D, Shepherd F, Dill J, Deboer G. VP-16 alone and in combination with cisplatin in previously treated patients with small cell lung cancer. Cancer 1984; 53:1461–1466.
9. Evans W, Osoba D, Feld R, Shepherd F, Bazos M, De Boer G. Etoposide (VP-16) and cisplatin: an effective treatment for relapse in small-cell lung cancer. J Clin Oncol 1985; 3:65–71.
10. Loehrer PS, Einhorn L, Greco F. Cisplatin plus etoposide in small cell lung cancer. Semin Oncol 1988; 15(suppl 3):2–8.
11. Einhorn L, Crawford J, Birch R, Omura G, Johnson D, Greco F. Cisplatin plus etoposide consolidation following cyclophosphamide, doxorubicin, and vincristine in limited small-cell lung cancer. J Clin Oncol 1988; 6:451–456.
12. Fukuoka M, Furuse K, Saijo N, et al. Randomized trial of cyclophosphamide, doxorubicin, and vincristine versus cisplatin and etoposide versus alternation of these regimens in small-cell lung cancer. J Natl Cancer Inst 1991; 83:855–861.
13. Roth BJ, DH, Einhorn L, Schacter L, et al. Randomized study of cyclophosphamide, doxorubicin, and vincristine versus etoposide and cisplatin versus alternation of these two regimens in extensive small-cell lung cancer: a phase III trial of the Southeastern Cancer Study Group. J Clin Oncol 1992; 10:282–291.
14. Veronesi A, Cartei G, Crivellari D, et al. Cisplatin and etoposide versus cyclophosphamide, epirubicin and vincristine in small cell lung cancer: a randomised study. Eur J Cancer 1994; 30A:1474–1478.

15. Hainsworth J, Levitan N, Wampler G, et al. Phase II randomized study of cisplatin plus eto-poside phosphate or etoposide in the treatment of small-cell lung cancer. J Clin Oncol 1995; 13:1436–1442.

16. Evans W, Eisenhauer E, Hughes P, et al. VP-16 and carboplatin in previously untreated pa-tients with extensive small cell lung cancer: a study of the National Cancer Institute of Canada Clinical Trials Group. Br J Cancer 1988; 58:464–468.

17. Kosmidis P, Samantas E, Fountzilas G, Pavlidis N, Apostolopoulou F, Skarlos D. Cisplatin/etoposide versus carboplatin/etoposide chemotherapy and irradiation in small cell lung can-cer: a randomized phase III study. Hellenic Cooperative Oncology Group for Lung Cancer Trials. Semin Oncol 1994; 21(suppl 6):23–30.

18. Skarlos D, Samantas E, Kosmidis P, et al. Randomized comparison of etoposide-cisplatin vs. etoposide-carboplatin and irradiation in small-cell lung cancer. A Hellenic Co-operative On-cology Group study. Ann Oncol 1994; 5:601–607.

19. Slevin M, Clark P, Joel S, et al. A randomized trial to evaluate the effect of schedule on the activity of etoposide in small-cell lung cancer. J Clin Oncol 1989; 7:1333–1340.

20. Maksymiuk A, Jett J, Earle J, et al. Sequencing and schedule effects of cisplatin plus eto-poside in small-cell lung cancer: results of a North Central Cancer Treatment Group ran-domized clinical trial. J Clin Oncol 1994; 12:70–76.

21. Hornback N, Einhorn L, Shidnia H, Joe B, Krause M, Furnas B. Oat cell carcinoma of the lung. Early treatment results of combination radiation therapy and chemotherapy. Cancer 1976; 37:2658–2664.

22. Johnson R, Brereton H, Kent C. Small-cell carcinoma of the lung: attempt to remedy causes of past therapeutic failure. Lancet 1976; 2:289–291.

23. Holoye P, Samuels M, Lanzotti V, Smith T, Barkley HJ. Combination chemotherapy and ra-diation therapy for small cell carcinoma. JAMA 1977; 237:1221–1224.

24. Jackson DJ, Case L, Zekan P, et al. Improvement of long-term survival in extensive small-cell lung cancer. J Clin Oncol 1988; 6:1161–1169.

25. Jett J, Everson L, Therneau T, et al. Treatment of limited-stage small-cell lung cancer with cyclophosphamide, doxorubicin, and vincristine with or without etoposide: a randomized trial of the North Central Cancer Treatment Group. J Clin Oncol 1990; 8:33–38.

26. Hong W, Nicaise C, Lawson R, et al. Etoposide combined with cyclophosphamide plus vin-cristine compared with doxorubicin plus cyclophosphamide plus vincristine and with high-dose cyclophosphamide plus vincristine in the treatment of small-cell carcinoma of the lung: a randomized trial of the Bristol Lung Cancer Study Group. J Clin Oncol 1989; 7:450–456.

27. Abratt R, Salton D, Malan J, Willcox P. A prospective randomised study in limited disease small cell carcinoma: doxorubicin and vincristine plus either cyclophosphamide or etopo-side. Eur J Cancer 1995; 31A:1637–1639.

28. Cullen M, Morgan D, Gregory W, et al. Maintenance chemotherapy for anaplastic small cell carcinoma of the bronchus: a randomised, controlled trial. Cancer Chemother Pharmacol 1986; 17:157–160.

29. Byrne M, van Hazel G, Trotter J, et al. Maintenance chemotherapy in limited small cell lung cancer: a randomised controlled clinical trial. Br J Cancer 1989; 60:413–418.

30. Party MRCLCW. Controlled trial of twelve versus six courses of chemotherapy in the treat-ment of small-cell lung cancer. Report to the Medical Research Council by its Lung Cancer Working Party. Br J Cancer 1989; 59:584–590.

31. Spiro S, Souhami R, Geddes D, et al. Duration of chemotherapy in small-cell lung cancer: a Cancer Research Campaign trial. Br J Cancer 1989; 59:578–583.

32. Giaccone G, Dalesio O, McVie G, et al. Maintenance chemotherapy in small-cell lung can-cer: long-term results of a randomized trial. J Clin Oncol 1993; 11:1230–1240.

33. Sculier J, Paesmans M, Bureau G, et al. Randomized trial comparing induction chemo-therapy versus induction chemotherapy followed by maintenance chemotherapy in small-cell lung cancer. European Lung Cancer Working Party. J Clin Oncol 1996; 14:2337–2344.

34. Beith J, Clarke S, Woods R, Bell D, Levi J. Long-term follow-up of a randomised trial of combined chemoradiotherapy induction treatment, with and without maintenance chemo-therapy in patients with small cell carcinoma of the lung. Eur J Cancer 1996; 32A:438–443.

35. Cohen M, Creaven P, Fossieck BJ, et al. Intensive chemotherapy of small cell bronchogenic carcinoma. Cancer Treat Rep 1977; 61:349–354.
36. Hande K, Oldham R, Fer M, Richardson R, Greco F. Randomized study of high-dose versus low-dose methotrexate in the treatment of extensive small cell lung cancer. Am J Med 1982; 73:413–419.
37. Johnson D, Einhorn L, Birch R, et al. A randomized comparison of high-dose versus conventional-dose cyclophosphamide, doxorubicin, and vincristine for extensive-stage small-cell lung cancer: a phase III trial of the Southeastern Cancer Study Group. J Clin Oncol 1987; 5:1731–1738.
38. Figueredo A, Hryniuk W, Strautmanis I, Frank G, Rendell S. Co-trimoxazole prophylaxis during high-dose chemotherapy of small-cell lung cancer. J Clin Oncol 1985; 3:54–64.
39. Souhami R, Finn G, Gregory W, et al. High-dose cyclophosphamide in small-cell carcinoma of the lung. J Clin Oncol 1985; 3:958–963.
40. Arriagada R, Le Chevalier T, Pignon J, et al. Initial chemotherapeutic doses and survival in patients with limited small-cell lung cancer. N Engl J Med 1993; 329:1848–1852.
41. Ihde D, Mulshine J, Kramer B, et al. Prospective randomized comparison of high-dose and standard-dose etoposide and cisplatin chemotherapy in patients with extensive-stage small-cell lung cancer. J Clin Oncol 1994; 12:2022–2034.
42. Spitzer G, Farha P, Valdivieso M, et al. High-dose intensification therapy with autologous bone marrow support for limited small-cell bronchogenic carcinoma. J Clin Oncol 1986; 4:4–13.
43. Postmus P, Mulder N, De Vries-Hospers H, et al. High-dose cyclophosphamide and high-dose VP-16-213 for recurrent or refractory small-cell lung cancer: a phase II study. Eur J Cancer Clin Oncol 1985; 21:1467–1470.
44. Sculier J, Paesmans M, Bureau G, et al. Multiple-drug weekly chemotherapy versus standard combination regimen in small-cell lung cancer: a phase III randomized study conducted by the European Lung Cancer Working Party. J Clin Oncol 1993; 11:1858–1865.
45. Miles D, Earl H, Souhami R, et al. Intensive weekly chemotherapy for good-prognosis patients with small-cell lung cancer. J Clin Oncol 1991; 9:280–285.
46. Souhami R, Rudd R, Ruiz de Elvira M, et al. Randomized trial comparing weekly versus 3-week chemotherapy in small-cell lung cancer: a Cancer Research Campaign trial. J Clin Oncol 1994; 12:1806–1813.
47. Gower N, Rudd R, Ruiz de Elvira M, et al. Assessment of 'quality of life' using a daily diary card in a randomised trial of chemotherapy in small-cell lung cancer. Ann Oncol 1995; 6:575–580.
48. Earl H, Rudd, RM, Spiro, SG, et al. A randomised trial of planned versus as required chemotherapy in small cell lung cancer: a Cancer Research Campaign trial. Br J Cancer 1991; 64:566–572.
49. Elliott J, Osterlind K, Hirsch F, Hansen H. Metastatic patterns in small-cell lung cancer: correlation of autopsy findings with clinical parameters in 537 patients. J Clin Oncol 1987; 5:246–254.
50. Littlewood T, Bentley D, Smith A. High-dose etoposide with autologous bone marrow transplantation as initial treatment of small cell lung cancer: a negative report. Eur J Respir Dis 1986; 68:370–374.
51. Ihde D, Deisseroth A, Lichter A, et al. Late intensive combined modality therapy followed by autologous bone marrow infusion in extensive-stage small-cell lung cancer. J Clin Oncol 1986; 4:1443–1454.
52. Humblet Y, Symann M, Bosly A, et al. Late intensification chemotherapy with autologous bone marrow transplantation in selected small-cell carcinoma of the lung: a randomized study. J Clin Oncol 1987; 5:1864–1873.
53. Souhami R, Harper P, Linch D, et al. High-dose cyclophosphamide with autologous marrow transplantation as initial treatment of small-cell carcinoma of the bronchus. Cancer Chemother Pharmacol 1982; 8:31–34.

54. Souhami R, Hajichristou H, Miles D, et al. Intensive chemotherapy with autologous bone marrow transplantation for small-cell lung cancer. Cancer Chemother Pharmacol 1989; 24:321–325.

55. Elias A, Ayash L, Skarin A, et al. High-dose combined alkylating agent therapy with autologous stem cell support and chest radiotherapy for limited small-cell lung cancer. Chest 1993; 103(suppl):433S–435S.

56. Pettengell R, Woll P, Thatcher N, Dexter T, Testa N. Multicyclic, dose-intensive chemotherapy supported by sequential reinfusion of hematopoietic progenitors in whole blood. J Clin Oncol 1995; 13:148–156.

57. Crawford J, Ozer H, Stoller R, et al. Reduction by granulocyte colony-stimulating factor of fever and neutropenia induced by chemotherapy in patients with small-cell lung cancer. N Engl J Med 1991; 325:164–170.

58. Trillet-Lenoir V, Green J, Manegold C, et al. Recombinant granulocyte colony-stimulating factor reduces the infectious complications of cytotoxic chemotherapy. Eur J Cancer 1993; 29A:319–324.

59. Miles D, Fogarty O, Ash C, et al. Received dose-intensity: a randomized trial of weekly chemotherapy with and without granulocyte colony-stimulating factor in small-cell lung cancer. J Clin Oncol 1994; 12:77–82.

60. Maher D, Lieschke G, Green M, et al. Filgrastim in patients with chemotherapy-induced febrile neutropenia. A double-blind, placebo-controlled trial. Ann Intern Med 1994; 121:492–501.

61. Woll P, Hodgetts J, Lomax L, et al. Can cytotoxic dose-intensity be increased by using granulocyte colony-stimulating factor? A randomized controlled trial of lenograstim in small-cell lung cancer. J Clin Oncol 1995; 13:652–659.

62. Fukuoka M, Masuda N, Negoro S, et al. CODE chemotherapy with and without granulocyte colony-stimulating factor in small-cell lung cancer. Br J Cancer 1997; 75:306–309.

63. Hamm J, Schiller J, Cuffie C, et al. Dose-ranging study of recombinant human granulocyte-macrophage colony-stimulating factor in small-cell lung carcinoma. J Clin Oncol 1994; 12:2667–2676.

64. Bunn PJ, Crowley J, Kelly K, et al. Chemoradiotherapy with or without granulocyte-macrophage colony-stimulating factor in the treatment of limited-stage small-cell lung cancer: a prospective phase III randomized study of the Southwest Oncology Group. J Clin Oncol 1995; 13:1632–1641.

65. Fanucchi M, Glaspy J, Crawford J, et al. Effects of polyethylene glycol-conjugated recombinant human megakaryocyte growth and development factor on platelet counts after chemotherapy for lung cancer. N Engl J Med 1997; 336:404–409.

66. Kudoh S, Sawa T, Kurihara N, et al. Phase II study of recombinant human interleukin 3 administration following carboplatin and etoposide chemotherapy in small-cell lung cancer patients. SDZILE964 (IL-3) Study. Cancer Chemother Pharmacol 1996; 38(suppl): S89–S95.

67. de Campos E, Radford J, Steward W, et al. Clinical and in vitro effects of recombinant human erythropoietin in patients receiving intensive chemotherapy for small-cell lung cancer. J Clin Oncol 1995; 13:1623–1631.

68. Goldie J, Coldman A. Quantitative model for multiple levels of drug resistance in clinical tumors. Cancer Treat Rev 1983; 67:923–931.

69. Wolf M, Pritsch M, Drings P, et al. Cyclic-alternating versus response-oriented chemotherapy in small-cell lung cancer: a German multicenter randomized trial of 321 patients. J Clin Oncol 1991; 9:614–624.

70. Aisner J, Whitacre M, Van Echo D, Wesley M, Wiernik P. Doxorubicin, Cyclophosphamide and VP16-213 (ACE) in the treatment of small cell lung cancer. Cancer Chemother Pharmacol 1982; 7:187–193.

71. Feld R, Evans W, Coy P, et al. Canadian multicenter randomized trial comparing sequential and alternating administration of two non-cross-resistant chemotherapy combinations in patients with limited small-cell carcinoma of the lung. J Clin Oncol 1987; 5:1401–1409.

72. Ettinger D. Evaluation of new drugs in untreated patients with small-cell lung cancer: its time has come. J Clin Oncol 1990; 8:374–377.
73. Wampler G, Heim W, Ellison N, Ahlgren J, Fryer J. Comparison of cyclophosphamide, doxorubicin, and vincristine with an alternating regimen of methotrexate, etoposide, and cisplatin/cyclophosphamide, doxorubicin, and vincristine in the treatment of extensive-disease small-cell lung carcinoma: a Mid-Atlantic Oncology Program study. J Clin Oncol 1991; 9:1438–1445.
74. Evans W, Feld R, Murray N, et al. Superiority of alternating non-cross-resistant chemotherapy in extensive small-cell lung cancer: a multicenter, randomized clinical trial by the National Cancer Institute of Canada. Ann Intern Med 1987; 107:451–458.
75. Goodwin P, Feld R, Evans W, Pater J. Cost-effectiveness of cancer chemotherapy: an economic evaluation of a randomized trial in small-cell lung cancer. J Clin Oncol 1988; 6:1537–1547.
76. Havemann K, Wolf M, Holle R, et al. Alternating versus sequential chemotherapy in small-cell lung cancer; a randomized German multicenter trial. Cancer 1987; 59:1072–1082.
77. Jensen P, Christensen I, Sehested M, Hansen H, Vindelev L. Differential cytotoxicity of 19 anti-cancer agents in wild type and etoposide resistant small-cell lung cancer cell lines. Br J Cancer 1993; 67:311–320.
78. Joss R, Bacchi M, Hurny C, et al. Early versus late alternating chemotherapy in small-cell lung cancer. Swiss Group for Clinical Cancer Research (SAKK). Ann Oncol 1995; 6:157–166.
79. James L, Gower N, Rudd R, et al. A randomised trial of low-dose/high-frequency chemotherapy as palliative treatment of poor-prognosis small-cell lung cancer: a Cancer Research Campaign trial. Br J Cancer 1996; 73:1563–1568.
80. Souhami R, Bradbury I, Geddes D, Spiro S, Harper P, Tobias J. Prognostic significance of laboratory parameters measured at diagnosis in small cell carcinoma of the lung. Cancer Res 1985; 45:2878–2882.
81. Osterlind K, Lassen U, Herrstedt J, Jorgensen M, Hansen H. Is intensive combination chemotherapy feasible in old patients with small-cell lung cancer (SCLC)? The Copenhagen group experience 1973–1987. Ann Oncol 1992; 3(suppl 5):37.
82. Radford J, Ryder W, Dodwell D, Anderson H, Thatcher N. Predicting septic complications of chemotherapy: an analysis of 382 patients treated for small-cell lung cancer without dose reduction after major sepsis. Eur J Cancer 1993; 29A:81–86.
83. Mead G, Thompson J, Sweetenham J, Buchanan R, Whitehouse J, Williams C. Extensive stage small cell carcinoma of the bronchus. A randomised study of etoposide given orally by one-day or five-day schedule together with intravenous adriamycin and cyclophosphamide. Cancer Chemother Pharmacol 1987; 19:172–174.
84. Smit E, Carney D, Harford P, Sleijfer D, Postmus P. A phase II study of oral etoposide in elderly patients with small-cell lung cancer. Thorax 1989; 44:631–633.
85. Einhorn L, Pennington K, McClean J. Phase II trial of daily oral VP-16 in refractory small cell lung cancer: a Hoosier Oncology Group study. Semin Oncol 1990; 17(suppl 2):32–35.
86. Carney D, Grogan L, Smit E, Harford P, Berendsen H, Postmus P. Single-agent oral etoposide for elderly small cell lung cancer patients. Semin Oncol 1990; 17(suppl 2):49–53.
87. Clark P, Cottier B. The activity of 10-, 14-, and 21-day schedules of single-agent etoposide in previously untreated patients with extensive small cell lung cancer. Semin Oncol 1992; 19(suppl 14):36–39.
88. Keane M, Carney D. Treatment of elderly patients with small-cell lung cancer. Lung Cancer 1993; 9(suppl. 1):S91–S98.
89. Carney D. Carboplatin/etoposide combination chemotherapy in the treatment of poor prognosis patients with small cell lung cancer. Lung Cancer 1995; 12(suppl 3):S77–S83.
90. Lee C, Nicholson P, Souhami R, Slevin M, Hall M, Deshmukh A. Patient compliance with prolonged low-dose oral etoposide for small cell lung cancer. Br J Cancer 1993; 67:630–634.

91. Cerny T, Lind M, Thatcher N, Swindell R, Stout R. A simple out-patient treatment with oral ifosfamide and oral etoposide for patients with small-cell lung cancer (SCLC). Br J Cancer 1989; 60:258–261.

92. Manegold C, Bucher M, Hug G, Drings P. Phase II study of oral ifosfamide/mesna in small cell lung cancer. Proc ASCO 1993; 12:346.

93. Miller A, Herndon JI, Hollis D, et al. Schedule dependency of 21-day oral versus 3-day intravenous etoposide in combination with intravenous cisplatin in extensive-stage small-cell lung cancer: a randomized phase III study of the Cancer and Leukemia Group B. J Clin Oncol 1995; 13:1871–1879.

94. Party MRCLCW. Comparison of oral etoposide and standard intravenous multidrug chemotherapy for small-cell lung cancer: a stopped multicentre randomised trial. Lancet 1996; 348:563–566.

95. Souhami R, Spiro S, Rudd R, et al. Five-day oral etoposide treatment for advanced small-cell lung cancer: randomised comparison with intravenous chemotherapy. J Natl Cancer Inst 1997; 89:577–580.

96. Aisner J, J A. Cisplatin for small-cell lung cancer. Semin Oncol 1989; 16(suppl 6):2–9.

97. Gatzemeier U, Hossfeld D, Neuhauss R, Reck M, Achterrath W, Lenaz L. Carboplatin in small cell lung cancer. Semin Oncol 1991; 18(suppl 2):8–16.

98. Moore T, Korn E. Phase II trial design considerations for small cell lung cancer. J Natl Cancer Inst 1992; 85:150–156.

99. Straus M, Selawry O, Wallach R. Chemotherapy in lung cancer. In: Straus M, ed. Lung Cancer: Clinical Diagnosis and Treatment. New York: Grune & Stratton, 1983:261–283.

100. Ettinger D. The place of ifosfamide in chemotherapy of small cell lung cancer: the Eastern Cooperative Oncology Group experience and a selected literature update. Semin Oncol 1995; 22(suppl 2):23–27.

101. Ettinger D. Ifosfamide in the treatment of small cell lung cancer. Semin Oncol 1996; 23(suppl 6):2–6.

102. Johnson D. New drugs in the management of small cell lung cancer. Lung Cancer 1989; 5:221–225.

103. Cantwell B, Bozzino J, P C, Harris A. The multidrug resistant phenotype in clinical practice; evaluation of cross resistance to ifosfamide and mesna after VP16-213, doxorubicin and vincristine (VPAV) for small cell lung cancer. Eur J Cancer Clin Oncol 1988; 24:123–129.

104. Blackstein M, Eisenhauer E, Wierzbicki R, Yoshida S. Epirubicin in extensive small-cell lung cancer: a phase II study in previously untreated patients: a National Cancer Institute of Canada Clinical Trials Group. J Clin Oncol 1990; 8:385–389.

105. Clark P, Slevin M, Joel S, et al. A randomized trial of two etoposide schedules in small-cell lung cancer: the influence of pharmacokinetics on efficacy and toxicity. J Clin Oncol 1994; 12:1427–1435.

106. Bork E, Hansen M, Dombernowsky P. Teniposide (VM-26), an overlooked highly active agent in small cell lung cancer: results of a phase II trial in untreated patients. J Clin Oncol 1986; 4:524–527.

107. Bork E, Ersboll J, Dombernowsky P, Bergman B, Hansen M, Hansen H. Teniposide and etoposide in previously untreated small-cell lung cancer: a randomized study. J Clin Oncol 1991; 9:1627–1631.

108. Nesbitt J, Lee J, Komaki R, Roth J. Cancer of the lung. In: Holland J, Bast RJ, Morton D, Frei EI, Kufe D, Weichselbaum R, eds. Cancer Medicine. Vol. 2. Baltimore: Williams & Wilkins, 1996:1723–1803.

39

Optimal Integration of Chemotherapy and Thoracic Irradiation in Limited-Stage Small-Cell Lung Cancer

NEVIN MURRAY

British Columbia Cancer Agency
Vancouver, British Columbia, Canada

I. Introduction

The marked regression of an advanced malignancy in response to treatment is a dramatic event in medicine. Physicians familiar with the treatment of limited-stage small-cell lung cancer (LSCLC) know that it is easy to produce highly satisfactory improvement in symptoms and chest radiographs within a short period of time with multiagent chemotherapy or thoracic irradiation. However, the natural history of LSCLC is that despite impressive remissions, the majority of patients harbor resistant elements of disease that persist after induction therapy and cause an incurable relapse. The challenge in the treatment of LSCLC is to combine chemotherapy and thoracic irradiation in an optimal fashion, resulting in an improvement in median survival and the proportion of long-term survivors.

The Veterans Administration Lung Group system (1) that divided patients into either limited or extensive stages has endured for SCLC because of its simplicity and reliable prognostic value (2,3). LSCLC is defined as tumor confined to one hemithorax and the regional lymph nodes, whereas extensive-stage small-cell lung cancer (ESCLC) patients have disease spread beyond this definition. The original operational definition of limited disease was tumor quantity and configuration that could be encompassed by a "reasonable" radiotherapy treatment volume. Because long-term survival is uncommon (7–9%) when chemotherapy alone is used to treat LSCLC (4,5), the reasonable radiotherapy port rule continues to be a practical guide in the design of combined-modality therapy.

Since tedious and expensive staging procedures delay symptom-relieving treatment, and because chemotherapy is recommended for all fit patients anyway, some clinicians prefer not to bother with standard staging procedures outside the context of clinical trials. This pattern of practice may not have been associated with serious negative consequences when the treatment paradigm consisted of initial treatment with multiple chemotherapy cycles followed sequentially by administration of consolidative thoracic irradiation after drug treatment was complete. However, patients with bona fide LSCLC, as proven by careful staging using modern technology, benefit from innovations in thoracic irradiation administration such as early delivery of radiotherapy with combination chemotherapy. The enhanced curative power of such integrated modality protocols justifies their increased complexity and toxicity in LSCLC but not ESCLC. Careful staging remains mandatory for both clinical trials and routine patient care.

II. Assembly of Effective Combined-Modality Therapy

Previous experience with treatment protocols for LSCLC make it difficult to explore the process of combining therapeutic modalities in an unprejudiced manner. In this section the basic reasoning for combining therapeutic modalities in various ways will be examined. The two major considerations that must be understood for the creation of effective multimodality protocols include strategic and logistical factors. Strategy refers to development of a clever plan to achieve a specific goal; the goal in the treatment of LSCLC is to increase the probability of elimination of the last clonogenic cancer cell, thereby attaining a durable complete remission. Logistics deal with feasibility and practical matters whereby the best strategic plan is deployed within the bounds of acceptable toxicity. As pragmatic clinical oncologists, we usually think of strategic and logistical considerations as inseparable concepts. It may be useful as a heuristic exercise to examine strategic and logistical considerations separately. This would allow one to conceptually address how therapeutic modalities could be deployed in the most efficacious way without limits imposed by toxicity. If a superior strategic plan emerged from this exercise, the next step would require determination of whether the strategic and logistical considerations were compatible. Synthesis of a workable protocol may involve compromises.

A simplified overview of strategic considerations for combined-modality therapy could identify two distinct plans for combining chemotherapy and thoracic irradiation (Table 1). The strategy of the first plan would be to destroy as many cancer cells as possible in the shortest period of time. Such front-end loaded therapy would involve using the most effective modalities early in the treatment program. The alternative approach would require rationalization of the strategic superiority of deploying modalities in a sequential fashion. Sequential rather than concurrent use

Table 1 Strategic Basis for Early Integration Versus Sequential Delivery of Therapeutic Modalities in the Assembly of Multimodality Cancer Treatment Programs

Early Integration of Modalities
Characteristics:
Eliminate as many cancer cells as possible in the shortest period of time
Deploy multiple modalities quickly
Rationale:
Decreased probability of metastatic events
Lower probability of chemotherapy resistance
Lower probability of resistance to radiotherapy
Minimize accelerated repopulation
Sequential Assembly of Therapy
Characteristics:
Modalities deployed with temporal separation
Tumor burden more effectively destroyed in phases
Rationale:
Originally impossible local therapy rendered feasible by neoadjuvant therapy
Reversible resistance

of modalities in oncology has been prevalent for obvious logistical reasons including simplicity and diminished toxicity. However, in this exercise the objective is to ponder strategy unfettered by logistics; logistic considerations are unavoidable but will be dealt with later. A superior strategy requires a sound scientific foundation. The scientific hypotheses in favor of early use of effective therapeutic modalities versus sequential use of effective therapeutic modalities are shown in Table 1. Four concepts support early integration of effective modalities including decreased probability of metastatic events, lower probability of development of chemotherapy resistance, lower probability of development of resistance to radiotherapy, and diminished accelerated repopulation. On the other hand, existence of reversible resistance is a concept that could support sequential therapy. If a definitive local therapy was originally impossible but was rendered feasible by neoadjuvant therapy, this concept would also support the sequential therapy model. The next section will deal with these ideas directly.

A. Strategic Concepts That Favor Early Integrated Combined-Modality Therapy

The concepts that scientifically favor early integration of effective therapeutic modalities have clear-cut characteristics. The probability of the occurrence of treatment failure events associated with these concepts must increase fairly quickly with the elapse of time. Therefore, the chance of avoiding treatment failure should be minimized with elimination of as many tumor cells as possible in the shortest period of time. Rapid eradication of tumor cells requires the early integration of definitive local treatment(s) with systemic chemotherapy.

Decreased Probability of Metastatic Events

Experimental work by Hill (6,7) indicates that tumor cells mutate spontaneously and randomly to acquire metastatic potential. Moreover, once tumors reach a critical size or volume, metastatic phenotypes are generated "explosively." The cumulative probability of the existence of metastases and the number of metastases increase in proportion to elapsed time. The best way to decrease metastatic events is to eliminate as much tumor as possible in the shortest time.

Lower Probability of Chemotherapy Resistance

A large body of experimental and clinical data exists that support the observation that variability exists for chemosensitivity within tumor cell populations (8,9). Moreover, tumor cells display a capacity to be resistant to many drugs concurrently (10). The biologic basis of this evolution of resistance originates during tumor growth from mutations in the cancer genome (11). The development of resistant mutants is a random process, and the probability of their appearance increases with time in proportion to the total number of cell divisions the neoplastic burden has undergone. The somatic mutation theory of drug resistance (12) predicts that once a tumor has reached a critical size, the probability of cure is lost over a small additional size increase in a short time period. The best way to minimize the probability of chemotherapy resistance is to eliminate as much tumor as possible in the shortest time.

Lower Probability of Resistance to Radiotherapy

Local control rates with radiotherapy are inversely related to tumor size (13,14). Although microenvironmental effects such as hypoxia (15) may be relevant, increasing evidence indicates that tumor cell populations are heterogeneous with respect to inherent radiosensitivity, and like chemotherapy resistance, resistance to ionizing radiation may be genetically determined and a stochastic process (16). SCLC is less responsive to irradiation when recurrent after chemotherapy, and mechanisms of resistance may overlap; however, cross-resistance is only partial (17). The probability of mutation to radiotherapy resistance should be minimized by the early deployment of radiotherapy.

Diminished Accelerated Repopulation

Accelerated proliferation of tumors undergoing radiotherapy has been proposed (18,19) to explain the clinical observation that extended therapy regimens often require increased radiation dosages to achieve an isoeffective result (20,21). Accelerated tumor growth has been reported after surgery (22) and chemotherapy (23) in animal models. Accelerated repopulation will decrease local control, but additionally increased mitotic activity with larger burden of residual tumor may also hasten the tempo of metastatic events and increase the probability of developing drug resistance. Noncurative perturbation of the primary tumor may have detrimental effects (possibly mediated by cytokines) on existing metastatic lesions (24). Accelerated repopulation is independent of modalities and an obvious form of cross-resistance. This phenomenon has not been mathematically modeled, but it appears to be well established within a few weeks after initiation of therapy (18). Rapid destruction of tumor by early integration of chemoradiation should minimize the amount of tumor capable of repopulation.

B. Strategic Concepts That Favor Sequential Application of Modalities

The strategic concepts favoring early combined modality have a simple rule for the timing of effective modalities; any delay is potentially detrimental because probability of treatment failure increases as a function of time. The rules are not as straightforward for concepts that favor sequential modalities because an additional element of information is required. It is necessary to understand the optimum delay necessary for the sequence of modalities. This crucial knowledge can only be acquired by precise data supplied by the concept or facts learned by the conduct of controlled clinical trials.

Originally Impossible Local Therapy Rendered Feasible by Neoadjuvant Therapy

An unambiguous scenario where sequential therapy would offer an advantage would be when a locally advanced tumor was originally untreatable by a definitive local therapy but such therapy could be rendered feasible by downstaging. This is a classic rationale for neoadjuvant chemotherapy before surgery. However, LSCLC is rarely considered for surgery, and the definition of this stage indicates that all original tumor should be encompassable within a reasonable radiotherapy treatment volume.

Reversible Resistance

Sequential application of modalities could be strategically superior if resistance to a particular therapy (chemotherapy or radiotherapy) was present at one point in the treatment program but reversed later, allowing successful use of that modality. Once genetically determined resistance to chemotherapy has been acquired by a tumor, it is improbable that such elements would disappear by spontaneous mutation (11). However, resistance to chemotherapy with an epigenetic basis could occur and would be a possible form of reversible resistance. Kinetic resistance is another type of reversible resistance. The potential superiority of sequential therapies as predicted by the Norton-Simon hypothesis (25) is based on the possible existence of kinetic resistance.

The arguments supporting either early integration of chemoradiation or sequential utilization of chemotherapy and thoracic irradiation are hypothetical and must be supported by clinical data. The clinical data from treatment of LSCLC patients requires that strategic concepts be compatible with logistics as evidenced by acceptable toxicity. Clinical data to be examined will be classified under the following categories: meta-analysis of randomized trials of chemotherapy versus chemoradiation, overview of large cooperative group trials of therapy for LSCLC, and randomized trials of thoracic irradiation timing.

III. Meta-Analyses of Phase III Trials of Chemotherapy With or Without Thoracic Irradiation

Many randomized studies investigated this question. Two meta-analyses have been published that examine the trials to determine the role of thoracic radiotherapy in LSCLC (4,5). One was based on published data (1911 patients) and looked at 2-year survival rates, local control, and toxicity (4). The other included 2140 patients and examined survival at 3 years and prognostic factors for survival (5). Because most data in each meta-analysis were derived from the same studies, the conclusions are consistent and complementary despite differences in the methods used in the meta-analyses. Both show a modest improvement in survival rates in those patients given thoracic radiotherapy. The survival benefit becomes evident at about 15 months after start of treatment and persists beyond 5 years. At 3 years, 8.9% of the chemotherapy-only group are alive, compared with 14.3% of the combined-modality group. The relative rate of death in the combined-modality group as compared with the chemotherapy group was 0.86 (95% confidence interval, 0.78–0.94; $p = 0.001$) corresponding to a 14% reduction in the mortality rate. The analysis of local control was based on 1521 patients for whom data were reported and showed a marked reduction in the absolute 2-year local failure rate comparing the irradiated patients (23%) to the nonirradiated patients (48%) ($p = 0.0001$). These benefits were obtained at the cost of an increase in treatment-related deaths of 1%.

Most of these studies were designed to permit a chemotherapy response evaluation, which allows the possibility of a reduction in the radiotherapy field size. The timing of thoracic irradiation was most often after three to six cycles of chemotherapy but was concurrent with the first cycle of chemotherapy in four studies. Most studies were initiated before 1981, and none delivered cisplatin and etoposide concurrent with thoracic irradiation. Treatment factors, such as radiotherapy timing and chemoradiation integration (sequential, concurrent, or alternating), were not significant in the meta-analyses, but the heterogeneity of trial design did not allow a precise assessment of these issues. An additional explanation for not demonstrating the importance of timing or integration of thoracic irradiation may be found in the shape of the survival curve and the statistical methodology used in this analysis. Initially, the overall survival graph begins in favor of chemotherapy, but the curves cross at about one year and later demonstrate a long-term survival advantage for chemoradiation. The initial separation of the curves is not large, but many events occur on this steep portion of the curves. Because thoracic irradiation adds toxicity, which may diminish chemotherapy delivery, the relative risk of death is not constant over time. The short-term mortality increase may cancel out the long-term survival gain as measured by relative risk. Reexamination of this data set for an effect of thoracic irradiation timing on long-term survival rather than relative risk of death may be useful. In the modern era, state-of-the-art thoracic irradiation concurrent with cisplatin and etoposide and proper supportive care should prevent any excess mortality from early chemoradiation and allow uncompromised administration of both modalities.

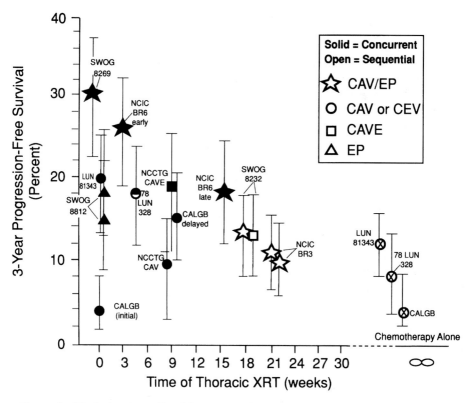

Figure 1 Limited stage small-cell lung cancer: 3-year progression-free survival versus time of thoracic irradiation relative to the beginning of chemotherapy. Solid symbols represent concurrent chemotherapy and thoracic irradiation. Open symbols represent sequential chemotherapy and thoracic irradiation. The half-solid symbol is alternating chemotherapy and split-course thoracic irradiation. Open symbols with an X indicate that thoracic irradiation was not given. Symbol shape indicates the type of chemotherapy: stars = CAV/EP (cyclophosphamide, doxorubicin, vincristine/etoposide, cisplatin); circles = CAV (cyclophosphamide, doxorubicin, vincristine); squares = CAVE (cyclophosphamide, doxorubicin, vincristine, etoposide); triangles = EP (etoposide/cisplatin). Study references: SWOG 8269 (29), LUN81343 (28), SWOG 8812 (34), CALGB (26,37), NCIC BR6 (30), NCCTG (31), SWOG 8232 (33), NCIC BR3 (32).

IV. Cooperative Group Experience Review

In an attempt to identify timing and integration factors associated with long-term survival, 18 arms of large (≥ 100 patients per arm) cooperative group trials (26–34) were reviewed (Fig. 1). In the figure, long-term survival rates are plotted against the timing of the initiation of thoracic irradiation relative to the initiation of chemotherapy (time 0). Three year progression-free survival was used as an estimation of long-term survival, as the "breakpoint" of progression-free survival curves for LSCLC trials typically occurs 2–3 years after the start of treatment (35). All studies used standard (36) chemotherapy regimens. The entire data set includes more than 2700 patients.

Examination of Figure 1 reveals a tendency for 3-year PFS to decrease as the time to the start of thoracic irradiation increases. Within the irradiated group, those receiving thoracic irradiation within 6 weeks of chemotherapy commencement appear to have an elevated 3-year PFS of 20.3% versus 13.2% for those irradiated later. Good survival rates from studies administering late thoracic irradiation (18–20 weeks from the beginning of systemic treatment) are conspicuous by their absence. The most unambiguous theme of this review of cooperative group experience is that the probability of cure deteriorates steadily as thoracic irradiation is progressively delayed in combined-modality LSCLC protocols. After about 20 weeks, thoracic irradiation may enhance palliation by increasing local control, but it makes little contribution to the cure rate.

V. Randomized Trials of the Timing of Thoracic Irradiation

The highest standard of evidence for the optimal timing of chemotherapy and thoracic irradiation for LSCLC comes from prospective randomized trials directly addressing this question. To date, five trials (26,30,37–40) of thoracic irradiation timing have been performed; three trials are published in peer-reviewed journals, and two are currently available as abstracts. Because of the importance of these data, each study is discussed separately, and the trials are summarized in Table 2.

A. The Cancer and Leukemia Group B Trial

This large trial (26,37), performed from 1981 to 1984, included 399 evaluable LSCLC patients distributed between three arms including chemotherapy alone (cyclophosphamide, etoposide, vincristine, and doxorubicin), initial chemoradiation (50 Gy thoracic irradiation and whole brain irradiation concurrently with the initial cycle of chemotherapy), and delayed chemoradiation (chest and brain irradiation concurrently with the fourth cycle of chemotherapy at week 9). Both arms that included thoracic irradiation had significantly superior response rates, time to progression, and overall survival rates compared with chemotherapy alone. However, no significant differences were found between the initial and delayed

Table 2 Randomized Trials of Thoracic Irradiation Timing in Limited Stage Small-Cell Lung Cancer

| Study (Ref.) | Drugs | Thoracic irradiation | | | Number of patients | | Survival, median (mo.) | | Survival, 5-year (%) | | p-value |
| | | Dose | Start Time | | | | | | | | |
			Early	Late	Early	Late	Early	Late	Early	Late	
1. CALGB (26,37)	CEVA	50Gy/25F/5wk	Week 1	Week 9	125	145	13.04	14.54	6.6	12.8	NS
2. Aarhus (38)	CAV/EP	40–45Gy/22F/6wk[a]	Week 1	Week 18	99	100	10.7	12.9	10.0	10.0	NS
3. NCIC (30)	CAV/EP	40/15F/3wk	Week 3	Week 15	155	153	21.2	16.0	22.0	13.0	0.013
4. Yugoslavian (39)	Carbo/EP	54Gy/36F/3 1/2wk	Week 1	Week 6	52	51	34	26	30	15	0.027
5. JCOG (40)	EP	45Gy/30F/3wk	Week 1	Week 15	114	114	31.3	20.8	30	15	<0.05

CALGB: Cancer and Leukemia Group B; NCIC: National Cancer Institute of Canada; JCOG: Japan Clinical Oncology Group; C: cyclophosphamide; E: etoposide; V: vincristine; A: doxorubicin; P: cisplatin; Carbo: carboplatin.
[a]Split course.

thoracic irradiation arms; the insignificant trend that existed favors the delayed thoracic irradiation arm. The rationale of a randomized trial is to hold all variables constant except the experimental one. Unfortunately, the interpretation of the CALGB study is confounded by the fact that, in addition to the differences in thoracic irradiation timing set by the protocol, myelosuppression from initial thoracic irradiation, brain irradiation, and concurrent CEV chemotherapy resulted in an unplanned attenuation (50% reduction) in subsequent doses of cyclophosphamide, etoposide, and doxorubicin. This trial clearly supports the addition of thoracic irradiation to chemotherapy in LSCLC, but the utility of the study to provide guidance for optimal integration of chemoradiation is doubtful. The long-term survival rates for chemoradiation in the CALGB study are <13% (37).

B. The Aarhus Lung Cancer Group Trial

In this Danish trial (38), performed between 1981 and 1989, 199 patients with LSCLC were randomly allocated to initial chest irradiation or late chest irradiation delayed by 18 weeks. Both groups received nine cycles of combination chemotherapy: three cycles of EP and six cycles of CAV. Initial thoracic irradiation was delivered sequentially rather than concurrently with EP. The timing of radiotherapy (40–45 Gy) had no significant effect on the median survival (about one year) or long-term survival (about 10%).

C. The National Cancer Institute of Canada Trial

In 1993, the NCIC published results of a randomized trial (30) (accrual period 1985–1988) comparing early versus late thoracic irradiation (Fig. 2) that demonstrated a significant improvement in survival for early thoracic irradiation in the combined modality therapy of LSCLC. All 308 eligible patients received CAV alternating with EP for three cycles of each regimen. Patients randomized to early thoracic irradiation received 40 Gy/15F to the primary site concurrent with the first cycle of EP (week 3), and the late thoracic irradiation arm received the same radiation concurrent with the last cycle of EP (week 15). Dose intensity and total dose of chemotherapy were uniform in both arms (85–90% delivery according to protocol).

Although complete response rates were not significantly different (CR early arm 64%, CR late arm 56%; $p = 0.14$), the overall survival was significantly superior ($p = 0.013$) in the early thoracic irradiation arm (Fig. 3). Median survival was 21.2 months in the early arm and 16.0 months in the late arm; actual survival at 5 years was 22% in the early arm and 13% in the late arm. A delay of thoracic irradiation by 12 weeks was associated with a 50% decrease in the probability of long-term survival. This was the first phase III study to demonstrate that actual 5-year survival rates of over 20% were achievable using early integrated chemoradiation in LSCLC.

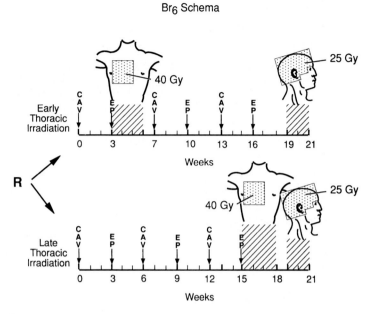

Figure 2   Schema of the National Cancer Institute of Canada BR6 trial. (From Ref. 30.)

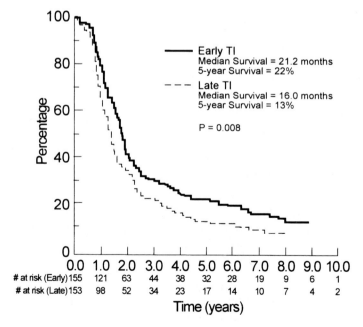

Figure 3   Final analysis for overall survival of the National Cancer Institute of Canada BR6 study. (From Ref. 30.)

D. The Yugoslavian Trial

This extraordinary phase III (39) study performed between 1988 and 1992 not only achieved outcomes in LSCLC that are superior to any other phase III study, but survival is also better than in any published phase II trial. All patients received accelerated hyperfractionated thoracic irradiation with 1.5 Gy twice daily to 54 Gy plus concurrent daily carboplatin/etoposide and four sequential cycles of EP. Early thoracic irradiation was delivered between weeks 1 and 4, and late thoracic irradiation patients received concurrent chemoradiation between weeks 6 and 9. The difference in timing of the initiation of thoracic irradiation between the two arms was only 6 weeks.

The median survival was 34 months for initial chemoradiation versus 26 months for delayed chemoradiation; 5-year survival was 30% and 15%, respectively. The difference was almost significant on univariate analysis ($p = 0.052$) and was significant on multivariate analysis ($p = 0.027$). This study by Jeremic and colleagues (39) shows that early integration of chemotherapy with intensive radiation for LSCLC may generate median survival times of almost 3 years, and long-term survival rates may approach 30%.

E. The Japan Clinical Oncology Group Trial

This study (40) also examined the optimal sequence of chemoradiation for LSCLC by randomizing patients to initial concurrent versus sequential chemoradiation. The chemotherapy prescription was EP (4 cycles), and thoracic irradiation consisted of 45 Gy over 3 weeks (2 daily fractions of 1.5 Gy). Two hundred and twenty-eight patients were entered between 1991 and 1995.

Initial concurrent chemoradiation was significantly superior ($p < 0.05$) to sequential therapy with median survivals of 31.3 and 20.8 months and projected 5-year survival rates of 30% and 15%, respectively. These results strengthen the conclusion that long-term survival rates of >20% for LSCLC are obtainable with early chemoradiation.

F. Why Are the Randomized Trials of Thoracic Irradiation Timing Discordant?

Of the five controlled trials of thoracic irradiation timing performed, three—NCIC (30), Yugoslavian (39), and JCOG (40)—support the concept that the optimal integration of chemotherapy and thoracic irradiation is early concurrent chemoradiation; the CALGB (26) and the Aarhus (38) studies suggest that the timing of thoracic irradiation does not change outcome. Why are the results discordant? There are three possible reasons:

1. The timing of thoracic irradiation is unimportant and the discordant results are due to the play of chance.
2. Delivery of chemotherapy or thoracic irradiation was compromised during early concurrent chemoradiation because of toxicity.
3. The patient populations differ.

Although the influence of chance cannot be discounted definitely, other explanations may be more credible. The CALGB study (26) may illustrate the detrimental effect of reduction in chemotherapy delivery below standard dosage. Concurrent chemoradiation with EP is clearly less toxic than with regimens based on cyclophosphamide. However, the most important reason for discordance of results probably is associated with differences in the patient populations. Thoracic irradiation improves the long-term prognosis of LSCLC only in cases in which the systemic therapy is successful at treating distant disease (where present) but fails to eliminate regional disease. The prevalence of metastatic drug-resistant tumor outside the thoracic irradiation volume creates an inherent statistical obstacle that makes it more difficult to show a survival advantage in clinical trials of thoracic irradiation (or an innovation of it such as timing or dose). If a poor-prognosis LSCLC population (as evidenced by short median survival) is studied, the prevalence of metastatic chemotherapy resistant disease must be high and the proportion of cases that can have their prognosis improved with optimal integration of chemoradiation is low. As demonstrated in Table 2, the median survival outcome is inferior in the CALGB (26) and Aarhus (38) trials, which fail to show superiority of early chemoradiation; long-term survival in these reports is also discouraging. The high proportion of incurable cases (defined by metastatic resistant elements) in these studies may "dilute out" the benefits of early chemoradiation. The NCIC (30), Yugoslavian (39), and JCOG (40) trials have better median and long-term survival because they have a higher proportion of patients that are potential beneficiaries of optimized chemoradiation. The benchmark for long-term survival in modern studies of chemoradiation for LSCLC should definitely be greater than 20%; delayed or consolidative thoracic irradiation protocols have never approached this milestone.

VI. Optimal Integration of Chemoradiation for LSCLC: Recommendations

After the diagnosis of SCLC, accurate staging should be completed as expediently as possible and therapy should begin without unnecessary delay. Patients with LSCLC should have consultation from both medical and radiation oncologists before commencing treatment. If an appropriate clinical trial is available, it should be offered to the patient. The ethics of phase II and III studies for LSCLC patients must consider that published integrated chemoradiation protocols reproducibly generate actual 5-year survival rates of at least 20% in patient populations eligible for such trials.

A. Integration of Chemotherapy and Thoracic Irradiation

The best results are obtained with a combination of multiagent chemotherapy and thoracic irradiation. Thoracic irradiation should be integrated with EP chemotherapy early (less than 6 weeks) (41) in a protocol that allows reliable delivery of both modalities.

B. The Chemotherapy Regimen

Sequential EP has become a widely accepted standard chemotherapy for LSCLC because it can be administered concurrently with thoracic irradiation with acceptable toxicity. Four cycles of EP appear to produce results as good as longer duration chemotherapy. Additionally, EP has been integrated with thoracic irradiation in a number of LSCLC trials that address thoracic irradiation questions, and early chemoradiation results (39,40,42) compare favorably with older data. However, it must be noted that no large LSCLC studies have directly compared the EP regimen to another chemotherapy regimen. Curiously, no randomized studies exist to demonstrate EP to be superior to any other regimen for any stage of SCLC. There is no proof that dose or dose intensity escalation above levels that produce moderately severe myelosuppression are more effective; however, trials examining more intensive therapy in SCLC have mainly been done in incurable ESCLC patients. The EP regimen has attained the status of standard chemotherapy for LSCLC by expert opinion rather than data from controlled trials; standard chemotherapy for a curable neoplasm should have better credentials (43).

C. Thoracic Irradiation

The radiotherapy volumes should encompass all areas of gross primary and mediastinal disease since there is no scientific rationale for the presumption that chemotherapy-resistant elements could be confined to a smaller volume. In the absence of evidence of infection, thoracic irradiation should not be interrupted for neutropenia, regardless of its severity. Dose fractionation regimens range from 40 Gy in 15 fractions to 50 Gy in 25 fractions. To date, there are no data from randomized trials to prove superiority of more intensive thoracic radiation. However, as more sensitive staging procedures select a more curable LSCLC patient population, the benefits of thoracic irradiation innovations such as altered fractionation may be more easily established.

VII. Moving Forward

Optimal integration of chemoradiation for LSCLC is an elusive goal that must be pursued with novel strategies. If current chemoradiation protocols are capable of generating a 20% long-term survival rate, lung cancer investigators must consider how much further improvement is important enough to warrant a clinical trial large enough to prove it. If a trial of a new therapy was proposed to declare significant (alpha = 0.05, power = 0.90) an increase in the long-term survival rate from 20 to 30%, the total sample size required would be 676 patients. An improvement from 20 to 25% would require over 2000 patients. The rationale for the creation of large intergroup trials is particularly strong in LSCLC, in which modest therapeutic advance seems possible. A substantial improvement from a succession of small advances is realistic.

References

1. Green RA, Humphrey E, Close H, et al. Alkylating agents in bronchogenic carcinoma. Am J Med 1969; 46:516–525.
2. Albain KS, Crowley JJ, LeBlanc M, et al. Determinants of improved outcome in small cell lung cancer: An analysis of the 2,580-patient Southwest Oncology Group data base. J Clin Oncol 1990; 8:1563–1574.
3. Rawson NSB, Peto J. An overview of prognostic factors in small cell lung cancer: a report from the Subcommittee for the Management of Lung Cancer of the United Kingdom Coordinating Committee on Cancer Research. Br J Cancer 1990; 61:597–604.
4. Warde P, Payne D. Does thoracic irradiation improve survival and local control in limited-stage small-cell carcinoma of the lung? A meta-analysis. J Clin Oncol 1992; 10:890–895.
5. Pignon JP, Arriagada R, Ihde DC, et al. A meta-analysis of thoracic radiotherapy for small cell lung cancer. N Engl J Med 1992; 327:1618–24.
6. Hill RP, Chambers AF, Ling V. Dynamic heterogeneity: rapid generation of metastatic variants in mouse B 16 melanoma cells. Science 1984; 224:998–1001.
7. Hill RP, Young SD, Ling V, et al. Metastatic cell phenotypes: quantitative studies using the experimental metastasis assay. Cancer Rev 1986; 5:118–151.
8. Claes Trope. Different susceptibilites of tumor cell subpopulations to cytotoxic agents and therapeutic consequences. In: Owens AH, Coffey DS, Baylin SB, eds. Tumor Cell Heterogeneity: Origins and Implications. New York: Academic Press, 1982:147.
9. Young RC. Drug Resistance: the clinical problem. In: Ozols RF, ed. Drug Resistance in Cancer Therapy. Norwell, MA: Kluwer Academic Publishers, 1989:1.
10. Cole SP, Bhardwaj G, Gerlach JH, et al. Overexpression of a transporter gene in a multidrug-resistant human lung cancer cell line. Science 1992; 258:1650–1654.
11. Goldie JH, Coldman AJ. Genetic origin of drug resistance in neoplasms. Cancer Res 1984; 44:3643–3653.
12. Goldie JG, Coldman AJ. A mathematical model for relating the drug sensitivity of tumors to their spontaneous mutation rate. Cancer Treat Rep 1979; 63:1727–1733.
13. Tubiana M. The role of local treatment in the cure of cancer. Eur J Cancer 1992; 28:2061–2069.
14. Suit H. Local control and patient survival. Int J Radiat Oncol Biol Phys 1992; 23:653–660.
15. Tomlinson RH, Gray LH. The histological structure of some human lung cancers and the possible implications for radiotherapy. Br J Cancer 1955; 9:539–549.
16. Yaes RJ. Tumor heterogeneity, tumor size, and radioresistance. Int J Radiat Oncol Biol Phys 1989; 17:993–1005.
17. Ochs JJ, Tester WJ, Cohen MH, et al. "Salvage" radiation therapy for intrathoracic small cell carcinoma of the lung progressing on combination chemotherapy. Cancer Treat Rep 1983; 67:1123–1126.
18. Withers HR, Taylor JMG, Maciejewski B. The hazard of accelerated tumor clonogen repopulation during radiotherapy. Acta Oncol 1988; 27:131–146.
19. Trott KR. Cell repopulation and overall treatment time. Int J Radiat Oncol Phys 1990; 19:1071–1075.
20. Maciejewski B, Preuss-Bayer G, Trott KR. The influence of the number of fractions and of overall treatment time on local control and late complication rate in squamous cell carcinoma of the larynx. Int J Radiat Oncol Biol Phys 1983; 9:321–328.
21. Holsti LR, Mantyla M. Split-course versus continuous radiotherapy. Analysis of a randomized trial from 1964 to 1967. Acta Oncol 1988; 27:153–161.
22. Simpson-Herren L, Sanford, AH, Holmquist JP. Effects of surgery on the cell kinetics of residual tumor. Cancer Treat Rep 1976; 60:1749–1760.
23. Stephens TC, Steel GG. Regeneration of tumors after cytotoxic treatment. In: Meyn RE, Withers HR, eds. Radiation Biology in Cancer Research. New York: Raven Press, 1980: 385–395.
24. Fisher B, Gunduz N, Coyle J, et al. Presence of a growth stimulating factor in serum following primary tumor removal in mice. Cancer Res 1989; 49:1996–2002.

25. Norton L, Simon R. Tumor size, sensitivity to therapy and design of treatment schedules. Cancer Treat Rep 1977; 61:1307–1317.
26. Perry MC, Eaton WL, Propert KJ, et al. Chemotherapy with or without radiation therapy in limited small-cell carcinoma of the lung. N Engl J Med 1987; 316:912–918.
27. Perez CA, Einhorn L, Oldham RK, et al. Randomized trial or radiotherapy to the thorax in limited small-cell carcinoma of the lung treated with multiagent chemotherapy and elective brain irradiation: a preliminary report. J Clin Oncol 1984; 2:1200–1208.
28. Johnson DH, Bass D, Einhorn LH, et al. Combination chemotherapy with or without thoracic radiotherapy in limited-stage small-cell lung cancer: a randomized trial of the Southeastern Cancer Study Group. J Clin Oncol 1993; 11:1223–1229.
29. McCracken JD, Janaki LM, Crowley JJ, et al. Concurrent chemotherapy/radiotherapy for limited small-cell lung carcinoma: a Southwest Oncology Group study. J Clin Oncol 1990; 8:892–898.
30. Murray N, Coy P, Pater J, et al. Importance of timing for thoracic irradiation in the combined modality treatment of limited-stage small-cell lung cancer. J Clin Oncol 1993; 11:336–344.
31. Jett JR, Everson L, Therneau TM, et al. Treatment of limited-stage small-cell lung cancer with cyclophosphamide, doxorubicin and vincristine with or without etoposide: a randomized trial of the North Central Cancer Treatment Group. J Clin Oncol 1990; 8:33–39.
32. Feld R, Evans WK, Coy P, et al. Canadian multicenter randomized trial comparing sequential and alternating administration of two non-cross resistant chemotherapy combinations in patients with limited small cell carcinoma of the lung. J Clin Oncol 1987; 5:1401–1409.
33. Goodman GE, Crowley JJ, Blasko JC, et al. Treatment of limited small cell lung cancer with etoposide and cisplatin alternating with vincristine, doxorubicin and cyclophosphamide versus concurrent etoposide, vincristine, doxorubicin, and cyclophosphamide and chest radiotherapy: A Southwest Oncology Group Study. J Clin Oncol 1990; 8:39–47.
34. Bunn P, Crowley J, Kelly K, Hazuka M, Beasley K, Upchurch C, Livingston R. Chemoradiotherapy with or without granulocyte-macrophage colony-stimulating factor in the treatment of limited-stage small-cell lung cancer: a prospective phase III randomized study of the Southwest Oncology Group 1995; 13:1632–1641.
35. Stephens R, Bailey A, Machin D. Long-term survival in small cell lung cancer: the case for a standard definition. Lung Cancer 1996; 15:297–309.
36. Ihde DH. Chemotherapy of lung cancer. N Engl J Med 1992; 327:1434–141.
37. Perry MC, Herndon JE, Eaton WL, Green MR. Thoracic radiation therapy added to chemotherapy in limited small cell lung cancer: an update of Cancer and Leukemia Group B study 8083 (abstr). Proc Am Soc Clin Oncol 1996; 15:384.
38. Nielsen OS, Fode K, Bentzen SM, Schultz HP, Steenholdt S, Palshof T. Timing of radiotherapy and chemotherapy in limited stage small cell lung cancer. Final analysis. Eur J Cancer 1991; suppl 2:S182.
39. Jeremic B, Shibamato Y, Acimovic L, Milisavljevic S. Initial versus delayed accelerated hyperfractionated radiation therapy and concurrent chemotherapy in limited small-cell lung cancer: a randomized study. J Clin Oncol 1997; 15:893–900.
40. Takada M, Fukuoka M, Furuse K, Ariyoshi Y, Ikegami H, Kurita Y, Nishiwaki Y, Nishikawa H, Wantanabe K, Noda K, Saijo N. Phase III study of concurrent versus sequential thoracic radiotherapy in combination with cisplatin and etoposide for limited-stage small cell lung cancer: preliminary results of the Japan Clinical Oncology Group (JCOG) (abstr). Proc Am Soc Clin Oncol 1996; 15:372.
41. Murray N, Coldman A. The relationship between thoracic irradiation timing and long-term survival in combined modality therapy of limited stage small cell lung cancer (abstr). Proc Am Soc Clin Oncol 1995; 14:360.
42. Johnson DH, Kim K, Sause W, Komaki R, Wagner H, Aisner S, Livingston R, Blum R, Turrisi AT. Cisplatin(P) & etoposide (E) + thoracic radiotherapy (TRT) administered once or twice daily (BID) in limited stage (LS) small cell lung cancer (SCLC): final report of intergroup trial 0096 (abstr). Proc Am Soc Clin Oncol 1996; 15:374.
43. Sackett DL. Rules of evidence and clinical recommendations on the use of antithrombotic agents. Chest 1989; 95(suppl):25–45.

40

Long-Term Survivors of Small-Cell Lung Cancer, Late Effects of Treatment, and Second Cancers

PASCALE JACOULET

Centre Hospitalier Universitaire
Besançon, France

DENIS MORO

Institut Albert Bonniot
Centre Hospitalier Universitaire
de Grenoble,
Grenoble, France

Since the introduction of chemotherapy, the prognosis of small-cell lung cancer (SCLC) has dramatically improved (1). Median survival increased from 3 months before the chemotherapy era to 12–16 months with the most recent treatment combinations. Matthews (2) in 1980 described the first report of long-term survivors (LTS) of SCLC. Since then, more than 111 publications have dealt with LTS of SCLC (3). LTS have been described in three different types of studies: analysis of prognostic factors in phase II and III chemotherapy trials (1,4–11), epidemiological studies (12), and medical registries of LTS (13,14). There is no consensus on the definition of long-term survival. Although the majority of studies have considered a duration of 2 years, the deadline chosen to define LTS could vary from 18 months to 5 years. Stephens (3) in a recent article studied the risk of death in a population of 2196 patients coming from 6 SCLC trials. The risk of death remains constant up to about 2 years and after a transition period decreases and remains constant for 3 years onwards. Thus, Stephens suggested that 3 years should be considered as the standard definition of LTS. Other authors (9,11,15) have noted the change in the causes of death occurring between 2 and 3 years.

The most frequent cause of mortality within the 2–3 first years is relapse of SCLC, while mortality thereafter is primarily due to second malignancies and intercurrent diseases (4,7).

I. Prognostic Factors of Long-Term Survival

A. Biological Prognostic Factors

Sloman (16) has compared the immunohistochemical characteristics of two groups of SCLC patients: LTS (>2 years) (13 patients) and a control group of short-term survivors (15 patients). The tumoral expression of corticotropin, bcl-2, *p*-glycoprotein, cathepsin B, cathepsin D, CD44, carcinoembryonic antigen, collagenase IV, Leu-7, neu oncoprotein, p53, S100, and synaptophysin was assessed. The tumors from prolonged survivors disclosed a relative absence of staining for cathepsin B (0/13 vs. 3/13 [23%]; p = 0.037), cathepsin D (5/13 [38%] vs. 13/15 [87%]; p = 0.006), carcinoembryonic antigen (5/13 [38%] vs. 11/15 [73%]; p = 0.047), and neu oncoprotein (5/13 [38%] vs. 14/15 [93%]; p = 0.0014).

Bobrow (17) compared the expression of immunohistochemical markers in biopsies taken from short- and long-term survivors. Neuroendocrine markers (NSE, chromogranin), adhesion molecules (N-CAM), carcinoembryonic antigen, S100 protein, cytokeratins, proliferating antigens, and mucins were not expressed differently in short- and long-term survivors.

B. Clinical Prognostic Factors

Clinical prognostic factors on survival have been largely studied from phase II or phase III trials (5,6,8,18). These factors, usually divided into three categories (tumor, patients' characteristics, therapy), show few differences from one author to another essentially due to various statistical methods (logistic regression, cox model, recursive partitioning). The strongest independent factor arising from all multivariate studies is always the stage. With a recursive partitioning method, the median survival was 15.5 months for limited SCLC, whereas it was 7.2 months for diffuse SCLC (p < 0.00005) (5). Other factors are then frequently studied in either limited or diffuse diseases.

In limited SCLC, performance status (PS) $\geq$ 2 and age $\geq$ 60 are unfavorable factors for survival (6,8). In a study by Albain et al., only PS was of significant importance for 5-year survival, but when biological parameters were added to the model, the lactate dehydrogenase (LDH) value became the most important factor to predict outcome at 5 years (6). The 2-year survival rate was 16% in case of normal LDH value versus 6% in case of elevated LDH value (18). Therapy played an important role as well, but only in short-term survival of limited SCLC: patients treated with chemoradiotherapy had a better 2-year survival rate than others, but there was no therapeutic factor of significant value in the 5-year survival of limited SCLC (6).

In diffuse SCLC, a bad PS is an unfavorable prognostic factor, whereas age is not (8). An elevated LDH value was the only independent prognostic factor to adversely affect one-year survival (6). Spiegelman pointed out the unfavorable effect of more than two metastatic sites (8).

Female gender was recognized as a favorable prognostic factor in both stages (8) as well as only in limited SCLC (5).

The above data were obtained from several thousand patients involved in clinical trials. In studies conducted by large cooperative American groups (CALGB, SWOG), the aim was to study not LTS but prognostic factors.

II. Long-Term Survivors

The studies of long-term survivors frequently took the form of descriptive analysis. The 5-year survival rates were similar, varying from 2.3 to 7.4% in different studies (7,11,18–20). In the SWOG analysis (6) 63 of 1363 limited SCLC patients (4.6%) were alive more than 5 years later, and the 2-year survival for diffuse SCLC patients was 4.4% (51/1138). The 10-year survival rate was 1.8% (limited: 2.5%; diffuse: 1.2%) in a study by Lassen et al. (11).

In the French database (21), 5- and 10-year survival rates were, respectively, 68% and 44% for patients having reached 30-month survival. In these patients, three independant factors were predictive of a survival longer *than* 5 years: age $\leq$ 60 at the time of diagnosis (OR = 2.85; IC 95% [1.23–6.6]; p = 0.01), chest radiotherapy (OR = 3.1; IC 95% [1.28–7.69]; p = 0.006), and absence of relapse (OR = 4.5; IC 95% [1.75–12.5]; p = 0.002).

A. Relapses

In the population of patients surviving longer than 5 years, the disease-free survival rates were 52% for limited disease (6) and 43% for both stages with a 9-year median time of follow-up (11). This means that relapse allows long-term survival for about one patient out of two. However, the absence of relapse was a predictive factor of a more than 5-year survival in the French multivariate study (21). The risk of relapse was estimated from 25 to 50% (4,7,9,21). Relapses can occur many years after the diagnosis of SCLC: the latest observed relapses were reported at 11 years (11,22). Nevertheless, the risk of relapse dramatically decreased from 32% at 2 years to 14% at 3 years in a study by Osterlind et al. (4). Relapse was more frequently responsible for death when it occurred in an initially diffuse SCLC: in the cohort of $\geq$5-year survivors, 49% of diffuse SCLC patients versus 5% of limited SCLC patients died from relapse (6). In the French data base of patients surviving longer than 30 months, 27% of patients relapsed, and the only independent risk factor for relapse was age $\geq$ 60 at the time of diagnosis (OR = 2.46; IC 95% [1.15–5.27]; p = 0.02). Sex, stage, tobacco smoking, cisplatin, number of cycles, and thoracic irradiation were not of significant value for the risk of relapse (21).

Retreatment of patients after relapse of SCLC is always debated. The majority of long-term survivors were initially treated with combination chemotherapy or combined radiation and chemotherapy. Thus, these patients have a reduced ability to tolerate retreatment with chemotherapy. Furthermore, some of these patients are unfit for retreatment. In a recent article, Chute et al. (23) reported that among 20 relapses of SCLC occurring in LTS, 25% had PS > 2. The objective response rate after second-line treatment was 56% in the NCI study (23) and 44% in the EORTC study (24). These results are in sharp contrast with those obtained in early relapses of SCLC. Albain et al. (25) reported a 4–13% response rate in a SWOG study of patients who relapsed within the first 6 months following completion of treatment. It must be stressed that in the NCI study the response rate increased to 69% in patients with PS = 0–2 and that none of the patients whose PS was greater than 2 had an objective response following retreatment (23). The response rate varied according to the type of retreatment with the best results obtained with etoposide-based regimens with or without cisplatinum. It has been demonstrated (26,27) that a late recurrence of SCLC (more than 1 year after first-line treatment) is often responsive to the same chemotherapy given as induction therapy. The survival duration after relapse seems to be improved by chemotherapy. The median survival in the NCI study was 6.5 months in the retreated patients (23). Sekine et al. (28), in a cohort of 13 patients, obtained a median survival of 7.4 months after retreatment of SCLC. In the French data base, the overall median survival was 12 months after relapse (range: 2–56+ months), and among the relapsing patients who received a second-line treatment, 21.8% survived longer than 30 months after retreatment.

B. Second Primary Tumors

The ability of developing a second primary tumor (SPT) has been widely recognized in long-term survivors of SCLC. The prolongation of survival has given these patients enough time to develop a second malignancy. The cumulative risk of SPT in long-term survivors may vary from 4 to 30% (4,6,7,9,11,13,21,29,30). The risk increases with time. The actuarial risk of developing a second aerodigestive cancer increases from 2% per patient per year to 14.4% over the course of 10 years (31). After 3 or 4 years, the risk of developing a SPT exceeds that of recurrent SCLC (9,32) and may reach 50% at 8 years.

Most of these SPT are smoking-related tumors, but in some reports the number of cancers not related to tobacco smoking seems more important than the number of smoking-related tumors (7,33). The predominant tumor types occurring in these patients are non–small-cell lung carcinomas, especially squamous cell carcinomas, head and neck, esophagus, and bladder cancers. It must be pointed out that some difficulties can be encountered in the differential diagnosis between a second primary non–small-cell lung cancer and a relapse of the initial SCLC. There is a real need for pathological confirmation. Martini and Melamed define SPT as histologically different tumors from the initial cancer occurring in a different site at least 2 years later in patients considered to be in complete remission (34). NSCLC occurring in LTS of SCLC or in LTS of Hodgkin's disease share the same type and frequency of mutations on *ras* and *p53* genes (35), suggesting the strong role of tobacco smoking in the development of these cancers.

In addition, it has been demonstrated that 30–38% of SCLC are in fact combined tumors, and NSCLC clones of cells are not always detected by small biopsies (36). Some second NSCLC could emerge belatedly from these combined tumors (37).

The relative importance of smoking-related tumors emphasizes the need for smoking cessation in patients in complete remission after chemotherapy or combined chemo-radiotherapy. Cigarette smoking cessation is associated with a decreasing risk of SPT (38,39).

Some tumors seem independent from tobacco carcinogens, such as gastrointestinal and prostate tumors. Acute leukemia and myelodysplasia have been described after chemotherapy, especially alkylating agents and epipodophyllotoxins (33). These hematological malignancies are well described in LTS of SCLC (40–42). However, their incidence has decreased in the last decade (7,9). No cases of secondary leukemias were observed by Lassen et al. or Rosti et al. (11,13) and only one by Jacoulet et al. (21). This might be explained by the limited number of cycles of chemotherapy as well as by the limited use of CCNU and procarbazine.

SPT were the cause of death in 35% of 5-year survivors (11). Median survival after SPT was 5.5 months in the French data base. In this study (21), a multiple regression analysis showed that risk factors for SPT were age > 60 (OR $= 2.92$; IC 95% $= [1.07–7.97]$; $p = 0.03$), and, as in Ihde and Tucker (32), number of chemotherapy cycles > 6 (OR $= 3.25$; IC 95% $= [1.08–9.8]$; $p = 0.02$). There was no influence by sex, stage, thoracic irradiation, CCNU, or cis DDP (21). Heyne et al. found that diffuse SCLC was a risk factor for SPT (9). SPT are probably favored by the addition of genetic predispositions, environmental carcinogens, and chemotherapy-induced immunosuppression. LTS of SCLC are appropriate patients for a secondary chemoprevention trial. A multicenter trial of *cis*-retinoic acid has been proposed (29).

C. Long-Term Behavior and Therapeutic Sequelae

Numerous sequelae have been described in long-term survivors of cancer (43).

Neuropsychological complications have been widely discussed and remain controversial. Two kinds of abnormalities have been reported: clinical ones include mental and cognitive impairment, strokes, ataxia, confusion, visual complaints, headaches, and memory loss (44). Cranial computer tomography and/or magnetic resonance imaging showed ventricular dilation, white matter abnormalities, and brain atrophy (44,45). The frequency of neurological abnormalities can be high: 13–86% (44–46). Prophylactic cranial irradiation and sometimes chemotherapy such as CCNU, procarbazine, methotrexate were thought to be responsible (45,47), but Komaki et al. (48) showed that 97% of patients had neurological impairment before treatment, and Lishner et al. (49) found no more neurological complications in patients who received PCI than in those who did not (18% and 20%, respectively). In the French data base, 13% of patients had neurological problems at 30 months not influenced by PCI (21). Van Oosterhout et al. concluded that cognitive impairment was partly disease related, probably due to emotional distress, aging, and deteriorated physical condition (50). Peripheral neuropathy, especially paresthesias, were noted in 40% at 18 months and 22% at 5 years by Lassen et al. (11).

Pulmonary sequelae were rarely mentioned. Blancke et al. pointed out the role of the combination of VP 16–cis DDP–thoracic irradiation on the occurrence of pulmonary fibrosis (51). This complication was encountered in 18% of patients in the French data base and had fair clinical impact in the majority of cases (21). Many other drugs have demonstrated pulmonary toxicity: e.g., CCNU, BCNU, alkylating agents (most noticeably cyclophosphamide) (43). Long-term outcome of pulmonary function will be determined by the severity of the acute injury and by the possible association to an underlying, tobacco-related chronic obstructive pulmonary disease.

Cardiac disorders have been classically described with anthracyclins, although cyclophosphamide and radiation therapy also may have profound effects (4,5,43,52). Patients with cardiac dysfunction occurring during or after completion of chemotherapy may stabilize or continue to have progressive deterioration. Steinherz noted a significant incidence of late cardiac decompensation (cardiac failure or arrhythmia) occurring 10–20 years after the administration of anthracyclins (53).

The risks of radiation are multiple, including valvular damage, pericardial thickening, and ischemic heart disease (54). These complications were especially described in patients with Hodgkin's disease. As for second malignancies, tobacco abuse can play a role in cardiovascular morbidity. In the French data base, 11% of long-term survivors developed a cardiomyopathy and/or a radiation-related pericardial effusion (21).

Despite all these late effects, the majority of patients can live a normal lifestyle: this concerns 50% of localized SCLC beyond 5 years who are free of late complications and recurrence (6) to 70% of patients beyond 2 years (4). Return to work was possible for 18–36% of patients after which the working capacity of LTS showed a declining tendency with time (4,11,21,55). The stage of the disease prior to treatment and the type of occupation seem to be major prognostic factors: patients with limited disease or light occupations more often returned to work than did patients with extensive disease or heavy occupations. Age, sex, and initial PS were less important factors, and patients with cardiac disturbances or SPT rarely returned to work (55). Among the French long-term survivors, return to work was possible in 31 of the 77 patients (40%) who had an occupation at the time of diagnosis and were less than 60 years old at 30 months. Return to work was not influenced by therapeutic sequelae, relapse, second primary tumors, or type of occupation (21).

III. Conclusion

There are three main issues in the outcome of long-term survivors: the relapse of SCLC, the occurrence of a SPT, and probably an excessive non–cancer-related mortality, which exceeds age-adjusted mortality up to the fourth year (56). This is probably attributable to many factors—therapeutic, individual, environmental, and genetic. However, long-term cure of SCLC is not as rare as once thought.

References

1. Ihde DC. Chemotherapy of lung cancer. N Engl J Med 1992; 12:1434–1140.
2. Matthews MJ, Rozencweig M, Staquet MJ, Minna JD, Muggia FM. Long term survivors with small cell carcinoma of the lung. Eur J Cancer 1980; 16:527–531.
3. Stephens RJ, Bailey AJ, Machin D, MRC. Lung Cancer Working Party. Long term survival in small cell lung cancer: the case for a standard definition. Lung Cancer 1996; 15:297–309.
4. Osterlind K, Hansen HH, Hansen M, Dombernowsky P, Andersen PK. Long-term disease-free survival in small-cell carcinoma of the lung: a study of clinical determinants. J Clin Oncol 1986; 4:1307–1313.
5. Albain KS, Crowley JJ, Leblanc M, Livingston RB. Determinants of improved outcome in small cell lung cancer: An analysis of the 2580 patient Southwest Oncology Group data base. J Clin Oncol 1990; 8:1563–1574.
6. Albain KS, Crowley JJ, Livingston RB. Long-term survival and toxicity in small-cell lung cancer: expanded Southwest Oncology Group experience. Chest 1991; 99:1425–1432.
7. Souhami RL, Law K. Longevity in small cell lung cancer—a report to the lung cancer sub-committee of the United Kingdom Coordinating Committee for cancer research. Br J Cancer 1990; 61:584–589.
8. Spiegelman D, Maurer LH, Ware JH, Perry MC, Chahinian AP, Comis R, Eaton W, Zimmer B, Green M. Prognostic factors in small cell carcinoma of the lung: an analysis of 1521 patients. J Clin Oncol 1989; 7:344–354.
9. Heyne KH, Lippman SM, Lee JJ, Lee JS, Hong WK. The incidence of second primary tumors in long-term survivors of small-cell lung cancer. J Clin Oncol 1992; 10:1519–1524.
10. Choi NC, Carey RW, Kaufman SD, Grillo HC, Younger J, Wilkins EW. Small cell carcinoma of the lung. A progress report of 15 years experience. Cancer 1987; 59:6–14.
11. Lassen U, Osterlind K, Hansen M, Dombernowsky P, Bergman B, Hansen HH. Long-term survival in small-cell lung cancer: posttreatment characteristics in patients surviving 5 to 18 years an analysis of 1,714 consecutive patients. J Clin Oncol 1995; 13:1215–1220.
12. Davis S, Wright PW, Schulman SF, Scholes D, Thorning D, Hammar S. Long term survival in small cell carcinoma of the lung: a population experience. J Clin Oncol 1985; 3:80–91.
13. Rosti G, Crino L, Tondini M, Scagliotti G, Favaretto M, Clerici M, Barni S, Marangolo M. Secondary malignant tumor affecting small cell lung cancer long survivors. Results of the Italian survey. Ann Oncol 1992; 3:66.
14. Moro D, Jacoulet P, Depierre A, Guerin JC, Quoix E, Lemarie E, Riviere A, Capron F, Ranfaing E, Lebeau B, Milleron B, Vincent J, Coetmeur D, Geraads A, Gouva S. Small cell lung cancer in patients surviving longer than thirty months: a multicenter study. Ann Oncol 1992; 3:37.
15. Armstrong JG. Long term outcome of small cell lung cancer. Cancer Treat Rev 1990; 17:1–13.
16. Sloman A, d'Amico F, Yousem SA. Immunohistochemical markers of prolonged survival in small cell carcinoma of the lung. An immunohistochemical study. Arch Pathol Lab Med 1996; 120:465–472.
17. Bobrow LG, Hirsh FR, Hay FG, Happerfield L, Skov BG, Law K, Leonard RCF, Souhami RL. An immunohistochemical investigation of diagnostic biopsy material taken from short and long term survivors with small cell lung cancer. Br J Cancer 1992; 66:547–551.
18. Sagman U, Feld R, Evans WK, Warr D, Shepherd FA, Payne D, Pringle J, Yeoh J, Deboer G, Malkin A, Ginsberg R. The prognostic significance of pretreatment serum lactate dehydrogenase in patients with small cell lung cancer. J Clin Oncol 1991; 9:954–961.
19. Szczepek B, Szymanska D, Decker E, Wasowska H, Slupek A, Rowinska-Zakrzewska E. Risk of late recurrence and/or second lung cancer after treatment of patients with small cell lung cancer (SCLC). Lung Cancer 1994; 11:93–104.
20. Crown JP, Chahinian AP, Jaffrey IS, Glidewell OJ, Kaneko M, Holland JF. Predictors of 5-year survival and curability in small-cell lung cancer. Cancer 1990; 66:382–386.

21. Jacoulet P, Depierre A, Moro D, Rivière A, Milleron B, Quoix E, Ranfaing E, Anthoine D, Lafitte JJ, Lebeau B, Kleisbauer JP, Massin F, Fournel P, Zaegel M, Leclerc P, Garnier G, Brambilla E, Capron F, on behalf of the Groupe d'Oncologie de Langue Française. Long-term survivors of small cell lung cancer (SCLC): a French multicenter study. Ann Oncol 1997; 8:1–6.
22. Fukuoka M, Masuda N, Matsui K, Makise Y, Takada M, Negoro S, Sakai N, Kusunoki Y, Kudoh S, Ryu S, Takifuji N. Combination chemotherapy with or without radiation therapy in small-cell lung cancer. An analysis of 5 year follow-up. Cancer 1990; 65:1678–1684.
23. Chute JP, Kelley MJ, Venzon D, Williams J, Roberts A, Johnson BE. Retreatment of patients surviving cancer-free 2 or more years after initial treatment of small cell lung cancer. Chest 1996; 110:165–171.
24. Postmus PE, Berendsen HH, Van Zandwijk N. Retreatment with the induction regimen in small cell lung cancer relapsing after an initial response to short term therapy. Eur J Cancer Clin Oncol 1987; 9:1409–1411.
25. Albain KS, Crowley JJ, Hutchins L. Predictors of survival following relapse or progression of small cell lung cancer: Southwest Oncology Group Study 8605 report and analysis of recurrent disease data base. Cancer 1993; 72:1184–1191.
26. Greco FA. Treatment options for patients with relapsed small-cell lung cancer. Lung Cancer 1993; 9:585–589.
27. Johnson DH. Treatment of relapsed small-cell lung cancer. Lung Cancer 1994; 11:142–143.
28. Sekine I, Nishiwaki Y, Kakinuma R, Kubota K, Hojo F, Matsumoto T, Ohmatsu H, Yokozaki M, Goto K, Kodama T. Late recurrence of small-cell lung cancer: treatment and outcome. Oncology 1996; 53:318–321.
29. Johnson BE. Second Cancers after Successful Treatment of Small Cell Lung Cancer. Los Angeles: ASCO Educational Book, 1995.
30. Yoshida T, Matsui K, Masuda N, Kusunoki Y, Takada M, Yana T. Risk of second primary cancer in two-year survivors of small-cell lung cancer. Nippon Kyobu Shikkan Gakkai Zasshi 1996; 34:741–746.
31. Johnson BE, Linnoila RI, Williams JP. Risk of second aerodigestive cancers increases in patients who survive free of small cell lung cancer for more than 2 years. J Clin Oncol 1995; 13:101–111.
32. Ihde DC, Tucker MA. Second primary malignancies in small-cell lung cancer—a major consequence of modest success. J Clin Oncol 1992; 10:1511–1513.
33. Sagman U, Lishner M, Maki E, Shepherd FA, Haddad R, Evans WK, DeBoer G, Payne D, Pringle JF, Yeah JL, Ginsberg R, Feld R. Second primary malignancies following diagnosis of small cell lung cancer. J Clin Oncol 1992; 10:1525–1533.
34. Martini N, Melamed M. Multiple primary lung cancers. J Thorac Cardiovasc Surg 1975; 70:606–612.
35. Kelley MJ, Williams J, Shaw EG, Longo DL, Duffey PL, Conrad NK, Duray P, LeRiche J, Murray N, Tucker MA, Johnson BE. TP53 and RAS mutations in metachronous Non-small cell lung cancers of patients with small cell lung cancer and hodgkin's disease. Proc Am Soc Clin Oncol 1995; 14:1073.
36. Sehested M, Hirsch FR, Osterlind K. Morphologic variations of small cell lung cancer: a histopathologic study of pretreatment and post treatment specimens in 104 patients. Cancer 1986; 57:804–807.
37. Brambilla E, Moro D, Gazzeri S, Brichon PY, Nagy-Mignotte H, Morel F, Jacrot M, Brambilla C. Cytotoxic chemotherapy induces cell differentiation in small cell lung carcinoma. J Clin Oncol 1991; 9:50–61.
38. Kawahara M, Furuse K, Kamimori T, Ushijima S, Matsui K, Takada M, Sofue T. Risk of second primary tumor in more than 2 years disease free survivors of small cell lung cancer in Japan. Proc Am Soc Clin Oncol 1995; 14:1070.
39. Richardson GE, Tucker MA, Venzon DJ, Linnoila RI, Phelps R, Phares JC, Edison M, Ihde DC, Johnson BE. Smoking cessation after successful treatment of small cell lung cancer is associated with fewer smoking-related second primary cancers. Ann Intern Med 1993; 119:383–390.

40. Chak LY, Sikic BI, Tucker MA. Increased incidence of acute non lymphocytic leukemia following therapy in patients with small cell carcinoma of the lung. J Clin Oncol 1984; 2: 385–390.

41. Pedersen-Bjergaard J, Osterlind K, Hansen M. Acute non lymphocytic leukemia, preleukemia and solid tumors following intensive chemotherapy of small cell lung cancer. Blood 1985; 66:1393–1397.

42. Johnson DH, Porter LL, List AF. Acute non lymphocytic leukemia after treatment of small cell lung cancer. Am J Med 1986; 81:962–968.

43. Schwartz CL. Late effects of treatment in long term survivors of cancer. Cancer Treat Rev 1995; 21:355–366.

44. Johnson BE, Patronas N, Hayes W. Neurologic computed cranial tomographic and magnetic resonance imaging abnormalities in patients with small-cell lung cancer. Further follow-up of 6- to 13-year survivors. J Clin Oncol 1990; 8:48–56.

45. Lee JS, Umsawasdi T, Lee YY, Barkley HT, Murphy WK, Welch S, Valdivieso M. Neurotoxicity in long-term survivors of small-cell lung cancer. Int J Radiat Oncol Biol Phys 1986; 12:313–321.

46. Frytak S, Shaw J, O'Neill B, Lee R, Eargan R, Shaw E, Richardson R, Coles D, Jett J. Leucoencephalopathy in small-cell lung cancer patients receiving prophylactic cranial irradiation. Am J Clin Oncol 1989; 12:27–33.

47. Livingston RB, Stephens RL, Bonnet JD, Grozea PN, Lehane DE. Long-term survival and toxicity in small-cell lung cancer. Am J Med 1984; 77:415–417.

48. Komaki R, Meyers CA, Shin DM, Garden AS, Byrne K, Nickens JA, Cox JD. Evaluation of cognitive function in patients with limited small-cell lung cancer prior to shortly following prophylactic cranial irradiation. Int J Radiat Oncol Biol Phys 1995; 33:179–182.

49. Lishner M, Feld R, Payne DG, Sagman U, Sculier JP, Pringle JF, Yeoh JL, Evans WK, Shepherd FA, Maki E, Warr D. Late neurological complications after prophylactic cranial irradiation in patients with small cell lung cancer: the Toronto experience. J Clin Oncol 1990; 8:215–221.

50. Van Oosterhout AG, Ganzevles PG, Wilmink JT, De Geus BW, Van Vonderen RG, Twijnstra A. Sequelae in long term survivors of small cell lung cancer. Int J Radiat Oncol Biol Phys 1996; 34:1037–1044.

51. Blancke C, De Vore R, Hande K, Murray M, Stewart J, Miller D, Lewis M, Johnson D. A pilot study of protracted low dose cisplatine and etoposide plus concurrent thoracic radiotherapy in stade III non small-cell lung cancer (abstract 1091). Am Soc Clin Oncol, 1995;

52. Skarin AT. Analysis of long-term survivors with small-cell lung cancer. Chest 1993; 103:440S–445S.

53. Steinherz KL. Cardiac toxicity 4 to 20 years after completing anthracycline therapy. JAMA 1991; 266:1672.

54. Stewart J, Fajardo L. Radiation induced heart disease: an update. Prog Cardiovasc Dis 1984; 27:173–194.

55. Bergman B, Sorenson S. Return to work among patients with small cell lung cancer. Eur J Respir Dis 1987; 70:49–53.

56. Brown B, Brauner C, Minnotte M. Noncancer deaths in white adult cancer patients. J Natl Cancer Inst 1993; 85:979–987.

41

New Drugs for New Chemotherapy Standards

GIORGIO V. SCAGLIOTTI and SILVIA NOVELLO

University of Turin
Turin, Italy

I. Introduction

Lung cancer is a major cause of death in most Western countries, it is an increasing health care problem in many developing nations, and establishing an effective treatment plan is a major public health priority and the subject of continuing debate.

Nowadays, patients who develop lung cancer are rarely cured, and the 5-year survival rate of 13% has remained unchanged for the last 20 years. The dismal survival rate is partially due to the fact that most patients with lung cancer initially present with advanced disease. In fact, 40% of patients with non–small-cell lung cancer (NSCLC) have distant metastases at the time of initial presentation. Similarly, the majority of small-cell lung cancer (SCLC) patients present with extensive disease, and their median survival, despite combination chemotherapy, is approximately 9–10 months.

When the role of chemotherapy in the management of advanced NSCLC was reviewed more than 10 years ago, ifosfamide, vindesine, cisplatin, and mitomycin C were identified as the agents with the greatest activity (>15% response rate as single agents) (1,2), and they still represent the nucleus of combination regimens. Two other drugs that have been frequently used in the treatment of advanced NSCLC are etoposide and carboplatin, although both of these agents have shown lower response rates than those of the established active agents. However, single-agent or combination chemotherapy yields only partial responses, and the duration of response is generally short.

There are a number of active single agents for the treatment of SCLC as well (for review, see Ref. 3). Many combination chemotherapy regimens have built on these single-agent activities to develop more effective treatments for SCLC. Still, despite these combination therapies, most patients with SCLC will eventually die of their disease. In the last 5–6 years we have seen a proliferation of new agents, some of which have novel mechanisms of action, with consistent activity as single agents in NSCLC as well as in SCLC and with promising results in terms of response rate and, occasionally, survival in initial combination regimens.

II. Antimetabolites

A. Gemcitabine

Gemcitabine (Gemzar®, difluorodeoxycytidine) is a nucleoside analog antimetabolite that differs from deoxycytidine by the presence of two fluorine atoms at the $2'$ position of the sugar. Gemcitabine exhibits multiple mechanisms of action: (1) it inhibits ribonucleotide reductase; (2) it causes masked DNA chain termination, whereby gemcitabine nucleotide is incorporated into the DNA chain but allows the insertion of one additional nucleotide before termination, making gemcitabine difficult to be detected and removed by proofreading exonucleases; and (3) it has at least three mechanisms of self-potentiation that serve to increase the formation of the active gemcitabine metabolites and decrease the elimination of the drug.

In preclinical studies gemcitabine has shown antitumor activity in a wide range of tumor xenografts including lung, ovarian, breast, head and neck, and colon cancers (4). Several phase II studies have demonstrated that gemcitabine is active against NSCLC, with an average response rate of 21% and consistent improvement in disease-related symptoms. At the dose and schedule chosen for these phase II studies—1000 mg/m^2 weekly × 3—toxicity was mild and mainly comprised myelosuppression (5).

Because of its unique mechanism of action, favorable adverse event profile, and lack of overlapping toxicity with other active agents, gemcitabine has been considered a good candidate for combination regimens. Preclinical models have demonstrated synergistic tumor killing when it is combined with cisplatin. Since the cytotoxic activity of cisplatin consists of the formation of DNA adducts and cancer cells may overcome this cisplatin effect because of excision-repair DNA mechanism, it has been hypothesized that gemcitabine inhibits this repair when used in combination with cisplatin, resulting in an apparently stabilized DNA. Indeed, gemcitabine induces depletion of both deoxyribonucleotide and ribonucleotide pools, which are the cornerstone elements for an adequate functioning of DNA repair mechanisms.

In the last few years several phase II studies have tested the combination of high-dose cisplatin and gemcitabine in unresectable locally advanced and metastatic NSCLC (6–11). All of these studies except one used a regimen of gemcitabine 1000 mg/m^2 weekly for 3 weeks and monthly cisplatin administered on day 15 (3 studies), day 2 (one study), and day 1 (one study) (Table 1). Although from experimental data there is no clear evidence of the superiority of a particular schedule, it seems likely that sequential administration of gemcitabine and cisplatin allowing some preincorporation of gemcitabine in the DNA could be most effective in achieving an interaction with cisplatin.

In all these studies gemcitabine was administered at full dose with enhancement of single-agent activity, reporting a response rate in the range of 30–54% while an acceptable toxicity profile was still maintained. Neutropenia and, in one study, thrombocytopenia grade 3 and 4 were the most common hematological side effects, which were usually short lived, mostly clinically asymptomatic, and not requiring hospitalization or hematopoietic growth factor support. Nonhematological toxicities were usually minimal and manageable.

The combination of gemcitabine and cisplatin appears promising in terms of response rate, excellent survival time, low hematological toxicity, and the absence of overlapping toxicity between the two agents. The regimen is currently being tested in phase III prospective randomized trials with cisplatin/etoposide and mitomycin C/ifosfamide/cisplatin as reference regimens. Recently two phase II randomized clinical trials evaluating the efficacy and the toxicity of gemcitabine versus the combination of cisplatin and etoposide have been finished. In both studies gemcitabine single agent was as effective as cisplatin/etoposide but with a better toxicity profile (12,13).

In extensive-stage SCLC, a phase II study was performed in 29 patients with previously untreated disease. The starting dose of gemcitabine was raised from

Table 1 Phase II Combination Studies of Gemcitabine and Cisplatin in Locally Advanced and Metastatic NSCLC[a]

Author (year)	No. of patients (evaluable)	Stage III/IV	Cisplatin dose (mg/m^2) and day of administration	% Response rate	MST (months)	% 1-year survival
Steward (1996)	66 (52)	43/23	100, day 15	38 (20 PR)	10.2	40
Crinò (1997)	48	22/26	100, day 2	54 (1 CR, 25 PR)	13	59
Sandler (1996)	31 (26)	5/26	100, day 1	42 (1 CR, 10 PR)	8.4	37
Abratt (1997)	53 (50)	33/20	100, day 15	52 (2 CR, 24 PR)	13	61
Shepherd (1996)	50 (47)	16/34	30, days 1-8-15	30 (14 PR)	8	N.E.
Anton (1996)	40 (37)	22/18	100, day 15	49 (18 PR)	10	N.E.

MST = Median survival time; CR = complete response; PR = partial response; NE = not evaluable.
[a] In all these studies gemcitabine has been administered at the dose of 1000 mg/m^2, days 1-8-15 in 4-week cycles.

1000 to 1250 mg/m^2/week because of lack of toxicity in the first 17 patients. An overall response rate of 27% was seen in 26 assessable cases (one complete response) with a median response duration of 12 weeks (14).

B. Edatrexate

Edatrexate (10-ethyl-10-deaza-aminopterin), an analog of methotrexate, is a folate antagonist that blocks the synthesis of nucleotides by competing stoiechiometrically for the folate-binding site of the enzyme dihydrofolate reductase. This binding and inhibition of dihydrofolate reductase leads to the depletion of reduced folates and inhibition of biochemical processes involving one-carbon transfer reactions, which are required for thymidine DNA synthesis and, to a lesser degree, for both RNA and protein synthesis. In in vivo preclinical studies edatrexate has demonstrated antitumor activity superior to that of methotrexate and the other antifolates tested. The improved therapeutic index of edatrexate appears to be related to its increased entry into and polyglutamylation within tumor cells and its relative exclusion and rapid elimination from sensitive host tissues compared to methotrexate.

Phase I and II clinical trials have primarily assessed the toxicity and activity of edatrexate on a weekly schedule of administration. In these trials the dose-limiting toxicity was mucositis, with leukopenia and thrombocytopenia being less prominent; activity has been seen against NSCLC, breast cancer, non-Hodgkin's lymphoma, and head and neck cancer. The recommended dose for phase II trials was 80 mg/m^2/week.

A pilot phase II study in NSCLC achieved a response rate of 32% in 19 evaluable patients (15), but two subsequent studies using different durations of therapy reported a 13% and 10% response rate in 45 and 30 evaluable patients, respectively (16,17).

Edatrexate has also been investigated in combination chemotherapy with cisplatin and cyclophosphamide (18) or ifosfamide (19). In both studies the addition of leucovorin rescue allowed a dose of 80 mg/m^2 to be given on days 1 and 8, without severe mucositis, yielding a response rate in excess of 40%.

The differing mechanisms of action, nonoverlapping toxicities, an in vitro synergistic effect, and the demonstrated single-agent activity of edatrexate and paclitaxel in NSCLC were the background to test the feasibility and the activity of the combination: in a phase I study the maximum tolerated dose was reached at the doses of edatrexate 120 mg/m^2 followed by paclitaxel 210 mg/m^2 every 2 weeks with a response rate of 60% (6 partial responses in 10 patients) (20).

III. Antimicrotubule Agents

A. Taxanes

The taxanes are an important new class of anticancer agent that exert their cytotoxic effects through a unique mechanism and are an exciting new class of cytotoxic agent which have been met with a great deal of enthusiasm because of the variety of antitumor responses seen in phase I and II testing of patients with refractory malignancies. Taxanes bind preferentially and reversibly to the β-subunit of tubulin in microtubules. This binding enhances tubulin polymerization and inhibits microtubule depolymerization, thereby inducing the formation of stable microtubule bundles. This disruption of the normal equilibrium ultimately leads to cell death.

B. Paclitaxel

In NSCLC several phase II studies testing paclitaxel (Taxol®) as single agent using 1-, 3-, and 24-hour infusion reported response rates of 22–38% and occasionally 1-year survival rates in excess of 40% (21–28) (Table 2). Using the 3-week schedule of administration, dose and infusion duration do not appear to influence efficacy of paclitaxel. However, in 25 evaluable patients with advanced NSCLC, a phase II study of weekly paclitaxel 175 mg/m^2 for 6 weeks of each 8-week cycle, a 56% response rate has been reported with 1-year survival rate of 53% (29). In these single-agent studies using the 24-hour infusion schedule, neutropenia was the most common dose-limiting toxicity, whereas myalgia/arthralgia and dose-dependent peripheral neuropathy were more frequent in the 3-hour infusion schedule.

Combination studies demonstrated that paclitaxel could be combined with either carboplatin or cisplatin at full doses using either a 3-hour or 24-hour infusion schedule (see Table 3). Response rates with these combinations have been high, usually 40–50%, which are higher than with any of the drugs used alone. In combination regimens neutropenia was again the most frequent toxicity and occurred less frequently with the 3-hour infusion schedule (30–36). Interestingly, neutropenia does not appear to be exacerbated by the combination of paclitaxel and carboplatin, whereas platelet toxicity is usually less than might expected with carboplatin alone (37), which could be attributed to a pharmacodynamic interaction. Two completed randomized clinical trials demonstrated that the paclitaxel/cisplatin regimen is superior to etoposide/cisplatin (38) or teniposide/cisplatin (39) regimens with respect to response rate and, in the ECOG study, to survival too (Table 4).

In SCLC, paclitaxel as monotherapy exhibits significant activity in untreated (40) as well as previously treated patients (41). Pilot studies in combination with cisplatin/etoposide (42) or carboplatin/oral etoposide (43) showed impressive results in terms of overall response rate (83–100%) without a significant increase in the percentage of complete responders.

Paclitaxel enhances the cytotoxic effects of ionizing radiation in vitro, possibly by inducing arrest in the premitotic G2 and mitotic phases of the cell cycle, which are the most radiosensitive phases (44). The feasibility of using paclitaxel alone or in combination with cisplatin or carboplatin administered concurrently with radiation to treat patients with locally advanced unresectable NSCLC has been proved (45), and excellent results have been reported (46,47).

Table 2 Phase II Studies of Paclitaxel Single Agent in NSCLC

Author (year)	No. of patients (evaluable)	Stage IIIB/IV	Schedule (mg/m^2) q3wks/infusion time	% Response rate	MST (months)	Main toxicities
Chang (1993)	25 (24)	0/24	250/24 h	21 (5 PR)	6.1 (1-yr surv. 42%)	Leukopenia G3–4 20%
Murphy (1993)	27 (25)	5/22	200/24 h	24 (1CR–5 PR)	10	Granulocytopenia dose-limiting
Gatzemeier (1995)	58 (50)	1642	225/3 h	24 (12 PR)	10	Polyneuropathy G3 2% Myalgia/arthralgia G3–4 14%
Hainsworth (1996)	59 (53)	Stage IV or relapsed	135–200/1 h	25 (13 PR)	7.8 (1-yr surv. 33%)	Leukopenia G3–4 12%
Alberola (1995)	50 (47)	23/27	210/3 h	36 (1 CR–16 PR)	N.E.	Neuropathy G3 2 cases
Tester (1996)	20 (19)	0/20	200/3 h	32 (6 PR)	6 (1-yr surv. 22%)	Neutropenia G3–4 20%
Millward (1996)	51 (51)	17/33	175/3 h	10% (5 PR)	6.7	Neutropenia G3–4 16% Myalgia/arthralgia G3–4 22%
Sekine (1996)	60	11/49	210/3 h	38 (23 PR)	11.2 (1-yr surv 48%)	Neutropenia G4 50%

G = WHO toxicity grade; CR = complete response; PR = partial response; NE = not evaluable.

Table 3 Phase II Combination Studies Including Taxanes with Cisplatin or Carboplatin

Author (year)	No. of patients (evaluable)	Stage IIIB/IV	Regimen (mg/m^2)	% Response rate	MST (months)	Main toxicities
Belli (1995)	32 (29)	9/23	P 135–225/3 h DDP 100–120 q3wks	38 (11 PR)	N.E.	Neutropenia G3–4 40% Neurotoxicity dose-dependent and cumulative
van Pawel (1996)	75 (67)	13/62	P 175/3 h DDP 75 q3wks	42 (3 CR–25 PR)	10	Neutropenia G3–4 50% Thrombocytopenia G3–4 2%
Georgiadis (1997)	42	12/30	P 100–180/96 h DDP 60–80 ± G-CSF	55 (2 CR–16 PR)	10	Cumulative peripheral neuropathy
Natale (1995)	41 (32)	19/22	P 150–250/24 h C AUC 6	62.5 (2 CR–18 PR)	N.E.	Arthralgia and neuropathy dose-limiting
Langer (1995)	54 (53)	4/50	P 135–215/24 h C AUC 7.5 q3wks	62 (5 CR–28 PR)	11.7	Neutropenia G3–4 51% (cycle 1) Thrombocytopenia 47%
Johnson (1996)	51	6/45	P 135–175/24 h C 300 or AUC 6 q4wks	27 (14 PR)	9.5	Neutropenia G-4 47% Thrombocytopenia G3–4 3%
Jagasia (1997)	63	10/53	P 175–200/1 h C AUC 6 q4wks	25 (3 CR–13 PR)	8.5	Neutropenia G3–4 T3% Neurotoxicity 41% Arthralgia/myalgia 28%
Millward (1997)	24 (18)	8/16	D 50–100/1 h DDP 75–100 q3wks	44 (8 PR)	7.9	Neutropenia diarrhea
Androulakis (1997)	52 (49)	27/25	D 100/1 h DDP 80 q3wks	47 (1 CR–22 PR)	6.0	Neutropenia G3–4 42% Feb. neutropenia 27%
Belani (1997)	47	0/47	D 100/1 h DDP 75 q3wks	21.3 (1 CR–9 PR)	10	Feb. neutropenia 8.5% Pulmonary tox. 4.3%

P = paclitaxel; D = docetaxel; C = carboplatin; DDP = cisplatin; AUC is expressed by plotting the plasma level of carboplatin over time and measuring the area beneath the plotted curve. The product of carboplatin concentration versus time constitutes the AUC (mg/ml/min); CR = complete response; PR = partial response; MST = median survival time; G = WHO toxicity grade; NE = not evaluable.

Table 4 Randomized Phase III Studies of Paclitaxel/Cisplatin Combination in NSCLC

Study	No. of patients	Treatment arms	% Response rate	MST (months)
EORTC 08925 (Giaccone, 1997)	162	Arm A: DDP 80 mg/m^2 d.1 Teniposide 100 mg/m^2 d1-3-5 q3wks	30	9.7
		vs.		
	155	Arm B: DDP 80 mg/m^2 d1 Paclitaxel 175 mg/m^2/3 h d1 q3wks	44	9.4
			($p = 0.02$)	($p = 0.971$)
ECOG 5592 (Bonomi, 1997)	194	Arm A: DDP 75 mg/m^2 d1 Etoposide 100 mg/m^2 d1-3-5 q3wks	12	7.4
		vs		
	187	Arm B: DDP 75 mg/m^2 d1 Paclitaxel 135 mg/m^2/24 h d1 q3wks	26.3	9.6
		vs.		
	190	Arm C: DDP 75 mg/m^2 d1 Paclitaxel 250 mg/m^2/24 h d1 q3wks + G-CSF	31.0	10.1
			($p = 0.01$ for B and C vs. A)	($p = 0.034$ for B and C vs. A)

G-CSF = Granulocyte colony-stimulating factor

C. Docetaxel

Docetaxel (Taxotere®) is a semisynthetic derivative of the European yew *Taxus baccata*. Its mechanism of action is similar to that of paclitaxel, but docetaxel is more water soluble and its cytotoxicity in vitro is higher at equimolar concentrations. Like paclitaxel, myelosuppression limits dose escalation on all schedules. In preclinical studies docetaxel has shown synergism with vinorelbine, etoposide, cyclophosphamide, 5-fluorouracil, and methotrexate against a variety of murine tumors.

Initial studies of docetaxel as a single agent in previously untreated locally advanced or metastatic NSCLC indicated efficacy at the doses of 100 mg/m^2 with response rates of about 30% and median survival times of 9 months (48–51). Further testing at 75 mg/m^2 (52) and at 60 mg/m^2 (53) have shown some decrease in response but preservation of median survival time (Table 5).

Table 5 Phase II Studies of Docetaxel Single Agent in NSCLC

Author (year)	No. of patients (evaluable)	Stage IIIB/IV	Schedule (mg/m²) q3 weeks/ infusion time	% Response rate	MST (months)	Main toxicities
Cerny (1994)	43 (35)	N.D.	100/1 h	23 (1 CR–7 PR)	11	Neutropenia G3–4 62%
Francis (1994)	29 (29)	4/24	100/1 h	38 (11 PR)	6.3	Neutropenia G3–4 76% Febrile neutropenia 41%
Fossella (1994)	41 (39)	4/37	100/1 h	33 (11 PR)	11.5	Neutropenia G3–4 97% HSRs 36% Dermatitis 74%
Miller (1995)	20 (20)	4/16	75/1 h	25 (5 PR)	9.1	Neutropenia G3–4 70%
Kunitoh (1996)	75 (72)	20/55	60/1–2 h	19 (14 PR)	9.7	Neutropenia G3–4 87%
Saarinen (1996)	29 (23)	N.E.	100/1 h	35 (8 PR)	N.E.	Neutropenic infections dose-limiting
Fossella (1995)[a]	44 (42)	4/40	100/1 h	21 (9 PR)	10.5	Neutropenia G3–4 85%
Burris (1995)[a]	44 (35)	N.E.	100/1 h	17 (6 PR)	5.8	Predominantly neutropenia Dermatitis
Gandara (1997)[2]	80	N.E.	100/1 h	16 (13 PR)	7.0 (1-yr surv. 25%)	Febrile neutropenia 14% Neuropathy 9%

[2]Studies performed in platinum-resistant (prior response to a platinum-containing regimen with subsequent progression) or platinum refractory (no response to, or progression on, a platinum-containing regimen) patients.
CR = Complete response; PR = partial response; MST = median survival time; G = WHO toxicity grade; NE = not evaluable.

Furthermore, it is certainly of interest that docetaxel retains its activity in second-line chemotherapy in patients resistant or refractory to platinum-containing regimens who generally have an extremely poor prognosis. Pooled response data from three different studies indicated an average response rate of 17% in 157 assessable patients (54–56) (Table 5). The apparent lack of cross-resistance between docetaxel and platinum implied by this observation could be predicted by the different mechanisms of action of the drugs and thus their different mechanisms of resistance (augmented DNA repair capability for platinum compounds, alteration in α- and β-tubulin, and overexpression of π-glycoprotein for docetaxel).

Grade IV neutropenia was the most common adverse events in all studies. This was generally of brief duration and well tolerated. Myelosuppression did not significantly compromise further docetaxel administration as relative dose intensity was maintained in excess of 0.92 in the chemotherapy-naive patients as well as in pretreated patients.

Other adverse events reported during these studies included infusion-associated hypersensitivity reactions, dermatitis, and alopecia. Fluid retention, characterized by peripheral edema, pleural effusions, and ascites and weight gain, was not reported in phase I studies but emerged after cumulative doses in phase II trials. The mechanism of this toxic effect is unknown, but results of capillary filtration tests with technetium 99m albumin and capillaroscopy suggested an abnormality in capillary permeability (57).

Fluid retention can respond to diuretics, including oral spironolactone, when these are administered promptly once symptoms are noted. Docetaxel dose reduction does not seem to lower the incidence of fluid retention, and the effect is reversible on docetaxel discontinuation. Premedication with corticosteroids may ameliorate fluid retention.

The association of docetaxel 75–100 mg/m^2 administered with cisplatin 75–100 mg/m^2 on day 1 in a 3-week cycle has been proved feasible with a substantial incidence of grade III and IV neutropenia, diarrhea, and, in some studies, febrile neutropenia, but with a consistent level of activity in excess of 40% (58–60) (Table 3).

Docetaxel also appears to be active in SCLC: 28 evaluable patients, most pretreated, received docetaxel 100 mg/m^2, which produced grade IV neutropenia in about 90% of the patients and clinically significant effusions, ascites, and edema in the minority of the patients. Seven patients achieved a partial response (25%) with a median duration of response of 4.7 months (61).

D. Rhizoxin

Rhizoxin, a novel tubulin-binding agent, was tested in a phase II study in 31 chemonaive patients with advanced NSCLC. Four partial responses have been reported in 27 accessable patients (15%), and the main toxic effects observed were stomatitis (34% of cycles) and neutropenia (41% of cycles) (62).

IV. Topoisomerase I Inhibitors (Camptothecins)

Camptothecin and its analogs are believed to exert cytotoxic effects through the inhibition of topoisomerase I, an essential nuclear enzyme that resolves topological problems in DNA, such as overwinding, underwinding, and catenation, which normally arises during replication, transcription, and perhaps other DNA processes.

The development of these agents was initially thwarted, owing to unpredictable and formidable toxicities, during early studies with camptothecin. Knowledge of the structure relationships of the parent compound has led to the recent development of effective soluble analogs with manageable toxicities. Broad antitumor activity shown in preclinical studies has been confirmed in phase I/II studies for irinotecan (CPT-11) and topotecan.

Interestingly, although camptothecin is a plant extract, it and most of its derivatives are not affected by the classic P-glycoprotein MDR1 mechanism of resistance, which may allow the development of novel combination chemotherapeutic regimens.

A. Irinotecan (CPT 11)

Irinotecan (Camptosar®) is in vivo converted by carboxylesterase enzymes of the liver to its active metabolite (SN 38), which has 100-fold or greater antitumor activity compared with the parent compound in vitro (63). Due to its novel mechanism of action, irinotecan has significant in vitro activity against a variety of solid tumors, including those particularly resistant to other cytotoxic agents. This activity has been confirmed in clinical trials of irinotecan as a single agent conducted in chemotherapy-naive patients with advanced NSCLC obtaining a response rate of 32–34% (64–66), and this has been improved to within the range of 43–54% using irinotecan in combination with cisplatin (for review, see Refs. 67, 68) (Table 6). Prior chemotherapy appears to reduce the response rate substantially in this setting, although the mechanisms of cross-resistance are partially unknown. Irinotecan is also active in SCLC with a single-agent response rate of 47–50% in patients previously treated with cisplatin (69,70). As might expected, irinotecan is more active when combined with cisplatin as first-line chemotherapy for SCLC, with a Japanese study reporting an average response rate of 85% (68).

In the irinotecan/cisplatin combination, the major dose-limiting toxicities of leukopenia and diarrhea were more pronounced than with irinotecan alone, suggesting that a pharmacodynamic interaction could exist between the two drugs. However, marked interpatient variability in these toxicities, which is a well-known feature of irinotecan, was observed during these trials.

In 61 metastatic NSCLC the combination of irinotecan and etoposide (a topisomerase II poison) with G-CSF support demonstrated feasible toxicity of moderate diarrhea and pulmonary toxicity but was marginally effective (21% response rate), equivalent to that expected with cisplatin-based chemotherapy or irinotecan alone (71).

Table 6 Phase II Studies of Irinotecan Single Agent in Lung Cancer

Author (year)	No. of patients	Type of cancer	Schedule	% Response rate	Main toxicities
Masuda (1992)	16	SCLC Relapsed or Refractory	100 mg/m^2 qwk	47	Leukopenia-diarrhea Pulmonary toxicity
Fujita (1995)	16 (4LD; 12 ED)	SCLC Refractory	100 mg/m^2 qwk	50	Leukopenia-diarrhea Pulmonary toxicity
Negoro (1991)	35	SCLC	100 mg/m^2 qwk	37	Leukopenia and diarrhea as dose-limiting toxicities
	67	NSCLC untreated		34	
	26	NSCLC pretreated		0	
Fukuoka (1992)	73	NSCLC	100 mg/m^2 qwk	32	Leukopenia G3–4 = 25% Diarrhea G3–4 = 21% Nausea and vomiting G3–4 = 21% Pneumonitis 3%
Baker (1997)	48	NSCLC	100 mg/m^2 qwk	15	Diarrhea G3–4 = 17% Neutropenia G3 = 15%

NSCLC = Non–small-cell lung cancer; SCLC = small-cell lung cancer; LD = limited disease; ED = extensive disease; G = WHO toxicity grade.

Because topoisomerase I may be important in the repair of potentially lethal damage, topoisomerase I inhibitors have been evaluated as potentiators of ionizing radiation. Both irinotecan and topotecan enhanced radiation-induced cytotoxicity in cell lines, and in a phase I/II study in locally advanced NSCLC the weekly administration for 6 weeks of irinotecan (30–45 mg/m^2) and simultaneous thoracic radiotherapy (total dose 60 Gy) was established to be feasible and highly active (76% response rate in 24 evaluable patients) (72).

Both early and late forms of irinotecan-induced diarrhea appear to be mediated from different mechanisms. Early diarrhea (within 24 hours), often preceded by diaphoresis and/or abdominal cramping, is believed to be cholinergic in nature and can be ameliorated by the administration of atropine. The physiologic mechanisms underlying late diarrhea (3–11 days posttherapy) are not fully understood and may be the result of the active metabolite SN38 on the gastrointestinal epithelium. Late diarrhea should be treated promptly with loperamide, which reduces the incidence of grade IV diarrhea from 30–40% to 10%.

B. Topotecan

Topotecan (Hycamtin®) is another semisynthetic camptothecin analog with improved water solubility. Phase I studies of topotecan as single-agent administered daily for 5 days every 21 days (maximum tolerated dose: 1.5–1.74 mg/m^2/daily) suggested that the dose-limiting toxicity is a short-lasting, noncumulative neutropenia, and the drug is almost devoid of any other side effect.

Topotecan as a single agent at the dose of 1.5–2.0 mg/m^2/daily for 5 days as well as administered by continuous infusion for 21 days every 4 weeks (0.5–0.6 mg/m^2/daily) has shown only marginal activity in patients with previously untreated NSCLC (73–75). Its activity seems to be mostly limited to patients with squamous cell carcinoma (76) (Table 7). In SCLC topotecan shows considerable activity in both previously treated "sensitive" (response to first-line chemotherapy and progression greater than 3 months after chemotherapy discontinuation) (77) and previously untreated patients with extensive disease (78), but a negative study in patients refractory to cisplatin and etoposide has been recently reported (79).

A major area of interest is the further development of topotecan combination using agent as paclitaxel and cisplatin. In a phase I study topotecan was administered on days 1–5 together with cisplatin given on day 1 of a 3-week cycle. The study revealed that the combination is feasible with a recommended phase II dose of topotecan of 1.0 mg/m^2/daily together with cisplatin 50–75 mg/m^2 with or without G-CSF (80). In another trial paclitaxel was combined with topotecan and the dose-limiting toxicity was neutropenia. The recommended dose of paclitaxel, 3-hour infusion, is 230 mg/m^2 and topotecan 1.0 mg/m^2/daily × 5 with G-CSF administration (81). In a subsequent randomized phase II trial using these recommended doses there was an unacceptable number of toxic deaths from neutropenic sepsis. The incidence of febrile neutropenia in these patients have been correlated with the duration of grade IV neutropenia (82).

C. Other Topoisomerase I Inhibitors Under Investigation

Other agents in development include 9-amino-camptothecin (9-AC) and GI 142742 (GG211). The drug 9-AC, a poorly soluble analog, has shown very promising preclinical and clinical activity. Early phase I trials using the intravenous formulation revealed that neutropenia is the principal dose-limiting toxicity. Other toxicities include thrombocytopenia, anemia, nausea, diarrhea, mucositis, and fatigue. The recommended phase II dose is 45 μg/m^2/hr as a 72-hour infusion every 3 weeks or 35 μg/m^2/hr every 2 weeks (83).

GG211 has a preclinical profile similar to that of topotecan but has a two- to five-fold increase in in vitro potency. Phase I trials of this agent reveal that the major dose-limiting toxicity is myelosuppression (84). A pilot study of GG211 at the dose of 1.2 mg/m^2/daily for 5 days every 3 weeks in 22 patients with advanced NSCLC has shown a good tolerability but only minor activity (9% response rate) (85).

V. New Vinca Alkaloids

Vinorelbine (Navilbine®; 5′norhydrovinblastine) is a relatively new semisynthetic vinca alkaloid that differs chemically from other vinca alkaloids by substitutions on the catharantine ring rather than on the vindoline ring of the molecule. Vinorelbine

Table 7 Phase II Studies of Topotecan Single Agent in Lung Cancer

Author (year)	No. of patients	Type of cancer	Schedule	% Response rate	Main toxicities
Lynch (1994)	20	NSCLC-Stage IV	2.0 mg/m^2/d×5 q3weeks	0	Neutropenia-rush
Perez-Soler (1996)	40	NSCLC-Stage IIIB/IV	1.5 mg/m^2/d × 5 q3weeks	15 (SCC-34%)	Granulocytopenia G3–4 = 76%
Kindler (1997)	26	NSCLC Stage IIIB/IV	0.5–0.6 mg/m^2 C.I. × 21 days q4wks	4%	Neutropenia G4 4% Thrombocytopenia G4 8%
Schiller (1996)	48	Extensive SCLC untreated	2.0 mg/m^2/d × 5 (35 with G-CSF d.10–14) q3 weeks	39	Neutropenia G3–4 without G-CSF = 92% with G-CSF = 29%
Perez-Soler (1996)	28	SCLC-refractory to DDP & ETO	1.25 mg/m^2/d q3weeks	11	Granulocytopenia G3–4 = 70%
Ardizzoni (1997)	92	SCLC 45 "sensitive" 47 "refractory"	1.5 mg/m^2/d × 5 q3 weeks	38 6.4	Granulocytopenia G3–4 = 74.8%

NSCLC = Non–small-cell lung cancer; SCLC = small-cell lung cancer; SCC = squamous cell carcinoma; DDP = cisplatin; ETO = etoposide; G-CSF = granulocyte colony-stimulating factor; "sensitive" = patients who responded to first-line treatment and progressed greater than 3 months after chemotherapy discontinuation; "refractory" = patients who failed first-line treatment ≤3 months from chemotherapy discontinuation; G = WHO toxicity grade.

also differs functionally from other vinca alkaloids by being relatively selective for mitotic microtubules with less toxicity to axonal microtubules, indicating that vinorelbine has a reduced potential for inducing neurotoxicity.

Indications from preclinical data suggesting that vinorelbine could show some activity against NSCLC (86) were subsequently supported by the observation that the drug was taken up into both normal lung tissue and tumor when surgical samples were examined from patients who had received vinorelbine 1–3 hours before surgery (87).

The significant single-agent activity of vinorelbine in initial phase II evaluations, in the range of 25–30% (for review, see Ref. 88), led to a European multicenter trial in which a total of 612 patients, previously untreated, were randomized to receive (1) vinorelbine 30 mg/m^2/week or (2) vinorelbine at the same dose and schedule along with cisplatin 120 mg/m^2 intravenously on day 1, day 29, then every 6 weeks, or (3) vindesine 3 mg/m^2/week intravenously for 6 weeks, then every other week along with cisplatin at the same dose and schedule mentioned above. The response rate produced by the combination of vinorelbine and cisplatin (30%) was significantly higher than the rates produced by vindesine and cisplatin (19%, $p = 0.03$) and vinorelbine alone (14%, $p < 0.01$), whereas the response rates for vindesine plus cisplatin and single agent vinorelbine were not significantly different. Vinorelbine plus cisplatin produced longer survival than vindesine plus cisplatin (median survival, 40 vs. 32 weeks, $p = 0.03$). The 1-year survival rates were 35% for vinorelbine plus cisplatin, 27% for vindesine plus cisplatin, and 30% for single agent vinorelbine (37). The incidence of severe (grades 3 and 4) neurotoxicity was higher in the cisplatin plus vindesine arm (17%) than the cisplatin plus vinorelbine arm (7%) (89). A detailed economic evaluation indicated that this combination provided benefit to the patients with a level of cost-effectiveness acceptable within conventional limits for medical intervention of this sort (90).

VI. Bioreductive Agents

Tirapazamine (SR 259075) is a benzotriazine compound exhibiting varying toxicity for hypoxic cells. Hypoxic human tumor cells tested were 15–50 times as sensitive as aerobic cells (91). Tirapazamine is a potent and selective hypoxic cytotoxic agent. In vitro the hypoxic cytotoxicity ratio (ratio of equitoxic doses under aerobic and hypoxic conditions) of tirapazamine is one to two times greater than nitroimidazole, mitomycin C, and porfiromycin.

Under hypoxic conditions, the drug undergoes one-electron reduction by cytochrome P450 and P450 reductase to a cytotoxic free radical (92). The free radical is believed to abstract hydrogen ions from DNA, resulting in DNA strand cleavage and selective hypoxic cell cytotoxicity. Acidic pH, expected in hypoxic tumor regions, increases the DNA-damaging activity of tirapazamine. In well-oxygenated tissues, the tirapazamine radical is rapidly back-oxidized to the inactive parent drug by molecular oxygen.

In a murine model implanted with RIF-1 tumor cells as well as in SCCVII tumor cells, the sequential administration of tirapazamine preceding 1–3 hours cisplatin demonstrated superadditive killing (93).

In two phase II trials performed in unresectable locally advanced and metastatic NSCLC, tirapazamine (260–390 mg/m^2) administered as 1- to 3-hour infusion followed 1–3 hours later by cisplatin (75 mg/m^2) produced a response rate of 23–29%. Major toxic effects included involuntary muscle contractions, vomiting, fatigue, diarrhea, and transient hearing loss (94,95).

VII. Conclusion

The results of more recent clinical trials provide some optimism that newly developed chemotherapeutic agents including taxanes, topoisomerase I inhibitors, and new antimetabolites are as active as or more active than previously available agents. Most of the clinical experience with these new agents has been obtained in the treatment of advanced NSCLC, in which until recently only a few standard chemotherapeutic agents have had activity in excess of 15%. These drugs can be combined with traditional agents such as cisplatin, carboplatin, and etoposide, as clearly shown by pilot phase II studies already performed, and encouraging results in terms of response rate (>50%) and, occasionally, of survival have been reported.

Two large multicenter cooperative group trials have evaluated the combination of paclitaxel and cisplatin versus a standard regimen (etoposide/cisplatin or teniposide/cisplatin) and concluded in favor of the experimental arm in terms of response rate and reduced toxicity. However, the impact on survival, a critical endpoint for this kind of trials, remains questionable.

Nevertheless, the availability of low-toxicity profile combinations resulting in tumor regression in about an half of treated patients could be of special value in unresectable locally advanced NSCLC, in which the integration of these new combinations in an aggressive combined modality therapeutic program will hopefully improve the outcome of this dismal disease. Alternatively, combination of thoracic radiotherapy with some of these new agents (taxanes, topoisomerase I inhibitors, and gemcitabine), which have been shown at noncytotoxic concentration to be radiosensitizers, could also be of relevance for patients with unresectable lung cancer confined to the chest where the local control of the neoplastic disease remains a critical issue.

Most of these agents have also been proved to be extremely active in SCLC: the encouraging results obtained with paclitaxel and topoisomerase I inhibitors confirm the need for additional randomized studies of the addition of these agents or their substitution for currently used agents as cisplatin, carboplatin, and etoposide.

References

1. Bakowski MT, Crouch JD. Chemotherapy of non-small cell lung cancer: a reappraisal and a look to the future. Cancer Treat Rev 1983; 10:159–172.
2. Joss RA, Cavalli F, Goldhirsh A, Mermillod B, Brunner KW. New agents in non-small cell lung cancer. Cancer Treat Rev 1984; 11:205–236.
3. Ihde DC. Chemotherapy of lung cancer. N Engl J Med 1992; 327:1434–1441.
4. Hertel LW, Boder GB, Kroin JS, Rinzel SM, Poore GA, Todd GC, Grindey GB. Evaluation of the antitunor activity of gemcitabine (2,2′-difluoro-2′-deoxycytidine). Cancer Res 1990; 50:4417–4442.
5. Kaye SB. Gemcitabine: current status of phase I and II trials. J Clin Oncol 1994; 12:1527–1531.
6. Abratt RP, Bezwoda WR, Goedhals L, Hacking DJ. Weekly gemcitabine with monthly cisplatin: effective chemotherapy for advanced non-small cell lung cancer. J Clin Oncol 1997; 15:744–749.
7. Steward WP, Dunlop DJ, Cameron C, et al. Gemcitabine combined with cisplatin in non-small cell lung cancer (NSCLC): a phase I/II study. Eur J Cancer 1995; 31A(5):225.
8. Crinò L, Scagliotti G, Marangolo M, Figoli F, Clerici M, De Marinis F, Salvati F, Cruciani G, Dogliotti L, Cocconi G, Paccagnella A, Adamo V, Incoronato P, Scarcella L, Mosconi AM, Tonato M. Gemcitabine-cisplatin combination in advanced non-small cell lung cancer: a phase II study. J Clin Oncol 1997; 15:297–303.
9. Sandler A, Ansari R, Mc clean J, Fisher W, Dorr FA, Einhorn LH. Gemcitabine plus cisplatin in non-small cell lung cancer: a phase II study. Eur J Cancer 1995; 31A(5):225.
10. Shepherd F, Burges R, Cormier Y, Crump M, Feld R, Strack T, Schulz M. Phase I dose-escalation trial of gemcitabine and cisplatin for non-small cell lung cancer: usefulness of mathematic modeling to determine maximum-tolerable dose. J Clin Oncol 1996; 14:1656–1662.
11. Anton A, Carrato A, Gonzales-Larriba JL, Vadell C, Masutti B, Montalar J, Aranda E, Barnetto J, Tarazona Y, Lopez Martin E. Phase II activity of gemcitabine in combination with cisplatin in advanced non-small cell lung cancer (NSCLC). Proc Am Soc Clin Oncol 1996; 15:380.
12. Perng R-P, Chen Y-M, Ming-Liu J, Tsai C-M, Lin W-C, Yang K-Y, Whang-Peng J. Gemcitabine versus the combination of cisplatin and etoposide in patients with inoperable non-small cell lung cancer in a phase II randomized study. J Clin Oncol 1997; 15:2097–2102.
13. Manegold C, Stahel R, Mattson K, Ricci S, van Walree NC, Bergman R, ten Bokkel Huinink WW. Randomized phase II study of gemcitabine monotherapy versus cisplatin plus etoposide in patients with locally advanced or metastatic non-small cell lung cancer (abstr). Proc Am Soc Clin Oncol 1997; 16:460a.
14. Cormier Y, Eisenhauer E, Muldal A, Gregg R, Ayoub I, Goss G, Steward D, Tarassoff P, Wong D. Gemcitabine is an active new agent in previously untreated extensive small cell lung cancer. A study of the National Cancer Institute of Canada Clinical Trials Group. Ann Oncol 1994; 5:283–285.
15. Shum KY, Kris Mg, Gralla RJ, Burke MT, Marks LD, Heelan RT. Phase II study of 10-ethyl-10-deaza-aminopterin in patients with stage III and IV non-small cell lung cancer. J Clin Oncol 1988; 6:446–450.
16. Souhami RL, Rudd RM, Spiro SG, Allen R, Lamond P, Harper PG. Phase II of edatrexate in stage III and IV non-small cell lung cancer. Cancer Chemother Pharmacol 1992; 30:465–468.
17. Lee JS, Libshitz HI, Murphy WK, Jeffries D, Hong WK. Phase II of 10-ethyl-10-deaza-aminopterin (10-EDAM, CGP 30694) for stage IIIB or IV non-small cell lung cancer. Invest N Drugs 1990; 8:299–304.
18. Lee JS, Libshitz HI, Fossella FV, Murphy WK, Pang AC, Lippman SM, Shin DM, Dimery IW, Glisson BS, Hong WK. Improved therapeutic index by leucovorin of edatrexate, cyclophosphamide and cisplatin regimen for non-small cell lung cancer. J Natl Cancer Inst 1992; 84:1039–1040.

19. Fossella FV, Lee JS, Winn R, Wester M, Graham S, Holder LW, Goodwin JW, Dakhil SR, Hong WK. Edatrexate, ifosfamide, cisplatin with leucovorin and mesna for advanced non-small cell lung cancer (abstr). Proc Am Soc Clin Oncol 1995; 14:336.

20. Fennelly DM, Rigas JD, Chou D, Miller VA, Pisters KMW, Grant SC, Tyson LB, Sirotnak F, Kris MG. Phase I trial of edatrexate plus paclitaxel using an administration schedule with demonstrated in vitro synergy (abstr). Proc Am Soc Clin Oncol 1994; 13:365.

21. Chang AY, Kim K, Glick J, Anderson T, Karp D, Johnson D. A phase II study of taxol, merbarone and piroxantrone in stage IV non-small cell lung cancer: the Eastern Cooperative Oncology Group results. J Natl Cancer Inst 1993; 85:388–394.

22. Murphy WK, Fossella FV, Winn RJ, Shin DM, Hynes HE, Gross HM, Cavilla E, Leimert J, Dhingra H, Raber MN, Krakoff IH, Hong WK. Phase II study of taxol in patients with untreated advanced non-small cell lung cancer. J Natl Cancer Inst 1993; 85:384–387.

23. Gatzemeier U, Heckmayer M, Neuhauss R, Schlauter I, von Pawel J, Wagner H, Dreps A. Chemotherapy of advanced inoperable non-small cell lung cancer with paclitaxel: a phase II trial. Semin Oncol 1995; 22(suppl.15):24–28.

24. Hainsworth JD, Thompson DS, Greco FA. Paclitaxel by 1-hour infusion: an active drug in metastatic non-small cell lung cancer. J Clin Oncol 1995; 13:1609–1614.

25. Alberola V, Rosell R, Gonzales-Larriba JL, Molina F, Ayala F, Garcia-conde J, Benito D, Perez JM. Single agent taxol, 3-hour infusion, in untreated non-small cell lung cancer. Ann Oncol 1995; 6(suppl.3):S49–S52.

26. Tester WJ, Jin PY, Reardon DH, Cohn JB, Cohen MH. Phase II study of patients with metastatic non-small cell carcinoma of the lung treated with paclitaxel by 3-hour infusion. Cancer 1997; 79:724–729.

27. Millward MJ, Bishop JF, Friedlander M, Levi JA, Goldstein D, Olver IN, Smith JG, Toner GC, Rischin D, Bell DR. Phase II trial of a 3-hour infusion of paclitaxel in previously untreated patients with advanced non-small cell lung cancer. J Clin Oncol 1996; 14:142–148.

28. Sekine I, Nishiwaki Y, Watanabe K, Yoneda S, Saijo N, Phase II study of 3-hour infusion of paclitaxel in previously untreated non-small cell lung cancer. Clin Cancer Res 1996; 2: 941–945.

29. Akerley W, Choy H, Glantz M, Safran H, Sikov W, Rege V, Sambandam S, Josephs J, Wittels E. Phase II trial of weekly paclitaxel for advanced non-small cell lung cancer (abstr). Proc Am Soc Clin Oncol 1997; 16:450a.

30. Belli L, Le Chevalier T, Goffried M, Adams D, Ruffie P, Le Cesne A, Tete L, Pellae-Cosset B. Phase I/II study of paclitaxel plus cisplatin as first-line chemotherapy for advanced non-small cell lung cancer: preliminary results. Semin Oncol 1995; 6(suppl.15):29–33.

31. von Pawel J, Wagner H, Niederle N, Heider A, Koschel G, Hecker D, Hanske M. Phase II study of paclitaxel and cisplatin in patients with non-small cell lung cancer. Semin Oncol 1996; 6(suppl 16):47–50.

32. Georgiadis MS, Schuler BS, Brown JE, Kieffer LV, Steinberg SM, Wilson WH, Takimoto CH, Kelley MJ, Johnson BE. Paclitaxel by 96-hour continuous infusion in combination with cisplatin. A phase I trial in patients with advanced lung cancer. J Clin Oncol 1997; 15: 735–743.

33. Natale RB. A phase I/II trial of combination paclitaxel and carboplatin in advanced or metastatic non-small cell lung cancer: preliminary results of an ongoing study. Semin Oncol 1995; 6(suppl.15):34–37.

34. Langer CJ, Leighton JC, Comis RL, O'Dwyer PJ, McAleer CA, Bonjo CA, Engstrom PF, Litwin S, Ozols RF. Paclitaxel and carboplatin in combination in the treatment of advanced non-small cell lung cancer: a phase II toxicity, response and survival analysis. J Clin Oncol 1995; 13:1860–1870.

35. Johnson DH, Paul DM, Hande KR, Shyr Y, Blanke C, Murphy B, Lewis M, De Vore RF. Paclitaxel plus carboplatin in advanced non-small cell lung cancer: a phase II trial. J Clin Oncol 1996; 14:2054–2060.

36. Jagasia M, Johnson D, Hande KR, Shyr Y, Blanke C, Chiappori A, Murphy B, Johnson DR, Butler TW, Schlabach L, McCullough N, Hughes D, Krozely P, Devore RF. Carboplatin and paclitaxel (1 and 24 hour infusion) in advanced non-small cell lung cancer: the results of sequential phase II trials (abstr). Proc Am Soc Clin Oncol 1997; 16:471a.

37. Jodrell DI, Egorin MJ, Canetta RM, Langenberg P, Goldbloom EP, Burroughs JN, Goodlaw JL, Tan S, Wiltshaw E. Relationship between carboplatin exposure and tumor response and toxicity in patients with ovarian cancer. J Clin Oncol 1992; 10:520–528.

38. Bonomi P, Kim K, Chang A, Johnson D. Cisplatin/etoposide vs paclitaxel/cisplatin/G-CSF vs paclitaxel/cisplatin in non-small cell lung cancer. Oncology 1997; 11(suppl. 3):9–10.

39. Giaccone G, Postmus P, Splinter TAW, Diaz Puente M, Van Zandwijk N, Scagliotti G, Ardizzoni A, De Bruyne C. Cisplatin/paclitaxel vs. cisplatin/teniposide for advanced non-small cell lung cancer. Oncology 1997; 11(suppl. 3):11–14.

40. Ettinger DS, Finkelstein DM, Sarma RP, Johnson DH. Phase II of paclitaxel in patients with extensive-disease small-cell lung cancer: an Eastern Cooperative Oncology Group study. J Clin Oncol 1995; 13:1430–1435.

41. Smit EF, Kloosterziel C, Groen HJM, Postmus PE, A phase II study of paclitaxel in heavily pretreated patients with small cell lung cancer: an Eastern Cooperative Oncology Group study. J Clin Oncol 1995; 13:1430–1435.

42. Bunn PA, Jr, Kelly K. Phase I study of cisplatin, etoposide, and paclitaxel in patients with extensive-stage, small-cell lung cancer: a University of Colorado Cancer Center study. Semin Oncol 1996; 23(suppl.16):11–15.

43. Greco FA, Hainsworth JD. Paclitaxel, carboplatin, and oral etoposide in the treatment of small cell lung cancer. Semin Oncol 1996; 23(suppl.16):7–10.

44. Tishler RB, Schiff PB, Geard CR, Hall EJ. Taxol: a novel radiation sensitizer. Int Radiat Oncol Biol Phys 1992; 22:613–617.

45. Choy H, Akerley W, Safran H, Clark J, Rege V, Papa A, Glantz M, Puthawada Y, Soderberg C, Leone L. Phase I trial of outpatients weekly paclitaxel and concurrent radiation therapy for advanced non-small cell lung cancer. J Clin Oncol 1994; 12:2682–2688.

46. Choy H, Akerley W, Safran H, Graziano S, Chang C, Cole B. Phase II of weekly paclitaxel and concurrent radiation therapy for locally advanced non-small cell lung cancer. Proc Am Soc Clin Oncol 1996; 15:371.

47. Greco FA, Stroup SL, Gray JR, Hainsworth JD. Paclitaxel in combination chemotherapy with radiotherapy in patients with unresectable stage III non-small cell lung cancer. J Clin Oncol 1996; 14:1642–1648.

48. Cerny T, Kaplan S, Pavlidis N, Schoffski P, Epelbaum R, van Meerbeeck J, Wanders J, Franklin HR, Kaye S. Docetaxel (Taxotere) is active non-small cell lung cancer: a phase II trial of the EORTC Early Clinical Trials Group (ECTG). Br J Cancer 1994; 70: 384–387.

49. Francis PA, Rigas JR, Kris MG, Pisters KMW, Orazem JP, Woolley KJ, Heelan RT. Phase II trial of docetaxel in patients with stage III and IV non-small cell lung cancer. J Clin Oncol 1994; 12:1232–1237.

50. Fossella FV, Lee JS, Murphy WK, Lippman SM, Calayag M, Pang A, Chasen M, Shin DM, Glisson B, Benner S, Huber M, Perez-Soler R, Hong WK, Raber M. Phase II of docetaxel for recurrent or metastatic non-small cell lung cancer. J Clin Oncol 1994; 12:1238–1244.

51. Saarinen A, Jekunen A, Halme M, Pyrhonen S, Tamminen K, Boyer R, Roubille N, Mattson K. A phase II trial of docetaxel in advanced non-small cell lung cancer. Anticancer Drugs 1996; 7:890–892.

52. Miller VA, Rigas R, Francis PA, Grant SC, Pisters KM, Venkatraman ES, Woolley K, Heelan RT, Kris MG. Phase II trial of a 75 mg/m2 dose of docetaxel with prednisone premedication for patients with advanced non-small cell lung cancer. Cancer 1995; 75:968–972.

53. Kunitoh H, Watanabe K, Onoshi T, Furuse K, Niitani H, Taguchi T. Phase II trial of docetaxel in previously untreated non-small cell lung cancer. J Clin Oncol 1996; 14:1649–1655.

54. Fossella FV, Lee JS, Shin DM, Calayag M, Huber M, Perez-Soler R, Murphy WK, Lippman S, Benner S, Glisson B, Chasen M, Hong WK, Raber M. Phase II of docetaxel for advanced or metastatic platinum refractory non-small cell lung cancer. J Clin Oncol 1995; 13: 645–651.

55. Burris HA, Eckardt J, Fields S, Rodriguez G, Smith L, Thurman A, Peacock N, Kahn J, Hodges S, Bellet R, Bayssas M, LeBail N, Von Hoff D. Phase II trials of taxotere in patients with non-small cell lung cancer (abstr). Proc Am Soc Clin Oncol 1993; 12:335.

56. Gandara DR, Vokes E, Green M, Bonomi P, Devore R, Comis R, Carbone D, Karp D, Belani C. Docetaxel (Taxotere) in platinum-treated non-small cell lung cancer: confirmation of prolonged survival in a multicenter trial (abstr). Proc Am Soc Clin Oncol 1997; 16:454a.

57. Oulid-Aissa D, Behar A, Spielmann M, Kayitalire L, Chau A, Plasse T, Le Bail N. Management of fluid retention syndrome in patients treated with Taxotere (docetaxel): effect of premedication (abstr). Proc Am Soc Clin Oncol 1994; 13:465.

58. Millward MJ, Zalcberg J, Bishop JF, Webster LK, Zimet A, Rischin D, Toner GC, Laird J, Cosolo W, Urch M, Bruno R, Loret C, James R, Blanc C. Phase I trial of docetaxel and cisplatin in previously untreated patients with advanced non-small cell lung cancer. J Clin Oncol 1997; 15:750–758.

59. Androulakis N, Dimopoulos AM, Kourousis C, Kakolyris S, Papadakis E, Apostolopoulou F, Papadimitriou F, Vossos A, Aggelidou M, Heras P, Tzannes S, Souklakos J, Hadzidaki D, Georgoulias V. First-line treatment of advanced non-small with docetaxel and cisplatin: a multicenter phase II study (abstr). Proc Am Soc Clin Oncol 1997; 16:461a.

60. Belani CF, Bonomi P, Dobbs T, Devore R, Ettinger D, Jett J, KozaK C, Cohen L, Capozzoli MJ. Multicenter phase II trial of docetaxel and cisplatin combination in patients with non-small cell lung cancer (abstr). Proc Am Soc Clin Oncol 1997; 16:462a.

61. Smyth JF, Smith IE, Sessa C, Schoffski P, Wanders J, Franklin H, Kaye SB. Activity of docetaxel in small cell lung cancer. Eur J Cancer 1994; 30A:1058–1060.

62. Kaplan S, Hanauske AR, Pavlidis N, Bruntsch U, Ten de Velde A, Wanders J, Heinrich B, Verweij J. Single agent activity of rhizoxin in non-small cell lung cancer: a phase II trial of the EORTC Early Clinical Trial Group. Br J Cancer 1996; 73:403–405.

63. Kawato J, Aonuma M, Hirota Y, Kuga H, Sato K. Intracellular roles of SN-38, a metabolite of the camptothecin derivative CPT-11, in the antitumor effect of CPT-11. Cancer Res 1991; 51:4187–4191.

64. Negoro S, Fukuoka M, Niitani H, Suzuki A, Nakabayashi T, Kimura M, Motomiya M, Kurita Y, Hasegawa K, Kuriyama T. A phase II study of CPT-11, a camptothecin derivative in patients with primary lung cancer. Gan To Kagaku Ryoho 1991; 18:1013–1019.

65. Fukuoka M, Niitani H, Suzuki A, Motomiya M, Hasegawa K, Nishiwaki Y, Kuriyama T, Ariyoshi Y, Negoro S, Masuda N. A phase II study of CPT-11, a new derivative of camptothecin for previously untreated non-small cell lung cancer. J Clin Oncol 1992; 10:16–20.

66. Baker L, Khan R, Lynch T, Savaraj N, Sandler A, Feun L, Schaser R, Hanover C, Petit R. Phase II of irinotecan in advanced non-small cell lung cancer (abstr). Proc Am Soc Clin Oncol 1997; 16:461a.

67. Fukuoka M, Masuda N. Clinical studies of irinotecan alone and in combination with cisplatin. Cancer Chemother Pharmacol 1994; 34(suppl):S105–S111.

68. Rothenberg ML. CPT-11: an original spectrum of clinical activity. Semin Oncol 1996; 23(suppl.3):21–26.

69. Masuda N, Fukuoka M, Kusunoki Y, Matsui K, Takifuji N, Kudoh S, Negoro S, Nishioka M, Nakagawa K, Takada M. CPT-11: a new derivative of camptothecin for the treatment of refractory or relapsed small cell lung cancer. J Clin Oncol 1992; 10:1225–1229.

70. Fujita A. Takabatake H, Tagaki S, Sekine K. Pilot study of irinotecan in refractory small cell lung cancer. Gan To Kagaku Ryoho 1995; 22:889–893.

71. Oshita F, Noda K, Nishiwaki Y, Fujita A, Kurita Y, Nakabayashi T, Tobise K, Abe S, Suzuki S, Hayashi I, Kawakami Y, Matsuda T, Tsuchiya S, Takahashi S, Tamura T, Saijo N. Phase II study of irinotecan and etoposide in patients with metastatic non-small cell lung cancer. J Clin Oncol 1997; 15:304–309.

72. Kudoh S, Kunhara N, Okishio K, Airata K, Yoshikawa J, Masuda N, Takada M, Takeda K, Negoro S, Fukuoka M. A phase I/II study of weekly irinotecan and simultaneous thoracic radiotherapy for unresectable locally advanced non-small cell lung cancer (abstr). Proc Am Soc Clin Oncol 1996; 15:372.

73. Lynch TJ, Jr., Kalish L, Strauss G, Elias A, Skarin A, Shulman LN, Posner M, Frei E, III. Phase II study of topotecan in metastatic non-small cell lung cancer. J Clin Oncol 1994; 12:347–352.

74. Perez-Soler R, Fossella FV, Glisson BS, Lee JS, Murphy WK, Shin DM, Kemp BL, Lee JJ, Kane J, Robinson RA, Lippman SM, Kurie JM, Huber MH, Raber MN, Hong WK. Phase II study of topotecan in patients with advanced non-small cell lung cancer previously untreated with chemotherapy. J Clin Oncol 1996; 14:503–513.

75. Kindler HL, Kris MG, Smith IE, Slevin ML, Krebs JB. Continuous infusion topotecan as first-line therapy in patients with non-small cell lung cancer: a phase II study (abstr). Proc Am Soc Clin Oncol 1997; 16:472a.

76. Perez-Soler R, Khurl F, Pisters C, Robinson R, Wimberly A, Fossella FV. Phase II study in patients with squamous cell carcinoma of the lung previously untreated with chemotherapy (abstr). Proc Am Soc Clin Oncol 1997; 16:450a.

77. Ardizzoni A, Hansen H, Dombernowsky P, Gamucci T, Kaplan S, Postmus P, Giaccone G, Schaefer B, Wanders J, Verweij J. Topotecan, a new active drug in the second line treatment of small-cell lung cancer: a phase II study in patients with refractory and sensitive disease. J Clin Oncol 1997; 15:2090–2096.

78. Schiller JH, Kim K, Hutson P, DeVore R, Glick J, Stewart J, Johnson D. Phase II study of topotecan in patients with extensive-stage small cell carcinoma of the lung: an Eastern Cooperative Oncology Group Trial. J Clin Oncol 1996; 14:2345–2352.

79. Perez-Soler R, Glisson BS, Lee JS, Fossella FV, Murphy WK, Shin DM, Hong WK. Treatment of patients with small-cell lung cancer refractory to etoposide and cisplatin with the topoisomerase I poison topotecan. J Clin Oncol 1996; 14:2785–2790.

80. Miller AA, Hargis JB, Lilenbaum RC, Fields JS, Rosnier GL, Schilsky RL. Phase I study of topotecan and cisplatin in patients with advanced solid tumors: a Cancer and Leukemia Group B study. J Clin Oncol 1994; 12:2743–2750.

81. Lilenbaum RC, Ratain MJ, Miller AA, Hargis JB, Hollis DR, Rosner GL, O'Brien SM, Brewster L, Green MR, Schilsky RL. Phase I study of paclitaxel and topotecan in patients with advanced tumors: a Cancer and Leukemia Group B study. J Clin Oncol 1995; 13:2230–2237.

82. Miller AA, Lilenbaum RC, Lynch TJ, Rosner GL, Ratain MJ, Green MR, Schilsky RL. Treatment-related fatal sepsis from topotecan/cisplatin and topotecan/paclitaxel. J Clin Oncol 1996; 14:1964–1965.

83. Dahut W, Brillart N, Takimoto C, Allegra JM, Hamilton JM, Sorenson JM, Arbuck S, Chen A, Grem J. A phase I trial of 9-aminocamptothecin in adult patients with solid tumors. Proc Am Soc Clin Oncol 1994; 13:138.

84. Eckardt JR, Rodriguez GI, Burris HA, Wissel PS, Fields SM, Rothenberg ML, Smith L, Thurman A, Kunka RL, DePee SP, Littlefield D, White LJ, Von Hoff DD. A phase I and pharmacokinetic study of the topoisomerase I inhibitor GG211. Proc Am Soc Clin Oncol 1995; 14:476.

85. Heinrich B, Lehnert M, Cavalli F, Pavlidis N, Wanders J, Hanauske AR. Phase II trial of GI147211 in locally advanced or metastatic non-small cell lung cancer: an EORTC-ECTG trial (abstr). Proc Am Soc Clin Oncol 1997; 16:470a.

86. Cros S, Wright M, Morimoto M, Lataste H, Couzinier JP, Krikorian A. Experimental antitumor activity of navilbine. Semin Oncol 1989; 16(suppl.4):15–20.

87. Leveque D, Quoix E, Dumont P. Pulmonary distribution of vinorelbine in patients with non-small cell lung cancer. Cancer Chemother Pharmacol 1993; 33:176–178.

88. Johnson SA, Harper P, Hortobagyi GN, Pouillart. Vinorelbine: an overview. Cancer Treat Rev 1996; 22:127–142.

89. Le.Chevalier T, Brisgard D, Douilliard JY, Pujol GL, Alberola V, Monnier A, Riviere A, Lianes P, Chomy P, Cigolari S, Ruffie P, Panizo A, Gaspard M-H, Ravaioli A, Besenval M, Besson F, Martinez A, Berthaud P, Tursz T. Randomised study of vinorelbine and cisplatin versus vindesine and cisplatin versus vinorelbine alone in advanced non-small cell lung cancer: results of a European multicentre trial including 612 patients. J Clin Oncol 1994; 12:360–367.

90. Smith TJ, Hillner BE, Neighbors DM, McSortey PA, Le Chevalier T. Economic evaluation of a randomised clinical trial comparing vinorelbine, vinorelbine plus cisplatin and vindesine plus cisplatin for non-small cell lung cancer. J Clin Oncol 1995; 13:2166–2173.

91. Zeman EM, Brown JM, Lemmon MJ, Hirst VK, Lee WW. SR-4233: a new bioreductive agent with high selective toxicity for hypoxic mammalian cells. Int J Radiat Oncol Biol Phys 1986; 12:1239–1242.

92. Keohane A, Godden J, Stratford IJ, Adams GE. The effects of three bioreductive drugs (mitomycin C, RSU-1069 and SR 4233) on cell lines selected for their sensitivity to mitomycin C or ionizing radiation. Br Cancer 1990; 61:722–726.

93. Dorie MJ, Brown JM. Tumor-specific, schedule-dependent interaction between tirapazamine (SR 4233) and cisplatin. Cancer Res 1993; 53:4633–4636.

94. Rodriguez GI, Valdivieso M, Von Hoff DD, Kraut M, Burris HA, Eckardt JR, Lookwood G, Kennedy H, von Roemeling R. A phase I/II trial of the combination of tirapazamine and cisplatin in patients with non small cell lung cancer (abstr). Proc Am Soc Clin Oncol 1996; 15:382.

95. Treat J, Haynes B, Johnson E, Belani C, Greenberg R, Rodriguez R, Drabbins P, Miller W, Meehan L, von Roemeling R. Tirapazamine with cisplatin: a phase II trial in advanced stage non-small cell lung cancer (abstr). Proc Am Soc Clin Oncol 1997; 16:455a.

42

Lung Metastases and Second Lung Cancer
Role of Surgery

UGO PASTORINO

European Institute of Oncology
Milan, Italy

FRANCESCO PEZZELLA

University College London
London, England

I. Clinical Relevance of Secondary Lung Tumors

A. Frequency and Clinical Presentation

The occurrence of pulmonary lesions in patients previously treated for a malignant tumor in other organs, or in the lung itself, represents a real challenge for the clinician in terms of detection, assessment, and proper management, but also for the experimental oncologist as a key to investigate the natural history of various neoplastic diseases.

The absolute frequency of secondary lung tumors depends on a number of factors, such as the type of primary tumor, the patient's life expectancy, and the intensity of follow-up. Surveillance programs adopted in comprehensive cancer centers, usually within prospective clinical trials testing different treatment modalities or adjuvant strategies, are more likely to detect new pulmonary opacities. The use of spiral computed tomography (CT) scan during routine follow-up has contributed to improve both early detection and clinical staging of these lesions, with a view to curative management. On the other hand, those clinicians who are in favor of more aggressive programs for salvage surgery have a practical justification to adopt a more intense follow-up.

B. Differential Diagnosis

In patients presenting with multiple lesions, the final diagnosis is almost invariably of metastatic disease. However, in occasional patients, multiple synchronous primaries or a single primary lung cancer associated with benign disease (hamartoma, granuloma, TB) may be detected.

The differential diagnosis between lung metastases and new primary tumors is more critical when the pulmonary lesion is solitary at CT scan examination. The radiological features are rarely helpful to make the distinction, while the pathological diagnosis may be missing or equivocal. In general, the likelihood of primary versus metastatic disease is mainly related to the type of prior cancer. As illustrated in Table 1, within a series of nearly 700 patients presenting with solitary lung opacities after a prior treatment for malignant tumors reported by Cahan et al. in 1972 (1), the overall frequency of new primary cancer was 73%, ranging from 8% in patients with a prior sarcoma to 92% in patients with lung cancer. These data are similar to our experience at the Istituto Nazionale Tumori of Milan, based on 464 cases of secondary lung tumors, where the frequency of new primaries was 30% overall but reached 95% among patients with a prior lung cancer. In practical terms, however, the difference may not be so relevant as both groups of patients are good candidates for salvage surgery.

Table 1   Probability of New Primary Cancer Versus Metastasis in Patients Presenting with Solitary Lung Opacity After Prior Treatment for Malignant Tumor

Prior tumor	New primary	Metastasis	Total
Wilms	0	8	8
Sarcoma	5 (8)	55	60
Melanoma	7 (19)	29	36
Testis	6 (33)	12	18
Kidney	11 (55)	9	20
Colon-Rectum	30 (58)	22	52
Breast	40 (63)	23	63
Ovary	6 (66)	3	9
Uterus	32 (74)	11	73
Bladder	25 (89)	3	28
Lung	47 (92)	4	51
Head and Neck	158 (94)	10	168
Other[a]	140 (100)	0	140
Total	**507 (73)**	**189**	**696**

[a]Esophagus, prostate, stomach, pancreas, skin, lymphoma/leukemia.
Source: Modified from Ref. 1.

II. Lung Metastases

A. Biology

Recent research on angiogenesis and growth factors has provided new insight into some aspects of distant tumor spread, but the basic mechanisms controlling the process of metastatic invasion remain largely unknown. In particular, we still have no biological explanation for the selectivity of distant metastases, summarized by the old "seed and soil" model.

We are currently investigating the role of biomarkers, such as p53, Bcl2, EGFR, hormone receptors, and angiogenesis, by comparing the features observed in resected lung metastases with those of the corresponding primary tumors in breast and colon cancer and soft tissue sarcomas. Preliminary data revealed very little variation in the expression of these proteins between primary and secondary foci. However, the analysis of breast tumors has shown that while the microvessel density was slightly lower in nodal metastases than in primary tumors (average count of hot spots by Chalkley camera = 15 vs. 17), the corresponding value of lung metastases was significantly higher (average count = 27) by the pool variance analysis. These findings suggest that, at least in breast cancer, the establishment of lung metastases is due to the selection of highly angiogenic clones, while nodal metastases appear to be independent from the angiogenic ability of the primary tumor.

Autopsy studies have shown in the past that a single filter organ, such as the lung, could represent the first site of distant spread, only later followed by systemic dissemination (2). The theory of organ-restricted spread was supported by the clinical evidence of natural history of sarcomas, where the lungs are often the only site of progression of the disease (3) and the ultimate cause of death in most patients (4–6). It appeared logical to hypothesize from these studies that complete removal of the lung deposits, whenever feasible, could prevent further spread to other sites and possibly eradicate the disease.

B. Diagnosis and Staging

Clinical staging of lung metastases should provide the most accurate information on several aspects concerning the nature, dimension and site of each individual lesion. These include a number of questions: probability of a false positive, single versus multiple lesions, unilateral versus bilateral disease, involvement of hilar or mediastinal lymphnodes and total required volume of lung resection.

CT and nuclear magnetic resonance (NMR) of the chest have significantly improved the quality of radiological diagnosis, particularly in the assessment of the number of lesions. The chest CT can identify up to 80% of all pulmonary nodules greater than 3 mm detected at surgical exploration, but a few such lesions may ultimately prove benign, while other radiologically occult nodules may be discovered. It has been estimated that the final diagnostic accuracy of radiological staging is in the order of 40% for plain chest x-rays and 60–80% for CT (7,8). The new developments of CT technology such as continuous spiral scanning have further improved the diagnostic yield of radiological staging, both in terms of minimum size parenchymal nodules (less than 3 mm) and significant hilar or mediastinal adenopathies. The data provided recently by the International Registry of Lung Metastases showed a 61% overall accuracy in the assessment of the number of metastases, with 25% of cases being underestimated and 14% overestimated (9). However, in patients who had bilateral surgical exploration, the radiological assessment was only accurate in 37% of cases and underestimated in 39%. Preclinical screening of occult extrapulmonary metastases (liver ultrasound, bone scan, and brain CT) is advisable in patients with multiple lesions.

The role of other diagnostic examinations such as PET scan is still under evaluation. Although the specificity of PET scan appears to be high, the minimum size of detectable pulmonary lesion may represent a critical factor.

C. Patient Selection

The eligibility criteria for curative resection of lung metastases can be summarized in four points: primary tumor previously cured or curable; no evidence of extrapulmonary metastases; complete resectability of all pulmonary metastases; planned resection volume tolerable by the patient. Although the majority of patients with metastatic disease are referred to the surgeon by medical oncologists after a selection based on prognostic factors such as number and disease-free interval, even patients presenting with synchronous metastases at the time of initial diagnosis or concurrent local relapse after the primary treatment and lung metastases may still be eligible for metastasectomy, provided that the primary tumor or local relapse are amenable to curative management. The most appropriate timing for surgery of primary tumors and metastases (simultaneous or sequential) as well as the need for primary chemotherapy have to be decided for each individual case with a multidisciplinary approach.

The range of application of metastasectomy is not the same for all primary tumors, but depends on the risk of metastases in other organs, the sensitivity to chemotherapy or hormone treatment, and the probability of new primary tumors (Table 2). The higher the probability of clinically occult extrapulmonary metastases, the

Table 2 Rationale of Metastasectomy in Different Primary Tumors

Primary site	Aim of metastasectomy	Application
Sarcomas	Permanent cure, better survival	Systematic
Teratoma	Confirm response, residual teratoma	Systematic
Colon-rectum	Permanent cure, ± liver resection	Selective
Kidney	Occasional cure, new primary	Highly selective
Melanoma	Occasional cure, new primary	Only single lesion
Breast	Hormone receptors, new primary	Only single lesion

more selective must be the use of lung metastasectomy. As a general rule, in bone and soft tissue sarcomas, salvage surgery is indicated whenever complete resection is technically feasible, and the goal is permanent cure. In nonsarcomatous tumors, the nature of the primary has a significant impact on the aim of salvage surgery as well as on the eligibility criteria.

D. Surgical Management

Extensive clinical experience has proved that only complete removal of all detectable lesions can achieve reliable prospect of long-term survival and cure. Incomplete resection with macroscopic or microscopic intrathoracic residual disease (debulking) does not improve survival, nor is it justifiable on the ground of palliative management. In order to achieve a macroscopically complete resection the surgeon must be able to palpate the lung, both in the inflated and deflated status, to detect any radiologically occult lesions and remove all of them with safe margins and appropriate surgical technique. In nonsarcomatous tumors, the unilateral or bilateral surgical approach is dictated by the radiological picture, while in sarcomas the optimal techniques is represented by sequential exploration of both lungs, even in case of single or unilateral metastases. In fact, it has been demonstrated that in 30–50% of cases presenting with unilateral lesions, median sternotomy revealed bilateral lung metastases (10–12).

In most cases, sublobar resection (atypical tangential or wedge resection) is generally adequate and preserves lung tissue with a view to future resections (13,14), while in solitary lesions a segmentectomy or lobectomy may be preferred when the disease is more likely to represent a primary lung tumor. The presence of nodal metastases may require a lobectomy or even a larger volume of resection, but such an event is rare in metastatic disease. For these reasons, we do not recommend the use of video-assisted thoracoscopy for metastasectomy as such technique precludes thorough palpation of the lungs and proper intraoperative staging and may result in inappropriate resection margins, with either insufficient or excessive resection volumes.

E. Long-Term Results

A more reliable assessment of long-term results of metastasectomy have been achieved recently through a multicentric data base. The International Registry of Lung Metastases has accrued 5206 cases from 18 departments of thoracic surgery in Europe, United States, and Canada (9). Of these patients, 4572 (88%) underwent complete surgical resection. Mean follow-up was 46 months. The overall perioperative mortality after complete resection was 0.8%.

The long-term results are illustrated in Table 3. In summary, the actuarial survival after complete resection was 36% at 5 years, 26% at 10 years, and 22% at 15 years (median 35 months); the corresponding values for incomplete resection were 13% at 5 years and 7% at 10 years (median 15 months). Among complete resections,

Table 3 The International Registry of Lung Metastases: Long-Term Survival After Complete Resection

		No.	5-year (%)	10-year (%)	Median (months)
Overall		4572	36	26	35
DFI	0–11 months	1384	33	27	29
	12–35 months	1662	31	22	30
	36+ months	1416	45	29	49
Number	1	2169	43	31	43
	2–3	1226	34	24	31
	4+	1123	27	19	27
	10+	342	26	17	26
Primary tumor	Germ cell	318	68	63	
	Epithelial	1894	37	21	40
	Sarcoma	1917	31	26	29
	Melanoma	282	21	14	19

the 5-year survival was significantly better for patients with a disease-free interval (DFI) of 36+ months or single lesions.

Such a large data base was used to set up a simplified system of prognostic grouping based on two elements: completeness of resection and poor risk factors (disease-free interval < 36 months or multiple metastases). Four clearly distinct prognostic groups could be identified: complete resection without risk factors, one risk factor only, two risk factors, and incomplete resections. Figure 1 shows the actuarial survival of the four prognostic groups. The difference among the curves was highly significant (log rank chi-square = 328.2); median survival was 61 months for group I, 34 months for group II, 24 months for group III, and 14 months for group IV. The discriminant power of this prognostic grouping was tested on different primary tumors and proved to be highly significant in each specific tumor type.

III. Second Primary Tumors

A. Biology

Multiple primary tumors may arise in the lung, as well as in the upper aerodigestive tract, due to a generalized exposure of this epithelium to a multiplicity of carcinogens contained in tobacco smoking, sometimes in association with other environmental risk factors. The theory of "field cancerization" indicates that repeated exposure of the entire epithelial surface to carcinogenic insults may result in the occurrence of multiple, independent premalignant or malignant foci (15). In support of this concept is the demonstration that significant genetic changes may be detectable, with various degrees of severity, in bronchial dysplasia as well as in pathologically normal mucosa of patients with lung cancer (16–18).

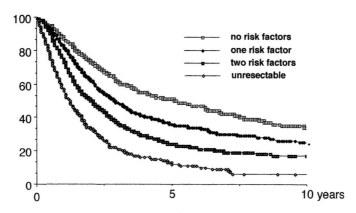

Figure 1 Results of the International Registry of Lung Metastases. Overall survival after lung metastasectomy by four main prognostic groups: resectable, no risk factors (DFI $\geq$ 36 months and single metastasis); resectable, 1 risk factor (DFI $<$ 36 months *or* multiple metastases); resectable, 2 risk factors (DFI $<$ 36 months and multiple metastases); and unresectable.

In a recently updated prospective series of 163 cases of resected non–small-cell lung cancer, we confirmed that the normal bronchial epithelium at distant sites from the primary tumor was affected by multiple genetic abnormalities, including a rearranged karyotype (mainly 3p, 7p, 17), microsatellite instability, overexpression of specific oncogenes (EGFR, HER2/NEU), or loss of RARbeta (19,20). The overall frequency of genetic changes in the normal epithelium was 55%, being significantly higher in patients with multiple tumors of the upper aerodigestive tract, as compared to those with single tumors (69% vs. 48%; $p = 0.019$; Fig. 2). These data suggest a new approach to the diagnosis and management of second primary tumors, based on specific genetic abnormalities detectable on the normal bronchial mucosa.

Whether these or other abnormalities detected in the distant bronchus of tumor-bearing patients are just an indicator of accumulated damage or may represent a specific marker of individual genetic predisposition to lung cancer remains to be clarified. In this respect, the interaction between exogenous carcinogens contained in tobacco smoking and individual tumor susceptibility is a crucial field of research. In Li-Fraumeni disease, an inherited autosomal dominant cancer syndrome where the germline p53 mutation confers a 50% risk of multiple cancers before the age of 30, lung cancers have been only occasionally reported (21). However, we have treated a 57-year-old woman with a familial germline p53 mutation who presented with multiple synchronous lung cancers. She had numerous prior cancers successfully resected (skin leiomyosarcoma, osteosarcoma of the ovary, breast carcinoma, endometrial adenocarcinoma, dermatofibrosarcoma protuberans of the mandible, and squamous skin cancer) and was asymptomatic when routine follow-up revealed a pulmonary opacity. As depicted in Figure 3, the CT and PET scan showed three independent neoplastic foci involving the right upper lobe and

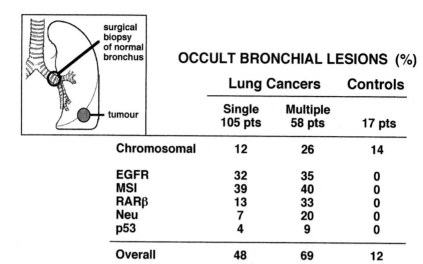

| | OCCULT BRONCHIAL LESIONS (%) | | |
| | Lung Cancers | | Controls |
	Single 105 pts	Multiple 58 pts	17 pts
Chromosomal	12	26	14
EGFR	32	35	0
MSI	39	40	0
RARβ	13	33	0
Neu	7	20	0
p53	4	9	0
Overall	48	69	12

Figure 2 Overall frequency of genetic changes in the normal bronchial epithelium of 163 patients resected for non–small-cell lung cancer; bronchial sample taken distant from the primary site of tumor.

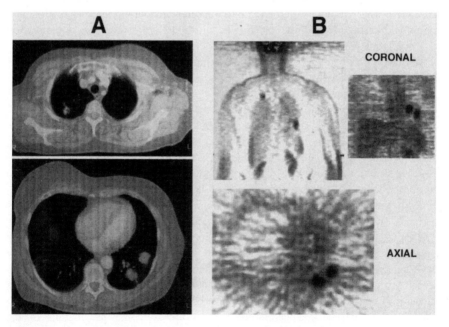

Figure 3 CT and PET scan appearance of three simultaneous primary lung adenocarcinomas within the right upper and left lower lobes in a 57-year-old woman with Li-Fraumeni syndrome.

left lower lobe. All lesions could be radically resected through median sternotomy, and the pathological examination revealed three well-differentiated adenocarcinomas (all T1N0) as well as a 2-mm focus of atypical adenomatous hyperplasia. As the patient was known to be a former moderate smoker, these findings suggest a possible synergistic effect of inherited p53 mutation and tobacco smoking.

B. Incidence

In lung cancer patients, the problem of second primary tumors has been underestimated for many years due to the limited expected survival, inaccurate follow-up and misclassification of solitary relapses in the lungs. Only a few careful clinical trials testing the efficacy of lung cancer–screening procedures or exploring the causes of failure after surgical treatment have contributed to clarify the magnitude of this problem (22–24). In patients cured for a cancer of the lung, the frequency of second primary tumors in all sites is 10–25%, depending on the intensity of follow-up, histologic type, and stage of the index tumor, and corresponds to an incidence of 2–3% per year. The majority of second primary tumors occur again in the lung (8–20% overall) and, particularly in patients with a good initial prognosis, may represent a relevant cause of mortality.

As a collateral effort to our prospective randomized trials on chemoprevention (25), we have kept under intense follow-up, with 4-monthly chest x-rays and sputum cytology, a cohort of Stage I lung cancers treated by surgery alone with the specific goal of assessing the frequency, clinical relevance, and curability of multiple primary cancers (26). The data summarized in Table 4 are relative to 659 patients, with a median observation time of 64 months overall but approaching 9 years in surviving patients. A total of 213 (32%) independent primary cancers were detected in 170 (26%) patients, either prior to (59), synchronous with (23), or after (131) resection of the index tumor. As for second primary tumors, the gross frequency was 20%

Table 4 Multiple Primary Tumors in a Series of Resected Stage I NSCLC: Site and Time of Appearance

Site	Before	Synchronous	After	Total
Lung	5	15	77	97
Larynx	17	1	10	28
Oral cavity	5	0	4	9
Esophagus	0	0	5	5
Bladder	6	2	11	19
Colon-Rectum	4	0	8	12
Breast	4	0	2	6
Lymphoma	6	3	0	9
Kidney	1	1	2	4
Other	11	1	12	24
Total	**59**	**23**	**131**	**213**

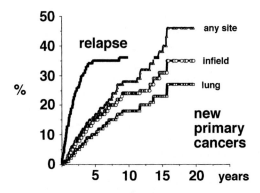

Figure 4 Long-term incidence of relapse and second primary tumors in a cohort of 659 patients who underwent resection for Stage I NSCLC.

(131/659). The large majority of metachronous tumors occurred in the tobacco-related field (107 or 82%), including lung (77), bladder (11), larynx (10), esophagus (5), and oral cavity (4). These figures are remarkably similar to those reported recently by Martini, based on 598 patients treated at Memorial Hospital (27). Figure 4 illustrates the long-term incidence of relapse and second primary tumors in this cohort of patients: while the vast majority of relapses occurred within the first 3 years from surgery, the incidence of second primaries was relatively constant over time up to 20 years. Of interest, all second primary lung cancers occurred in the group of patients that were either current or former smokers at the time of surgery (Fig. 5). Such observation reinforces the concept of tobacco-related field cancerization effect.

C. Differential Diagnosis

The differential diagnosis between locoregional recurrence and second primary lung cancer may be extremely difficult on clinical grounds. Traditional criteria based on the anatomic site (distance from prior cancer), histologic type (same vs. different),

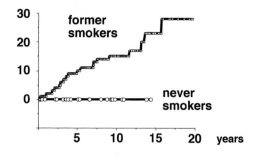

Figure 5 Incidence of second primary lung cancers according to prior smoking: current or former smokers versus life-long nonsmokers.

and temporal sequence (time elapsed from prior cancer) are invariably influenced by individual cultural biases and limited specificity of routine histopathology. As a matter of fact, in our experience 60% of new primaries showed the same histological type as the prior lung cancer.

Recent studies suggest that biologic markers such as P53 mutations may improve the differential diagnosis of multiple primary tumors occurring in the same area (28). Genetic evidence for an independent origin of multiple preneoplastic and neoplastic lung lesions was also provided by our experience with multiple synchronous lung cancers, where a different pattern of genetic abnormalities was found in the various neoplastic foci (29). The observed discordance involved at least one of the following markers: 3p deletion, loss of heterozygosity (LOH 3p), P53 mutation, and K-ras mutation. Interestingly, these data were obtained from tumors with identical histologic type and/or occurring in the same pulmonary lobe. These studies have provided unequivocal evidence that second cancers arise as independent events regardless of site, type, and temporal sequence and that genetic markers are superior to clinical or pathologic assessment in the differential diagnosis of multiple primary tumors.

D. Surgical Management

As a result of intense clinical follow-up, the applicability of salvage surgery was relatively high in our cohort. Out of 70 patients who developed 77 metachronous lung cancers, 35 or 50% achieved a complete resection. These figures compare well with the overall resectability rate of non–small-cell lung cancer, which usually ranges between 10 and 20%. One patient had four sequential lung cancers resected. The perioperative mortality rate was 9% (3/35)—not surprisingly higher than average, due to limited cardiopulmonary function and technical difficulties of redo surgery, sometimes requiring completion pneumonectomy. Thirteen patients (19%) were not eligible for curative surgery, mostly on a functional basis, but received radical radiotherapy.

The overall 5-year survival from the time of diagnosis of metachronous tumor was 27%. Patients treated by salvage surgery experienced a 45% survival at 5 years, being significantly better ($p < 0.01$) than nonsurgical treatment. The long-term survival after radiotherapy was 16%, while none of the 22 patients receiving palliative treatment survived more than 3 years. Again our resectability and survival data were very similar to the one reported by other cancer centers (30).

Such a broad clinical experience justifies the use of long-term follow-up after curative resection of primary lung cancer, particularly in the case of early stage disease, for the screening of multiple primary lung carcinomas and complete resection whenever possible.

IV. Conclusion

Secondary lung tumors have emerged as an important field of research, with potential clinical implications in many areas: preclinical events in lung carcinogenesis, mechanisms of tumor progression, screening and early diagnosis, biological classification, salvage surgery, and/or chemo-radiotherapy and chemoprevention. Second primary lung cancers are an optimal endpoint to test the efficacy of chemopreventive agents, such as retinoids, vitamins, and antioxidants. In fact, patients cured for a prior cancer show a higher motivation to accept the extra burden of a chemoprevention plan, compared to healthy subjects. Side effects are better tolerated, and higher doses can be given in order to achieve a potential adjuvant effect against primary cancer relapse.

References

1. Cahan WG, Shah JP, Castro EB. Benign solitary lung lesions in patients with cancer. Ann Surg 1978; 187:241–244.
2. Viadana E, Bross IDJ, Pickren JW. Cascade spread of blood-borne metastadses in solid and nonsolid cancers of humans. In: Weiss L, Gilbert HA, eds. Pulmonary Metastasis. Boston: GK Hall & Co, 1978:142–167.
3. Weiss L, Gilbert HA, eds. Pulmonary Metastasis Boston: GK Hall & Co, 1978:100.
4. Friedman MA, Carter SK. The therapy of osteogenic sarcoma: current status and thoughts for the future. J Surg Oncol 1972; 4:482–510.
5. Weiss L, Gilbert HA, eds. Pulmonary Metastasis. Boston: GK Hall & Co, 1978:100.
6. Marcove R, Mike V, Hajek JV, Levin AG, Hutter RVP. Osteogenic sarcoma under the age of 21: a review of 145 operative cases. J Bone Joint Surg 1970; 52A:411–418.
7. Chang AE, Schaner EG, Conkle DM, Flyle MW, Doppmann YJL, Rosemberg SA. Evaluation of Computed Tomography in the detection of pulmonary metastases. Cancer 1979; 43:913.
8. Muller NL, Gamsu G, Webb WR. Pulmonary nodules: detection using magnetic resonance and computed tomography. Radiology 1985; 155:687.
9. The International Registry of Lung Metastases. Long-term results of lung metastasectomy: prognostic analyses based on 5,206 cases. J Thorac Cardiovasc Surg 1997; 113:37–49.
10. Roth JA, Pass HI, Wesley MN, White D, Putnam JB, Seipp C. Comparison of median sternotomy and thoracotomy for resection of pulmonary metastases in patients with adult soft-tissue sarcomas. Ann Thorac Surg 1986; 42:134–138.
11. Johnston MR, et al. Median sternotomy for resection of pulmonary metastases in patients with soft-tissue sarcomas. Arch Surg 1986; 121:1248–1252.
12. Pastorino U, Valente M, Gasparini M, Azzarelli A, Santoro A, Tavecchio L, Casali P, Ravasi G. Median sternotomy and multiple lung resections for metastatic sarcomas. Eur J Cardiothorac Surg 1990; 4(9):477–481.
13. McCormack P. Surgical treatment of pulmonary metastases: Memorial Hospital experience. In: Weiss L, Gilbert HA, eds. Pulmonary Metastasis. Boston: GK Hall & Co, 1978.
14. Mountain CF, McMurtrey MJ, Hermes KE. Surgery for pulmonary metastasis: a 20-year experience. Ann Thorac Surg 1984; 38:323–330.
15. Slaughter DP, Southwick HW, Smejkal W. "Field cancerization" in oral stratified squamous epithelium: clinical implications of multicentric origin. Cancer 1953; 6:963–968.
16. Sozzi G, Miozzo M, Tagliabue E, Calderone C, Lombardi L, Pilotti S, Pastorino U, Pierotti MA, Della Porta G. Cytogenetic abnormalities and overexpression of receptors for growth factors in normal bronchial epithelium and tumor samples of lung cancer patients. Cancer Res 1991; 51:400–404.
17. Sundaresan V, Ganly P, Hasleton P, Rudd R, Sinha G, Bleehen NM, Rabbitts P. p53 and chromosome 3 abnormalities, characteristic of malignant lung tumours, are detectable in preinvasive lesions of the bronchus. Oncogene 1992; 7:1989–1997.
18. Sozzi G, Miozzo M, Donghi R, Pilotti S, Cariani CT, Pastorino U, Della Porta G, Pierotti MA. Deletions of 17p and p53 mutations in preneoplastic lesions of the lung. Cancer Res 1992; 52:6079–6082.

19. Pastorino U, Sozzi G, Miozzo M, Tagliabue E, Pilotti S, Pierotti MA. Genetic changes in lung cancer. J Cell Biochem 1993; 17F:237–248.
20. Xu XC, Sozzi G, Lee JS, Lee JJ, Pastorino U, Pilotti S, Kurie JM, Hong WK, Lotan R. Suppression of retinoic acid receptor beta in non small cell lung cancer in vivo: implications for lung cancer development. JNCI 1997;
21. Malkin D, Li FP, Strong LC, Fraumeni JF Jr, Nelson CE, Kim DH, Kassel J. Germ line p53 mutations in a familial syndrome of breast cancer, sarcomas, and other neoplasms. Science 1990; 250:1233–1238.
22. Fontana RS. Early diagnosis of lung cancer. Am Rev Respir Dis 1977; 116:399–402.
23. Pairolero P, Williams DE, Bergstrahl EJ, Piehler JM, Bernatz PE, Payne SP. Postsurgical stage I bronchogenic carcinoma: morbid implications of recurrent disease. Ann Thorac Surg 1984; 38:331–338.
24. Shields TW, Robinette CD. Long-term survivors after resection of bronchial carcinoma. Surg Gyn Obst 1973; 136:759–768.
25. Pastorino U, Infante I, Maioli, M, Chiesa G, Buyse M, Firket P, Rosmentz N, Clerici M, Soresi E Valente M, Belloni PA, Ravasi G. Adjuvant treatment of stage I lung cancer with high dose vitamin A. J Clin Oncol 1993; 11:1216–1222.
26. Andreani S, Pastorino U, Ante M, Tavecchio L, Valente M, Sozzi G, Pilotti S, Ravasi G. Second primary tumours in resected stage I lung cancer (abstr). Lung Cancer 1994; 11:167.
27. Martini N, Bains MS, Burt ME, Zakowski MF, McCormack P, Rush VW, Ginsberg RJ. Incidence of local recurrence and second primary tumors in resected stage I lung cancer. J Thorac Cardiovasc Surg 1995; 109:120–129.
28. Chung KY, Mukhopadhyay T, Kim J, Casson A, Ro JY, Goepfert H, Hong WK, Roth JA. Discordant p53 gene mutations in primary head and neck cancers and corresponding second primary cancers of the upper aerodigestive tract. Can Res 1993; 53:1676–1683.
29. Sozzi G, Miozzo M, Pastorino U, et al. Genetic evidence for an independent origin of multiple preneoplastic and neoplastic lung lesions. Cancer Res 1995; 55:135–140. 1995.
30. Rosengart TK, Martini N, Ghosn P, Burt M. Multiple primary lung carcinomas: prognosis and treatment. Ann Thorac Surg 1991; 52:773–778.

43

Occupational Lung Cancer

**YVES MARTINET, PHILIPPE
SCHEID, JEAN-MICHEL VIGNAUD
and NADINE MARTINET**

Université Henri-Poincaré
Vandoeuvre-les-Nancy, France

JEAN-JACQUES MOULIN

INRS
Vandoeuvre-les-Nancy, France

I. Introduction

Due to its high frequency and poor treatment efficiency, lung cancer is the most common cause of death by cancer in western countries and will be in developing countries within the foreseeable future. Obviously, active smoking is the most important cause of lung cancer and the elimination of tobacco still stands as the highest priority (1–3). However, tobacco consumption is far from being the only cause of lung cancer. Indeed, several other factors can contribute to lung cancer occurrence, including individual genetic susceptibility, nutritional habits, socioeconomic status, environmental factors, and occupational exposures. All these factors can interact with each other and with tobacco exposure, and several (mainly environmental and occupational) are closely related, the main difference being the magnitude of exposure.

The role of nonoccupational factors is intimately intricated with those of tobacco consumption and occupational exposures. If, strictly speaking, no genetic factor for lung cancer has yet been described (4), an individual susceptibility to toxic substances present in tobacco smoke has been found to be related to the P450 cytochrome system (aryl hydrocarbon hydroxylase, debrisoquine metabolisms), suggesting that high metabolizers, if they smoke, have a higher risk of lung cancer than

693

low metabolizers who smoke (5). Interestingly, everyday behavior is also important, since smokers can expect a protective effect against lung cancer from high fruit and vegetable (and possibly aspirin) intake (6,7). In other respects, a strong inverse relationship between social class and lung cancer has been observed and is likely to be related, at least in part, to the actual manner of smoking. The magnitude and role of most environmental risk factors in lung cancer incidence are mainly suggested, but not yet precisely characterized, due to the usually low levels of exposure, which require large epidemiological studies. At present, the most evidence for their deleterious role comes from extrapolations of occupational exposures. The most common of these hazards are due to residential radon (8), air pollution (9,10), urbanization, asbestos, diesel exhaust, and passive smoking.

II. Importance of Occupational Exposure in Lung Cancer Incidence

Since Paracelsus' description in 1531 of lung cancers in Schneeberg cobalt miners in Erzgebirge (now known to be related to radium inhalation), numerous compounds have been shown, or suggested, to contribute to lung cancer occurrence. They can act as isolated agents (or group of agents) or mixtures; where it is not possible to isolate an agent or a mixture, lung cancer is then related to an exposure circumstance. Several factors prevent an accurate evaluation of the global importance of occupational risks in lung cancer incidence, including (11): (1) the overwhelming importance of tobacco consumption, (2) the limited number of studies trying to take into account all occupational risks together and not only one specific risk, (3) the poor evaluation of agricultural risks, (4) the variability of occupational risks from one place to another, (5) the difficulties in describing and quantifying each risk exposition (e.g., type of exposure, duration), (6) the long delay between exposure and cancer occurrence, (7) the evolution over years of the risks and protection against them, (8) the continuous emergence of new risks and the evolution of our understanding of their role, and (9) the difficulties in pooling in a prospective fashion all workers exposed to lung carcinogens.

Despite these limitations, several authors have published estimates of the portion of lung cancer that is due to occupational exposure. The estimate by Doll and Peto (12) that approximately 15% of male lung cancer and 5% of female lung cancer could be due to occupational carcinogens (12), lies in the center of a wide range of previous estimates (13). In addition, a meta-analysis of several case-control studies carried out by Simonato et al. showed that the attributable lung cancer risk in the male population ranged between 0.6 and 35% according to studies using job-exposure matrices, and between 2.4 and 40% according to studies focused on recognized carcinogenic exposure (14). Most of the studies reviewed by Simonato et al. gave results adjusted for smoking. In addition, Simonato et al. showed that tobacco smoking had a very limited confounding effect on the results (14).

It is noteworthy that the results obtained by Simonato et al. agree with the estimate by Doll and Peto, which did not use any formal methodology. This strengthens the estimate by Doll and Peto of 15% for male lung cancer due to occupational exposure.

III. Epidemiological Studies on Occupational Lung Cancer Risks

The identification of occupational lung cancer risks results largely from a review, for a given substance, of published data provided by three sets of studies: in vitro tests, animal bioassays, and epidemiological studies. Experimental studies relying on animal models, cell transformation in culture, microorganism mutation, etc. can strengthen epidemiological data when they correlate with them. However, some substances can induce cancer in animals but not in humans, and thus, epidemiological data are central to the identification of human carcinogens.

Case reports are generally based on clinical experience: when some cases of lung cancer have occurred, more frequently than would be expected by chance, in an exposed population or among men involved in the same occupation. Case reports do not belong to epidemiology, but they generate hypotheses for epidemiology.

Definite evidence of carcinogenicity in humans is provided only by epidemiological studies. These studies may be cohort studies or case-control studies, and they can be carried out either in the general population ("population-based" epidemiological studies) or in cohorts selected among workers employed in one factory or in an industry ("industry-based" epidemiological studies):

> Cohort studies consist in comparing the observed lung cancer mortality (or incidence) in an occupational cohort, i.e., the "exposed" workers, to that of a "nonexposed" population, which is usually the general population of the country, or the district, where the factory is located (national or regional references, respectively). The relative risk is adjusted for sex, age, and year of death: standardized mortality ratio (SMR) or standardized incidence ratio (SIR).
>
> Case-control studies consist in comparing occupational histories collected by interview of patients having lung cancer, i.e., the "cases," to that of a random sample of subjects free of this disease at the date of diagnosis of corresponding cases, i.e., the "controls." Age, sex, and smoking, along with other potential confounding factors, can be taken into account when calculating relative risks: odds ratios (OR).

The aim of epidemiological studies is to detect a statistically significant association, after controlling for confounding factors, between lung cancer occurrence and an occupation or occupational exposure, including a dose-response relationship:

> The dose-response relationship is based on an assessment of past and present occupational exposure, using (1) exposure measurements in the study fac-

tories or in similar factories, and (2) the development of job-exposure matrices by qualified experts to provide information on exposure throughout the whole study period.

Smoking is a major confounding factor, since (1) tobacco smoke is an etiological factor of lung cancer and (2) exposed workers may have smoked more than nonexposed workers used as reference. Case-control studies can easily deal with this problem, since data concerning smoking habits are systematically collected when interviewing cases and controls. As a result, relative risks are computerized after adjustment on smoking. Conversely, smoking is a problem for cohort studies, since most of the study populations are historical cohorts for which many subjects have left the factory before the data collection, so that little or no information on smoking habits is available (15). Axelson and Steenland have proposed an indirect method to assess the degree of confounding that could result from a possible tobacco overconsumption in the study cohort as compared to the reference population (15). They showed that, when comparing lung cancer mortality (or incidence) of an occupational cohort to that of a general population used as reference, lung cancer excess due to smoking cannot be higher than 1.40–1.50 (15). This means that even if no information is available on smoking habits in a cohort study, any lung cancer excess over 1.50 is very unlikely to be due to smoking.

Numerous epidemiological studies have been conducted in industrialized countries during the last five decades. Their results have led to the current knowledge on occupational risks for lung cancer.

IV. Identification of Occupational Lung Cancer Risks

Evidence of the carcinogenicity of any substance, for animals or for humans, can be classified as "sufficient," "limited," or "inadequate." Using this method, experts at the International Agency for Research on Cancer (IARC) have defined five types, according to the probability, of substances (16,17):

Group 1—The agent (mixture) is carcinogenic to humans. The exposure circumstances entail exposures that are carcinogenic to humans.

Group 2A—The agent (mixture) is probably carcinogenic to humans. The exposure circumstance entails exposures that are probably carcinogenic to humans.

Group 2B—The agent (mixture) is possibly carcinogenic to humans. The exposure circumstance entails exposures that are possibly carcinogenic to humans.

Group 3—The agent (mixture or exposure circumstance) is not classifiable as to its carcinogenicity to humans.

Group 4—The agent (mixture) is probably not carcinogenic to humans.

Table 1 contains a list of the recognized lung carcinogens for humans according to the present knowledge. The list is limited to agents classified in Groups 1, 2A, and 2B by the IARC. The carcinogens are classified as (1) "agents," when a single agent has been demonstrated as causative for lung cancer in humans (e.g., chromium VI compounds, crystalline silica), (2) "mixtures," when complex simultaneous exposures are considered responsible for lung cancer occurrence (e.g., diesel fumes, coal tar pitches), and (3) "exposure circumstances," when an occupation or an industrial process is associated with a lung cancer without any specific single agent having been identified as causative factor (e.g., iron and steel founding, welding fumes).

Several good reviews have been published on these different agents (18–30), and only very limited information will be given here about the most frequently involved and evaluated carcinogens, including the main exposed occupations, interaction with smoking, and some specific comments.

A. Arsenic and Arsenic Compounds

Main occupations: metalliferous ore miners, vineyard workers, pesticide manufacture and application, nonferrous smelters, fur handlers, manufacturers of sheep-dip compounds.

Interaction with smoking: not well characterized.

Specific comments: Suggested histologic specificity not confirmed (see below).

Arsenic interferes with the DNA replication process (DNA polymerase).

Relationship exists between lung cancer incidence and arsenic levels in urine.

B. Asbestos

Main occupations: asbestos miners, manufacturing of asbestos, construction workers, insulation, mechanics (brakes), shipyard workers.

Interaction with smoking: multiplicative synergistic relationship with cigarette smoking (see below).

Specific comments: Relationship with lung fibrosis (asbestosis), discussed below.

All types of asbestos, serpentine (chrysotile) and amphibole (e.g., amosite, tremolite), can cause lung cancer.

Clear dose-response relationship, but accurate estimate of exposure levels is often difficult to define.

C. Beryllium and Beryllium Compounds

Main occupations: mining, refining, manufacture of ceramics, electronic and aerospace equipment.

Table 1   IARC Classification of Main Occupational Lung Carcinogens, February 1997

Group 1	
Agents and groups of agents	Arsenic and arsenic compounds
	Asbestos
	Beryllium and beryllium compounds
	Bis (chloromethyl) ether and chloromethyl methyl ether (technical-grade)
	Cadmium and cadmium compounds
	Chromium(VI) compounds
	Mustard gas (sulfur mustard)
	Nickel compounds
	Radon and its decay products
	Silica, crystalline (inhaled in the form of quartz or cristobalite from occupational sources)
	Talc-containing asbestiform fibers
Mixtures	Coal tar pitches
	Coal tars
	Mineral oils, untreated and mildly treated
	Soots
Exposure circumstances	Aluminum production
	Boot and shoe manufacture and repair[a]
	Coal gasification
	Coke production
	Furniture and cabinet making[a]
	Hematite mining (underground) with exposure to radon
	Iron and steel founding
	Painter (occupational exposure a)
	Rubber industry[a]
Group 2A	
Agents and groups of agents	Acrylonitrile
	Benz(a)anthracene
	Benzo(a)pyrene
	Dibenz(a,h)anthracene
	Nitrogen mustard
Mixtures	Diesel engine exhaust
	Nonarsenical insecticides (occupational exposures in spraying and application of)[a]
Exposure circumstances	Art glass, glass containers, and pressed ware (manufacture of)[a]
	Petroleum refining (occupational exposure in)
Group 2B	
Agents and groups of agents	Carbon black
	Ceramic fibers
	Cobalt and cobalt compounds
	Glass wool
	Lead and lead compounds, inorganic[a]
	Nickel, metallic, and alloys
	Rock wool
	Slag wool

Table 1 Continued

Mixtures	Bitumens, extracts of steam-refined and air-refined
	Diesel fuel, marine
	Engine exhaust, gasoline
	Welding fumes

[a]Occupations and industries reported to present a cancer risk, but for which the assessment of lung cancer risk is not definitive.

Interaction with smoking: not well characterized.

Specific comments: plants with high SMR for berylliosis also have high SMR for lung cancer, but beryllium exposure is then usually high.

D. Bis(chloromethyl)ether (BCME) and Chloromethyl Methyl Ether (CMME), Technical Grade

Main occupations: manufacture and use of BCME and CMME.

Interaction with smoking: conflicting results.

Specific comments: high incidence of small-cell lung carcinoma.

E. Cadmium and Cadmium Compounds

Main occupations: cadmium smelter, nickel-cadmium battery workers, electroplating, manufacture of plastics and pigments (stabilizer).

Interaction with smoking: not well characterized.

Specific comments: the usual concurrent use of arsenic and nickel is a limit to the definition of cadmium carcinogenicity.

F. Chromium(VI) Compounds

Main occupations: stainless steel manufacturing and welding, chrome alloys, chrome-containing pigments, chrome plating.

Interaction with smoking: not well characterized.

Specific comments: Only hexavalent chrome is carcinogenic.

G. Mustard Gas (Sulfur Mustard)

Main occupations: manufacture and exposure to bis(β-chloroethyl) sulfide.

Interaction with smoking: addition of risks with cigarette smoking.

Specific comments: increased risk of larynx, lip, tongue, salivary gland, and pharynx carcinoma.

H. Nickel Compounds

Main occupations: production of stainless steel, nonferrous alloys, electroplating, manufacture of batteries, nickel roasting, smelting, refinery.

Interaction with smoking: not well characterized.
Specific comments: increased risk of sinonasal carcinoma.

I. Radon and Its Decay Products

Main occupations: uranium hematite and other metals miners, processing of
    ore and radioactive materials.
Interaction with smoking: multiplicative synergistic relationship with cigarette
    smoking.
Specific comments: carcinogenicity due to α-particle ionizing radiation;
                    clear-cut dose-response relationship.

J. Silica, Crystalline (Inhaled in the Form of Quartz or
Cristobalite Form Occupational Sources) (31,32)

Main occupations: miners, foundry workers, granite cutters, ceramic workers,
    pottery, masonry, stonework.
Interaction with smoking: not well characterized.
Specific comments: relationship with silicosis is discussed below.

K. Polycyclic Aromatic Hydrocarbons

Main occupations: coal gasification, coke production, gas-retort house pro-
                    cess,
                    aluminum production through the Söderberg process,
                    chimney sweeping (soot),
                    printing industry,
                    diesel exhaust fume exposure (professional drivers, rail-
                        road workers),
                    roofing, asphalt industry.
Interaction with smoking: not well characterized.
Specific comments: dose-response relationship is well established for differ-
                    ent types of exposure;
                    cigarette smoke contains several carcinogenic polycyclic
                    aromatic hydrocarbons, including benzo(α)pyrene.

L. General Comments

In some exposure circumstances inducing a high incidence of lung cancer, it is difficult to pinpoint the actual toxic substances involved. For example, in iron and steel
founding, potential carcinogens include silica, metal fumes, formaldehyde, and
polycyclic aromatic hydrocarbons. In a similar fashion, welders are exposed to
metal fumes and asbestos. A similar problem exists for the rubber industry, boot and
shoe manufacturing and repair, painters, and furniture and cabinet makers.

  Table 2 shows the combined relative risks given by the literature regarding the
most important carcinogens for humans. Some combined relative risks were pub-

Table 2 Risks for Lung Cancer in Association with Selected Occupational Exposures

Exposure or agent	IARC classification	Studies (nb)	Relative risks	Ref.
Agents				
Arsenic	1	6	3.69[a]	28
Asbestos	1	20	2.00[a]	28
Beryllium	1	4	1.49[a]	28
Cadmium	1	1	1.49	28
Chromium (VI)[b]	1	10	2.78[a]	28
Nickel	1	13	1.56[a]	28
Silica	1	13	1.33[a]	28
Mixtures				
Coal tar and coal tar pitches	1	6	1.38[c]	21
Soots and PAHs	1	8	1.22[c]	21
Diesel fumes	2A	6	1.31[a]	28
Welding fumes	2B	49	1.38[a]	30
Exposure circumstances				
Aluminum production	1	10	1.18[c]	21
Coal gasification	1	3	2.17[c]	21
Coke production	1	9	1.71[c]	21
Iron and steel founding	1	10	1.40[c]	21
Painting	1	7	$\cong 1.40$	23
Interaction between smoking and asbestos				
Asbestos	1	1	5.2	33
Smoking	1	1	10.9	33
Asbestos and smoking		1	53.2	33

[a]Published meta-analysis or combination of results.
[b]Chromium and chromate production, chromium plating.
[c]Combined relative risks calculated from data presented in Ref. 21.
PAHs: polycyclic aromatic hydrocarbons.

lished earlier by Steenland et al. and Moulin for exposure to arsenic, asbestos, beryllium, cadmium, chromium VI, nickel, silica, and welding (28,30). The other summary risks were calculated on the basis of studies reviewed by Boffetta et al. in their tables (19). These combined relative risks and their variances were calculated through a logarithm transformation of relative risk values reported by Boffetta et al. (19) and a weighing using the inverted variance of each relative risk.

Table 2 shows that the relative risks obtained for arsenic, asbestos, chromium(VI), nickel, coal gasification, and coke production are beyond the approximately 40–50% excess that might be expected due to positive confounding by smoking (15). Although the other relative risks are lower, the corresponding agents have been classified as carcinogens for humans by the IARC, since several studies have shown either elevated relative risks after adjusting for smoking or clear dose-response relationships or high relative risks using internal references.

Table 2 also provides the results of the study by Hammond et al. demonstrating the interaction between asbestos exposure and smoking in lung cancer occurrence, the relative risks being 5.2 for asbestos-exposed workers versus nonexposed workers, 10.9 for smokers versus nonsmokers, and 53.2 for smokers exposed to asbestos versus nonsmokers not exposed to asbestos (33).

V. Lung Cancer/Lung Fibrosis Relationships

Several interstitial (granulomatous and nongranulomatous) lung diseases leading to a diffuse lung fibrosis are characterized by an abnormally high incidence of lung cancer. In some instances, the etiologic cause of the disease is unknown, as is the case in idiopathic pulmonary fibrosis (and in pulmonary histiocytosis X; but, in this case, smoking may be important), or very well known and related to the inhalation of, for example, asbestos, crystalline silica, beryllium, cobalt, or iron.

The main question, in this respect, is to know if lung cancer occurrence is a consequence of lung fibrosis or if both diseases develop in an independent fashion. If the answer is positive, then (1) both fibrosis and cancer processes must share some pathogenic pathway, and fibrosis could be described as a preneoplastic disorder of the lung, and (2) it could be argued that only patients with characterized lung fibrosis should be recognized as having an occupationally related lung cancer. Obviously, this chapter does not tackle the question of tumor stroma formation in lung cancer. In this case, the fibrotic process is local, due to the presence of cancer cells, and is tightly controlled and involved with tumor development (34).

The suggested relationship between fibrosis and cancer evolves from clinical and epidemiological studies. One of the first models is asbestos exposure, in which lung cancer may be related to asbestosis (35). Besides the epidemiological evidence of asbestos and lung cancer in exposed subjects, two observations have been used to try to establish a correlation between lung fibrosis and lung cancer: (1) the specific incidence of lung adenocarcinoma in asbestos-exposed workers (lung fibrosis being a parenchymal disease, and adenocarcinoma being frequently peripheral tumors) and (2) the frequent colocalization of asbestos-related lung cancer and asbestosis to the lower lobes. However, evidence for the frequency of adenocarcinoma in asbestos-exposed workers is currently thought to be weak (see below), and thus, the current understanding is that asbestos (mainly amphibole) inhalation, with or without evidence of lung fibrosis, contributes to lung cancer, and that cigarette smoking markedly increases this risk.

In respect to crystalline silica exposure, it is acknowledged that "silicosis produces an increased risk for bronchogenic carcinoma" (ATS) and this risk is likely to be increased by smoking (31). For nonsmoking exposed workers, the specific risk of lung cancer is currently difficult to confirm and quantify. For silica exposure, but also for asbestos exposure, it is clear that subjects who develop silicosis or asbestos are usually exposed to high levels of toxic substances. It is thus not surprising that these patients develop more lung cancer than less exposed individuals.

One obvious difficulty, however, in defining this relationship is that, while it is usually easy to diagnose a lung cancer, lung fibrosis is more difficult to define and recognize. Indeed, fibrosis is a pathological process characterized by the replacement of normal tissue by mesenchymal cells and the extracellular matrix produced by these cells (36). This definition is a pathological one and, thus, requires lung parenchyma observation. This can be easily carried out for patients undergoing surgery for lung cancer, but in most epidemiological studies, fibrosis is suggested on chest x-ray and, less often, on CT scan, with obvious limitations to the specificity of this type of evaluation.

Both lung cancer and fibrosis result from a local and repeated injury. In respect to the biological phenomena leading to fibrosis and cancer, a major contradiction exists with, on one hand, fibrosis essentially being a pathological process that relies on normal biological mechanisms but expressed in an exuberant fashion (36), while on the other hand, cancers result from the sequential accumulation of gene mutations (37). Beside this major difference, the lung fibrotic process mainly involves the alveolar space and its interstitial surrounding with little bronchial involvement, whereas lung cancer results from bronchial cell transformation. However, some of the biological processes observed in fibrosis and cancer require the involvement of some identical molecules, such as growth factors and cytokines, these mediators playing a role in inflammation and cell replication regulation.

VI. Histological Type

Several histological types are comprised under the term "lung cancer," and the actual classification includes more than 15 subtypes (38). However, from a practical (clinical) point of view, two main types of lung cancer cell types are opposed: small-cell carcinoma and non–small-cell carcinoma (including squamous cell carcinoma, adenocarcinoma, and large-cell carcinoma). This complexity is increased by the not so rare observation of composite carcinomas characterized by the simultaneous presence in one tumor of different histological types.

Despite major efforts over the last 10 years to better understand the biology of early stages of bronchial cell transformation, it is not yet clear which type(s) of bronchial cell transform into lung cancer and if one type of cell specifically gives rise to one type of cancer. It is currently accepted that all types of lung cancer derive from a bronchial stem cell called "totipotent," and that bronchial cell transformation is a multistep process clinically characterized by the occurrence of preneoplastic lesions. While these lesions are well described for squamous cell lung carcinoma, very little is known in this respect concerning adenocarcinoma and small-cell carcinoma.

It is generally accepted that tobacco smoking can induce all different types of lung cancer, and the question remains as to whether some occupational exposures can induce one specific histological type of lung cancer. This question is important for several reasons: (1) if one specific type of lung cancer occurs in occupationally exposed individuals, the follow-up of these individuals would be a good model for the study of the biology of this type of lung cancer and its preneoplastic lesions; (2) the histological specificity would be an argument for a relationship with an occupational exposure.

The answer to this question is problematic because of smoking as a major confounding factor and because conclusions can only be drawn from studies in which one exposure dominates (39). In two instances, epidemiological data are quite convincing and suggest that one type of cancer, namely, small-cell lung carcinoma, is specifically induced in the workplace by chloromethyl ether and radon inhalation. In respect to radon, the combined effect of smoking is difficult to suppress, but it is likely that small-cell carcinoma incidence is increased in both smokers and non-smokers.

More frequent incidence of squamous cell carcinoma has been suggested in subjects exposed to chromium and nickel compounds, as well as in arsenic-exposed smelters, although new studies tend to question this statement.

Finally, in respect to asbestos exposure, several papers have suggested the predominance of lung adenocarcinoma. However, more recent studies, taking into account the importance of associated cigarette smoking, suggest that both squamous cell and adenocarcinoma incidence is increased by asbestos (40).

VII. Prevention and Early Cancer Detection

Death by lung cancer will markedly increase in the years to come in developing countries, while decreasing tobacco consumption should eventually lessen its incidence in developed countries. However, the long delay before cancer occurrence after toxic exposure means that this disease will still be a major health problem in most countries at least for the next 20 years (3).

In respect to early cancer detection, several large trials have shown that radiographic screening does not bring any significant clinical benefit and that simultaneous sputum cytology does not add any improvement in terms of cancer mortality. Hopefully, a better understanding of lung cancer biology and of its preneoplastic stages is likely to lead to the description of new detection methods. However, the evaluation of any such methods will require large epidemiological studies to define its efficiency.

Since lung cancer treatment and early detection are so difficult, prevention should be the focus in the future. This is a wide field and, again, tobacco control should rank first in the order of priority. In respect to occupational exposures, all exposure levels should be brought down—if possible, to zero. However, if this cannot be done, an accurate quantification of the risk should be carried out in a prospective fashion, and workers should be specifically informed about the risks and the possible protective actions and their efficiency, as well as about the smoking/occupational exposure relationship. When people seek such a job, a phenotyping in respect to gene susceptibility (P450 cytochrome system) to lung cancer has been suggested, leading to screening before hiring. However, no real data exist about the possible involvement of P450 in non–smoking-related lung cancer, and, furthermore, subjects with more favorable phenotypes may wrongly believe they are immune to this disease.

Once workers have been exposed, a prospective clinical follow-up must be undertaken. In parallel, it would be of interest to offer them chemoprevention. Oral retinoid chemoprevention was initially suggested to prevent lung cancer. However, large trials using oral retinoids and/or antioxidants (e.g., β-carotene) failed to show any protective effect against lung cancer. Thus, at this stage, the only efficient way to decrease lung cancer deaths is to prevent exposure to carcinogens.

VIII. Conclusion

Despite its clear significance, it is difficult to accurately quantify the contribution of occupational exposure to lung cancer incidence and mortality. Currently, some carcinogenic agents or exposure circumstances are well described and do require a firm and prospective attitude in order to reduce them. In the future, it is likely that among new industrial processes, as well as new agricultural compounds, some will be toxic for bronchial cells and induce mutations and cancer. With this in mind, beside the justified fight against tobacco use, more energy should be put into this field.

Acknowledgments

This work was supported, in part, by grants from Ligue Nationale contre le Cancer (comités de Moselle, Meurthe-et-Moselle et Meuse). We want to thank Nathalie Thomas for her patient and talented typing.

References

1. American Thoracic Society. Cigarette smoking and health. Am J Respir Crit Care Med 1996; 153:861–865.
2. Doll R. Introduction and overview. In: Samet JM, ed. Epidemiology of Lung Cancer. New York: Marcel Dekker, 1994:1–14.
3. Mulshine JL, Zhou J, Treston AM, Szabo E, Tockman MS, Cuttitta F. New approaches to the integrated management of early lung cancer. Hematol/Oncol Clin North Am 1997; 11: 235–252.
4. Schwartz AG, Young P, Swanson GM. Familial risk of lung cancer among nonsmokers and their relatives. Am J Epidemiol 1996; 144:554–562.
5. Economou P, Lechner JF, Samet JM. Familial factors in the pathogenesis of lung cancer. In: Samet JM, ed. Epidemiology of Lung Cancer. New York: Marcel Dekker, 1994:359–363.
6. Byers T. Diet as a factor in the etiology and prevention of lung cancer. In: Samet JM, ed. Epidemiology of Lung Cancer. New York: Marcel Dekker, 1994:335–352.
7. Schreinemachers DM, Everson RB. Aspirin use and lung, colon, and breast cancer: incidence in a prospective study. Epidemiology 1994; 5:138–146.

8. Pershagen G, Åkerblom G, Axelson O, Clavensjö B, Damber L, Desai G, Enflo A, Lagarde F, Mellander H, Svartengren M, Swedjemark GA. Residential radon exposure and lung cancer in Sweden. N Engl J Med 1994; 330:159–164.
9. Cislaghi C, Nimis PL. Lichens, air pollution and lung cancer. Nature 1997; 387:463–464.
10. Dockery DW, Pope III CA, Xu X, Spengler JD, Ware JH, Fay ME, Ferris BG, Speizer FE. An association between air pollution and mortality in U.S. cities. N Engl J Med 1993; 329:1753–1759.
11. Morabia A, Markowitz S, Garibaldi K, Wynder EL. Lung cancer and occupation: results of a multicentre case-control study. Br J Ind Med 1992; 49:721–727.
12. Doll R, Peto R. The causes of cancer: quantitative estimates of avoidable risks of cancer in the United States today. J Natl Cancer Inst 1981; 66:1193–1309.
13. Kogevinas M, Boffetta P. Occupational exposure to carcinogens and cancer occurrence in Europe. Med Lav 1995; 86:236–262.
14. Simonato L, Vineis P, Fletcher AC. Estimates of the proportion of lung cancer attributable to occupational exposure. Carcinogenesis 1988; 9:1159–1165.
15. Axelson O, Steenland K. Indirect methods of assessing the effects of tobacco use in occupational studies. Am J Ind Med 1988; 13:105–118.
16. IARC Monographs on the Evaluation of Carcinogenic Risks to Humans. Lyon: International Agency for Research on Cancer, 1997.
17. Tomatis L, Aitio A, Day NE. Cancer: Causes, Occurrence and Control. Lyon: IARC Scientific Publications, 1990.
18. Harrington JM, Levy LS. Lung cancer. In: Parkes WR, ed. Occupational Lung Disorders. Oxford: Butterworth-Heinemann, 1995:644–666.
19. Boffetta P, Saracci R. Occupational factors of lung cancer. In: Hirsch A, Goldberg M, Martin JP, Masse R, eds. Prevention of Respiratory Diseases. New York: Marcel Dekker, 1995: 37–63.
20. Steenland K, Stayner L. Silica, asbestos, man-made mineral fibers, and cancer. Cancer Causes Control 1997; 8:491–503.
21. Boffeta P, Jourenkova N, Gustavsson P. Cancer risk from occupational and environmental exposure to polycyclic aromatic hydrocarbons. Cancer Causes Control 1997; 8: 444–472.
22. Dich J, Zahm SH, Hanberg A, Adami HO. Pesticides and cancer. Cancer Causes Control 1997; 8:420–443.
23. Lynge E, Anttila A, Hemminki K. Organic solvents and cancer. Cancer Causes Control 1997; 8:406–419.
24. Tolbert PE. Oils and cancer. Cancer Causes Control 1997; 8:386–405.
25. Hayes RB. The carcinogenicity of metals in humans. Cancer Causes Control 1997; 8: 371–385.
26. Boice JD, Lubin JH. Occupational and environmental radiation and cancer. Cancer Causes Control 1997; 8:309–322.
27. Takkouche B, Gestal-Otero JJ. The epidemiology of lung cancer: review of risk factors and Spanish data. Eur J Epidemiol 1996; 12:341–349.
28. Steenland K, Loomis D, Shy C, Simonsen N. Review of occupational lung carcinogens. Am J Ind Med 1996; 29:474–490.
29. Harrington JM, Levy LS. Lung cancer. In: Parkes WR, ed. Occupational Lung Cancer. Oxford: Butterworth-Heinemann, 1994:644–666.
30. Moulin JJ. A meta-analysis of epidemiologic studies of lung cancer in welders. Scand J Work Environ Health 1997; 23:104–113.
31. American Thoracic Society. Adverse effects of crystalline silica exposure. Am J Respir Crit Care Med 1997; 155:761–765.
32. Weill M, Mc Donald JC. Exposure to crystalline silica and risk of lung cancer: the epidemiological evidence. Thorax 1996; 51:97–102.
33. Hammond EC, Selikoff IJ, Seidman H. Asbestos exposure, cigarette smoking and death rates. Ann NY Acad Sci 1979; 473–490.

34. Vignaud JM, Marie B, Picard E, Nabil K, Siat J, Galateau-Salle F, Borrelly J, Martinet Y, Martinet N. Tumor stroma formation in lung cancer. In: Martinet Y, Hirsch F, Martinet N, Vignaud JM, Mulshine J, eds. Clinical and Biological Basis of Lung Cancer Prevention. Basel: Birkhäuser, 1998:75–93.
35. Hugh-Jones P. Controversy: asbestos, asbestosis and lung cancer. Eur Respir Topic 1996; 2:6–8.
36. Martinet Y, Ménard O, Vaillant P, Vignaud JM, Martinet N. Cytokines in human lung fibrosis. Arch Toxicol 1995; 18:127–139.
37. Varmus H, Weinberg RA. Genes and the Biology of Cancer. New York: Scientific American Library, 1993.
38. World Health Organization. The World Health Organization histological typing of lung tumors. Am J Clin Pathol 1982; 77:123–129.
39. Churg A. Lung cancer cell type and occupational exposure. In: Samet JM, ed. Epidemiology of lung cancer. New York: Marcel Dekker, 1994:413–436.
40. De Klerk NH, Musk AW, Eccles JL, Hansen J, Hobbs MST. Exposure to crocidolite and the incidence of different histological types of lung cancer. Occup Environ Med 1996; 53: 157–159.

44

Lung Cancer Cell Immunogenicity and Immunotherapy

PATRICK WEYNANTS

Université Catholique de Louvain
Yvoir, Belgium

I. Introduction

The rationale behind the use of immunotherapy in cancer is based on the possibility of increasing the antitumor defenses of the host. This approach was applied to lung cancer in 1972; the authors reported improved survival in lung cancer patients who developed postoperative empyemas as compared with noninfected patients, suggesting an adjuvant immunostimulatory effect of bacterial products (1). These results raised a key question: does immunotherapy in cancer enhance the immunocompetence of the host or the antigenicity of tumor cells, or both?

By 1957, Burnet had already suggested that tumor cells have antigenic properties and that the development of cancer is linked to a defect of the immune system, thereby leading to an inappropriate tumor rejection response (2). Immunosuppression is generally associated with advanced cancer, however. Thus, both in vitro and in vivo immune responses have been found to be reduced in cancer patients (3). The immunosuppressive response includes a decrease of delayed-type hypersensitivity reactions, abnormal distribution of T-lymphocyte subsets, reduced cytolytic activity of peripheral blood mononuclear cells, and impaired proliferative response of lymphocytes to various mitogens (4–6). Recently, defects in cytokine production have also been reported in cancer patients (3,6). The precise mechanisms of the immunosuppression still remain uncertain, but a multiplicity of factors have been postulated, including tumor-derived suppressor molecules such as transforming growth factor beta (TGF-β) and interleukin-10 (IL-10) (3). By contrast, a number of studies have documented the activation of immune processes in patients with cancer, including lung carcinoma. In particular, the lymphocytes infiltrating the tumor appear to be activated and high levels of interleukin-2 (IL-2) receptors are observed in the peripheral blood of patients with limited bronchial tumors when compared with patients with advanced disease (7,8). Furthermore, patients whose preoperative peripheral blood lymphocytes demonstrate autologous tumor killing activity [ATK(+)] survive significantly longer than ATK-negative patients (9,10). It is reasonable to assume that, at an early stage of their disease, lung cancer patients are immunocompetent and that their immunocompetence decreases as their disease progresses. External factors such as cachexia and chemo- and radiotherapy are likely to contribute to this immunosuppression.

The counterpart of the immunocompetence of the host is the antigenicity and the immunogenicity of cancer cells. This necessarily implies that cancer cells are not only "antigenic," i.e., express antigens, but that these antigens are also "immunogenic," that is, able to be recognized and rejected by the immune system if appropriately presented and processed.

It is a long-standing dream of immunologists to demonstrate antigenicity and to identify the relevant antigens to render them immunogenic and induce tumor rejection. We will review the most relevant studies of the humoral (production of an-

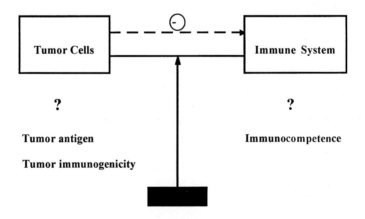

Figure 1 Schematic presentation of immunologic aspects and immunotherapy trials in lung cancer. (1) Passive immunotherapy: monoclonal antibodies; (2) adoptive immunotherapy: LAK cells, TIL cells + cytokines; (3) active nonspecific immunotherapy: BCG, cytokines (IL-2, IFN); (4) active specific immunotherapy: tumor vaccine, anti-diotypic vaccine.

tibodies) and cellular immune response directed against lung cancer cells and their application in immunomodulatory clinical trials (Fig. 1).

II. Monoclonal Antibodies in Therapeutic Applications

Circulating antibodies against autologous tumor cell proteins have been identified in lung cancer (LC) patients. Antibodies against p53 proteins have been detected in the sera of small-cell lung cancer (SCLC) patients, and anti-HU, anti-JO, and anti-RI neuronal antibodies have been identified in the sera of SCLC patients with neurologic paraneoplastic syndromes (11,12). One recent study confirmed that the sera of LC patients frequently contain antibodies against several tumor cell proteins. In SCLC patients, the presence of these circulating antibodies was associated with improved survival. Moreover, patients with limited disease were more likely to demonstrate such a humoral response (13). However, the epitopes recognized by these antibodies have not yet been identified. In contrast, one study observed that the presence of anti-p53 antibodies in the serum of SCLC patients was not of prognostic value (14). Interestingly, it was observed recently that the serum of cancer patients including LC contains antibodies that recognize intracellular proteins encoded by several genes with tumor-specific expression (15). Throughout the past decade, numerous monoclonal antibodies (MAb) have been generated against tumor LC cells. These MAb have been classified into 15 different clusters according to their pattern of reactivity (16). Antigenic targets for these antibodies include neural cell adhesion molecules, carbohydrate antigens, high molecular weight mucins, or blood group antigens. Some are highly specific for neuroendocrine cells, while others demonstrate cross-reactivity with epithelial cells. None of the antigens studied are specific to the LC subset, nor are they universally present on all LC specimen. Thus, these antigens recognize markers of differentiation rather than specific tumor markers and therefore represent lung cancer–associated antigens (LCAA) rather than tumor-specific antigens (TSA) (16).

MAb are investigated as therapeutic tools in four different applications: (1) mediators of immune effector function; (2) carriers of cytotoxic agents; (3) agents to block growth factors or their receptors; and (4) anti-idiotype vaccines (Fig. 2). Despite the important information obtained with these models, results should be analyzed with caution, since animal models as well as in vitro binding studies do not necessarily predict the efficacy of MAb in humans trials. Phase I clinical studies have only recently been initiated to evaluate the toxicity, the pharmacology, and the biological effects of MAb.

A. Mediators of Immune Effector Function

MAb directed against LCAA have been selected to mediate effector mechanisms, including complement-induced cytotoxicity and cellular cytotoxicity. For instance, a combination of antibody and human complement can be used for selective eradication of SCLC from bone marrow in vitro. More recently, a phase I/II study using

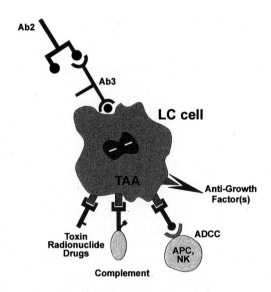

Figure 2   Potential mechanisms for lung cancer (LC) cell killing mediated by humoral host immunity. APC: Antigen-presenting cells; TAA: tumor-associated antigen; ADCC: antibody-dependent cytotoxicity (see text for details).

the MAb ABL 364 directed against the cluster 6 antigens has been initiated in refractory SCLC (17). If this type of therapy proves efficient, it will provide alternative treatments for tumors resistant to conventional therapy.

B. Immunoconjugates

Clinical trials with naked MAb, i.e., nonconjugated with drugs, toxins, or isotopes, have generally demonstrated limited responses, if any. A partial explanation for this resides in the observation that most murine antibodies do not activate human effector cells or have direct cytotoxic effects (18). Moreover, the cytotoxicity of MAb has only been demonstrated in vitro in conditions where MAb, complement, or effector cells were present in large excess (19). To increase their biological activity, MAb have subsequently been used as a vehicle for site-directed delivery of toxic substances. These immunoconjugates tested in vitro have demonstrated their potential value in therapy.

A blocked ricin immunoconjugate N 901-b R (an anti-NCAM MAb) (CD56) has recently been evaluated against relapsing SCLC. The preliminary phase I study demonstrated a partial response in one patient, and further studies are currently underway (20). Preclinical studies have documented an antitumor effect of antibody-drug conjugates in lung adenocarcinoma and squamous cell carcinoma (21). These reports indicate significant tumor regression compared to free drug or free MAb administered either singly or in combination.

C. MAb Antigrowth Factor

The ability of cancer cells to produce, secrete, and respond to several growth factors has become a central theme for studying the mechanism of growth regulation of tumor cells. Several of such autocrine growth factors have been described in SCLC and NSCLC (22). Bombesin/GRP, insulin-like growth factor 1 (IGF 1), or somatomedin and transferrin have been identified as growth factors in SCLC, while epithelial growth factor (EGF), IFG-1 and transforming growth factor alpha (TGF-α) are involved in NSLC cell proliferation (22). A better knowledge of their mechanisms of action could provide us with alternative therapeutic approaches in the management of patients with LC. These include the use of MAb directed against growth factors and/or against their receptor, the use of polypeptide antagonist for growth factors, and, finally, the disruption of the signal pathway after internalization of these factors within cells. Preclinical studies have clearly shown that a MAb (2 A11) with specificity for the carboxy-terminal portion of bombesin is able to block the binding of bombesin/GRP to its receptor and to inhibit the clonal growth of SCLC cell lines in vitro. The growth of some SCLC xenografts can be significantly inhibited by this MAb (23). Unfortunately, these interesting observations have not been further documented using other cancer cell lines. Nevertheless, preclinical phase I/II studies using the injection of MAb anti-GRP have recently been started at the National Cancer Institute. So far, only low doses have been used and, except in one patient, no evidence of objective tumor regression in advanced SCLC patients has been observed (24,25). Among other MAb against tumor growth factors, MAb directed against the EGF receptor conjugated with ricin A chain have also been found to be selectively cytotoxic for NSCLC tumors when injected in nude mice xenografts (26).

More recently, Divgi et al. reported a preliminary phase I study with a labeled anti-EGF receptor MAb in patients with squamous cell LC (27). Several drawbacks are likely to interfere with optimal response. First, it is uncertain whether the antibody penetration into the tumor bed is adequate, and second, it is likely that a particular tumor produces and responds to more than one single growth factor, underlying the necessity of a panel of antigrowth MAb. Finally, the heterogeneity of lung tumors suggests that no single antiproliferative agent will be curative (22).

D. Anti-Idiotype Vaccine

The immunization of patients with anti-idiotypic antibodies (Ab2), which carry the functional image of tumor antigens (TA), can elicit an immune response mediated by anti-anti-idiotypic antibodies (Ab3) directed against the tumor carrying the corresponding antigen, and this represents an alternative approach for specific immunotherapy in patients with cancer (28). Previous studies in animal models have demonstrated the validity as well as the efficacy of the immunization with Ab2 to induce immunity against tumor cells (28). Clinical trials with Ab2 anti-TA are presently ongoing in patients with colorectal carcinoma and melanoma, and preliminary reports in advanced melanoma suggest clinical response with increased survival (29). In this regard, monoclonal Ab2 elicited with a MAb against a cluster 5 and 5a antigen (TA sialoglycoprotein) have recently been reported (30). Their injection in mouse and rat species produces an Ab3 response effective against SCLC cell lines sharing the cluster 5a antigen. One of these Ab2 antibodies, LY 8-229, was found to be the most effective to induce an Ab3 response. In addition, an idiotype-specific antibody reactivity was recently reported against this Ab2 in the sera of SCLC patients. This suggests that this Ab2 (LY 8-229) represents a nominal SCLC antigen and therefore should be a candidate for active immunotherapy in SCLC patients (30).

Active immunotherapy with Ab2 antibodies has several theoretical advantages when compared to passive immunization with Ab1: (1) lower doses are required; (2) the stimulated immune cells cross the endothelial barrier and reach the tumor more easily; (3) this type of immune response could generate permanently activated immune B and T cells.

The progress in molecular biology techniques could also provide new approaches for anti-idiotypic immunotherapy. For instance, messenger RNA sequence analysis of the "internal image" of murine monoclonal anti-idiotypic antibodies may identify regions of sequence critical to antigen mimicry. Therefore, peptides corresponding to these sequences could provide useful reagents for synthetic vaccines in active immunotherapy against TAA (28).

In summary, with the advances of MAb technology, new approaches for the therapy of LC are now available. Preclinical studies have demonstrated the potential therapeutic effects of these agents in in vitro and in vivo models, but several problems need to be solved before clinical therapeutic benefits can be reached (31). These include: (1) cross-reactivity with normal tissue; (2) inadequate tumor penetration; (3) heterogeneity of antigen expression and antigenic modulation; (4) development of a human antibody response against the mouse monoclonal protein; and (5) discovery of true specific tumoral antigens.

III. Immune Cells of Tumor Cytolysis and Cytokine-Adaptive Therapy

The cellular immune response against tumor can be mediated by four types of cells: natural killer (NK) cells, lymphokine-activated killer cells (LAK), cytotoxic T lymphocytes (CTL), and activated macrophages (Fig. 3).

A. Natural Killer Cells

NK cells represent a third lineage of lymphocytes in addition to T and B cells (32). They are not target-specific but exhibit a more potent cytotoxic activity against tumor cells and virus infected cells than normal cells in the absence of prior sensitization. Phenotypically, NK cells are large granular lymphocytes that express neither α/β nor γ/δ T-cell receptors nor CD3 on their surface. NK cells are present in the peripheral blood of normal and cancer individuals and mediate non–HLA-restricted cytotoxic activity. The majority of NK cells possess low-affinity receptors for the Fc

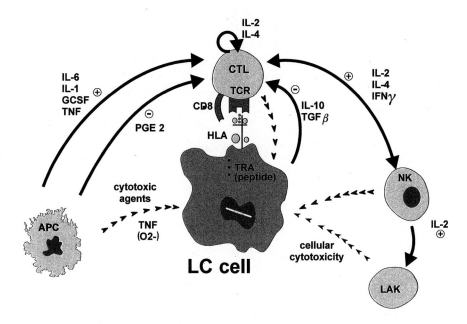

Figure 3 The potential effectors involved in cellular host immunity that could be involved in tumor cell killing. CTL: Cytolytic T lymphocytes; TCR: T-cell receptor; MHC: major histocompatibility complex; NK: natural killer cells; LAK: lymphokine-activated killer cells; APC: antigen-presenting cells (see text for details).

portion of IgG and therefore are also capable of mediating ADCC. Interestingly, the cytotoxic activity of NK cells is rapidly enhanced by IL-2 and the three types of interferons. In addition to cytotoxic activity, NK cells produce various lymphokines, such as IFN-γ, TNF, and GM-CSF. However, there is no convincing evidence yet that NK cells play a significant role in surveillance against LC, even through these cells are particularly effective in lysing targets devoid of HLA class I molecules. Moreover, despite the fact that peripheral blood from patients with large tumors or advanced cancer exhibit reduced NK activity, attempts to correlate low NK cell activity with tumor development have not been successful (33,34). Finally, conflicting results have been reported concerning pulmonary NK cells in patients with LC (35,36). Discrepancies in these reports could be due partially to different sampling compartments: Weissler et al. (35) reported a reduction in NK cell activity of cells obtained from lung tissue, whereas Pitchenic et al. (36) found an increase in NK function of cells recovered from the lavage fluid.

B. LAK Cells

The culture of leukocytes with high doses of IL-2 for a few days induces the generation of a broadly reactive cytotoxic population able to lyse not only target cells sensitive to NK cells but also targets that are resistant to NK cells, such as fresh tumor cells. These effector cells have been designated lymphokine-activated killer cells (LAK) (37). It is now clear that LAK cell activity is primarily mediated by IL-2–activated NK cells. Both SCLC and NSCLC cell lines are sensitive to LAK activity (38,39). LAK cells are usually derived from peripheral blood, but lymph node and tumor infiltrating lymphocytes represent an additional source of LAK cells (40) as well as pleural cells.

C. Specific Cytotoxic T Lymphocytes

In mice, T lymphocytes were shown to be the cells of the immune system that constitute the specific component of tumor rejection responses and that carry long-term memory of tumor rejection response. The observation that tumor cells that escaped rejection in vivo were resistant to antitumor CTL demonstrated that the antigen recognized in vitro by the CTL could be effective targets in vivo (41). It is now a common observation that T lymphocytes of cancer patients can be stimulated in vitro to produce CTL that show specificity for autologous tumor cells (42). Most of the antitumor CTL clones that specifically recognize the autologous tumor cells, in so far as they do not lyse autologous EBV-transformed B cells or K562 cells (the prototype target of NK-like cytolytic effector cells), have been generated against melanomas (43). Peripheral blood lymphocytes are the major source of lymphocytes for study of anti-tumor CTL, but CTL have also been generated from invaded lymph node, malignant pleural effusions, and tumor-infiltrating lymphocytes (TIL) (44). CTL response to human tumors is mainly mediated by CD8+ T cells. The antigen recognized by a CD8+ CTL consists of a complex between a peptide of 9–10 amino acids and a human leukocyte antigen (HLA) class I molecule (HLA-A, -B, or -C).

The antigenic peptides are produced inside the cell, mostly through degradation of endogenous cellular protein (Fig. 3). Gene transfection was used to identify the genes that encode the antigenic peptides or tumor rejection antigens (TRA) recognized by such anti-tumor CTL (45). The genes that have been identified so far fall into three groups (46). The first group includes genes such as MAGE-1, MAGE-3, BAGE, and GAGE, which are not expressed in the normal tissues except testis, but are expressed in significant proportions of different types of tumors including NSCLC and SCLC (47). The second group comprises genes tyrosinase, Mela-A^{MART-1}, gp^{100} Pme117, and gp^{75}, which are only expressed in melanocytes and in melanoma cells. The third group contains genes which are mutated in tumor cells, such as MUM-1, CDK-4, or HLA-A2 molecule (47–49). In lung cancer, oligoclonal T-cell populations isolated from either TIL or draining lymph nodes of advanced NSCLC can be expanded in vitro in the presence of IL-2 and have the capability of lysing autologous cancer cells (50–52). Some MHC class I–restricted CTL lines or clones that show specificity for autologous NSCLC cells or SCLC cells have been obtained from peripheral blood lymphocytes. Their target antigens have yet to be identified (53–56). SCLC cells have been shown to be poorly labeled with anti-HLA class I antibodies, and SCLC cell lines could neither stimulate nor be lysed by autologous cytolytic T lymphocytes unless they had been incubated with IFN-γ in order to increase the expression of HLA class I molecules (57). However, CTL derived from lymphocytes infiltrating NSCLC were shown to recognize a peptide encoded by the HER-2/neu gene and presented by HLA-A2 molecules (58). This gene is overexpressed in several types of tumors, including NSCLC and ovarian cell lines.

D. Cytokine Associated or Not with Adaptive Immunotherapy

The discovery that immune cells produce cytokines involved in regulation of the immune response and the ability to produce large quantities of the human cytokines by recombinant techniques has expanded their use as potential anticancer agents. The effects of IL-2 and IFNs, either alone or in combination with immune cells, other cytokines, or cytostatic agents, have been studied in lung cancer.

IL-2 promotes the growth of activated lymphocytes, increases their cytolytic activities against tumor cells, and induces the generation of LAK cells that are cytotoxic against autologous, syngenic, and allogenic tumor cells (37). IL-2 associated or not with LAK or TIL was found to produce encouraging results in melanomas and renal cell carcinomas (59,60). However, in advanced lung cancer patients, the results obtained with adaptive immunotherapy (high doses of IL-2 alone or in combination with LAK cells or TIL) were disappointing. Thus, in patients with advanced SCLC who did not achieve a complete response after chemotherapy, IL-2 infusion could induce either complete remission or additional tumor regression in almost 20% of the cases (61). By contrast, marginal responses were achieved in patients with ad-

Table 1 Cytokine (IL-2/IFN) Phase I/II in LC Combined or Not with Immune Cells

Histology	No. of patients	Agents	Results	Ref.
Advanced NSCLC	1	IL-2 alone	NR	60
	5	IL-2/LAK	NR	60
	1	IL-2/IFN-a	NR	64
	11	IL-2/LAK	1 PR	64
	16	IL-2/TNF-a	1 PR	63
			3 MR	
	11	IL-2/IFN-a	NR	65
	5	IL-2/IFN-a Continuous infusion	1 PR	59
	11	IL-2 Continuous infusion	NR	66
	8	IL-2 intralesional + systemic	2 PR	67
	11	IL-2/TIL	NR	62
SCLC	24	IL-2 postchemotherapy	5 OR	61

NR: No response; PR: partial response; MR: minor response; OR: objective response; according to the WHO criteria for tumor response.
IL-2: Interleukin-2; LAK: lymphokine-activated killer cells.

vanced NSCLC, a majority experiencing severe toxicity (59–67). However, the therapeutic response appears to vary according to the anatomical site suggesting a different susceptibility according to the location of the tumor. Thus, in LC patients, pleural infusion of IL-2 induces the disappearance of malignant effusion (68) or objective tumor response in 10 out of 22 patients (69).

Moreover, it remains uncertain whether the administration of LAK cells plus IL-2 provides a therapeutic benefit compared with IL-2 alone (60). The mechanism of response and the reasons for variable response to immunotherapy within groups of patients with similar disease is not clear. Parmiani (70) proposes that successful adoptive immunotherapy is more dependent on the recruitment of activated host antitumor-specific CTL than on the presence of LAK cells. Therefore, we could hypothesize that the number of circulating T cells specific against LC cells is too low to provide a sufficient amount of specific antitumor effector cells for adoptive immunotherapy. Furthermore, the majority of clinical trials were phase I or II studies including patients with advanced refractory LC. This represents a major limitation to the appropriate evaluation of the efficacy of immunotherapeutic agents, since evidence from animal models and clinical experience indicates that immunotherapy will best benefit cancer patients at an early stage of the disease with minimal tumor burden. Thus, two recent studies have evaluated the feasibility and the efficacy of IL-2/LAK or IL-2/TIL as adjuvant therapy after resection of locally advanced LC (71,72), and Kimura and Yamaguchi (71) reported that the 7-year survival rate was greater in the immunotherapy group than in the control group (39% vs. 12.7%).

IFNs are a family of three (α, β, and γ) cytokines demonstrating potent antiproliferative and immunomodulatory activities. Although these mediators have proved to be effective in some malignancies, their activity in NSCLC seems to be rather marginal (73–76). In SCLC, a recently published phase III study did not confirm the positive role of IFN-α and -γ as maintenance therapy in complete responder patients (77). However, complete tumor responses were observed after intrapleural injection of IFN-γ in stage I and II mesothelioma patients (78). In addition, an in vitro study suggested that IFN could potentiate the cytotoxic effect of cisplatin; but here again, despite encouraging phase II clinical studies, IFNs offered no survival benefit over chemotherapy alone in phase III studies (79,80).

E. Macrophages

The relevance of macrophages in cancer is supported by recent reports documenting that the majority of tumor-infiltrating cells are in fact macrophages (81). The precise role of these macrophages needs to be clarified, however. The mononuclear phagocytes, and in particular the tumor-associated macrophages (TAM), are often considered as major defenders of the host against tumors, but there is now evidence to support that TAM can also promote tumor growth (82). TAM, including lung macrophages, contain several secretory products potentially toxic for tumor cells, and among these products, oxygen metabolites, IFN-α, TNF-α, IL-1, and IL-6 have been investigated most. In addition, macrophages can also play an indirect role in the antitumoral immune response through the recruitment and activation of leukocytes to the tumor site.

In addition, alveolar macrophages can kill sensitized tumor cells through their Fcg receptors, which trigger an ADCC. Efforts to activate the tumoricidal properties of macrophages in vivo with lymphokines including IFN-γ have so far provided disappointing results. More recently, synthetic macrophage activators such as muramyl di- or tripeptide (MTP) were entrapped within liposomes in order to prolong their life and improve their targeting (83). Phase I clinical studies using intravenous liposome-encapsulated MTP demonstrated that antitumoral properties of blood monocytes from cancer patients are upregulated, but no significant reduction in tumor size was observed.

The role of tumor cells in the control of the macrophage response appears equally important. Indeed secretory products of the tumor can influence macrophage functions. Among these secretory products, IL-10 and TGF-β are potent immunosuppressive agents for macrophages. In addition, TGF-β is a fibroblast activator and could therefore participate in the remodeling of the extracellular matrix during the process of tumor progression.

IV. Tumor Antigen and Active Specific Immunotherapy

The concept of vaccination against cancer (active immunotherapy) is not new and mainly originates from the success of vaccines in infectious diseases. Unfortunately, despite the thousands of patients injected with various types of tumor vaccines during the last 50 years, only occasional clinical responses have been monitored (84). The most important prerequisite for any conventional vaccine approach depends on the ability to identify specific antigens associated with neoplasia and to elicit an appropriate protective host immune response to those antigens. The strongest evidence for the existence of such antigens comes from the study of transplanted tumors in inbred animals. Some of these tumors express antigens that elicit T-cell–mediated immune rejection responses in syngeneic host. These antigens, called transplanted specific tumor antigens (TSTA), can be either specific for individual tumors (usually tumors induced by chemical or physical carcinogen) or common to a class of tumors (virus-induced tumors) (85).

In human LC, early studies focused on boosting immune response against putative tumor antigens with adjuvants such as BCG (bacille Calmette-Guérin), *Corynebacterium parvum,* and levamisole, each known to stimulate either cellular and or humoral immune response. All these trials are classified as active nonspecific immunotherapy. The most commonly tested adjuvant was BCG, which was administered by various routes (intrapleural, intratumoral, interdermal, or aerosol) (86). It is difficult to compare all these trials because of differences in strain, viability, concentration, dose, as well as the heterogeneity of population, stage of disease, or time of therapy. However, two recent important randomized studies failed to show an additional survival benefit as compared to conventional treatment alone (87,88).

As opposed to passive immunization, active specific immunotherapy involves immune stimulation with tumor vaccines containing irradiated autologous or allogeneic tumor cells obtained from the tumor specimens. These tumor vaccines have been administered through different routes such as intradermal, intralesional, intralymphatic, or subcutaneous injection and have occasionally been combined with adjuvant products such as BCG, complete Freund, or lytic virus. For lung tumors, despite several studies, no clear benefit has been reported so far (86,89,90). Moreover, all trials share two characteristic features: therapeutic effect is either not observed or cannot be confirmed independently since no information is provided regarding the presence of tumor antigens in the vaccine. A partial reason for failure in tumor vaccine immunotherapy may have been due to the previous impossibility of matching immunogens to patients. Indeed, even when autologous tumor cells were used, there was no way to ascertain that a tumor antigen was expressed by these cells. The recent identification of tumor rejection antigens (TRA) and their encoding genes should shed new light on active specific immunotherapy in cancer patients (46). It is now obvious that patients must be selected for antitumor antigen immunization on the basis of the expression of the relevant antigen(s) by their tumor. Thus, eligibility criteria should include analysis of expression by the tumor of the gene encoding defined antigens (Fig. 4). This can be easily performed by reverse transcription-PCR on a small tumor sample correctly frozen and preserved. The patient must also be

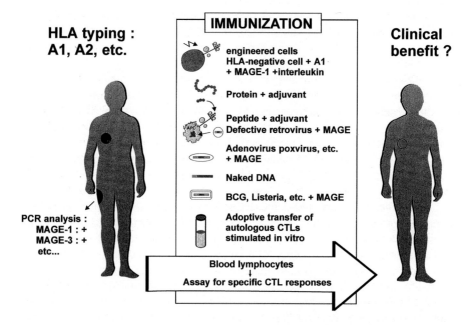

Figure 4   Examples of specific immunotherapy of lung cancer using defined tumor antigens (see text for details).

typed for HLA. Thus, one should know whether a tumor expresses a peptide-HLA combination corresponding to a known tumor antigen recognized by CTL. The number of NSCLC patients eligible for immunotherapy with one of the tumor antigens identified so far can be determined according to the percentage of tumors expressing the gene encoding defined antigens and the frequence of the given HLA class I molecule expression. At this time, it has been possible to include 49% of NCSLC patients in immunotherapy trials with a tumor rejection antigen (Table 2). Once the patient becomes eligible, we must choose a mode of immunization. To immunize against defined antigens recognized by T cells, there is a vast array of different modalities, but at this time it is unknown which one of them will be optimal in cancer patients. A first possibility is the inoculation of irradiated allogenic cells expressing the relevant antigen, but they will also induce an allogenic response preventing effective immunization against the tumor antigen. If this approach is feasible, it may be possible to build cells expressing only the relevant HLA class I molecules. To improve the immunogenecity of these cells, one could engineer them to produce cytokines that play a role in the development of a CTL response such as IL-2, IL-6 or IL-12, IFN-γ, GM-CSF. Transfecting the gene of the costimulatory molecule B7 may also prove very useful (92–94). A second possibility is the inoculation of patient with antigenic peptide or with the protein containing peptides. Peptides or proteins can be endocytosed by antigen-presenting cells and be presented by the relevant HLA class I molecules at the cell surface. The ability of peptides to prime CD8+ T cells in vivo has been demonstrated for viral antigens and rodent tumor antigens. The success of this approach may depend on the adjuvant formulations. However, tumor regression responses in melanoma patients treated with a peptide encoded by gene MAGE-3 have recently been recorded (95). Another mode of immunization is the use of autologous specialized antigen-presenting cells such as macrophages or dendritic cells that can be isolated from the blood, pulsed in vitro with proteins or peptides, and inoculated back into the patient (96,97). Recombinant viruses (adenovirus, vaccinia, retrovirus) or bacteria (BCG, *Salmonella*) carrying a gene coding for antigenic peptides can also be tested as immunogens. Intramuscular inoculation of DNA encoding the antigen is yet another possibility. The injected DNA can be integrated into the genome of muscle cells, which will synthesize the protein encoded by the DNA vaccine. Last but not least, an alternative approach is adoptive transfer of autologous T cells stimulated in vitro with the antigen.

All these immunogens have to be tested and evaluated in prospective clinical studies to determine which are the best. The evaluation of immunization can be made by clinical observation showing the regression of tumor or prolonged disease-free survival if the vaccine is given as adjuvant therapy. It will also be very important to evaluate whether immunization results in increased production of CTL precursors (98). To summarize, the main task is to demonstrate that effective immunogens can be derived with the available tumor rejection antigens. Furthermore, several drawbacks may limit the efficacy of immunization, for example, the heterogeneity of tumor cells combined with the possible presence of tumor cells

Table 2 Percentage of NSCLC-Expressing Antigens Encoded by MAGE, BAGE, or GAGE Genes

HLA frequency (Caucasians)	Percentage of MAGE-BAGE-GAGE expressing tumors								
	MAGE 1 45%	MAGE 2 49%	MAGE 3 49%	MAGE 6 52%	BAGE 5%	GAGE 19%	BAGE 5%	BAGE 5%	GAGE 19%
A1 (26%)	12	13							
A2 (49%)		24							
B44 (22%)		11							
CW16 (8%)	4		4						
CW6 (16%)									3

n = 104 patients.

% of eligible patients: Total—71%; in practice—49%, according to tumor specimens expressing several antigens.

Source: Ref. 91.

lacking antigen expression. Unfortunately, this heterogeneity cannot be evaluated by RT-PCR. It could be tested by immunochemical staining or in situ hybridization, but at this time appropriate antibodies are not available. However, if immunity can be raised against different tumor antigens, the loss of one of them would not necessarily result in tumor escape. Another problem is the loss of a molecule involved in the presentation pathway of the antigenic peptide such as HLA class I, β_2-microglobulin, TAP protein (99). Perhaps such HLA-negative cells could still be eliminated by NK cells, which appear to display specificity for cells having lost expression of HLA class molecules supporting the concept of combined immunological pathways to efficiently eradicate the tumor (100).

V. Conclusion

An increased knowledge of the mechanisms involved in both humoral and cellular immune response against lung cancer as well as the recent identification of genes coding for human tumor antigens have initiated a new phase in the search for an effective specific immunotherapy for lung cancer.

References

1. Ruckdeschel JC, Codis SD, Stranahan A, McKneally MF. Postoperative empyema improves survival in lung cancer. N Engl J Med 1972; 287:1013–1017.
2. Burnet FM. Cancer, a biological approach. Br Med J 1957; 1:844–852.
3. Sulitzeanu D. Immunosuppressive factors in human cancer. Adv Cancer Res 1993; 60: 247–267.
4. Dillman RO, Koziol JA, Zavanelli MI, Beauregard JC, Halliburton BL, Glassy MC, Royston I. Immunoincompetence in cancer patients. Cancer 1984; 53:1481–1491.
5. Nakaruma H, Ishiguro K, Mori T. Different immune functions of peripheral blood, regional lymph node, and tumor infiltrating lymphocytes in lung cancer. Cancer 1988; 62:2489–2497.
6. Masumo T, Ikeda T, Yokota S, Komuta K, Ogura T, Kishimoto S. Immunoregulatory T-lymphocyte functions in patients with small cell lung cancer. Cancer Res 1986; 46:4195–4199.
7. Wei YQ, Hang ZB. In situ observation of lymphocyte-tumor interaction in human lung carcinoma. Immunol Invest 1989; 18:1095–1105.
8. Ginns LO, De Hoyos A, Brown MC, Gaumon GR. Elevated concentration of soluble interleukine-2 receptors in serum of smokers and patients with lung cancer. Am Rev Respir Dis 1990; 142:398–402.
9. Vanky F, Klein E, Willems J, Willems J, Book K, Ivert T, Peterffy A, Nilsonne U, Kreicbergs A, Aparisi T. Lysis of autologous tumor cells by blood lymphocytes tested at time of surgery. Cancer Immunol Immunother 1986; 21:69–76.
10. Uchida A, Kariya Y, Okamoto N, Sugie K, Fujimoto T, Yagita M. Prediction of post-operative clinical course by autologous tumor killing activity in lung cancer patients. J Natl Cancer Inst 1990; 82:1697–1701.
11. Winter SF, Minna JD, Johnson BE, Takahashi T, Gazdar AF, Carbone DP. Development of antibodies against p53 in lung cancer patients appears to be dependent on the type of p53 mutation. Cancer Res 1992; 52:4168–4174.

12. Drlicek M, Grisold W, Liszka U. Correlation of circulating antineuronal antibodies (CANA) with paraneoplastic syndromes in lung cancer. Lung Cancer 1993; 8:245–258.

13. Winter SF, Sekido Y, Minna JD, McIntiner D, Johnson BE, Gazdar AF, Carbone DP. Antibodies against autologous tumor cell proteins in patients with small-cell lung cancer: association with improved survival. J Natl Cancer Inst 1993; 85:2012–2018.

14. Rosenfeld MR, Malats N, Schramm L, Graus F, Cardenal F, Vinolas N, Rosell R, Tora M, Real FX, Posner JB, Dalmau J. Serum anti-p53 antibodies and prognosis of patients with small-cell lung cancer. J Natl Cancer Inst 1997; 89:381–385.

15. Sahin U, Tureci O, Schmitt H, Cochlovius B, Johannes T, Schmits R, Stenner F, Luo G, Schobert I, Pfreundschuh M. Human neoplasms elicit multiple specific immune responses in the autologous host. Proc Natl Acad Sci USA 1995; 92:11810–11813.

16. Stahel RA, Gilks WR, Schenker T. Antigens of lung cancer: results of the third international workshop on lung tumor and differentiation antigens. J Natl Cancer Inst 1994; 86:669–672.

17. Stahel RA, Lacroix H, Sculier JP, Morant R, Richner J, Janzek E, Loibner H, Blythman H. Phase I/II study of monoclonal antibody against Lewis Y hapten in relapsed small-cell lung cancer. Ann Oncol 1992; 3:319–320.

18. Foon KA. Biological response modifiers: the new immunotherapy. Cancer Res 1989; 49:1621–1639.

19. Mach JP, Pelegrin A, Buchegger F. Imaging and therapy with MoAb in non hematopoietic tumors. Curr Opin Immunol 1991; 3:685–693.

20. Lynch TJ Jr. Immunotoxin therapy of small-cell lung cancer—N901-blocked ricin for relapsed small-cell lung cancer. Chest 1993; 103:436S–439S.

21. Bumol TF, Deherdt SV, Zimmerman DL, Apelgren LD. Monoclonal antibody-oncolytic drug conjugates for site-directed therapy of human adenocarcinomas. Proc Am Assoc Cancer Res 1989; 30:647–648.

22. Woll PJ. Growth factors and lung cancer. Thorax 1991; 46:924–929.

23. Cuttitta F, Carney DN, Mulshine J, Moody TW, Fedorko J, Fischler A, Minna JD. Bombesin-like peptides can function as autocrine growth factors in human small-cell lung cancer. Nature 1985; 316:823–826.

24. Avis IL, Kovacs TO, Kasprzyk PG. Preclinical evaluation of an anti-autocrine growth factor monoclonal antibody for treatment of patients with small-cell lung cancer. J Natl Cancer Inst 1991; 83:1470–1476.

25. Mulshine JL, Shuke H, Daghighian F, Carrasquillo J, Ghosh B, Walsh T, Avis I, Reynolds JC, Cuttitta F, Larson SM. The correct dose: pharmacologically guided end point for anti-growth factor therapy. Cancer Res 1992; 52:2743s–2746s.

26. Masui H, Kamrath H, Apell G. Cytotoxicity against human tumor cells mediated by the conjugate of anti-epidermal growth factor receptor monoclonal antibody to recombinant ricin a chain. Cancer Res 1989; 49:3482–3488.

27. Divgi CR, Welt S, Kris M. Phase I and imaging trial of indium 111 labelled anti-epidermal growth factor receptor monoclonal antibody 225 in patients with squamous cell lung carcinoma. J Natl Cancer Inst 1991; 83:97–104.

28. O'Connell MJ, Chen ZJ, Yang H. Active specific immunotherapy with antiidiotypic antibodies in patients with solid tumors. Sem Surg Oncol 1989; 5:441–447.

29. Quan WDY Jr, Dean GE, Spears L, Spears CP, Groshen S, Merritt JA, Mitchell MS. Active specific immunotherapy of metastatic melanoma with an antiidiotype vaccine: a phase I/II trial of I-Mel-2 plus SAF-m. J Clin Oncol 1997; 15:2103–2110.

30. Lehmann HP, Zwicky C, Waibel R, Stahel RA. Tumor-antigen-specific humoral immune response of animals to anti-idiotypic antibodies and comparative serological analysis of patients with small-cell lung carcinoma. Int J Cancer 1992; 50:86–92.

31. Kuzel TM, Rosen ST. Antibodies in the treatment of human cancer. Curr Opin Oncol 1994; 6:622–626.

32. Whiteside TL, Herberman RB. Human natural killer cells in health and disease. Biology and therapeutical potential. Clin Immunother 1994; 1:56–66.

33. Sibbitt WL, Bankhurst AD, Jumonville AJ, Saiki JH, Saiers JH, Doberneck RC. Defects in natural killer cell activity and interferon response in human lung carcinoma and malignant melanoma. Cancer Res 1984; 44:852–856.

34. Ching-Chi L, Yuh-Chi K, Wen-Chu H, Ching-Yuang L. Natural killer cell activity in lung cancer patients. Chest 1987; 92:1022–1024.

35. Weissler JC, Nicod LP, Lipscomb MF, Toews GB. Natural killer cell function in human lung is compartmentalized. Am Rev Respir Dis 1987; 135:941–949.

36. Pitchenik AE, Guffee J, Stein-Streilein J. Lung natural killer and Interleukin-2 activity in lung cancer. Am Rev Respir Dis 1987; 136:1327–1332.

37. Grimm EA, Mazumder A, Zhang HZ, Rosenberg SA. Lymphokine-activated killer cell phenomenon: lysis of natural killer-resistant fresh solid tumor cells by interleukin 2-activated autologous human peripheral blood lymphocytes. J Exp Med 1982; 155:1823–1841.

38. Robinson BWS, Morstyn G. Natural killer (NK)-resistant human lung cancer cells are lysed by recombinant interleukin-2-activated NK cells. Cell Immunol 1987; 106:215–222.

39. Lagadec PF, Saraya KA, Balkwill FR. Human small-cell lung cancer cells are cytokine-resistant but NK/LAK-sensitive. Int J Cancer 1991; 48:311–317.

40. Yano T, Yasumoto K, Nomoto K. Generation and expansion of lymphokine-activated killer cells from lymph node lymphocytes in human lung cancer. Eur J Cancer Clin Oncol 1989; 25:201–208.

41. Boon T, Cerottini JC, Van den Eynde B, van der Bruggen P, Van Pel A. Tumor antigens recognized by T lymphocytes. Annu Rev Immunol 1994; 12:337–365.

42. Anichini A, Fossati G, Parmiani G. Clonal analysis of the cytolytic T-cell response to human tumors. Immunol Today 1987; 8:385–389.

43. Hérin M, Lemoine C, Weynants P, Vessière F, Van Pel F, Knuth A, Devos R, Boon T. Production of stable cytolytic T-cell clones directed against autologous human melanoma. Int J Cancer 1987; 39:390–396.

44. Hainaut P, Weynants P, Coulie PG, Boone T. Antitumor T-lymphocyte responses. Immunol Allergy Clin North Am 1990; 10:639–662.

45. Boon T, Coulie P, Marchand M, Weynants P, Wölfel T, Brichard V. Genes coding for tumor rejection antigens: perspectives for specific immunotherapy. In: DeVita V, ed. Important Advances in Oncology. Philadelphia: JB Lippincott Company, 1994:53–69.

46. Van den Eynde B, Brichard VG. New tumor antigens recognized by T cells. Curr Opin Immunol 1995; 7:674–681.

47. Weynants P, Lethé B, Brasseur F, Marchand M, Boon T. Expression of MAGE genes by non-small-cell lung carcinomas. Int J Cancer 1994; 56:826–829.

48. Coulie P, Lehmann F, Lethé B, Herman J, Lurquin C, Andrawiss M, Boon T. A mutated intron sequence codes for an antigenic peptide recognized by cytolytic T lymphocytes on a human melanoma. Proc Natl Acad Sci USA 1995; 92:7976–7980.

49. Brändle D, Brasseur F, Weynants P, Boon T, Van den Eynde B. A mutated HLA-A2 molecule recognized by autologous cytotoxic T lymphocytes on a human renal cell carcinoma. J Exp Med 1996; 183:2501–2508.

50. Yoshino I, Yano T, Yoshikai Y, Murata M, Sugimachi K, Kimura G, Nomoto K. Oligoclonal T lymphocytes infiltrating human lung cancer tissues. Int J Cancer 1991; 47:654–658.

51. Melioli G, Ratto G, Guastella M, Meta M, Biassoni R, Semino C, Casartelli G, Pasquetti W, Catrullo A, Moretta L. Isolation and in vitro expansion of lymphocytes infiltrating non-small cell lung carcinoma: functional and molecular characterisation for their use in adoptive immunotherapy. Eur J Cancer 1994; 30A(1):97–102.

52. Meta M, Ponte M, Guastella M, Semino C, Pietra G, Ratto GB, Melioli G. Detection of oligoclonal T lymphocytes in lymph nodes draining from advanced non-small-cell lung cancer. Cancer Immunol Immunother 1995; 40:235–240.

53. Vose BM, Bonnard GD. Specific cytotoxicity against autologous tumour and proliferative responses of human lymphocytes grown in interleukin-2. Int J Cancer 1982; 29:33–39.

54. Slingluff CL, Cox AL, Stover JM, Moore MM, Hunt DF, Engelhard VH. Cytotoxic T-lymphocyte response to autologous human squamous cell cancer of the lung: epitope reconstitution with peptides extracted from HLA-Aw68. Cancer Res 1994; 54:2731–2737.

55. Nakao M, Yamana H, Imai Y, Toh Y, Toh U, Kimura A, Yanoma S, Kakegawa T, Itoh K. HLA A2601-restricted CTLs recognize a peptide antigen expressed on squamous cell carcinoma. Cancer Res 1995; 55:4248–4252.

56. Weynants P, Marchand M, Baurain TF, Deloos M, Boon Th, Coulie PG. Production of cytolytic T cell (CTL) clones directed against autologous small cell and non-small cell lung cancer cell lines (abstr). Lung Cancer 1997; 18:147.

57. Weynants P, Wauters P, Coulie PG, Van Den Eynde B, Symann M, Boon T. Cytolytic response of human T cells against allogeneic small cell lung carcinoma treated with interferon gamma. Cancer Immunol Immunother 1988; 27:228–232.

58. Yoshino I, Goedegebuure PS, Peoples GE, Parikh AS, DiMaio JM, Lyerly HK, Gazdar AF, Eberlein TJ. HER2/neu-derived peptides are shared antigens among human non-small cell lung cancer and ovarian cancer. Cancer Res 1994; 54:3387–3390.

59. West WH, Tauer KW, Yannelli JR, Marshall GD, Orr DW, Thurman GB, Oldham RK. Constant-infusion recombinant interleukin-2 in adoptive immunotherapy of advanced cancer. N Engl J Med 1987; 316:898–905.

60. Rosenberg SA, Lotze MT, Yang JC, Aebersold PM, Marston Lineham W, Seipp CA, White DE. Experience with the use of high-dose Interleukin-2 in the treatment of 652 cancer patients. Ann Surg 1989; 210:474–483.

61. Clamon G, Herndon J, Perry MC, Ozer H, Kreisman H, Maher T, Ellerton J, Green MR. Interleukin-2 activity in patients with extensive small-cell lung cancer: a phase II trial of cancer and leukemia group B. J Natl Cancer Inst 1993; 85:316–320.

62. Kradin RL, Lazarus DS, Dubinett SM, Gifford J, Grove B, Kurnick JT, Preffer FI, Pinto CE, Davidson E, Callahan RJ, Strauss HW. Tumour-infiltrating lymphocytes and interleukin-2 in treatment of advanced cancer. Lancet 1989; i:577–580.

63. Yang SC, Owen-Schaub L, Mendiguren-Rodriguez A, Grimm EA, Hong WK, Roth JA. Combination immunotherapy for non-small cell lung cancer. Results with interleukin-2 and tumor necrosis factor-α. J Thorac Cardiovasc Surg 1990; 99:8–13.

64. Bernstein ZP, Goldrosen MH, Vaickus L, Friedman N, Watanabe H, Rahman R, Park J, Arbuck SG, Sweeney J, Vesper DS, Takita H, Zeffren J, Dennin RA, Foon KA. Interleukin-2 with ex vivo activated killer cells: therapy of advanced non-small-cell lung cancer. J Immunother 1991; 10:383–387.

65. Jansen RLH, Slingerland R, Hoo Goey S, Franks CR, Bolhuis RLH, Stoter G. Interleukin-2 and Interferon-a in the treatment of patients with advanced non-small-cell lung cancer. J Immunother 1992; 12:70–73.

66. Ardizzoni A, Bonavia M, Viale M, Baldini E, Mereu C, Vera A, Ferrini S, Cinquegrana A, Molinari S, Mariani GL, Roest GJ, Sharenberg J, Palmer PA, Rosso R, Ropolo F, Raso C. Biologic and clinical effects of continuous infusion Interleukin-2 in patients with non-small cell lung cancer. Cancer 1994; 73:1353–1360.

67. Scudeletti M, Filaci G, Imro MA, Motta G, Di Gaetano M, Pierri I, Tongiani S, Indiveri F, Puppo F. Immunotherapy with intralesional and systemic Interleukin-2 of patients with non-small-cell lung cancer. Cancer Immunol Immunother 1993; 37:119–124.

68. Yasumoto K, Miyazaki K, Nagashima A, Ishida T, Kuda T, Yano T, Sugimachi K, Nomoto K. Induction of lymphokine-activated killer cells by intrapleural instillations of recombinant Interleukin-2 in patients with malignant pleurisy due to lung cancer. Cancer Res 1987; 47:2184–2187.

69. Astoul Ph, Viallat JR, Laurent JC, Brandely M, Boutin C. Intrapleural recombinant IL-2 in passive immunotherapy for malignant pleural effusion. Chest 1993; 103:209–213.

70. Parmiani G. An explanation of the variable clinical response to interleukin 2 and LAK cells. Immunol Today 1990; 11:113–115.

71. Kimura H, Yamaguchi Y. Adjuvant immunotherapy with interleukin-2 and lymphokine-activated killer cells after noncurative resection of primary lung cancer. Lung Cancer 1995; 13:31–44.

72. Ratto GB, Melioli G, Zino P, Mereu C, Mirabelli S, Fantino G, Ponte M, Minuti P, Verna A, Noceti P, Tassara E, Rovida S. Immunotherapy with the use of tumor-infiltrating lympho-cytes and interleukin-2 as adjuvant treatment in stage III non-small-cell lung cancer. A pilot study. J Thorac Cardiovasc Surg 1995; 109:1212–1217.

73. Olesen BK, Ernst P, Nissen MH, Hansen HH. Recombinant interferon A (IFL-rA) therapy of small cell and squamous cell carcinoma of the lung. A phase II study. Eur J Cancer Clin Oncol 1987; 23:987–989.

74. van Zandwijk N, Jassem E, Dubbelmann R, Braat P, Rumke P. Aerosol application of Interferon-alpha in the treatment of bronchialveolar carcinoma. Eur J Cancer 1990; 26: 738–740.

75. Wheeler RH, Herndon JE, Clamon GH, Green MR. A phase II study of recombinant b-interferon at maximum tolerated dose in patients with advanced non-small cell lung can-cer: a cancer and leukemia group B study. J Immunother 1994; 15:212–216.

76. Jassem J. Biological treatment of NSCLC. The need for conclusive studies. Chest 1996; 109:119S–124S.

77. Jett JR, Maksymiuk AW, Su JQ, Mailliard JA, Krook JE, Tschetter LK, Kardinal CG, Twito DI, Levitt R, Gerstner JB. Phase III trial of recombinant interferon gamma in complete re-sponders with small-cell lung cancer. J Clin Oncol 1994; 12:2321–2326.

78. Boutin C, Viallat JR, Van Zandwijk N, Douillard JT, Paillard JC, Guerin JC, Mignot P, Migueres J, Varlet F, Jehan A, Delepoulle E, Brandely M. Activity of intrapleural recombi-nant gamma-interferon in malignant mesothelioma. Cancer 1991; 67:2033–2037.

79. Kajata V, Yap A. Combination of cisplatin and interferon-a 2a (Roferon®-A) in patients with non-small cell lung cancer (NSCLC). An open phase II multicentre study. Eur J Cancer 1995; 31A(1):35–40.

80. Schiller JH, Storer B, Dreicer R, Rosenquist D, Frontiera M, Carbone PP. Randomized phase II–III trial of combination beta and gamma interferons and etoposide and cisplatin in inoperable non-small cell cancer of the lung. J Natl Cancer Inst 1989; 81:1739–1743.

81. Mantovani A, Botazzi B, Colotta F. The origin and function of tumor-associated macro-phages. Immunol Today 1992; 13:265–270.

82. Mantovani A. Biology of disease. Tumor-associated macrophages in neoplastic progression: a paradigm for the In vivo function of chemokines. Lab Invest 1994; 71:5–16.

83. Fidler IJ, Sone S, Fogler WE. Eradication of spontaneous metastases and activation of al-veolar macrophages by intravenous injection of liposomes containing muramyl dipeptide. Proc Natl Acad Sci USA 1981; 78:1680–1684.

84. Livingston Ph. Active specific immunotherapy in the treatment of patients with cancer. Im-munol Allergy North Am 1991; 11:401–423.

85. Boon Th. Tum-variants: immunogenic variants obtained by mutagen treatment of tumor cells. Immunol Today 1985; 6:307–311.

86. Fishbein GE. Immunotherapy of lung cancer. Semin Oncol 1993; 20:351–358.

87. LLCSG. Immunostimulation with intrapleural BCG as adjuvant therapy in resected non-small cell lung cancer. Cancer 1986; 58:2411–2416.

88. Matthay RA, Mahler DA, Beck GJ, Loke J, Baue AE, Carter DC, Mitchell MS. Intratumoral Bacillus Calmette-Guérin immunotherapy prior to surgery for carcinoma of the lung: results of a prospective randomized trial. Cancer Res 1986; 46:5963–5968.

89. Takita H, Hollinshead AC, Adler RH, Bhayana J, Ramundo M, Moskowitz R, Rao UNM, Raman S. Adjuvant, specific, active immunotherapy for resectable squamous cell lung car-cinoma: a 5-year survival analysis. J Surg Oncol 1991; 46:9–14.

90. Price-Evans DA, Roberts HL, Hewitt S, Walsh D, Donohoe WTA, Lambourne A. A trial of adjuvant immunotherapy for bronchial carcinoma with irradiated autochthonous tumor cells. Int J Immunother 1987; 3:293–305.

91. Weynants P, Marchand M, Brasseur F, Boon Th. Expression by 104 non-small cell lung car-cinomas of defined antigens recognized by T lymphocytes: perspectives for anti-cancer vac-cines (abstr). Lung Cancer 1997; 18:S158.

92. Fearon ER, Pardoll DM, Itaya T. Interleukin-2 production by tumor cells bypasses T helper function in the generation of antitumor response. Cell 1990; 60:397–403.

93. Watanabe Y, Kuribayashi K, Mitadabe S. Exogenous expression of mouse interferon gamma cDNA in mouse neuroblastoma C1300 cells results in reduced tumorigenicity by augmented anti-tumor immunity. Proc Natl Acad Sci USA 1989; 86:9456–9460.

94. Townsend S, Allison JP. Tumor rejection after direct costimulation of CD8+ T cells by B7-transfected melanoma cells. Science 1993; 259:368–370.

95. Marchand M, Weynants P, Rankin E, Arienti F, Belli F, Parmiani G, Cascinelli N, Bourlond A, Vanwijck R, Humblet Y, Canon JL, Laurent C, Naeyaert JM, Plagne R, Deraemaeker R, Knuth A, Jäger E, Brasseur F, Herman J, Coulie PG, Boon T. Tumor regression responses in melanoma patients treated with a peptide encoded by gene MAGE-3. Int J Cancer 1995; 63:883–885.

96. Mayordoma JI, Zorina T, Storkus WJ, Celluzi C, Falo LD, Melief CJ, Ildstad T, Kast WM, DeLeo AB, Lotze MT. Bone marrow-derived dendritic cells pulsed with synthetic tumor peptides elicit protective and therapeutic antitumor immunity. Nature Med 1995; 1:1297–1302.

97. Celuzzi CM, Mayordomo JI, Storkus WJ, Lotze MT, Falo LD. Peptide-pulsed dendritic cells induce antigen-specific, cytotoxic T lymphocyte-mediated protective immunity. J Exp Med 1996; 183:283–287.

98. Coulie P, Somville M, Lehmann F. Precursor frequency analysis of human cytolytic lymphocytes directed against autologous melanoma cells. Int J Cancer 1992; 50:289–297.

99. Korkolopoulou P, Kaklamanis L, Pezzella F, Harris AL, Gatter KC. Loss of antigen-presenting molecules (MHC class I and TAP-1) in lung cancer. Br J Cancer 1996; 73:148–153.

100. Ljunggren HG, Kärre K. In search of the "missing self": MHC molecules and NK cell recognition. Immunol Today 1990; 11:237–244.

45

Gene Therapy

CHRISTIAN BRAMBILLA, ADRIEN NEGOESCU, MARIE FAVROT, AND JEAN-LUC COLL

Institut Albert Bonniot
Centre Hospitalier Universitaire de Grenoble
Grenoble, France

The promising antitumor effects observed in animal models suggest that gene therapy could be a very attractive approach for the treatment of cancer. So far, phase I and II trials indicate that gene therapy is safe. However, none of the current clinical strategies has demonstrated real efficacy (for review see Ref. 1).

The first challenge for gene therapy concerned congenital diseases. At that time, it appeared that the correction of a single lost function was a simple matter. Actually, it turned out to be a very complicated problem, requiring long-term expression of the transgene, targeted delivery, and very often a correct "natural" regulation of this gene. Researchers were then kindly asked to return to the bench to improve their gene transfer systems. At the same time, more and more investigators were considering cancer as a suitable target for gene therapy. Integration of the transgene was no longer necessary, since a short burst of expression providing therapeutic levels during a brief period of time was sufficient. In addition, the immunogenicity of the vector was more acceptable if one could achieve a satisfying gene transfer efficacy after a single injection.

Transformation of a normal cell to its malignant counterpart is the result of the acquisition of a series of genetic lesions. Nonetheless, it has been shown that the correction of a single mainstream genetic alteration can be sufficient to reduce significantly tumorigenicity, but other approaches are also very promising, including activation of the immune system or destruction of the neo-angiogenesis.

Several recent reviews summarize the different strategies currently developed and present a summary of the ongoing clinical protocols. The aim of this chapter is to focus particularly on lung cancer.

I. Drug Sensitization/Drug Resistance

Lung cancer is a highly metastatic disease. Metastasis represents one of the major challenges for gene therapy, since it is not possible to reach every single tumor cell. One possibility to address this question is to treat a primary target and to induce a bystander effect able to amplify the antitumor response. One of the first systems known to be associated with a bystander effect is the thymidine kinase/ganciclovir (TK/GCV) couple.

The TK gene encodes for an enzyme involved in the phosphorylation of an antiviral nucleoside, ganciclovir, that is not metabolized by mammalian cells. Thus, GCV is not toxic under normal conditions, while triphosphorylated GCV can be incorporated into nascent DNA of the cycling cell and eventually results in its death. GCV toxicity is not restricted to TK-expressing cells, and several studies have reported the existence of a "bystander" effect where only a small percentage of cells need to be transduced with the TK gene to achieve effective tumor eradication (2–5). This is usually explained by the diffusion of the toxin from one cell to another through gap junctions, but some studies suggest that it may also be due to an activation of the immune system. It has been established that transfer of a plasmid encoding for IL-2 into the tumors was synergistic with TK and induced a systemic antitumor immunity that resulted in the regression of tumors as well as protection against challenges of parental tumor cells (6,7). These authors established that the antitumor activity was mediated by $CD8^+$ T lymphocytes, but that this immunity rapidly waned over time, resulting in the death of the animals after tumor recurrence.

Twenty-one clinical protocols using TK/GCV are underway (1); one of them concerns the treatment of pleural mesothelioma (8). Despite the very encouraging results obtained in animals studies (9), the adeno-mediated TK treatment was unsuccessful in humans (8). Eight patients with pleural mesothelioma were injected with doses of TK-expressing adenovirus ranging from 10^9 to 10^{10} PFU. No tumor regression was noticed, as well as no toxicity beyond a mild fever. Gene transfer was extremely low; it was documented by in situ hybridization in only a few cells of one pleural biopsy 3 days after injection.

Different studies demonstrated the existence of a powerful TK/GCV antitumor activity in murine models (6–11). All of them established a pronounced decrease in tumor size after TK/GCV treatments, but the gain in survival time was very small. This clearly suggests that even if a strong reduction in the tumor burden is achieved by TK/GCV treatment, other parameters like the clinical presentation, variations of sensitivity, and/or immunogenicity will render the recovery a gamble. Our group demonstrated that in vitro analysis can help to anticipate the opportunity to start a TK treatment, and that the combination of suicide effect and immunostimulation was recommended (5). Thus it is reasonable to assume that the poor efficiency of the human clinical protocol can be attributed to the low sensitivity of the patients' cells to adenovirus gene transfer, but also to a low efficiency of TK/GCV antitumor activity. In addition, the doses of GCV commonly used in animal models are usually much higher than the maximum tolerated dose in humans. Thus, the GCV treatment in humans cannot be really adapted. Several groups are trying to circumvent this problem by creating a new TK enzyme with improved enzymatic activities.

Other suicide genes are emerging, like cytosine deaminase, nitroreductase, and cytochrome P415. Some of them may have interesting properties for the treatment of lung cancer, but still need further testing.

II. Immunopotentiation

As mentioned before, the induction of a bystander effect able to destroy metastatic cells is of primary importance. The immune system is normally able to play this role, but cancer cells very often developed sophisticated strategies to avoid detection. Indeed, most of the malignant cells are HLA negative (12), but also frequently present very low levels of costimulatory molecules like B7 on their surface. These costimulatory molecules are responsible for the T-cell receptor-mediated recognition of the abnormal cells. Thus, cancer cells devoid of recognition molecules are almost undetectable by the immune system. In addition, tumor cells frequently overexpress soluble factors able to decrease the antigen presentation and the lymphocyte activation. Nevertheless, a weak immune response against tumor cells does exist, but is unable to stop the tumor progression. Thus the idea emerged to consolidate this response by increasing the local concentration of cytokines and/or to facilitate the detection of tumor cells by adding a flag on their surface.

The first attempts consisted in the local secretion of cytokines by tumor infiltrating lymphocytes (TIL) (13). TIL were purified from the patient tumor, cultivated and expanded in vitro, infected by a retrovirus expressing the cytokine of interest (IL-2 or TNF), and infused into the patient blood stream. Using tagged TIL, it has been demonstrated that these lymphocytes could be detected up to 300 days after their infusion in the patient blood, but no particular homing in the tumor was observed (14).

The next step was to transduce a cytokine gene into tumor cells to increase their immunogenicity and the activation of surrounding T lymphocytes. This could be performed ex vivo on autologous tumor cells using liposome or retroviral vectors or directly in vivo using an adenoviral vector (15–17). While about 45 such protocols are ongoing, mainly on melanoma and renal cancer, there is only one on small-cell lung cancer (no result available). Another approach is to restore the immunogenicity of the tumor cells by transfection of B7 (18), which is, however, only one of the components of immune recognition loss of the tumor cells. There is no clinical trial with this technique on lung cancer. The last approach is the induction of specific cytocytic T lymphocytes (CTL) (19). Several clinical trials of vaccination by a recombinant vaccine virus expressing CEA (in Roth) has begun and could be applied in lung cancer expressing CEA, particularly adenocarcinoma, but no results are available yet.

Expression of MAGE antigen by small cell lung cancer could be another approach to induce specific CTL (see previous chapter). One of the promising methods of vaccination involves using the genetic abnormalities of the cell cycle control genes to elicit CTL in a kind of boomerang effect. However, to be efficient in vivo at the human scale the pathway of immunodepression has to be efficiently disrupted.

III. Gene Replacement

Since cancer cell proliferation is the result of an activation of oncogenes and inactivation of tumor suppressor genes, blocking the former by an anti-sense oligonucleotides (20) or restoring the normal function of the latter was used in vitro to exhibit the function of a cell cycle control gene (21). In vitro and animal experiments (22) blocking the activity of ras (23) was shown to reduce growth of lung tumor in nude mice. A clinical protocol has been approved with this technique severely hampered by the required duration of expression and efficiency of transfection (24).

The same restrictions applied to the transfection of tumor suppressor genes such as p53. Several studies showed that transfection of wild-type p53 decreases the tumor growth in vitro and in vivo on xenografts (25–28) and reduces the tumorigenicity of explanted tumor (29,30). It was shown that overexpression of p53 induced apoptosis (31–33) in the transduced cells bearing complex abnormalities. Thus p53 expression could correct or reverse the malignant phenotype. In addition, p53-induced bystander effect as well as its low toxicity for the surrounding normal tissues render this approach suitable for clinical trials. Five clinical trials are underway, two by Roth et al. (34). The first used a retroviral vector expressing p53 directly injected in the tumor through a fiberoptic bronchoscope in patients out of reach for conventional treatment. Three out of nine patients were stabilized, one had partial regression, while a complete regression was observed in the last one (34). Since overexpression of p53 was associated with an increased sensitivity to cisplatin (35), a second protocol has begun to compare the action of adenovirus-mediated p53 gene transfer plus or minus cisplatin (10^7–10^{11}) (36). Seven patients were included (37). Posttreatment tumor biopsies demonstrated the presence of the vector DNA after polymerase chain reaction (PCR), of p53 transgene expression by reverse transcriptase–PCR and immunohistochemistry. This was associated with increased necrosis on H and E sections and increased apoptosis after in situ TUNEL staining. Transgene expression occurred in posttreatment tumor biopsies in patients with circulating antibodies to adenovirus. There was no change in the inflammatory cells infiltrating the tumor, suggesting that nonspecific inflammation was not responsible for the therapeutic effects. These results suggest that adenoviral mediated p53 gene transfer can be successfully achieved with minimal toxicity in patients with lung cancer. Adeno-p53 clinical activity appears improved at higher doses of vector and when used in combination with CDDP. Clinical protocols are already underway and preliminary results appearing; nevertheless, the nature of p53 antitumor activity needs to be extensively investigated now in order to better understand the mechanism(s) of tumor cell death.

Tumor progression or regression is the final result of proliferation and cell death. Necrosis mostly resulting from hypoxia is the most visible pattern of cell death but may not be the most efficient. Apoptosis, although conspicuous (visible on less than 5% of cells) may be quantitatively more important. The term apoptosis describes genetically driven active cell death (ACD). Apoptotic cells undergo separation form their neighbors, membrane blebbing, chromatin condensation, nuclear breakdown into micronuclei within 2–5 minutes, and cytolysis into condensed apoptotic bodies, which undergo phagocytosis and digestion by the surrounding cells within 3 hours without inflammatory reaction. Tumor cells are protected from apoptosis by overexpression of survival genes such as bcl2 or deregulation of p53, and or rb functions (see corresponding chapters). Conversely, tumor cells with wild-type p53 functions are also more susceptible to apoptosis. Several types of oncogene activations (myc, E2F, cyclin D1) may induce p53-dependent apoptosis. Margins between tumor growth and regression could be crossed by a relatively minor augmentation in the rate of highly inducible ACD.

Indeed, for the last 15 years, a general concept has emerged that all nonsurgical modalities of cancer therapy act primarily via the induction of apoptosis, as do chemotherapy and radiotherapy but also immunotherapy or hormone ablation (38–42). Though mechanisms involved in therapy-induced ACD are only partially elucidated, a general property that provides the therapeutic window appears to be the apoptosis threshold, which is higher in normal as opposed to neoplastic cells. Thus, surrounding normal tissues may arrest in G1 and repair the damage induced by therapy while tumor cells die through apoptosis (43).

Since p53 has a major role to play in both cell proliferation and apoptosis induction, it has been extensively used in gene therapy. Nonetheless, other important genes also involved in these processes may have important properties to consider for gene therapy applications.

Concerning growth arrest induction, different genes including Rb, P21/Waf1, and P16^{INK4A} were studied. The first tumor suppressor gene described, retinoblastoma gene, is able to reverse the tumorigenic phenotype when reexpressed in Rb-negative tumors (44,45). Because Rb expression is mainly associated with a transient growth arrest (cytostatic) rather than a long-lasting, nonreversible activity, its use in gene therapy of lung cancer has not been proposed, even if most of the SCLC are known to be Rb deficient.

Waf1 (Cip1, P21) is a known mediator of p53-induced growth arrest. It is a cyclin-dependent kinase (cdk) inhibitor controlling cdk-mediated Rb phosphorylation and cell cycle progression (46). P21 transfection gave conflicting results in different tumors (47). As observed with Rb, P21/Waf1 expression induced a G1 arrest in lung cancer cell lines but no ACD, thus lowering its level of priority in the list of interesting therapeutic genes.

Adeno-mediated gene transfer of P16^{INK4A}, another cdk inhibitor frequently inactivated in lung cancer, did not per se induce a significant tumor regression in vivo. Nevertheless, this gene may have some potential therapeutic value when used in association with p53 in hepatocellular and colon carcinoma (48).

Concerning apoptotic genes, a model progressively emerged giving the central position to the members of the bcl2 gene family (49,50). As described in various solid tumors, transregulatory mechanisms can be responsible for the high levels of Bcl2 protein (50). Bcl2 heterodimerizes with Bax, a protein of the same family sharing 21% homology with Bcl2. Bax can be considered as the main effector of apoptosis. Its function in active cell death as a homodimer Bax-Bax is opposed by heterodimerization with Bcl2 (Bax-Bcl2). This model was substantiated by results showing that Bax also heterodimerizes with other ACD-inhibiting members of the Bcl2 family such as BclXL, Mcl-1, A-1 (51); it is also corroborated by the correlation between Bcl2 expression and both low spontaneous ACD in tumors and general resistance to cancer therapy (50,52,53). Conversely, Bax expression is correlated with high incidence of apoptosis in lung and stomach cancers (52,54), and low Bax levels are associated with poor response to chemotherapy in breast and ovary tumors (55,56). As recently demonstrated, lack of Bax protein in cancer cells can be the result of mutations in the bax gene (57).

BclX is another member of the bcl2 gene family. Due to alternate mRNA splicing, bclX is transcribed into long (bclXL) and short (bclXS) forms. The BclXL protein functions as an inhibitor of apoptosis. In contrast, the BclXS is an inducer of ACD (58). However, BclXS acts as a monomer and does not show the ability to form heterodimers with other Bcl2 family members (59), which makes it potentially active when transfected in cells overexpressing Bcl2. The final step of apoptosis induction, termed "executioner" by Martin and Green (60), is represented by proteases of the interleukin-1β converting enzyme (ICE) family, which directly generate cell destruction; they have recently been grouped under the term "caspases" for "cysteine-aspartic acid specific proteinase" (61). Caspases are most probably stimulated by the Bax-Bax homodimer, and the process can be opposed by heterodimerization with Bcl2 (Bax-Bcl2) producing caspase blocking and cell survival (62). Recent results indicate that Bax can induce apoptosis independently of dimerization processes (63,64) and, furthermore, without caspase activation (65); caspase-independent execution was also described for another death-inducing homolog of Bax, Bak (66). This would imply that Bax and Bak are not merely inducers of the executioner, but, together with caspases, components of it.

This model proved useful to tentatively explain the function of many ACD regulators. The first among these is the P53 protein. Wild-type (wt) P53 accumulates if DNA is damaged and blocks the cell cycle to allow DNA repair. If repair fails, P53 triggers apoptosis. Thus, tumor cells lacking normal P53 function will accumulate mutations and chromosome rearrangements leading to selection of highly malignant clones. This "guardian of the genome" model for P53 function (67) is strongly supported by the lack of normal p53 in more than half of all tumor cell types (68). Because P53 is the main known downregulator of bcl2, its mutations could result in elevated production of Bcl2. In addition, P53 strongly induces the expression of bax (69). Thus, P53 appears to be an important regulator of apoptosis through the Bax-Bcl2 balance, and any type of P53 inactivation could abrogate cell death through Bax/Bcl2 dysbalance, as recently confirmed in vivo (70). Accordingly, the survival advantage conferred by the absence of normal P53 in malignant cells may explain their increased drug resistance. Similarly, radiation-induced ACD is P53-dependent and is inhibited by Bcl2 and BclXL (71–73).

Caspase activation can also occur directly, without mediation by Bax homodimers. Such a mechanism is best illustrated by the tumor necrosis factor receptor (TNFR) family members, such as Fas (specific for the Fas ligand) and TNFR1 (which binds TNF-α) (74).

The main approach of survival-gene inactivation was targeted on bcl2, and antisense strategies have been developed to lower bcl2 expression. They potentiated spontaneous apoptosis and chemotherapy-induced ACD of lymphoma cell lines or of acute myeloid leukemia patient–derived cells, both in vitro and in vivo. The likely explanation is that, by downregulating bcl2 (about 30% reduction as compared to control) in a cell that is heavily dependent on Bcl2 for survival, the cell is committed to ACD (75,76). Bcl2 antisense strategy formed the basis of a first clinical protocol for non-Hodgkin's lymphoma (77). An 18-base antisense oligonucleotide was subcutaneously administered for 2 weeks to nine patients. In two of these tumors regressed, and in two others the number of circulating lymphoma cells decreased. Eight patients received further chemotherapy, six of them exhibiting favorable evolution.

BclXS efficiency as an antitumoral agent has been recently tested. In vitro, its expression constantly induced growth arrest via apoptosis induction in cell lines originating in tumors of breast, stomach, colon, and neuroblastoma. In accordance with its probable dimerization-independent apoptotic action, BclXS was strongly efficient even in the presence of high levels of Bcl2 or BclXL. Moreover, BclXS potentiated chemotherapy-induced apoptosis in cultured breast cancer cells. In vivo, BclXS suppressed growth of mammary tumor cells implanted in nude mice via apoptosis induction. Antitumoral activity was greater than predicted from the percentage of transduced cells, which raises the possibility of a BclXS-mediated bystander apoptosis (78–81). Bax in vitro transduction of breast and ovarian cancer cells did not affect viability but increased chemo- and radio-induced apoptosis (82,83). During the last year, our team concentrated upon comparing therapeutic effects of p53, bax, and bclXS in H322 (mutated p53) and H358 (p53-null) bronchioloalveolar carcinoma cells (84). Our results demonstrated an important advantage for bax in terms of apoptosis-based cytotoxicity over both p53 and bclXS, the latter two providing almost identical effects (Fig. 1). Therefore, it is conceivable that transfection-induced Bax expression acts by enriching the cellular pool of Bax-Bax homodimers,

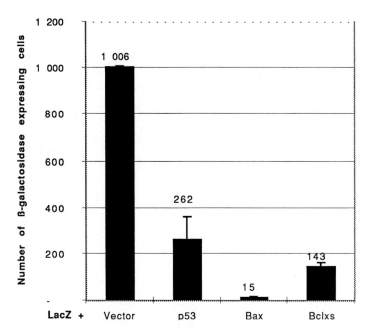

Figure 1   In vitro toxicity of p53, bax, or bclxs expression in NSCLC. Subconfluent H322 cells were transfected with 2 μg of a solution of DNA containing one-fifth of pLacZ and four-fifths of an empty vector, p53, bax, or bclxs plasmids. Forty eight hours later, the number of LacZ expressing cells was determined. This number reflects the number of viable transfected cells. Expression of p53 or bclxs greatly reduced the number of live transfected cells by approximately 75%. This effect was even stronger after expression of bax, since only 1% of the LacZ positive cells were still alive. Thus, bax is more cytotoxic than p53 or bclxs in this model.

which readily turns on caspases and initiates the execution of the cell. Such a mechanism could be more immediate and thus more efficient than ACD induction by P53. This interpretation is supported by the difference we observed in Bax cytotoxicity between H322 cells (about 70% of Bax-expressing cells died) and H358 cells (more than 90% cytotoxicity). Indeed, blot experiments revealed undetectable levels of Bcl2 in H-358 cells as opposed to a notable expression of this protein in H322 cells. Since P53 regulates the Bax-Bcl2 balance by repressing bcl2 and transactivating bax (69), bax-p53 co-transfections would be expected to enhance the apoptotic effect of bax by favoring the liberation of Bax from heterodimers with endogenous Bcl2 and the accumulation of ACD-inducing Bax-Bax homodimers. We were not able to identify such a cytotoxic advantage for bax-p53 co-transfections, possibly because there was little enhancement to be gained beyond the strong effect of bax acting alone. Our results showed poor, if any, bystander killing and growth inhibition after p53 or bax transfer in vitro. Finally, work in progress in our laboratory indicates that the in vivo antitumoral effect of bax is as strong than that of p53 and that bax delays in vivo tumor growth via induction of apoptosis, but also by the activation of poorly understood bystander mechanisms (Fig. 2).

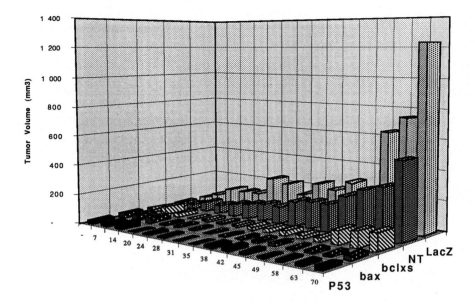

Figure 2 Antitumor activity of p53, bax, and bclxs gene transfer. H322 NSCLC cells were implanted subcutaneously in nude mice. When the tumor size reached an average diameter of at least 5 mm, they were treated twice a week with 10 μg of DNA injected intratumoraly. Nontreated (NT) or moked treated (LacZ) tumors progressed rapidly while, in contrast, p53 or bax treated tumors remained very small in 50% of the animals. The other 50% did not present any detectable tumors and were considered as tumor-free.

IV. P53-Based Gene Therapy

Because of its high frequency of genetic alterations and its central role in the control of cell proliferation and apoptosis, P53 has been widely used in gene therapy. In addition, recent studies suggest that p53-mediated antitumoral activity may not be the sole result of wild-type P53 control on cell growth or death (85), but presumably involve many other mechanisms like angiogenesis or activation of the immune system. Indeed, wild-type P53 can transactivate the expression of thrombospondin 1 (86), an inhibitor of angiogenesis, whereas mutant p53 augments the expression of VEGF, which is an activator of angiogenesis (87). Thus, overexpression of wild-type P53 can prevent the neovascularization of the tumors (Fig. 3).

P53 gene transfer could also induce a vaccination against p53. Using recombinant canary pox virus expressing wild-type or mutated p53, it was shown (88) in a mouse model that animals can be vaccinated against a lethal injection of tumorigenic cells expressing high levels of mutant p53. The tumor protection was equally effective regardless of whether wild-type or mutant p53 was used for the immunization. It remains to be demonstrated that vaccination induces a tumor regression and not only a prevention of tumor uptake. One advantage of this technique is that

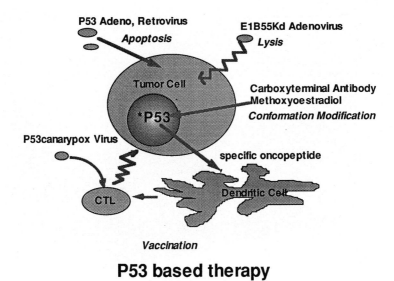

P53 based therapy

Figure 3 Different ways of including an antitumor response using the expression of P53.

the nature of the p53 mutation present in the tumor is not important. This is not the case when induction of a specific cellular immunity is induced by injection of on-copeptides derived from a specific mutant form of p53 (89). Nevertheless, antigenic peptide are sometimes more efficient than the whole protein, since the protein located in the nucleus needs to be processed and exported into the endoplasmic reticulum by transporters of antigen presentation (TAP), where they will form complexes with major histocompatibility class 1 heavy chain and β_2-microglobulin (light chain) before being exposed on the cell surface. Tumors may acquire the ability to mask these neoantigens by altering their pathway of presentation (TAP or MHC expression) (90). In lung tumors, professional antigen-presenting cells, the dendritic cells (DC), are impaired in their capacity to mature by the presence of VEGF secreted by the tumor (91). A clinical trial of peptide immunization using activated dendritic cells pulsed with oncopeptide has begun. Forty percent of the 30 patients included in this protocol presented a good immunological response (89).

Thus, overexpression of wild-type P53 can activate several pathways. Interestingly, stabilization of the endogenous P53 in tumors expressing wild-type P53 can also lead to the induction of apoptosis. This stabilization of the wild-type conformation of P53 is observed after treatment of the tumors by a metabolite of estradiol (methoxyoestradiol) (92). Also, a mutant P53 protein can recover a wild-type conformation in the presence of geldanamycin (93) or of antibodies directed against its carboxy-terminal domain (94) and reacquire its normal functions.

The presence of a mutant form of P53 can also be use to selectively kill the tumor cells harboring it. The early viral gene E1B of adenoviruses encodes a 55 kDa protein that inhibits apoptosis by inactivating wild-type p53. Bischoff and colleagues constructed an E1B-55-kDa–deficient adenovirus unable to replicate in cell expressing a wild-type p53 but able to replicate into cells expressing an inactive form of p53 (as well as p53-null cells). This virus is thus a selective killer of tumor cells. It was tested in animal models, in which complete tumor regression was observed. Clinical trials are on their way.

V. Future Development

Amelioration of vector design, length, level of gene expression, cell targeting, and regulation of transcription associated with a control of toxicity are the goals of future development. Viral and nonviral vectors are far from ideal (for review, see Refs. 1, 12). Amelioration of now classical vectors (retrovirus and adenovirus) should allow repeated injection without immunologic reaction with high viral titers. Major advantages of recombinant adeno associated virus (AAV) vectors (95) include lack of pathogenicity, ability of wild-type AAV to integrate the chromosome 19, potential ability to infect nondividing cells, broad range of infectivity, high titers (up to 10^{12} infection units/ml) and weak immunogenicity. However, several problems still preclude AAV vector from being ideal: variation of integration on chromosome 19 of recombinant virus, need of adenovirus for production of AAV with the risk of contamination, and the difficulty of obtaining high titers.

Canary pox virus also seems to be a good candidate for immunization purposes. Although restricted to avian species for its replication, canary pox virus functions effectively as an immunization vehicle, since it infects mammalian cells nonproductively and express foreign antigens (88). It has already been demonstrated to work safely in humans.

Different approaches to improve nonviral vectors are currently being investigated. The first one concerns the screening of new molecules coming out every day (96). Very efficient molecules, mainly cationic lipids, are now available. But although their ability to transfect cells in vitro is clearly established, their performances in vivo are not. Another way to improve nonviral vectors is to enhance their specificity for their target by covalently associating a specific ligand to a polycation, as demonstrated by our group (97) and others. The first example was described by Wu and Wu, who used an asialoglycoprotein covalently linked to polylysine and incorporated into a DNA-polylysine-AsOr complex in order to target hepatocytes (98). Other ligands, like antibodies (97,99), lectine (100), or surfactant-associated proteins (101) have been described. Ferkol and coworkers described the obtention of complexes in which the ligand (an antipolymeric immunoglobulin receptor Fab fragment) was able to target airway epithelial cells (102). The specificity of each of these different kinds of complexes was clearly demonstrated, but their efficiency was rather low in vivo, certainly because of the poor activity of polylysine to protect the DNA from degradation once internalized.

In parallel, targeting was also considered from the DNA's point of view by adapting the promoters to the tissue of interest. Numerous candidates were studied, including the carcinoembryonic antigen (CEA) (103), neuron-specific enolase (NSE) (104), and prostate-specific antigen promoters (105). The EGFR gene is also very interesting since its overexpression is very commonly observed in lung cancers. Moreover, expression of the EGFR is activated by both wild-type or mutant p53, but specific DNA sequences were found in this promoter responsible for its transactivation by the mutant p53 only. Such a promoter would then be tumor specific. Furthermore, other investigators took advantage of the high level of expression of the EGFR protein to create a targeted DNA delivery device by coupling EGF to polylysine. Thus, the overexpression of the EGFR gene in lung cancer can be used in two different ways to target these malignant cells. Finally, we will just mention the elegant work of Kumagai et al. (106), who created a TK construct driven by a Myc-responsive promoter. This plasmid was thus particularly efficient to kill Myc-overexpressing tumor cells, especially SCLC cells.

References

1. Roth JA, Cristiano RJ. Gene therapy for cancer: what have we done and where are we going? J Natl Cancer Inst 1997; 89:21–39.
2. Freeman SM, Whartenby KA, Koeplin DS, Moolten FL, Abboud CN, Abraham GN. The "bystander effect": tumor regression when a fraction of the tumor mass contains the HSV-TK gene. J Cell Biochem 1992; 16F:47.
3. Elshami AA, Saavedra A, Zhang H, et al. Gap junctions play a role in the "bystander effect" of the herpes simplex virus thymidine kinase/ganciclovir system in vitro. Gene Ther 1996; 3:85–92.
4. Beck C, Cayeux S, Lupton SD, Dörken B, Balnkestein T. The thymidine kinase-ganciclovir-mediated "suicide" effect is variable in different tumor cells. Hum Gene Ther 1995; 6:1525–1530.
5. Coll JL, Mesnil M, Lefèvre M-F, Lancon A, Favrot MC. Long term survival of immuno-competent rats with intraperitoneal colon carcinoma tumors using herpes simplex thymidine kinase/ganciclovir and IL-2 treatments. Gene Ther 1997 (in press).
6. Chen S-H, Chen XHL, Wang Y, Kosai K-I, Finegold MJ, Rich SS, Woo SLC. Combination gene therapy for liver metastasis of colon carcinoma in vivo. Proc Natl Acad Sci USA 1995; 92:2577–2581.
7. Caruso M, Pham-Nguyen K, Kwong Y-L, Xu B, Kosai K-I, Finegold M, Woo SLC, Chen S-H. Adenovirus-mediated interleukin-12 gene therapy for metastatic colon carcinoma. Proc Natl Acad Sci USA 1996; 93:11302–11306.
8. Hwang HC, Smythe WR, Elshami AA, et al. Gene therapy using adenovirus carrying the herpes simplex thymidine kinase gene to treat in vitro models of human malignant mesothelioma and lung cancer. Am J Respir Cell Mol Biol 1995; 13:7–16.
9. Elshami AA, Kucharczuk JC, Zhang HB, Smythe WR, Hwang HC, Litzky LA, Kaiser LR, Albelda SM. Treatment of pleural mesothelioma in an immunocompetent rat model utilizing adenoviral transfer of the herpes simplex virus thymidine kinase gene. Hum Gene Ther 1997; 7:141–148.
10. Yee D, McGuire SE, Brünner N, Kozelsky TW, Allred DC, Chen S-H, Woo SLC. Adenovirus-mediated gene transfer of herpes simplex virus thymidine kinase in an ascites model of human breast cancer. Hum Gene Ther 1996; 7:1251–1257.
11. Smythe WR, Kaiser LR, Hwang HC, Amin KM, Pilewski JM, Eck SL, Wilson JM, Albelda SL. Successful adenovirus-mediated gene transfer in an in vivo model of human malignant mesothelioma. Ann Thor Surg 1994; 57:1395–1401.

12. Whartenby KA, Abboud CN, Marrogi AJ, Ramesh R, Freeman SM. The biology of cancer gene therapy. Lab Invest 1995; 72:131–145.
13. Schendel DJ, Gansbacher B. Tumor specific lysis of human renal cell carcinomas by tumor infiltrating lymphocytes: modulation of recognition through retroviral transduction of tumor cells with interleukin 2 complementary DNA and exogenous alpha interferon treatment. Cancer Res 1993; 53:4020–4025.
14. Merrouche Y, Négrier S, Bain C, Combaret V, Mercatello A, Coronel B, Moskovtchenko JF, Tolstoshev P, Moen R, Philip T, Favrot MC. Clinical application of retroviral gene transfer in oncology: Results of a French study with tumor infiltrating lymphocytes transduced with the gene of resistance to neomycin. J Clin Oncol 1995; 13:410–418.
15. Han SK, Brody SL, Crystal RG. Suppression of in vivo tumorigenicity of human lung cancer cells by retrovirus-mediated transfer of the human tumor necrosis factor-α cDNA. Am J Respir Cell Mol Biol 1994; 11:270–278.
16. Fearon ER, Pardoll DM, Itaya T, Golumbek P, Levitsky HI, Simons JW, et al. Interleukin-2 production by tumor cells bypasses T helper function in the generation of an antitumor response. Cell 1990; 60:397–403.
17. Golumbek PT, Lazenby AJ, Levitsky HI, Jaffe LM, Karasuyama H, Baker M, et al. Treatment of established renal cancer by tumor cells engineered to secrete interleukin-4. Science 1991; 254:713–716.
18. Gaken J, Hollingsworth S, Darling D, Hirst W, Peakman M, Kuiuiper M, et al. Treatment of tumour bearing mice with autologous tumour cells expressing combination B7.1 and IL-2. Cancer Gene Ther 1994; 1:310.
19. Mandelboim O, Berke G, Fridkin M, Feldman M, Eisenstein M, Eisenbach L. CTL induction by a tumor-associated antigen octapeptide derived from a murine lung carcinoma. Nature 1994; 369:67–71.
20. Thompson JD, Macejak D, Couture L, Stinchcomb DT. Ribozymes in gene therapy. Nature Med 1995; 1:277–278.
21. Zhang Y, Mukhopadhyay T, Donehower LA, Georges RN, Roth JA. Retroviral vector-mediated transduction of K-ras antisense RNA into human lung cancer cells inhibits expression of the malignant phenotype. Hum Gene Ther 1993; 4:451–460.
22. Georges RN, Mukhopadhyay T, Zhang Y, Yen N, Roth JA. Prevention of orthotopic human lung cancer growth by intratracheal instillation of a retroviral antisense K-ras construct. Cancer Res 1993; 53:1743–1746.
23. Mukhopadhyay T, Tainski M, Cavender AC, Roth JA. Specific inhibition of K ras expression and tumorigenicity of lung cancer cells by antisense DNA. Cancer Res 1991; 51:1744–1748.
24. Roth JA. Modification of mutant K-ras gene expression in non-small cell lung cancer (NSCLC) with an adenovirus vector expressing wild-type p53 and cisplatin. Hum Gene Ther 1996; 7:875–889.
25. Takahashi T, Carbone D, Takahashi T, Nau MM, Hida T, Linnoila I, Ueda R, Minna JD. Wild-type but not mutant p53 suppresses the growth of human lung cancer cells bearing multiple genetic lesions. Cancer Res 1992; 52:2340–2343.
26. Cai DW, Mukhopadhyay T, Liu Y, Fujiwara T, Roth JA. Stable expression of the wild-type p53 gene in human lung cancer cells after retrovirus-mediated gene transfer. Hum Gene Ther 1993; 4:617–624.
27. Zhang WW, Fang X, Mazur W, French BA, Georges RN, Roth JA. High-efficiency gene transfer and high-level expression of wild-type p53 in human lung cancer cells mediated by recombinant adenovirus. Cancer Gene Ther 1994; 1:5–13.
28. Liu TJ, Zhang WW, Taylor DL, Roth JA, Goepfert H, Clayman GL. Growth suppression of human head and neck cancer cells by the introduction of a wild-type p53 gene via a recombinant adenovirus. Cancer Res 1994; 54:3662–3667.
29. Fujiwara T, Cai DW, Georges RN, Mukhopadhyay T, Grimm EA, Roth JA. Therapeutic effect of a retroviral wild-type p53 expression vector in an orthotopic lung cancer model. J Natl Cancer Inst 1994; 86:1458–1462.
30. Clayman GL, El-Naggar AK, Roth JA, Zhang WW, Goepfert H, Taylor DL, Liu TJ. In vivo molecular therapy with p53 adenovirus for microscopic residual head and neck squamous carcinoma. Cancer Res 1995; 55:1–6.

31. Fujiwara T, Grimm EA, Mukhopadhyay T, Cai DW, Owen-Schaub LB, Roth JA. A retroviral wild-type p53 expression vector penetrates human lung cancer spheroids and inhibits growth by inducing apoptosis. Cancer Res 1993; 53:4129–4133.
32. Radinski R, Fidler IJ, Price JE, Esumi N, Tsan R, Petty CM, Bucana CD, Bar-Eli M. Terminal differentiation and apoptosis in experimental lung metastases of human osteogenic sarcoma cells by wild-type p53. Oncogene 1994; 9:1877–1883.
33. Adachi JI, Ookawa K, Shiseki M, Okazaki T, Tsuchida S, Morishita K, Yokota J. Induction of apoptosis but not G_1 arrest by expression of the wild-type p53 gene in small cell lung carcinoma. Cell Growth Diff 1996; 7:879–886.
34. Roth JA, Nguyen D, Lawrence DD, Kemp BL, Carrasco CH, Ferson DZ, Hong WK, Komaki R, Lee JJ, Nesbitt JC, Pisters KMW, Putnam JB, Schea R, Shin DM, Walsh GL, Dolormente MM, Han CI, Martin FD, Yen N, Xu K, Stephens LC, McDonnel TJ, Mukhopadhyay T, Cai D. Retrovirus-mediated wild-type p53 transfer to tumors of patients with lung cancer. Nature Med 1996; 2:985–991.
35. Fujiwara T, Grimm EA, Mukhopadhyay T, Zhang WW, Owen-Schaub LB, Roth JA. Induction of chemosensitivity in human lung cancer cells in vivo by adenovirus-mediated transfer of the wild-type p53 gene. Cancer Res 1994; 54:2287–2291.
36. Roth JA. Modification of tumor suppressor gene expression and induction of apoptosis in non-small cell lung cancer (NSCLC) with an adenovirus vector expressing wild-type p53 and cisplatin. Hum Gene Ther 1996; 7:1013–1030.
37. Roth JA, Swisher DD, Lawrence BL, Kemp CH, Carrasco AK, El-Naggar AK, Fossela FV, Glisson BS, Hong WK, Khuri FR, Nesbitt JC, Pisters K, Putnam JB, Schrump DS, Shin DM, Walsh GL. Gene replacement for lung cancer. Lung Cancer 1997; 18(suppl2):76.
38. Green DR, Bissonnette RP, Cotter TG. Apoptosis and cancer. In: DeVita VT, Hellman S, Rosenberg SA, ed. Important Advances in Oncology. Philadelphia: J.B. Lippincott, 1994:37–52.
39. Hannun YA. Apoptosis and the dilemma of cancer chemotherapy. Blood 1997; 89:1845–1853.
40. Lennon SV, Martin SJ, Cotter TG. Dose-dependent induction of apoptosis in human tumour cell lines by widely diverging stimuli. Cell Prolif 1991; 24:203–214.
41. McDonnell TJ, Meyn RE, Robertson LE. Implications of apoptotic cell death regulation in cancer therapy. Semin Cancer Biol 1995; 6:53–60.
42. Tenniswood MP. Active cell death in hormone—dependent tissues. Cancer Metast Rev 1992; 11:197–220.
43. Fisher DE. Apoptosis in cancer therapy: crossing the threshold. Cell 1994; 78:539–542.
44. Ookawa K, Shiseki M, Takahashi R, Yoshida Y, Terada M, Yokota J. Reconstitution of the RB gene suppresses the growth of small-cell lung carcinoma cells carrying multiple genetic alterations. Oncogene 1993; 8:2175–2181.
45. Antelman D, Machemer T, Huyghe BG, Shepard HM, Maneval D, Johnson DE. Inhibition of tumor cell proliferation in vitro and in vivo by exogenous p110^{RB}, the retinoblastoma tumor suppressor protein. Oncogene 1995; 10:697–704.
46. El-Deiry WS. WAF1/Cip1 is induced in p53-mediated G1 arrest and apoptosis. Cancer Res 1994; 54:1159–1174.
47. Katayose D, Wersto R, Cowan KH, Seth P. Effects of a recombinant adenovirus expressing WAF1/Cip1 on cell growth, cell cycle, and apoptosis. Cell Growth Diff 1995; 6:1207–1212.
48. Sandig V, Brand K, Herwig S, Lukas J, Bartek J, Strauss M. Adenovirally transfected p16 INK4/CDKN2 and p53 genes co-operate to induce apoptotic tumor cell death. Nature Med 1997; 3:313–319.
49. Oltvai ZN, Milliman CL, Korsmeyer SJ. Bcl2 heterodimerizes in vivo with a conserved homolog, Bax, that accelerates programed cell death. Cell 1993; 74:609–619.
50. Yang E, Korsmeyer S. Molecular thanatopsis: a discourse on the bcl2 family and cell death. Blood 1996; 88:386–401.
51. Sedlak TW, Oltvai ZN, Yang E, Wang K, Boise LH, Thompson CB, Korsmeyer SJ. Multiple Bcl2 family members demonstrate selective dimerizations with Bax. Proc Natl Acad Sci USA 1995; 92:7834–7838.

52. Brambilla E, Negoescu A, Gazzeri S, Lantuejoul S, Moro D, Brambilla C, Coll JL. Apoptosis-related factors P53, Bcl2, and Bax in neuroendocrine lung tumors. Am J Pathol 1996; 149:1941–1952.

53. Kernohan NM, Cox LS. Regulation of apoptosis by Bcl2 and its related proteins: immunocytochemical challenges and therapeutic implications. J Pathol 1996; 179:1–3.

54. Koshida Y, Saegusa M, Okayasu I. Apoptosis, cell proliferation and expression of Bcl2 and Bax in gastric carcinomas: immunohistochemical and clinicopathological study. Br J Cancer 1997; 75:367–373.

55. Krajewski S, Blomqvist C, Franssila K, Krajewska M, Wasenius VM, Niskanen E, Nordling S, Reed JC. Reduced expression of proapoptotic gene bax is associated with poor response rates to combination chemotherapy and shorter survival in women with metastatic breast adenocarcinoma. Cancer Res 1995; 55:4471–4487.

56. Perego P, Giarola M, Righetti SC, Supino R, Caserini C, Delia D, Pierotti MA, Miyashita T, Reed JC, Zunino F. Association between cisplatin resistance and mutation of p53 gene and reduced bax expression in ovarian carcinoma cell systems. Cancer Res 1996; 56: 556–562.

57. Rampino N, Yamamoto H, Ionov Y, Li Y, Sawai H, Reed J. C, Perucho M. Somatic frameshift mutations in the bax gene in colon cancers of the microsatellite mutator phenotype. Science 1997; 275:967–969.

58. Boise LH, Gonzàlez-Garcia H, M, Postema CE, Ding L, Lindsten T, Turka LA, Mao X, Nunez G, Thompson CB. BclX, a bcl2-related gene that functions as a dominant regulator of apoptotic cell death. Cell 1993; 74:597–608.

59. Minn AJ, Boise LH, Thompson CB. BclX S antagonizes the protective effects of BclX L. J Biol Chem 1996; 271:6306–6312.

60. Martin SJ, Green DR. Protease activation during apoptosis: death by a thousand cuts? Cell 1995; 82:349–352.

61. Alnemri ES, Livingston DJ, Nicholson DW, Salvesen G, Thornberry NA, Wong WA, Yuan J. Human ICE/CED3 protease nomenclature. Cell 1996; 87:171.

62. Wyllie AH. Death gets a brake. Nature 1994; 369:272–273.

63. Simonian PL, Grillot DAM, Merino R, Nunez G. Bax can antagonize BclX L during etoposide and cisplatin-induced cell death independently of its heterodimerization with BclX L. J Biol Chem 1996; 271:22764–22772.

64. Simonian PL. Bax homodimerization is not required for Bax to accelerate chemotherapy-induced cell death. J Biol Chem 1996; 271:32073–32077.

65. Xiang J, Chao DT, Korsmeyer SJ. Bax-induced cell death may not require ICE enzyme-like proteases. Proc Natl Acad Sci USA 1996; 93:14559–14563.

66. McCarthy NJ, Whyte MKB, Gilbert CS, Evan GE. Inhibition of CED3/ICE proteases does not prevent cell death induced by oncogenes, DNA damage or the Bcl2 homologue Bak. J Cell Biol 1997; 136:215–227.

67. Lane DP. P53, guardian of the genome. Nature 1992; 358:15–16.

68. Ko JK, Prives C. P53: puzzle and paradigm. Genes Dev 1996; 10:1054–1072.

69. Miyashita T, Reed JC. Tumor suppressor p53 is a direct transcriptional activator of the human bax gene. Cell 1995; 80:293–299.

70. Yin C, Knudson CM, Korsmeyer SJ, van Dyke T. Bax suppresses tumorigenesis and stimulates apoptosis in vivo. Nature 1997; 385:637–640.

71. Lowe SW, Ruley HE, Jacks T, Housman DE. P53-dependent apoptosis modulates the cytotoxicity of anticancer agents. Cell 1993; 74:957–967.

72. Lowe SW. P53 is required for radiation-induced apoptosis in mouse thymocytes. Nature 1993; 362:847–848.

73. Clarke AR, Purdie CA, Harriso DJ, Morris RG, Bird CC, Hooper ML, Wyllie AH. Thymocyte apoptosis induced by P53-dependent and independent pathways. Nature 1993; 362:849–852.

74. Strasser A, Harris AW, Huang DCS, Krammer PH, Cory S. Bcl2 and Fas/Apo1 regulate distinct pathways to lymphocyte apoptosis. EMBO J 1995; 14:6136–6147.

75. Keith FJ, Bradbury DA, Zhu YM, Russell NH. Inhibition of bcl2 with antisense oligonucleotides induces apoptosis and increases the sensitivity of AML blasts to Ara-C. Leukemia 1995; 9:131–138.
76. Kitada S, Takayama S, de Riel K, Tanaka S, Reed JC. Reversal of chemoresistance of lymphoma cells by antisense-mediated reduction of bcl2 gene expression. Antisense Res Dev 1994; 4:71–79.
77. Webb A, Cunningham D, Cotter F, Clarke PA, di Stefano F, Ross P, Corbo M, Dziewanowska Z. Bcl2 antisense therapy in patients with non-Hodgkin lymphoma. Lancet 1997; 349:1137–1141.
78. Clarke MF, Apel IJ, Benedict MA, Eipers PG, Sumantran V, Gonzàlez-Garcia M, Doedens M, Fukunaga N, Davidson B, Dick JE, Minn AJ, Boise LH, Thompson CB, Wicha M, Nunez G. A recombinant bclXS adenovirus selectively induces apoptosis in cancer cells but not in normal bone marrow cells. Proc Natl Acad Sci USA 1995; 92:11024–11028.
79. Dole MG, Clarke MF, Holman P, Benedict M, Lu J, Jasty R, Eipers P, Thompson CB, Rode C, Bloch C, Nunez G, Castle VP. BclXS enhances adenoviral vector-induced apoptosis in neuroblastoma cells. Cancer Res 1996; 56:5734–5740.
80. Ealovega MW, McGinnis PK, Sumantran VN, Clarke MF, Wicha MS. BclXS gene therapy induces apoptosis of human mammary tumors in nude mice. Cancer Res 1996; 56:1965–1969.
81. Sumantran VN, Ealovega MW, Nunez G, Clarke MF, Wicha MS. Overexpression of bclX S sensitizes MCF7 cells to chemotherapy-induced apoptosis. Cancer Res 1995; 55:2507–2510.
82. Sakakura C, Sweeney EA, Shirayama T, Igarashi Y, Hakomori SI, Nakatani H, Tsujimoto H, Imanishi T, Ohgaki M, Ohyama T, Yamazaki J, Hagiwara A, Yamaguchi T, Sawai K, Takahashi T. Overexpression of bax sensitizes human breast cancer MCF7 cells to radiation-induced apoptosis. Int J Cancer 1996; 67:101–105.
83. Strobel T, Swanson L, Korsmeyer S, Cannistra SA. Bax inhances paclitaxel-induced apoptosis through a P53-independent pathway. Proc Natl Acad Sci USA 1996; 93:14094–14099.
84. Negoescu A, Louis N, Sachs L, Tenaud C, Girardot V, Gazzeri S, Demeinex B, Brambilla E, Brambilla C, Favrot M, Coll JL. Apoptosis induction by lipid-delivered bax and p53 genes in non small cell lung cancer cell lines. Gene Ther, in press.
85. Werthman PE, Drazan KE, Rosenthal JT, Khalili R, Shaked A. Adenoviral-p53 gene transfer to orthotopic and peritoneal murine bladder cancer. J Urol 1996; 155:753–756.
86. Dameron KM, Volpert OV, Tainsky MA, Bouck N. Control of angiogenesis in fibroblasts by p53 regulation of thrombospondin-1. Science 1994; 265:1582.
87. Van Meir EG, Polverini PJ, Chazin VR, et al. Release of an inhibitor of angiogenesis upon induction of wild type p53 expression in glioblastoma cells. Nat Genet 1994; 8:171–176.
88. Roth J, Dittmer D, Rea D, Tartaglia J, Paoletti E, Levine AJ. P53 as a target for cancer vaccines: recombinant canarypox virus vectors expressing p53 protect mice against lethal tumor cell challenge. Proc Natl Acad Sci 1996; 93:4781–4786.
89. Gabrilovich D, Kavanaugh D, Ishida T, Oyama T, Lee CT, Nadaf S, Sepetavec T, Jensen R, Gazdar A, Ciernik IF, Corak J, Bersofsky J, Carbone DP. Induction of p53/ras specific cellular immunity in patients with common solid tumors. Lung Cancer 1997; 18(suppl2): 190–91.
90. Chen HL, Gabrilovich D, Tampe R, Girgis KR, Nadaf S, Carbone DP. A functionally defective allele of TAP1 results in loss of MHC class 1 antigen presentation in a human lung cancer. Nature Genetics 1996; 13:210–213.
91. Gabrilovich DI, Chen HL, Girgis KR, Cunningham Y, Meny G, Nadaf S, Kavanaugh D, Carbone DP. Production of vascular endothelial growth factor by human tumors inhibits the functional maturation of dendritic cells. Nature Med 1996; 2:1096–1103.
92. Mukhopadhyay T, Roth JA. Induction of apoptosis in human lung cancer cells after wild-type p53 activation by methoxyestradiol. Oncogene 1997; 14:379–384.
93. Blagosklonny MV, Toretsky J, Neckers L. Geldanamycin selectively destabilizes and conformationally alters mutated p53. Oncogene 1995; 11:933–939.

94. Mundt M, Hupp T, Fritsche M, Merkle F, Hansen S, Lane D, Groner B. Protein interactions at the carboxyl terminus of p53 result in the induction of its in vitro transactivation potential. Oncogene 1997; 15:237–244.

95. Qazilbash MH, Xiao X, Seth P, Cowan KH, Walsh CE. Cancer gene therapy using a novel adeno-associated virus vector expressing human wild-type p53. Gene Ther 1997; 4:675–682.

96. Gao X, Huang L. Cationic liposome-mediated gene transfer. Gene Ther 1995; 2:710–722.

97. Coll JL, Wagner E, Combaret V, et al. In vitro targeting and specific transfection of human neuroblastoma cells by chCE7 antibody-mediated gene transfer. Gene Ther 1997; 4:156–161.

98. Wu GY, Wu CH. Receptor-mediated in vitro gene transformation by a soluble DNA carrier system. J Biol Chem 1987; 262:4429–4432.

99. Buschle M, Cotten M, Kirlappos H, et al. Receptor-mediated gene transfer into human T lymphocytes via binding of DNA/CD3 antibody particles to the CD3 T cell receptor complex. Hum Gene Ther 1995; 6:753–761.

100. Batra RK, Wang-Johanning F, Wagner E, et al. Receptor-mediated gene delivery employing lectin-binding specificity. Gene Ther 1994; 1:255–260.

101. Baatz JE, Bruno MD, Ciraolo PJ, et al. Utilization of modified surfactant-associated protein B for delivery of DNA to airway cells in culture. Proc Natl Acad Sci USA 1994; 91:2547–2551.

102. Ferkol T, Kaetzel CS, Davis PB. Gene targeting into respiratory epithelial cells by targeting the polymeric immunoglobulin receptor. J Clin Invest 1993; 92:2394–2400.

103. Richards CA, Austin EA, Huber BE. Transcriptional regulatory sequences of carcinoembryonic antigen: identification and use with cytosine deaminase for tumor-specific gene therapy. Hum Gene Ther 1995; 6:881–893.

104. Colucci-D'Amato GL, Santelli A, D'alessio G, et al. Dbl expression driven by the neuron specific enolase promoter induces tumor formation in transgenic mice with a p53(+/−) genetic background. Biochem Biophys Res Commun 1995; 216:762–770.

105. Lee CH, Liu M, Sie KL, et al. Prostate-specific antigen promoter driven gene therapy targeting DNA polymerase-alpha and topoisomerase II alpha in prostate cancer. Anticancer Res 1996; 16:1805–1811.

106. Kumagai T, Tanio Y, Osaki T, et al. Eradication of Myc-overexpressing small cell lung cancer cells transfected with herpes simplex virus thymidine kinase gene containing Myc-Max response elements. Cancer Res 1996; 56:354–358.

AUTHOR INDEX

Italic numbers give the page on which the complete reference is listed.

D

D'Agay, MF, 456, *467*

D'Alessio, G, 739, *745*

D'Amato, RJ, 352, *362*, 375, *381*

D'Amico, D, 144, *154*, 177, *186*, 293, *300*, 458, 460, *469*

D'Amico, F, 50, *58*, 648, *653*

D'Amore, PA, 348, 357, 358, *360*, *363*, 366, 367, *377*

D'Angeli, B, 504, 505, 507, 511, *518*

D'Souza, T, 311, *319*

Da Costa, P, 109, *124*

Dabouis, G, 569, 570, 573, 574, *577*, *578*, 586, 587, 588, 589, 590, *592*, *593*

Dachowski, L, 527, *534*

Daghighian, F, 713, *724*

Dahlbom, M, 494, *500*

Dai, HB, 30, *53*

Daikuhara, Y, 408, *420*

Dail, DH, 101, *108*

Dakhil, SR, 660, *674*

Dalamau, J, 711, *724*

Dalesio, O, 52, *58*, 140, 141, *152*, 289, *299*, 322, 329, *332*, *334*, 557, 558, *563*, *564*, 571, *579*, 603, *608*, 614, *626*

Dalphin, JC, 90, 91, *103*, 569, 573, 574, *577*

Dalquen, P, 178, *187*, 460, *469*

Dalton, Rj, 570, *579*

Daly, BDP, 491, *497*

Daly, M, 158, *167*

Damber, L, 436, *446*, 694, *706*

Dameron, KM, 183, *188*, 393, *396*, 737, *744*

Damico, D, 293, *301*

Damjanov, I, 512, *520*

Damjanovich, L, 424, *432*

Damon, DH, 348, 358, *360*

Damstrup, L, 554, *561*

Dan-Aouta, M, 442, *450*

Dang, P, 613, *625*

Daniel, G, 513, *520*

Daniels, GL, 159, *168*

Dano, K, 403, 404, *418*

Dar, AR, 599, *607*

Dardi, LE, 22, *27*

Dardick, I, 21, *27*

Darling, D, 731, *741*

Dartvelle, PG, 384, 387, *395*

Darwish, S, 557, *563*, 570, *578*

Daryalova, SL, 558, *564*

Dass, KK, 544, 549, *551*

Dassonville, O, 572, *580*

Daugaard, G, 128, *136*

Daures, JP, 429, *433*, 442, *448*, 589, *593*

Dautzenberg, B, 570, *578*

Daven, A, 589, *593*

Daver, A, 442, *448*

David, G, 350, *360*

Davidoff, AM, 456, *467*

Davidson, AG, 178, *187*, 217, *224*

Davidson, B, 735, *744*

Davidson, E, 718, *726*

Davidson, NE, 228, 229, *233*, *234*

Davis, BH, 40, 50, *56*

Davis, BT, 307, *317*

Davis, M, 544, *550*

Davis, MB, 158, 159, *167*, *168*

Davis, MD, 367, *377*

Davis, MP, 123, *126*

Davis, PB, 739, *745*

Davis, RW, 339, 340, *344*

Davis, S, 370, *379*, 558, *564*, 570, *578*, 600, *607*, 647, *653*

Davis, TP, 309, *318*

Davis, WB, 91, *104*

Davis, B, 40, *56*

Davis-Smyth, T, 358, *361*

Davison, AM, 109, *124*

Dawsey, S, 330, *333*

Dawson, MI, 306, *316*

Day, IN, 231, *235*

Day, NE, 696, *706*

Day, RP, 90, *104*

Day, RS, 200, 203, *208*, 216, *223*

Daya, M, 141, *153*

Dayagrosjean, L, 458, *469*

Dayananth, P, 203, *209*

Dazin, P, 195, *206*, 219, *225*

Dazord, L, 504, 507, *517*, *522*

De Angelis, G, 441, *451*

De Anta, JM, 140, 141, 150, *152*

De Benedetti, VMG, 464, *470*

De Bries, N, 329, *334*

De Bruyne, C, 661, *675*

De Camp, M, 237, 238, *252*

De Campos, E, 621, *628*

De Campos, JM, 158, *166*

De Chadarevian, JP, 101, *107*

De Cremoux, H, 557, 558, *563*, 597, *607*

De Geus, BW, 651, *655*

De Gregorio, L, 73, 80, *85*, 140, *153*, 159, 164, 165, *169*, *170*, *171*, 281, *285*, 314, *319*

De Greve, L, 557, *562*

De Grossouvre, D, 405, *420*

Fujino, S, 357, *363*, 490, *497*
Fujisawa, M, 504, 514, *518*
Fujishiro, S, 403, *419*
Fujita, A, 667, *676*
Fujita, M, 488, *497*
Fujita, T, 375, *381*
Fujiwara, S, 413, 415, 416, *422*
Fujiwara, T, 454, 465, *466*, 471, 494, *500*, 732, *741*, *742*
Fujiwara, Y, 586, 587, *591*
Fujoka, S, 445, *449*
Fujta, RM, 404, *419*
Fukayama, M, 101, *107*
Fuks, Z, 605, *608*
Fukuda, H, 494, *500*
Fukuda, K, 488, *497*
Fukuoka, M, 445, *452*, 475, *479*, 559, *564*, 570, *579*, 613, 620, *625*, *628*, 638, 642, 644, *646*, 649, *654*, 667, 668, *676*
Fuller, JC, 401, 404, 408, *418*
Fumoleau, P, 504, 516, *518*, *521*
Funa, K, 350, 352, *361*
Funa, R, 19, *27*
Funae, Y, 6, *10*, 75, 77, 80, *86*
Fung, YK, 219, *225*
Fung, YKT, 191, 192, 195, 198, *204*, *206*, 207
Funk, WD, 271, *277*
Furcht, LT, 354, 357, *362*, *363*
Furman, M, 436, 438, 439, 440, 442, *446*, *447*, *448*
Furnas, B, 613, *626*
Furuse, K, 475, *479*, 559, *564*, 569, 570, 573, *577*, *578*, *580*, 613, *625*, 638, 642, 644, *646*, 651, *654*, 664, *675*
Fusco, V, 570, *578*
Fusenig, NE, 413, *421*
Futcher, AB, 269, *276*
Fuwa, N, 596, 598, *607*
Fuykunaga, N, 735, *744*

G

Gabrielson, E, 198, 201, 204, *207*, *208*, 216, *223*, 291, *300*
Gabrilovich, D, 737, 738, *744*
Gabrys, T, 570, 572, *578*
Gack, S, 409, *420*
Gadek, JE, 91, *104*
Gadgeel, S, 305, *316*
Gaeta, J, 129, *136*
Gaffey, MJ, 121, *126*, 215, *223*
Gaiccone, G, 259, *266*
Gail, M, 330, *333*

Gail, MH, 438, 442, *450*, 560, *564*
Gailani, M, 457, *469*
Gaillard, C, 456, *467*
Gaire, M, 413, 415, 416, *422*
Gais, P, 50, *58*
Gaken, J, 731, *741*
Gal, A, 33, 35, 36, 38, 39, 40, 42, 46, 51, 52, *54*, *55*, *56*, *57*, 121, *126*
Galanski, M, 483, *497*
Galateau, F, 90, 92, 93, *103*
Galateau-Salle, F, 33, *54*, 703, *707*
Gale, M, 586, 588, *592*
Galey, WT, 504, 505, 511, *518*
Gallager, HS, 13, 17, *26*
Gallagher, J, 350, *360*
Galli, J, 215, *223*
Galli, SJ, 368, *377*
Gallie, BL, 191, 193, 194, *204*, *206*, 217, *224*
Gallinger, S, 269, *276*
Gallo Curcio, C, 570, *578*
Gamble, AR, 128, *136*
Gamble, G, 158, *167*
Gamson, J, 525, *532*
Gamsu, G, 681, *690*
Gamucci, T, 669, *677*
Gandara, DR, 440, *450*, 560, *565*, 572, *579*, 666, *676*
Ganderton, RH, 231, *235*
Ganguly, J, 308, *317*
Ganju, RK, 404, 405, 408, 413, *419*
Ganly, P, 23, *27*, 73, *85*, 159, *169*, 184, *189*, 258, *266*, 280, *284*, 290, *300*, 314, *319*, 409, *421*, 465, *471*, 684, *690*
Gansbacher, B, 731, *741*
Ganz, A, 568, *577*
Ganz, PA, 568, *577*
Gao, HG, 146, *155*
Gao, X, 739, *745*
Garay, E, 456, *468*
Garcia, AJ, 174, *185*
Garcia, DK, 158, 159, *167*, *168*
Garcia, M, 357, *363*
Garcia, R, 544, 546, *551*
Garcia-Asenjo, JA, 440, *447*
Garcia-Conde, J, 661, *674*
Garcia-Viera, M, 110, 115, *125*
Garden, AS, 651, *655*
Gardner, WN, 527, *534*
Garewal, H, 141, 148, 149, *153*
Garfinkel, I, 183, *189*
Garfinkel, L, 62, 63, *84*, 255, 257, *265*, *266*, 272, *277*, 280, *284*, 409, *418*
Garibaldi, K, 694, *706*

N

SUBJECT INDEX